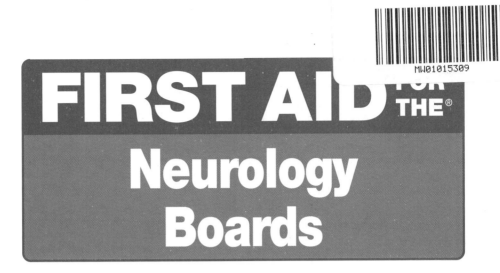

Second Edition

MICHAEL S. RAFII, MD, PhD
Director, Memory Disorders Clinic
Medical Director, Alzheimer's Disease Cooperative Study
Director, Neurology Residency Training Program
Assistant Professor of Neurosciences
University of California San Diego Health System
La Jolla, California

THOMAS I. COCHRANE, MD, PhD
Assistant Professor of Neurology
Division of Neuromuscular Disease
Department of Neurology
Harvard Medical School
Brigham and Women's Hospital
Boston, Massachusetts

SERIES EDITOR:

TAO LE, MD, MHS
Assistant Clinical Professor of Medicine and Pediatrics
Chief, Section of Allergy and Immunology
Department of Medicine
University of Louisville
Louisville, Kentucky

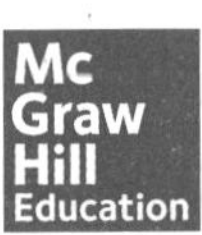

New York / Chicago / San Francisco / Athens / London / Madrid / Mexico City
Milan / New Delhi / Singapore / Sydney / Toronto

First Aid for the® Neurology Boards, Second Edition

1 2 3 4 5 6 7 8 9 0 DOW DOW 19 18 17 16 15

ISBN 978-0-07-183741-5
MHID 0-07-183741-8

NOTICE

Medicine is an ever-changing science. As new research and clinical experience broaden our knowledge, changes in treatment and drug therapy are required. The authors and the publisher of this work have checked with sources believed to be reliable in their efforts to provide information that is complete and generally in accord with the standards accepted at the time of publication. However, in view of the possibility of human error or changes in medical sciences, neither the authors nor the publisher nor any other party who has been involved in the preparation or publication of this work warrants that the information contained herein is in every respect accurate or complete, and they disclaim all responsibility for any errors or omissions or for the results obtained from use of the information contained in this work. Readers are encouraged to confirm the information contained herein with other sources. For example and in particular, readers are advised to check the product information sheet included in the package of each drug they plan to administer to be certain that the information contained in this work is accurate and that changes have not been made in the recommended dose or in the contraindications for administration. This recommendation is of particular importance in connection with new or infrequently used drugs.

This book was set in Electra LT Std by Rainbow Graphics.
The editors were Catherine A. Johnson and Cindy Yoo.
The production supervisor was Jeffrey Herzich.
Project management was provided by Rainbow Graphics.
RR Donnelley was printer and binder.
This book is printed on acid-free paper.

Library of Congress Cataloging-in-Publication Data

Rafii, Michael S., author.
First aid for the neurology boards / Michael S. Rafii, Thomas I. Cochrane. – Second edition.
p. ; cm.
Includes index.
ISBN 978-0-07-183741-5 (paperback : alk. paper) — ISBN 0-07-183741-8 (paperback : alk. paper)
I. Cochrane, Thomas I., author. II. Title.
[DNLM: 1. Neurology—United States—Outlines. 2. Specialty Boards—United States—Outlines. WL 18.2]
RC343.5
616.80076—dc23

2015008755

DEDICATION

To the contributors to this and future editions, who took time to share their knowledge, insight, and humor for the benefit of residents and clinicians.

and

To our families, friends, and loved ones, who endured and assisted in the task of assembling this guide.

Contents

Contributing Authors

WILLIAM Z. BARNARD, MD
Clinical Fellow in Psychiatry
Beth Israel Deaconess Medical Center
Harvard Medical School
Boston, Massachusetts
Chapter 15/Delirium
Chapter 19/Major Depressive Disorder

BEAU B. BRUCE, MD, PhD
Assistant Professor of Ophthalmology, Neurology, and Epidemiology
Departments of Ophthalmology and Neurology
Emory University School of Medicine
Atlanta, Georgia
Chapter 8/Neuro-ophthalmology and Neuro-otology

W. BRYAN BURNETTE, MD, MS
Associate Professor
Pediatrics and Neurology
Vanderbilt University School of Medicine
Nashville, Tennessee
Chapter 12/Pediatric Neurology and Neurogenetics

DAVID W. CHEN, MD
Instructor
Department of Neurology
Harvard Medical School
Massachusetts General Hospital
Boston, Massachusetts
Chapter 6/Headache and Pain

THOMAS I. COCHRANE, MD, PhD
Assistant Professor of Neurology
Division of Neuromuscular Disease
Department of Neurology
Harvard Medical School
Brigham and Women's Hospital
Boston, Massachusetts
Chapter 1/Guide to the ABPN Examination
Chapter 11/Neuromuscular Disease

RONALD COHN, MD, PhD
The Hospital for Sick Children
Chief, Clinical and Metabolic Genetics
Associate Professor of Pediatrics
University of Toronto
Toronto, Canada
Chapter 12/Pediatric Neurology and Neurogenetics

SAURAV DAS, MBBS
Visiting International Physician
Banner Alzheimer's Institute
Phoenix, Arizona
Stanley Medical College
Chennai, Tamilnadu, India
Chapter 5/Neurodegenerative Disorders

JAN DRAPPATZ, MD
Associate Director
Adult Neuro-oncology Program
Associate Professor
Departments of Neurology and Medicine
University of Pittsburgh
Pittsburgh, Pennsylvania
Chapter 7/Neuro-oncology

ADAM FLEISHER, MD, MAS
Associate Director of Brain Imaging
Banner Alzheimer's Institute
Phoenix, Arizona
Chapter 5/Neurodegenerative Disorders

RYAN C. W. HALL, MD
Assistant Professor of Psychiatry
Department of Medical Education
University of Central Florida College of Medicine
Orlando, Florida
Affiliated Assistant Professor
Department of Psychiatry
University of South Florida
Tampa, Florida
Chapter 17/Somatic Symptom and Related Disorders (formerly Somatoform Disorders)

MARIA K. HOUTCHENS, MD, MMSCI
Staff Neurologist
Partners Multiple Sclerosis Center
Brigham and Women's Hospital
Harvard Medical School
Boston, Massachusetts
Chapter 4/Neuroimmunology

LORI C. JORDAN, MD, PhD
Assistant Professor of Pediatrics and Neurology
Vanderbilt University School of Medicine
Nashville, Tennessee
Chapter 12/Pediatric Neurology and Neurogenetics

MATTHEW A. KOENIG, MD, FNCS
Associate Medical Director of Neurocritical Care
The Queen's Medical Center
Assistant Professor of Medicine
University of Hawaii
John A. Burns School of Medicine
Honolulu, Hawaii
Chapter 9/Stroke and Neurocritical Care

DEVIN D. MACKAY, MD
Assistant Professor of Neurology, Ophthalmology, and Neurosurgery
Indiana University
Indianapolis, Indiana
Chapter 8/Neuro-ophthalmology and Neuro-otology

TRACEY A. MILLIGAN, MD, MS
Assistant Professor of Neurology
Harvard Medical School
Brigham and Women's Hospital
Boston, Massachusetts
Chapter 13/Seizures, Epilepsy, and Sleep Disorders

PRITI OJHA, MD
Resident Physician
Department of Psychiatry
University of California San Diego School of Medicine
San Diego, California
Chapter 18/Bipolar Disorder
Chapter 20/Primary Psychotic Disorders

KATHERINE B. PETERS, MD, PhD
Assistant Professor of Neurology
The Preston Robert Tisch Brain Tumor Center at Duke
Duke University Medical Center
Durham, North Carolina
Chapter 2/Neuroanatomy

IRFAN QURESHI, MD
Instructor
The Saul R. Korey Department of Neurology
Albert Einstein College of Medicine
Bronx, New York
Chapter 3/Neuropharmacology

MICHAEL S. RAFII, MD, PhD
Director, Memory Disorders Clinic
Medical Director, Alzheimer's Disease Cooperative Study
Director, Neurology Residency Training Program
Assistant Professor of Neurosciences
University of California San Diego Health System
La Jolla, California
Chapter 1/Guide to the ABPN Examination
Chapter 5/Neurodegenerative Disorders
Chapter 10/Neurological Infections

TIMOTHY SCARELLA, MD
Clinical Fellow in Psychiatry
Harvard Longwood Psychiatry Training Program
Harvard Medical School
Boston, Massachusetts
Chapter 14/Substance Abuse and Dependence
Chapter 16/Anxiety and Related Disorders

Reviewers

VALERIE BIOUSSE, MD
Professor of Ophthalmology and Neurology
Cyrus H. Stoner Professor of Ophthalmology
Emory University
Atlanta, Georgia

JEFFREY GOLD, MD, PhD
Associate Professor of Neurosciences and Pediatrics
University of California, San Diego
San Diego, California

JONG WOO LEE, MD, PhD
Division of EEG, Epilepsy, and Sleep Medicine
Brigham and Women's Hospital
Harvard Medical School
Boston, Massachusetts

JOSHUA R. LEO, MD, MPH
Instructor in Psychiatry
Harvard Medical School
Staff Psychiatrist
Beth Israel Deaconess Medical Center
Boston, Massachusetts

SANJAI RAO, MD
Assistant Clinical Professor of Psychiatry
Associate Residency Training Director
University of California, San Diego
Veterans Administration Medical Center
San Diego, California

Preface

With *First Aid for the Neurology Boards, Second Edition*, we hope to provide residents and clinicians with the most useful and up-to-date preparation guide for the American Board of Psychiatry and Neurology (ABPN) certification and recertification exams. This second edition represents an outstanding effort by a talented group of authors and includes the following:

- A practical exam preparation guide with resident-proven test-taking and study strategies
- Concise summaries of thousands of board-testable topics
- Hundreds of high-yield tables, diagrams, and illustrations
- Key facts in the margins highlighting "must know" information for the boards
- Mnemonics throughout, making learning memorable and fun

We invite you to share your thoughts and ideas to help us improve *First Aid for the Neurology Boards, Second Edition*. See How to Contribute, p. xiii.

La Jolla	Michael S. Rafii
Boston	Thomas I. Cochrane
Louisville	Tao Le

Acknowledgments

This has been a collaborative project from the start. We gratefully acknowledge the thoughtful comments and advice of the residents, international medical graduates, and faculty who have supported the authors in the development of *First Aid for the Neurology Boards, Second Edition.*

Thanks to our publisher, McGraw-Hill, for the valuable assistance of their staff. For enthusiasm, support, and commitment to this challenging project, thanks to our editor, Catherine Johnson. A special thanks to Rainbow Graphics for remarkable production work.

La Jolla	Michael S. Rafii
Boston	Thomas I. Cochrane
Louisville	Tao Le

How to Contribute

To continue to produce a high-yield review source for the ABPN exam, you are invited to submit any suggestions or corrections. Please send us your suggestions for

- Study and test-taking strategies for the ABPN
- New facts, mnemonics, diagrams, and illustrations
- Low-yield topics to remove

For each entry incorporated into the next edition, you will personal acknowledgment in the next edition. Diagrams, tables, partial entries, updates, corrections, and study hints are also appreciated, and significant contributions will be compensated at the discretion of the authors. Also let us know about material in this edition that you feel is low yield and should be deleted.

The preferred way to submit entries, suggestions, or corrections is via electronic mail. Please include name, address, institutional affiliation, phone number, and e-mail address (if different from the address of origin). If there are multiple entries, please consolidate into a single e-mail or file attachment. Please send submissions to:

firstaidteam@yahoo.com

NOTE TO CONTRIBUTORS

All entries become property of the authors and are subject to editing and reviewing. Please verify all data and spellings carefully. In the event that similar or duplicate entries are received, only the first entry received will be used. Include a reference to a standard textbook to facilitate verification of the fact. Please follow the style, punctuation, and format of this edition if possible.

CHAPTER 1

Guide to the ABPN Examination

Michael S. Rafii, MD, PhD
Thomas I. Cochrane, MD, PhD

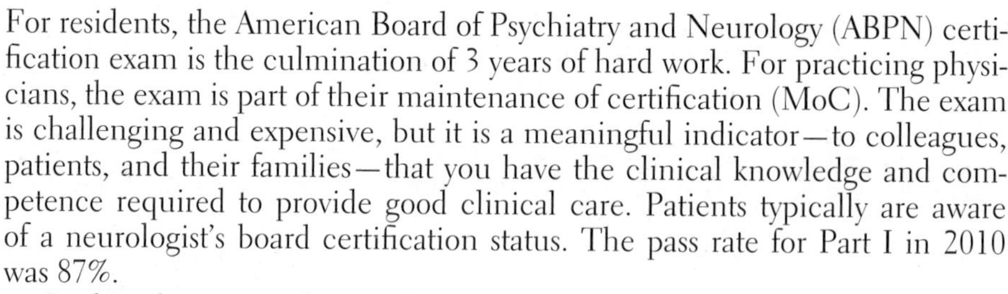

For residents, the American Board of Psychiatry and Neurology (ABPN) certification exam is the culmination of 3 years of hard work. For practicing physicians, the exam is part of their maintenance of certification (MoC). The exam is challenging and expensive, but it is a meaningful indicator—to colleagues, patients, and their families—that you have the clinical knowledge and competence required to provide good clinical care. Patients typically are aware of a neurologist's board certification status. The pass rate for Part I in 2010 was 87%.

In this chapter we discuss the ABPN exam and provide you with proven approaches to conquering the exam. For a detailed and official description of the exam visit the ABPN web site at **www.abpn.com** and refer to the *Booklet of Information (ABPN Policies and Procedures)*.

KEY FACT

Most patients will be aware of your certification status. Many hospitals and potential employers insist on board certification as a condition of employment.

ABPN—The Basics

HOW DO I REGISTER TO TAKE THE EXAM?

You can register online at www.abpn.com. The application fee in 2014 was $700, and the examination fee $1810. The regular registration deadline is typically in February of that year. If you miss the application deadline, a $500 nonrefundable late fee is also tacked on. Check the ABPN web site for the latest registration deadlines, fees, and policies.

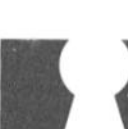

KEY FACT

Register before March to avoid the late fee.

HOW IS THE ABPN TEST STRUCTURED?

The initial certification examination is a 1-day test, administered on computers at Pearson VUE testing centers (www.vue.com). It is composed of 2 sections: a morning session and an afternoon session. Both sessions are $3\frac{1}{2}$ hours long, and there is a mandatory 1-hour break between the morning and afternoon sessions, totaling 8 hours for the entire examination.

The ABPN divides the test content into 3 groupings: Neurology A: Basic Neuroscience; Neurology B: Behavioral Neurology, Cognition, and Psychiatry; and Neurology C: Clinical Neurology. The subtopics in each of these categories are shown in Table 1.1. The content outlines can also be obtained at www.abpn.com/content_outlines.htm.

Morning Session

The morning session consists of 210 questions drawn from the Neurology A and Neurology B content outlines. Each item is a stand-alone multiple-choice question. You will have the opportunity to "flag" questions for review as you go and can return to difficult questions later.

Afternoon Session

The afternoon session consists of 210 questions derived from the Neurology C content outline and includes 60% adult neurology questions and 40% child neurology questions. Most questions in this section refer to case presentations. These may be presented in a 30- to 90-second video clip, or as a text vignette, with or without images (eg, CT, MRI, pathology). A single case may have 5 or 6 associated questions. Answers to already completed questions are sometimes revealed in subsequent questions, so you will not be able to flag items for review in the afternoon session.

TABLE 1.1. Initial Certification Examination Sections and Content

Neurology A: Basic Neuroscience
I. Neuroanatomy
II. Neuropathology
III. Neurochemistry
IV. Neurophysiology
V. Neuroimmunology/neuroinfectious disease
VI. Neurogenetics/molecular neurology, and neuroepidemiology
VII. Neuroendocrinology
VIII. Neuropharmacology
Neurology B: Behavioral Neurology, Cognition, and Psychiatry
I. Development through the life cycle
II. Behavioral and social sciences
III. Diagnostic procedures
IV. Clinical and therapeutic aspects of psychiatric disorders
V. Clinical and therapeutic aspects of behavioral neurology
Neurology C: Clinical Neurology (Adult and Child)
I. Headache disorders
II. Pain disorders
III. Epilepsy and episodic disorders
IV. Sleep disorders
V. Genetic disorders
VI. Congenital disorders
VII. Cerebrovascular disease
VIII. Neuromuscular diseases (adult and child)
IX. Cranial nerve palsies

Scoring

Your score report will indicate your overall percentage of correct responses and the percentage of correct responses within each subtopic. Subtopic scores are provided primarily for your learning and information. Your overall score percentage of correct responses is what determines whether you pass or fail.

WHAT TYPES OF QUESTIONS ARE ASKED?

All questions are **single best answer.** Most questions on the exam are vignette based. You will be presented with a scenario, then a question followed by 5 options. Extraneous information is often included, and some questions can be answered without actually reading the case. Like other board exams, there is no penalty for guessing. Between 5% and 10% of the questions require interpretation of photomicrographs, radiology studies, photographs of physical findings, and the like. It is your job to determine which information is superfluous and which is pertinent to the case at hand.

KEY FACT

Most questions are case-based.

CLINICAL EXAMINATION/ORAL BOARDS

If you entered neurology or child neurology residency **on or after July 1, 2005**, the clinical skills evaluations (previously conducted as the Part II examination) now takes place during residency. These evaluations are performed at your home institution, and you will have to submit documentation of satisfactory performance in the 5 required clinical skills evaluations. These evaluations must be completed in an Accreditation Council for Graduate Medical Education (ACGME)-accredited training program and are required as part of the ABPN credentialing process.

As of 2010, the Part II examination was no longer required for first-time takers (there will no longer be a Part I and Part II).

THE RECERTIFICATION EXAM

The recertification exam is one part of the Maintenance of Certificate Program (MCP). This 200-item, multiple-choice examination is administered on computer for 5 hours. The exam fee in 2014 was $1500. Historically, pass rates range from 92% to 100%.

TEST PREPARATION ADVICE

Candidate knowledge is assessed in headache and other pain syndromes; epilepsy; cerebrovascular disease; aging, dementia, and degenerative diseases; spinal cord and nerve root disorders; neuromuscular disorders; movement disorders; demyelinating disorders; critical care and trauma; neurology of systemic disease; neuro-ophthalmology/neuro-otology; neurogenetics/neurometabolic disorders; neuro-oncology; infectious diseases; cognitive neurology; neurologic disorders presenting with psychiatric symptoms; neurotoxicology; sleep disorders; ethics and professionalism; and neurorehabilitation.

The ABPN exam tends to focus on the diagnosis and management of diseases and conditions that you have seen during your training, so *First Aid* and a good source of practice questions may be all you need. But most residents should consider using *First Aid* as a **guide.** Like any review book, *First Aid* is not comprehensive, and should be supplemented by textbooks, practice questions with explanations, review articles, and a concise electronic text such as *UpToDate*. Original research articles are low yield, and very new research (ie, less than 1–2 years old) will not be tested. There are a number of high-quality board review courses offered around the country. Board review courses are expensive but can help those who need some focus and discipline.

KEY FACT

Use a combination of *First Aid*, textbooks, journal reviews, and practice questions such as the RITE exam.

The American Academy of Neurology (AAN) Residency In-service Training Exam (RITE) is a self-assessment tool designed to gauge knowledge of neurology and neuroscience, identify areas for potential growth, and provide references and discussions for each. This exam has been considered a very helpful tool in preparing for the Neurology Board examination.

Ideally, you should start your preparation early in your **last year of residency,** especially if you are starting a demanding job or fellowship right after residency. Cramming in the period between end of residency and the exam is **not advisable.**

For **common diseases,** learn both the common and **uncommon presentations;** for **uncommon diseases,** focus on the **classic presentations** and manifestations. Draw on the experiences of your residency training to anchor some of your learning. When you take the exam, you will realize that you've seen most of the clinical scenarios in your 3 years of wards, clinics, morning report, case conferences, or grand rounds.

Comprehensive understanding of a subject is by far the best way to perform well on a test, and translates directly into better real-world performance. But when preparing for a high-stakes test with limited preparation time, rote memorization of high-yield facts can be a smart strategy. Know your own learning style—there is no single best way to prepare.

OTHER HIGH-YIELD AREAS

Focus on topic areas that are typically not emphasized during residency training but are board favorites. These include:

- Topics in outpatient specialties (eg, movement disorders, epilepsy, dementia, pediatric neurology, neuromuscular disease).
- Neuropathology and neuroradiology (eg, classic pathology of meningiomas, MRI of cortical tubers of tuberous sclerosis, angiogram of carotid dissection).
- Adverse effects of drugs.
- Anatomy of the peripheral nervous system. Rememorize the brachial and lumbosacral plexuses (know the roots, trunks, cords, and nerve for each commonly tested muscle!). Getting this "down cold" just before the test won't take long and will yield many free points on the exam.

TEST-TAKING ADVICE

You've probably taken so many tests by now that you need little advice from us. But under pressure, it's easy to forget the basics. Here are a few tips to keep in mind when taking the exam:

- For long vignette questions, read the question stem and scan the options, **then** go back and read the case. You may get your answer without having to read through the whole case.
- There's no penalty for guessing, so you should **never** leave a question blank.
- Pacing is key to getting through all the questions. Even though you have 2 minutes per question on average, you should aim for a pace of 90–100 seconds per question. If you don't know the answer within a short period, make an educated guess and move on.
- In the morning session, make use of the option to flag questions for review. Take an educated guess, flag the question, and come back at the end if you have time.
- It's okay to **second-guess** yourself. Contrary to popular wisdom, "second hunches" tend to be better than first guesses.
- Don't panic over "impossible" questions—no one will get every question. Take your best guess and move on.
- Note the age and race of the patient in each clinical scenario. When ethnicity or race is given, it is often relevant. Know the associations between disease, sex, and race, especially for more common diagnoses.
- Eponyms are used rarely in the test—most questions simply describe clinical findings.

TESTING AND LICENSING AGENCIES

American Board of Psychiatry and Neurology, Inc.
2150 E. Lake Cook Road, Suite 900
Buffalo Grove, IL 60089
Phone: (847) 229-6500
Fax: (847) 229-6600

American Academy of Neurology
1080 Montreal Avenue
Saint Paul, MN 55116
Phone: (800) 879-1960 or (651) 695-2717
Fax: (651) 695-2791

Educational Commission for Foreign Medical Graduates (ECFMG)
3624 Market Street, Fourth Floor
Philadelphia, PA 19104-2685
Phone: (215) 386-5900 or (202) 293-9320
Fax: (215) 386-9196
www.ecfmg.org

Federation of State Medical Boards (FSMB)
P. O. Box 619850
Dallas, TX 75261-9850
Phone: (817) 868-4000
Fax: (817) 868-4099
www.fsmb.org

SECTION I

Neurology Topics

CHAPTER 2

Neuroanatomy

Katherine B. Peters, MD, PhD

Central Nervous System

GROSS ANATOMY

The central nervous system (CNS) is enclosed in the meninges. It contains the majority of the nervous system and consists of the brain and the spinal cord. The CNS is divided into divisions and the brain into lobes.

- Ridges = gyrus
- Each groove = sulcus
- Very deep sulcus = fissure

Divisions of CNS	Components
Cerebrum	Hemispheres, basal ganglia
Diencephalon	Thalamus, hypothalamus
Brain stem	Midbrain, pons, medulla
Cerebellum	
Spinal cord	

Lobes of the Brain (Figures 2.1 and 2.2)

Frontal Lobe

Extends from the frontal pole to the central sulcus and the lateral fissure.

- Central sulcus
- Precentral gyrus
- Precentral sulcus
- Cingulate gyrus
- Superior frontal gyrus
- Middle frontal gyrus
- Inferior frontal gyrus

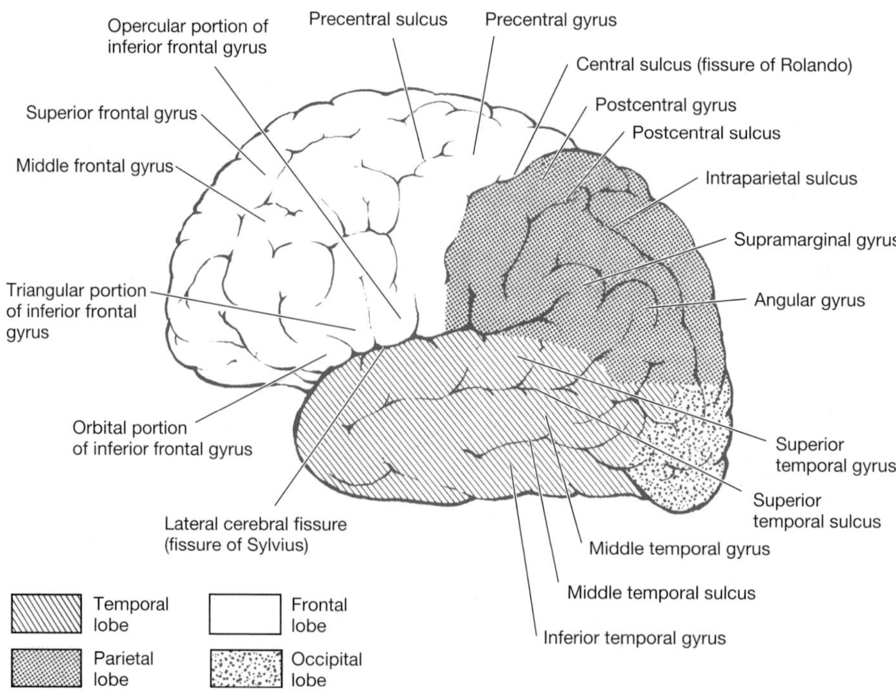

FIGURE 2.1. Lateral view of left hemisphere. (Reproduced, with permission, from Waxman SG. *Clinical Neuroanatomy*, 25th ed. New York: McGraw-Hill, 2003: Figure 10-6.)

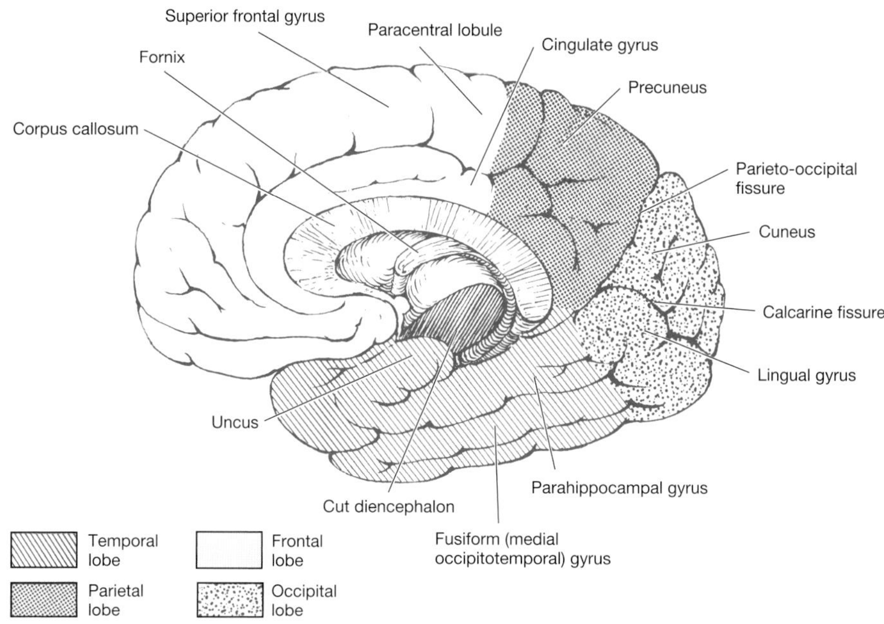

FIGURE 2.2. Medial view of right hemisphere. (Reproduced, with permission, from Waxman SG. *Clinical Neuroanatomy*, 25th ed. New York: McGraw-Hill, 2003: Figure 10-6.)

Parietal Lobe

Extends from the central sulcus to the parieto-occipital fissure.

- Central sulcus
- Postcentral gyrus
- Postcentral sulcus
- Supramarginal gyrus (follow lateral fissure)
- Angular gyrus (follow the superior temporal sulcus)
- Occipital lobe

Situated behind the parieto-occipital.

- Parieto-occipital fissure
- Cuneus
- Calcarine fissure
- Lingual gyrus

Temporal Lobe

Lies below the lateral cerebral fissure and extends back to the level of the parieto-occipital fissure on the medial surface of the hemisphere.

- Lateral cerebral fissure (fissure of Sylvius)
- Superior temporal gyrus
- Superior temporal sulcus
- Middle temporal gyrus
- Middle temporal sulcus
- Inferior temporal sulcus
- Uncus
- Parahippocampal gyrus

Other Stuctures

Diencephalon

Buried in the middle of the brain.

- Thalamus
- Interthalamic adhesion
- Hypothalamus
- Habenula
- Pituitary
- Mammillary bodies
- Infundibular stalk: Stalk connecting the pituitary to the hypothalamus
- Pineal gland (called the "seat of the soul" by Descartes; secretes melatonin)

Brain Stem

- Medulla
- Pons
- Midbrain

Meninges

See Table 2.1.

EPIDURAL AND SUBDURAL SPACES

- **Epidural space:** Between bone and dura, potential space in brain, but actual space in spinal cord (contains fat).
  - **Epidural hematoma** (Figure 2.3): Accumulation of blood in the epidural space. Shape is convex lens.
  - Usually see associated skull fracture due to torn meningeal vessel (usually middle meningeal artery).
  - Uncontrolled arterial bleeding may lead to compression of the brain and subsequent herniation.
- **Subdural space:** Between dura and arachnoid, potential space.
  - **Subdural hematoma** (Figure 2.4): Accumulation of blood in the subdural space. Shape is concave lens.
  - Tearing of bridging veins between the brain surface and dural sinus (can shear when the brain is jostled).
  - Children (because they have thinner veins) and adults with brain atrophy (because they have longer bridging veins) are at greatest risk. Alcoholics are also at risk because of brain atrophy.
  - Bleeding can recur; subdural blood can be reabsorbed or encapsulated or calcified.

TABLE 2.1. Components of the Meninges

Dura Mater	Arachnoid	Pia
■ Periosteal layer: Fused to the bone. ■ Meningeal layer: Inner. ■ **Falx cerebri:** Separates the two cerebral hemispheres. ■ **Tentorium cerebelli:** Separates the inferior occipital lobe from the cerebellum. ■ **Falx cerebelli:** Separates the two cerebellar hemispheres.	■ Thin membrane that appears transculent. ■ **Arachnoid villi:** Small protrusions of the arachnoid, allow one-way efflux of the cerebrospinal fluid into the sinus. ■ **Arachnoid granulations:** Large groupings of arachnoid villi along the superior sagittal sinus.	■ Delicate membrane that is one cell layer thick. ■ Covers the brain. ■ **Denticulate ligament:** Pial extension that penetrates the dura in the spinal cord to provide horizontal support. ■ **Filum terminale:** Thin pial extension that attaches to the coccyx. Provides vertical support.

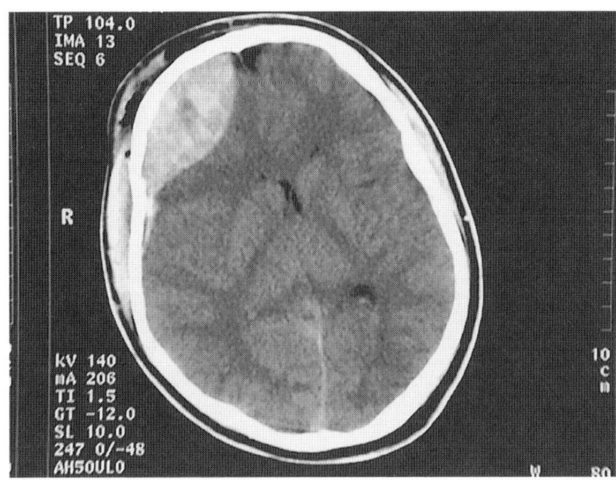

FIGURE 2.3. Epidural hematoma. (Reproduced, with permission, from Stone CK, Humphries RL. *Current Diagnosis & Treatment: Emergency Medicine*, 6th ed. New York: McGraw-Hill, 2008: Figure 20-3.)

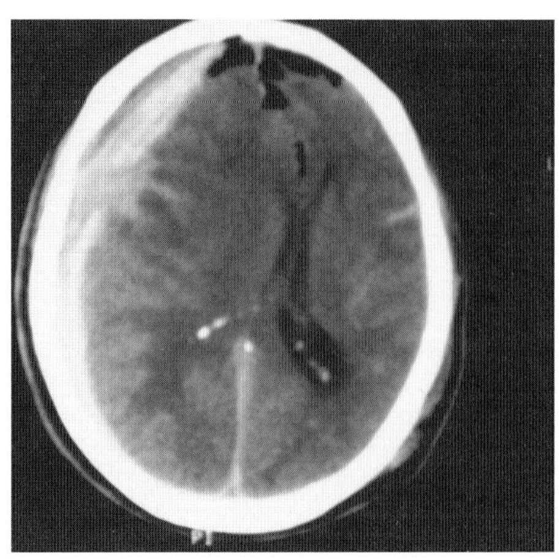

FIGURE 2.4. Subdural hematoma. (Reproduced, with permission, from Brunicardi FC, Anderson DR, Billiar TR, Dunn DL, Hunter JG, Matthews JB, Poliok RE, Schwartz ST. *Schwartz's Principles of Surgery*, 8th ed. New York: McGraw-Hill, 2005: 138.)

- **Subarachnoid space:** Between arachnoid and pia, actual space.
  - **Subarachnoid hemorrhage** (Figure 2.5): Bleed into the subarachnoid space due to ruptured aneurysms or vascular malformations.
  - Berry aneurysm (congenital).
  - Mycotic aneurysm (infection).
  - Vascular malformations.

VENTRICLES/CEREBROSPINAL FLUID (CSF)

Flow of CSF

- **Flow of CSF is unidirectional** (Figure 2.6): Lateral ventricles → **interventricular foramina of Monro** → third ventricle → **cerebral aqueduct** → fourth ventricle → **foramina of Luschka** and **foramen of Magendie**

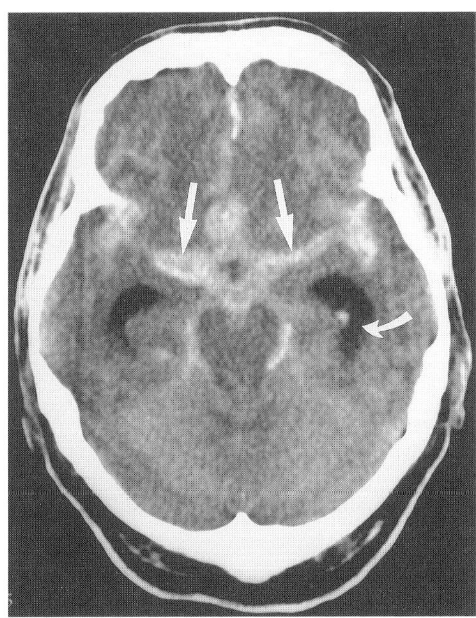

FIGURE 2.5. Subarachnoid hemorrhage. (Reproduced, with permission, from Tintinalli JE. *Tintinalli's Emergency Medicine: A Comprehensive Study Guide*, 6th ed. New York: McGraw-Hill, 2004: 1445.)

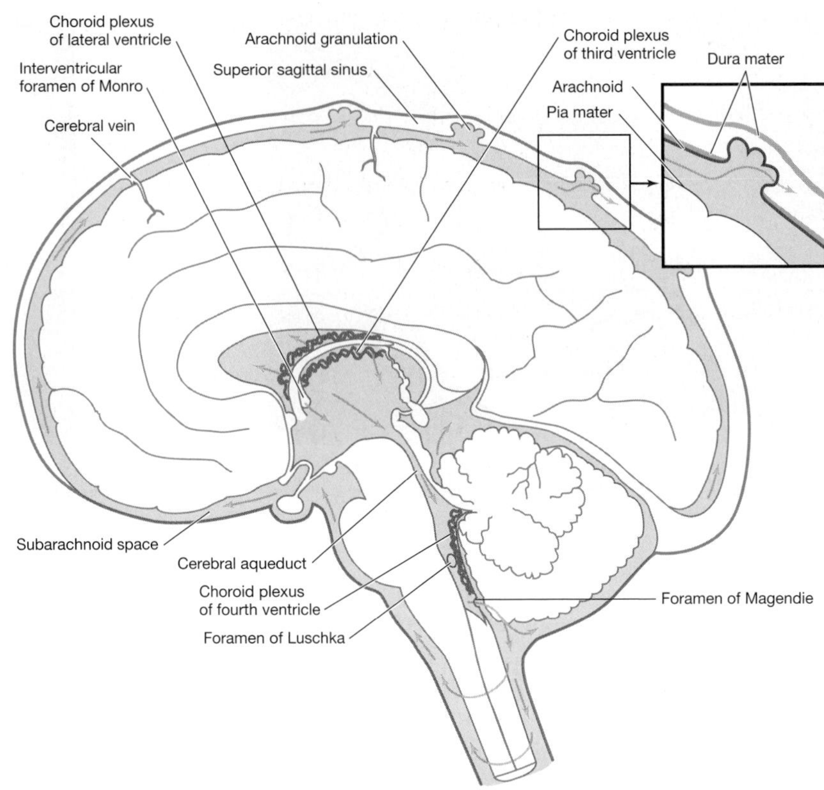

FIGURE 2.6. Flow of cerebrospinal fluid. (Reproduced, with permission, from Aminoff MJ, Simon RP. *Clinical Neurology*, 6th ed. New York: McGraw-Hill, 2005: Figure 1-14.)

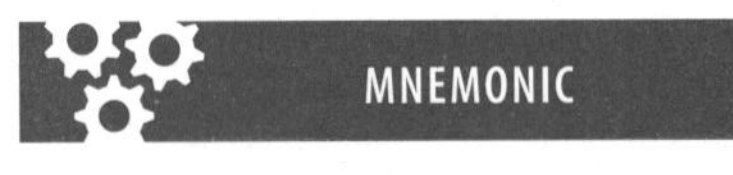

L—**L**ateral for **L**uschka
M—**M**edial for **M**agendie

→ cisterna magna (subarachnoid space) → arachnoid granulation → superior sagittal sinus.

- Volume of CSF: 70–160 mL.
- Normally, CSF is produced at the rate of 0.3 cc/min (or 400–500 cc/day).
- CSF pressure: 80 to 180 mm H_2O.

Hydrocephalus

There are 2 types of hydrocephalus: Communicating and noncommunicating (obstructive). See Table 2.2.

Genetic/congenital conditions associated with **noncommunicating hydrocephalus** include:

TABLE 2.2. Hydrocephalus

Type	Cause	Effect
Noncommunicating (obstructive): ■ From blockage within the system ■ Can be due to a congenital malformation, trauma, tumors, hemorrhages, or infections	Obstruction of interventricular foramen Obstruction of cerebral aqueduct Obstruction of outflow foramens of fourth ventricle	Enlargement of lateral ventricle Enlargement of lateral and third ventricles Enlargement of all ventricles
Communicating: From prior bleeding or meningitis	Obstruction of perimesencephalic cistern Obstruction of subarachnoid CSF flow over the cerebral convexities	Enlargement of all ventricles; widening of posterior fossa cisterns Enlargement of all ventricles; widening of all basal cisterns

- Chiari I: Due to adhesions occluding fourth ventricular foramina.
- Chiari II: Cerebral aqueductal stenosis.
- Dandy Walker: Atresia of the foramina of Luschka and Magendie.
- Bickers-Adams syndrome: X-linked recessive, mutation in L1 cell adhesion molecule (L1CAM), characterized by stenosis of cerebral aqueduct, severe mental retardation, and in 50% by an adduction-flexion deformity of the thumb.

Genetic conditions associated with **communicating hydrocephalus** include:

- Hunter syndrome: Mucopolysaccharoidosis type II, iduronate-2-sulfatase deficiency, X-linked recessive.
- Hurler syndrome: Mucopolysaccharoidosis type I, alpha L-iduronidase deficiency, autosomal recessive.

VASCULAR STRUCTURES

Arterial System (Figure 2.7)

Branches from Interal Carotid Artery (ICA)

1. **Ophthalmic artery:** Supplies the eye and adjacent structures. Branches of the ophthalmic artery include the central retinal artery and ciliary arteries.
   - Central retinal artery occlusion: Sudden painless loss of vision.
2. **Anterior choroidal artery:** Supplies most of the optic tracts, choroid plexus of the lateral ventricles, internal globus pallidus, hippocampus, amygdala, lateral geniculate nucleus, crus cerebri, posterior limb of the internal capsule, and anteromedial portion of the head of the caudate.
   - Stroke: Contralateral hemiplegia, hemihypesthesia, homonymous hemianopsia.

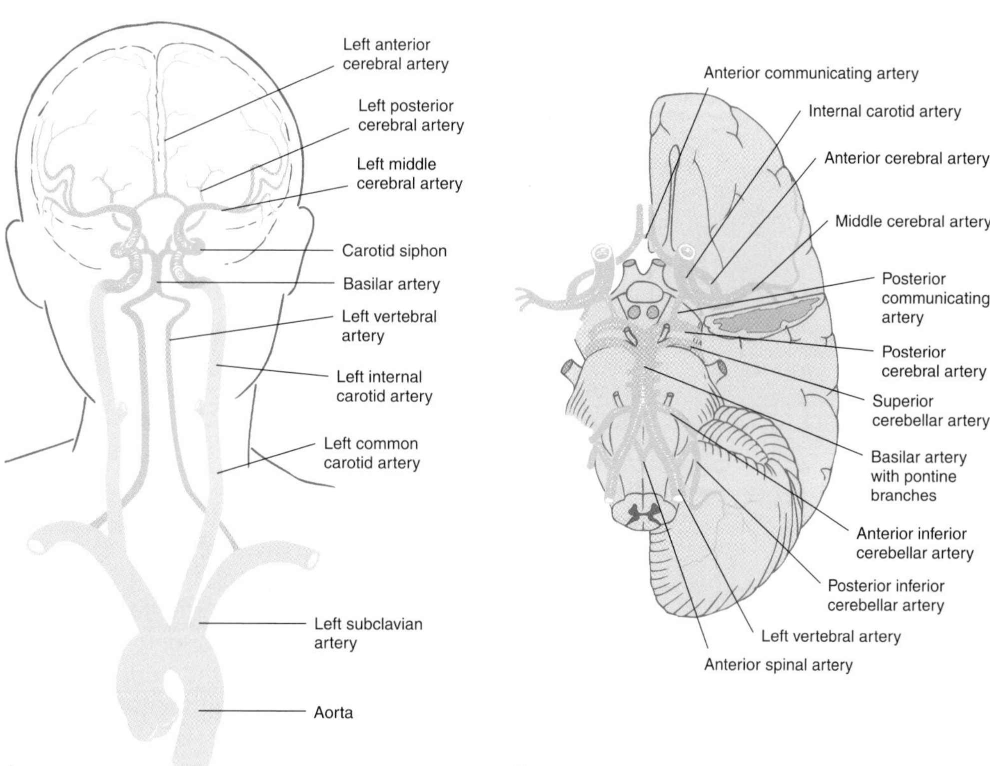

FIGURE 2.7. **Major cerebral arteries. (A)** Anterior view. **(B)** Inferior view showing the circle of Willis and principal arteries of the brain stem.

(Reproduced, with permission, from McPhee SJ, Ganong WF. *Pathology of Disease: An Introduction to Clinical Medicine*, 5th ed. New York: McGraw-Hill, 2006: Figure 7-33.)

3. **Posterior communicating arteries (PCoA):** Connects internal carotid artery to posterior cerebral arteries. Supplies arteries to the thalamus with the polar arteries.
   - Aneurysm of posterior communicating artery: Second most common aneurysm. Leads to ipsilateral oculomotor palsy (with pupillary involvement).
4. **Anterior cerebral artery (ACA):** Supplies the medial surface of the cerebral hemispheres for anterior pole of the brain, anterior corpus callosum, anterior limb of the internal capsule, and inferior part of the caudate anterior globus pallidus.
   - Recurrent artery of Heubner: Supplies head of caudate and anteroinferior internal capsule.
5. **Anterior communicating artery (ACoA):** Connects the 2 anterior cerebral arteries. Common site for aneurysms. Anterior cerebral artery supplies the medial part of the frontal and parietal lobes.
6. **Middle cerebral artery (MCA):** Supplies the majority of the lateral surface of the cerebral hemispheres. Divided into 4 segments. Supplies lateral portions of frontal and parietal lobes, superior parts of the temporal lobe, insula, putamen, outer globus pallidus, posterior limb of internal capsule, body of caudate, and corona radiata.
   - M1: Main MCA trunk with deep penetrating vessels and lenticulostriate arteries.
   - M2: Located in the Sylvian fissure.
   - M3: Cortical branches.
   - M4: More cortical branches over the surface.
7. **Lenticulostriate arteries:** small perforating arteries that supply the basal ganglia and internal capsule. **Stroke:** contralateral face and arm >> leg weakness, homonymous hemianopsia, frontal eye field deviation toward stroke, aphasia (left hemisphere), and neglect (right hemisphere).

Branches from Vertebrobasilar System

1. Vertebral artery:
   - **Posterior spinal arteries:** Supply posterior one-third of the spinal cord.
   - **Anterior spinal arteries:** Supply anterior two-thirds of the spinal cord.
   - **Posterior inferior cerebellar artery (PICA):** Supplies all of the posteroinferior cerebellum, cerebellar tonsil, inferior vermis, posterolateral medulla, and choroid plexus of fourth ventricle.
   - **Lateral medullary syndrome/Wallenberg syndrome:** Vertigo, nystagmus, nausea/vomiting, ipsilateral Horner syndrome, dysphagia, hoarsness, ipsilateral ataxia, loss of pain and temperature on contralateral body but ipsilateral face, and vertical diplopia.
2. Basilar artery:
   - **Anterior inferior cerebellar artery (AICA):** Supplies the inferior surface of the cerebellum, cerebellar flocculus, middle cerebellar peduncle, and caudal part of the pons.
   - **Lateral inferior pontine syndrome:** Horizontal/vertical nystagmus, vertigo, nausea, deafness, ipsilateral facial paralysis, ipsilateral ataxia, loss of pain and temperature on the contralateral body but ipsilateral face, and paralysis of conjugate gaze to the side of the lesion.
   - **Superior cerebellar artery:** Supplies superior portion of the cerebellum, superior aspect of the pons, and the midbrain.
   - **Perforating pontine branches:** Most of the pons.
   - **Basilar artery thrombosis:** "Locked-in syndrome" due to a complete blockage of the basilar artery. Usually starts in a stuttering course with some signs/symptoms referable to the brain stem. If stroke completes before treatment, then it can lead to bilateral corticospinal and corticobulbar weakness → resultant quadriplegia. Patient can be awake and

have complete cognition. Somatosensory pathways are usually spared; therefore, patients can sense their surroundings. Only motor modality spared is vertical eye movements. Acute treatment within 0–3 hours is IV tissue plasminogen activator (tPA), but intra-arterial tPA can be given up to 48 hours. Very poor prognosis.

3. **Posterior cerebral arteries (PCA):** Supply parts of the midbrain, the subthalamic nucleus, the thalamus, the mesial inferior temporal lobe, and the occipital and occipitoparietal cortices. Posterior cerebral artery supplies most of the blood to the thalamus.
   - Interpeduncular branches: Supplies red nucleus, substantia nigra, medial cerebral peduncles, medial longitudinal fasciculus, and medial lemnicus.
   - Thalamoperforate/paramedian thalamic arteries: Supplies inferior, medial, and anterior thalamus.
   - Thalamogenticulate branches: Supplies posterior thalamus.
   - Medial branches: Supplies lateral cerebral peduncles, lateral tegmentum, corpora quadrigeminal, pineal gland.
   - Posterior choroidal: Supplies posterosuperior thalamus, choriod plexus, posterior hypothalamus, hippocampus, subthalamic nucleus.
   - Cortical branches: Inferomedial temporal lobes, medial occipital.
   - Infarctions in the PCA distribution are prone to occur in patients with increased intracranial pressure. With increased intracranial pressure, the PCA can be compressed against the tentorium cerebelli as it crosses from the infratentorial region to the supratentorial region.

Vascular Supply to the Thalamus

- PCoA → polar arteries → reticular, ventral anterior, medial nuclei.
- Basilar artery → paramedian thalamesencephalic arteries → reticular, ventrolateral, medial, midline, centromedian nuclei.
- PCA → thalamogenticulate pedicle → ventral caudal nuclei.
- vPCA → posterior choroidal arteries → centromedian, ventroposteromedial, medial geniculate, pulvinar, medial, anterior, lateral geniculate, laterodorsal.

Circle of Willis: Provides anastomotic flow for the brain. Only approximately 30% of people have complete circle of Willis.

Venous System (Figure 2.8)

- **Dural venous sinuses:** Venous channels lined by mesothelium that lie between the inner and outer layers of dura.

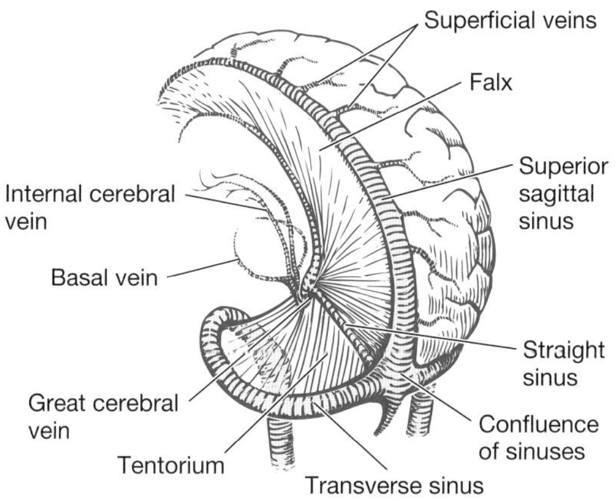

FIGURE 2.8. Venous sinuses. (Reproduced, with permission, from Waxman SG. *Clinical Neuroanatomy*, 25th ed. New York: McGraw-Hill, 2003: Figure 12-9.)

- Superior sagittal sinus: Between the falx and the inside of the skullcap.
- Inferior sagittal sinus: Below the falx.
- Straight sinus: In the seam between the falx and tentorium.
- Transverse sinuses: Between the tentorium and its attachment on the skullcap.
- Sigmoid sinuses: S-curved continuations of the transverse sinuses into the jugular veins.
- Cavernous sinus: On either side of the sella turcica. Blood leaves the cavernous sinus via the petrosal sinuses.
- Inferior petrosal sinus: From the cavernous sinus to the jugular foramen.
- Superior petrosal sinus: From the cavernous sinus to the beginning of the sigmoid sinus.
- **Venous sinus thrombosis:** Thrombosis within the venous sinus system. Risk factors include inherited hypercoagulable states, pregnancy, oral contraceptives, malignancy, infections, inflammatory conditions, dehydration, trauma. Leads to focal neurologic deficits (can be hemorrhagic or ischemic infarcts) and/or signs of increased intracranial pressure. Can present like pseudotumor cerebri. Diagnosis can be obtained with magnetic resonance venogram (MRV)/computed tomographic venography (CTV). Treatment is anticoagulation.

- Other venous structures:
  - **Great cerebral vein (vein of Galen):** A vein formed by the junction of the 2 internal cerebral veins and passes between the corpus callosum and the pineal gland to continue into the straight sinus.
  - **Vein of Galen malformation:** This congenital vascular malformation involves a direct connection between a cerebral artery and cerebral vein. The malformation develops during weeks 6–11 of fetal development as a persistent embryonic prosencephalic vein of Markowski. It is the most frequent arteriovenous malformation in neonates. In neonates, it presents as congestive heart failure (shunt effect), and in older infants, it can present with hydrocephalus, seizures, headache, development delay and heart failure. Hydrocephalus occurs because the malformation compresses the cerebral aqueduct. Initial diagnosis can be obtained with cranial ultrasound, but if surgery is considered, other imaging including magnetic resonance imaging and angiogram are useful. Treatment includes cardiovascular support for congestive heart failure, surgery, and embolization.
  - **Cavernous sinus** (Figure 2.9): Channel of venous blood by the sphe-

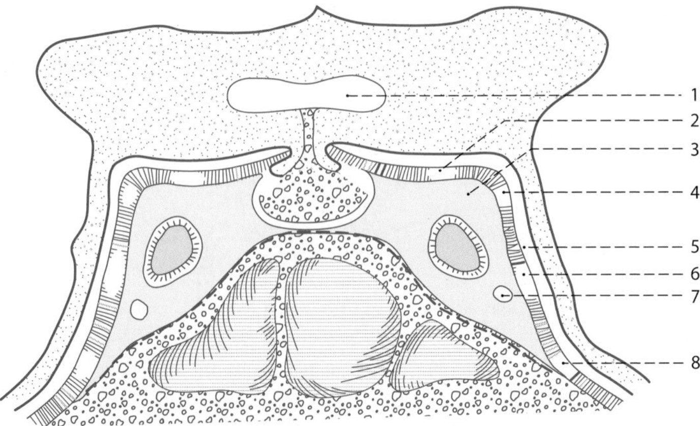

FIGURE 2.9. Diagram of the cavernous sinus. (1) Optic chiasm; (2) oculomotor nerve; (3) cavernous sinus; (4) trochlear nerve; (5) internal carotid artery; (6) ophthalmic nerve; (7) abducens nerve; (8) maxillary nerve. (Reproduced, with permission, from Ropper AH, Brown RH. *Adams and Victor's Principles of Neurology*, 8th ed. New York: McGraw-Hill, 2005: 735.)

noid and temporal bones. Many important structures, including the ICA and multiple cranial nerves, travel through the cavernous sinus.
- **Cavernous sinus syndrome:** Superfluous, and mildly inaccurate (can be caused by infection or clot in the cavernous sinus). Usually due to a tumor (eg, nasopharyngeal carcinoma, pituitary tumor, craniopharyngioma), aneurysm, or infection. Leads to ophthalmoplegia (involvement of CN III, CN IV, and CN VI), visual loss (involvement of optic chiasm), and sensory loss in distribution of maxillary nerve.

MNEMONIC

Structures in the Cavernous Sinus—
Oh, TOMCAt:
Oculomotor nerve (CN III)
Trochlear nerve (CN IV)
Ophthalmic nerve (CN V1)
Maxillary nerve (CN V2)
Carotid
Abducens nerve (CN V1)

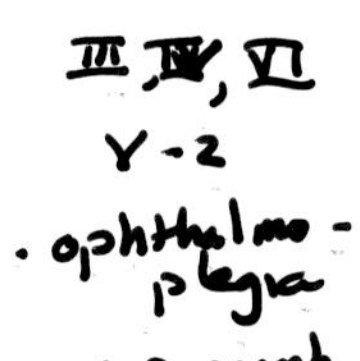

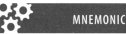

SPINAL CORD (FIGURE 2.10)

- Extends caudally to vertebral level L1–L2.
- Functional segmented (31 total):
  - 8 cervical
  - 12 thoracic
  - 5 lumbar
  - 5 sacral
  - 1 coccygeal

Important Anatomical Structures

- **Conus medullaris:** Conical distal end of the spinal cord.
- **Filum terminale:** Extends from the tip of the conus and attaches to coccygeal ligament (made of pia).
- **Denticulate ligaments:** Pial extensions anchor the cord to dura to provide lateral support.
- **Cervical enlargement:** C5–T1, nerves of the brachial plexus.
- **Lumbar enlargement:** L2–S3, nerves of the lumbosacral plexus.
- **Cauda equina:** Lower lumbar, sacral, and coccygeal spinal nerves that extend after the end of spinal cord; travel in the subarachnoid space (lumbar cistern). See Table 2.3 for a comparison of cauda equina syndrome and conus medullaris syndrome.
- **Dorsal medial fissure:** Shallow.
- **Ventral medial fissure:** Deeper.
  - **Posterolateral sulcus** → dorsal roots (inputs enter the cord). Aα: largest fibers from muscle spindles and spinal cord reflexes. Aβ: from mechanoreceptors in skin and joints. C and Aδ: small, noxious, and thermal stimuli.
  - **Anterolateral sulcus** → ventral roots (outputs leave through this area). Aα motor neuron axons to extrafusal striated muscles. Aγ motor neuron axons to intrafusal muscle of muscle spindles. Preganglionic autonomic fibers at thoracic, upper lumbar, and midsacral. Few afferent, small-diameter axons from thoracic and abdominal viscera.
- **Arterial supply:**
  - **Anterior spinal artery:** Fusion of vertebral, anterior median fissure, supplies anterior two-thirds of spinal cord.
  - **Posterior spinal arteries:** Smaller, from PICA, much less, forms plexus, supplies posterior one-third of spinal cord.
  - **Radicular arteries:** From aorta, send collaterals to spinal cord; although in early embryonic development every segment of spinal cord receives paired radicular arteries, these disappear, leaving 1 or 2 cervical, 2 or 3 throacic, and 1 or 2 lumbar arteries.
  - **Artery of Adamkiewicz:** Largest radicular artery (forms the caudal-most portion of anterior spinal artery); arises from the left side at T10 in approximately 80% of people.
  - **Anterior spinal artery syndrome:** Below the level of the lesion → bilateral weakness, loss of pain and temperature sensation; loss of bowel and

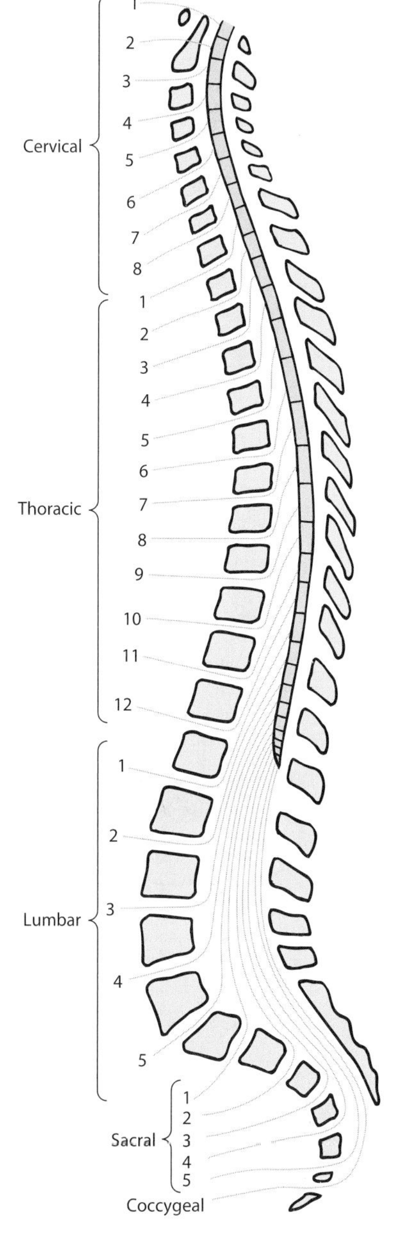

FIGURE 2.10. Spinal cord. (Reproduced, with permission, from Waxman SG. *Clinical Neuroanatomy*, 25th ed. New York: McGraw-Hill, 2003: Figure 5-4.)

TABLE 2.3. Cauda Equina Syndrome versus Conus Medullaris Syndrome

	Level of Lesion	Weakness	Sensory Deficit	Reflexes	Bowel/Bladder Involvement
Cauda equina Onset: Gradual Asymmetric	L4, L5, or S1	Asymmetric	Asymmetric saddle anesthesia in all modalities	Ankle jerk absent Knee jerk absent	Retention, develops later Decreased rectal tone
Conus medullaris Onset: Sudden Bilateral	L1, L2	Symmetric	Symmetric saddle anesthesia in small fibers	Ankle jerk absent Knee jerk preserved	Incontinence develops early

bladder control; preservation of proprioception and vibration sensation. Seen after aortic injury (eg, surgery, atherosclerosis, dissection), spinal trauma, vasculitis, or infection. Can be caused by a thrombosis to the artery of Adamkiewicz.
  - **Primary watershed areas:** Midthoracic region of the spinal cord. Levels T1–T4 and T8–T9 are prone to ischemic damage during thoracic surgery or hypotension because only a few radicular arteries persist in this region as an adult.
- **Venous drainage:** Diffuse → epidural space → empty into vena cavae.
- **Central canal:** Lined with ependymal cells, filled with CSF, opens upward into the inferior portion of the fourth ventricle, only in cervical levels.
- **Myxopapillary ependymoma:** Ependymal tumor that presents at the lumbar cistern. Arises from a remnant of ependymal cells from the central canal (that recedes to the cervical region during development).

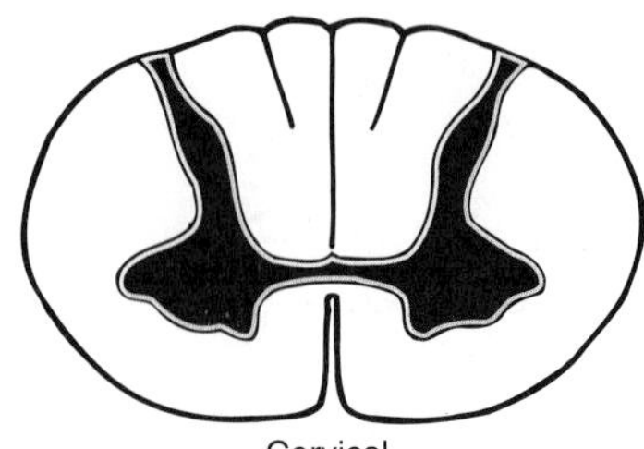

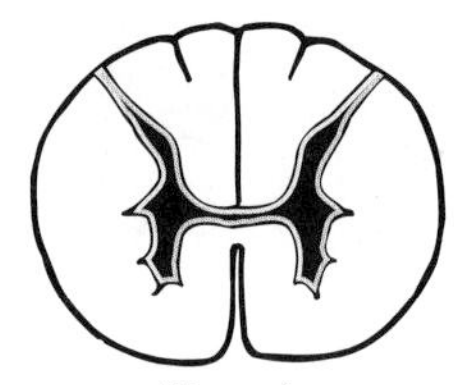

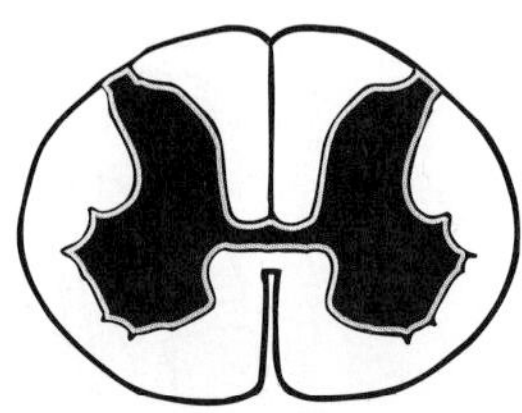

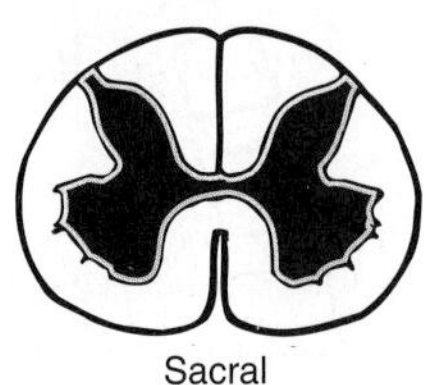

FIGURE 2.11. Levels of spinal cord. (Reproduced, with permission, from Waxman SG. *Clinical Neuroanatomy,* 25th ed. New York: McGraw-Hill, 2003: Figure 5-10.)

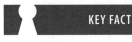

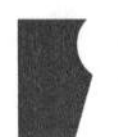
KEY FACT

Cervical gray matter looks like "baby booties"; thoracic gray matter looks like a "Honda" symbol.

Organization of Spinal Cord Segments

Gray Matter

- H-shaped internal mass surrounded by white matter.
  - Dorsal horn.
  - Intermediolateral gray column.
  - Ventral horn.
- Proportion of gray to white is greatest in the lumbar and cervical enlargements (Figure 2.11).
- In thoracic region, both the dorsal and ventral columns are narrow, lateral columns.
- In lumbar region, dorsal and ventral columns are broad and expanded.

Rexed Laminae (Figure 2.12)

Layers of nerves cells in the spinal cord gray matter. In motor neuron pools (IX), the neurons are somatotopically organized as follows: flexor muscles close to the central canal, extensor muscles located more peripherally. Medial neurons → proximal muscles; lateral neurons → distal muscles.

Gray Matter Laminae

See Table 2.4.

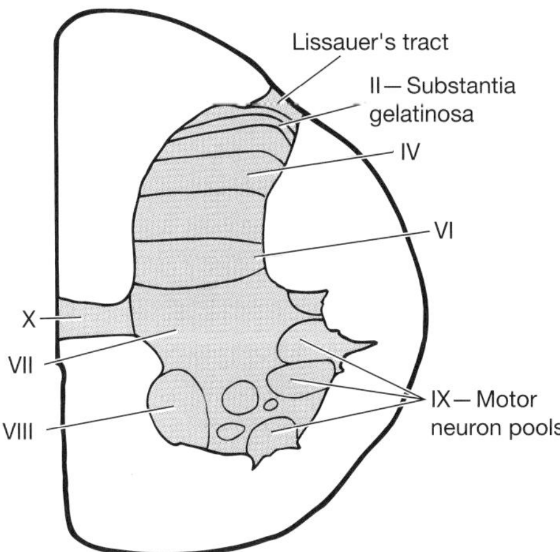

FIGURE 2.12. Laminae of the gray matter of the spinal cord (only one-half shown).
(Reproduced, with permission, from Waxman SG. *Clinical Neuroanatomy*, 25th ed. New York: McGraw-Hill, 2003: Figure 5-11.)

TABLE 2.4. Gray Matter Laminae

Lamina	Common Name	Function
I	Marginal zone	Thin marginal layer contains neurons that respond to noxious stimuli and send axons to contralateral spinothalamic tract.
II	Substantia gelatinosa	Interneurons; respond to noxious stimuli, sensibility to pain. ■ Release naturally occurring opiates, thereby limiting release of substance P from pain-sensitive dorsal root fibers.
III, IV, V, VI	Nucleus proprius	Neurons that receive inputs from large fibers, which mediate finely localized touch, stereognosis, proprioception, vibration sense. ■ Secrete γ-aminobutyric acid (GABA).
VII	Clarke's column	From T1–L2, receives inputs on joint position and sends info to the cerebellum via the dorsal spinocerebellar tract.
VII	Intermediolateral cell column	From T1–L2, preganglionic neurons project to sympathetic ganglia.
VIII	Ventral horn interneurons	Involved in reflexes, main target of descending motor commmands from motor/premotor cortex and brain stem. ■ All inhibitory, use glycine > GABA. ■ 1a interneurons: Inhibit motor neurons of antagonist muscle; receive sensory input from agonist muscle's spindle afferents. ■ 1b interneurons: Inhibit motor neurons of agonist muscle; receive sensory input from agonist muscle's Golgi tendon organs. ■ Renshaw cells: Have direct input agonist muscle, inhibits agonist motor neuron and the interneurons of antagonist muscles → increases antagonist muscle tone.
IX	Ventral horn motor neurons	Pools of motor neurons that innervate skeletal musculature. ■ α_I: Innervate fatigable and fatigue-resistant fast-twitch muscles. ■ α-II: Innervate fatigue-resistant slow-twitch muscles. ■ γ: Innervate intrafusal muscle fibers of muscle spindles.
X	Central gray	Small neurons, no known function.

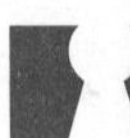

KEY FACT

Big 4: Sensory modalities that are transmitted on large diameter myelinated fibers.

- Light touch
- Stereognosis
- Vibration sense
- Proprioception

KEY FACT

Little 3: Sensory modalities that are transmitted on small unmyelinated (sometimes myelinated fibers).

- Pain
- Temperature
- Crude touch

White Matter (Figure 2.13)

Ascending (see Table 2.5) and descending white matter pathways in the spinal cord. They are also somatotopically organized.

Descending Pathways

Corticospinal Tract

- Neurons in motor and premotor cortical areas descend in cerebral peduncles as pyramidal tract.
- Fibers cross in medulla at the decussation of the pyramids and descend down the spinal cord in lateral corticospinal tract.
- Terminate on neurons of the ventral horn.
- Only 1% of these neurons make a direct 1:1 connection with primary motor neurons.
- About 15% of corticospinal fibers do not cross in pyramidal decussation and descend anteriorly and medially in anterior corticospinal tract (usually contribution to the flexors of the upper extremities and extensors of the lower extremities).

Other Descending Tracts

- Lateral vestibulospinal tract: Controls postural reflexes—lateral vestibular nucleus → travels in ventral column → descends uncrossed to the anterior horn interneurons and motor neurons (for extensors).
- Medial vestibulospinal tract: Controls postural reflexes—medial vestibular nucleus → travels in ventral column → descends crossed and uncrossed to the anterior horn interneurons and motor neurons.
- Rubrospinal tract: Motor function—red nucleus → travels in lateral column → immediately crosses and terminates in the contralateral ventral horn interneurons.
- Medial reticulospinal tract: Motor function (excitation of flexor and proximal trunk and axial motor neurons)—pontine reticular formation → travels in lateral column → descends uncrossed to the ventral horn.
- Lateral reticulospinal tract: Modulation of sensory transmission and spinal reflexes; excitation and inhibition of axial (neck and back) motor neurons—medullary reticular formation → travels in lateral column → descends crossed and uncrossed to most of the ventral horn and the basal portion of the dorsal horn.
- Tectospinal tract: Reflex head turning—superior colliculus → travels in ventral column → contralateral ventral horn interneurons.

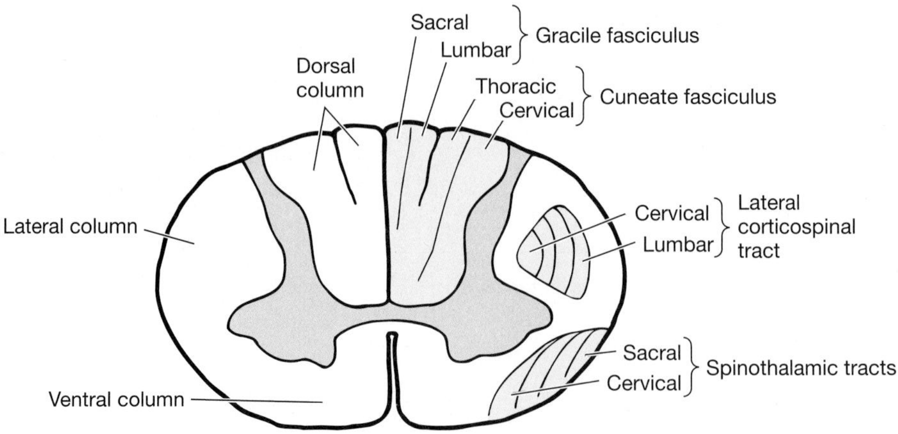

FIGURE 2.13. Somatotopic organization (segmental arrangement) in the spinal cord. (Reproduced, with permission, from Waxman SG. *Clinical Neuroanatomy*, 25th ed. New York: McGraw-Hill, 2003: Figure 5-15.)

TABLE 2.5. Ascending Pathways

NAME	FUNCTION	ORIGIN	TARGET
Dorsal column/medial lemniscal tract (Figure 2.14)	Light touch Stereognosis Vibration sense Proprioception	Encapsulated mechanoreceptors in skin, joints, tendons (afferent limb of large-diameter Aα or Aβ axon)	Dorsal column nuclei in brainstem (2° contralateral ventral posterior lateral [VPL] thalamus)
Anterolateral system (spinothalamic and spinoreticulothalamic) tract (Figure 2.15)	Pain Temperature Crude touch	Free nerve endings	Substantia gelatinosa (2° contralateral reticular formation or direct to contralateral VPL thalamus)
Dorsal spinocerebellar/ cuneocerebellar tracts (Figure 2.16)	Movement and joint position (unconscious)	Muscle spindles and Golgi tendon organs	Clarke's nucleus (T1–L2) or accessory cuneate nucleus (2° ipsilateral cerebellum via inferior cerebellar peduncle)
Ventral spinocerebellar tract (Figure 2.16)	Movement and joint position (unconscious)	Muscle spindles and Golgi tendon organs	Laminae V, VI, VII in sacral and lumbar levels (2° anterior cerebellum via superior cerebellar peduncle)

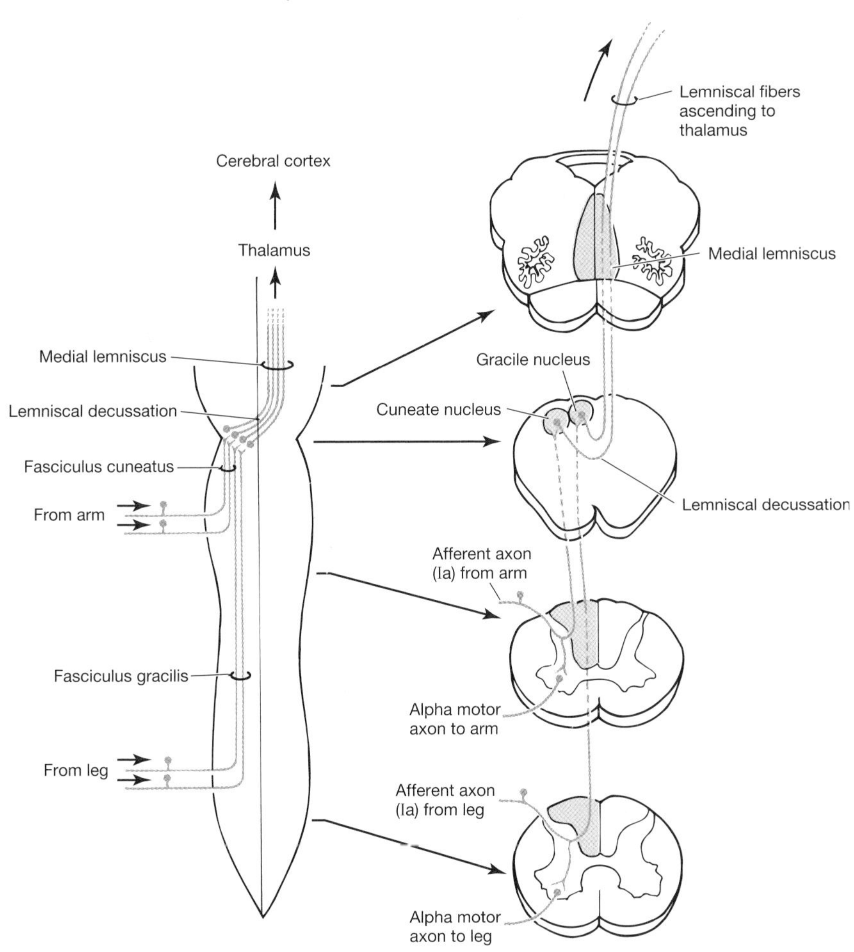

FIGURE 2.14. Dorsal column pathway. (Reproduced, with permission, from Waxman SG. *Clinical Neuroanatomy*, 25th ed. New York: McGraw-Hill, 2003: Figure 5-14.)

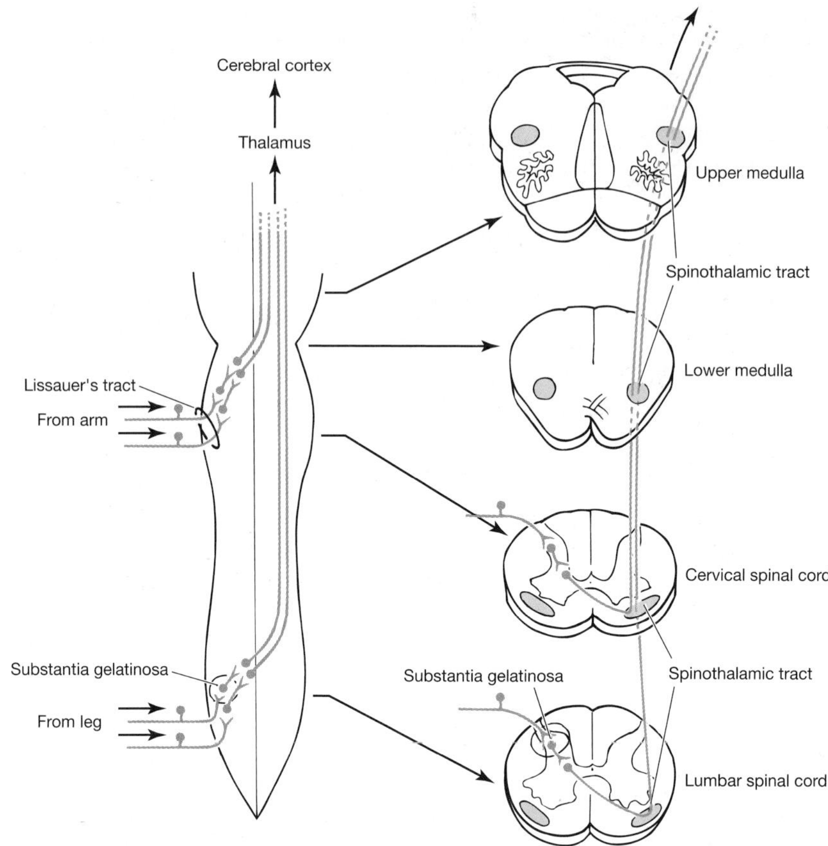

FIGURE 2.15. Anterolateral system pathway. (Reproduced, with permission, from Waxman SG. *Clinical Neuroanatomy*, 25th ed. New York: McGraw-Hill, 2003: Figure 5-16.)

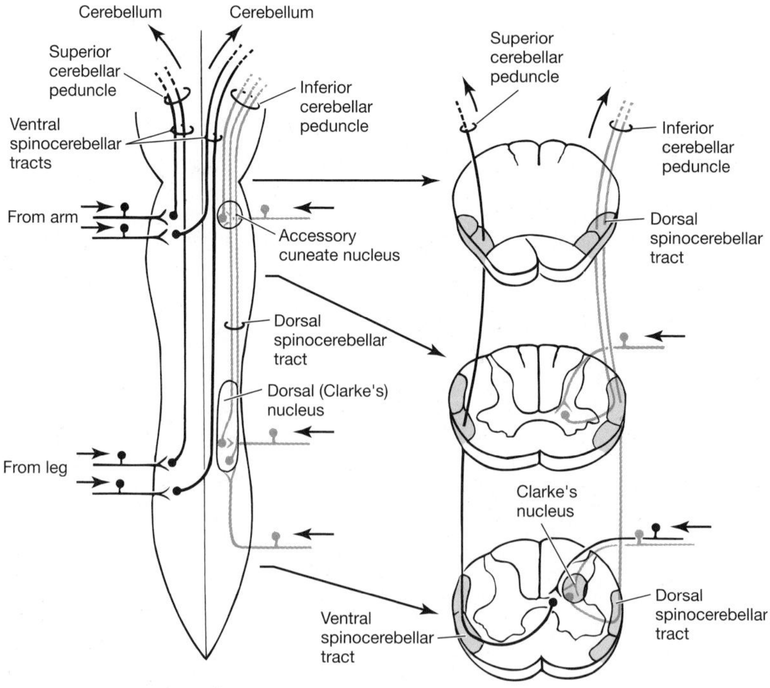

FIGURE 2.16. Spinocerebellar pathway. (Reproduced, with permission, from Waxman SG. *Clinical Neuroanatomy*, 25th ed. New York: McGraw-Hill, 2003: Figure 5-17.)

- Medial longitudinal fasciculus: Coordination of head and eye movements—vestibular nuclei → travels in ventral column → cervical gray matter motor neurons.

Classical Lesions/Diseases of the Spinal Cord (Table 2.6)

Syringomyelia

Capitation of spinal cord (usually cervical). Expansion of the central canal. If it involves the brain stem, it is called *syringobulbia.*

- Can be associated with Chiari malformation; also associated with tumors, trauma, inflammation.
- Causes central cord syndrome.
- Affects fibers from the anterolateral system that are crossing in the anterior white commissure; can also affect lateral corticospinal tract and anterior horn cell motor neurons; dorsal columns are usually spared.
- Bilateral loss of temperature, pain, and crude touch sensation at the level of the lesion.
- Lower motor neuron weakness in hands and upper motor neuron weakness/hyperreflexia in legs.

Brown-Séquard Syndrome

Complete transverse hemisection of spinal cord. Rare to have a complete hemisection of the cord; most examples are incomplete.

- Can be due to trauma (eg, stab wounds to the neck), tumors, inflammation/infection, hematomas, degenerative disk disease.
- Contralateral loss of pain, temperature, and crude touch below the level of the lesion.
- Ipsilateral loss of proprioception, light touch, and vibration sense below the level of the lesion.
- Motor paralysis on the ipsilateral side (UMN pattern below the lesion and LMN pattern at the level of the lesion).
- Some ipsilateral sensory loss at level of the lesion.

Tabes Dorsalis

Neurologic sequalae associated with tertiary syphilis.

- Degeneration of dorsal columns.
- Loss of proprioception, light touch, and vibratory sensation.

TABLE 2.6. Clinical Localization of Spinal Cord Lesions

	Lower Motor Neuron (LMN) Lesion	Upper Motor Neuron (UMN) Lesion
Weakness	Flaccid paralysis	Spastic paralysis
Deep tendon reflexes	Decreased or absent	Increased
Babinski reflex	Absent	Present
Atrophy	May be present	Absent or due to disuse
Fasciculations and fibrillations	May be present	Absent

Friedreich Ataxia

Autosomal recessive spinocerebellar ataxia.

- Mutations in fraxatin gene on chromosome 9; trinucleotide repeat disease (GAA repeat).
- Slow degeneration of dorsal columns, spinocerebellar tracts, corticospinal tracts, and dentate nucleus projections.
- Present usually in ages 5–15; death by 40 years of age.
- Leads to ataxia, nystagmus, dysarthria, loss of proprioception, spastic weakness in legs, hyporeflexia; Babinski reflex is upgoing.
- Patients also suffer from diabetes and cardiomyopathy.

Subacute Combined Degeneration

Traditionally associated with vitamin B_{12} deficiency.

- Degeneration of the lateral and dorsal columns of the spinal cord.
- Progressive disease with ataxia (loss of spinocerebellar tracts), loss of proprioception and vibratory sense (loss of dorsal columns), and weakness in lower > upper extremities (loss of corticospinal tract).
- Can look like copper deficiency or folate deficiency.

Amyotrophic Lateral Sclerosis (ALS; Lou Gehrig Disease)

- Most cases are sporadic; 10% are genetic (autosomal dominant), and a subset of those is associated with superoxide dismutase (SOD-1) gene mutation.
- Gradual degradation of the motor neurons in the ventral horns and the corticospinal tracts in the lateral columns of spinal cord.
- Progressive weakness with fasciculations and cramping.
- Both upper and lower motor neurons are affected in spinal cord, resulting in both muscular atrophy and hyperreflexia.

Spinal Muscular Atrophy (SMA)

Heterogenous group of genetic disorders with progressive LMN weakness.

- Most are autosomal recessive.
- Time of presentation varies as SMA I (Werdnig-Hoffman disease) presents at birth, whereas SMA IV can present in adulthood.
- Degeneration of ventral horn motor neurons.

Poliomyelitis

Infection by enterovirus that directly infects the ventral horn motor neurons; LMN pattern.

- Rare in developed countries, but can still be seen in developing countries.
- Gastrointestinal virus followed by asymmetric weakness and fasciculations (lower extremities > upper extremities; can rarely affect the bulbar musculature).
- Postpolio syndrome: Increased weakness in previously affected muscles several years after initial infection.

CRANIAL NERVES (CNs) (FIGURE 2.17)

CN I: Olfactory—Sensory

Component: Special sensory (special afferent).
Function: Olfactory sensation.
Outlet: Cribriform plate of ethmoid bone. Emerges from olfactory bulb.

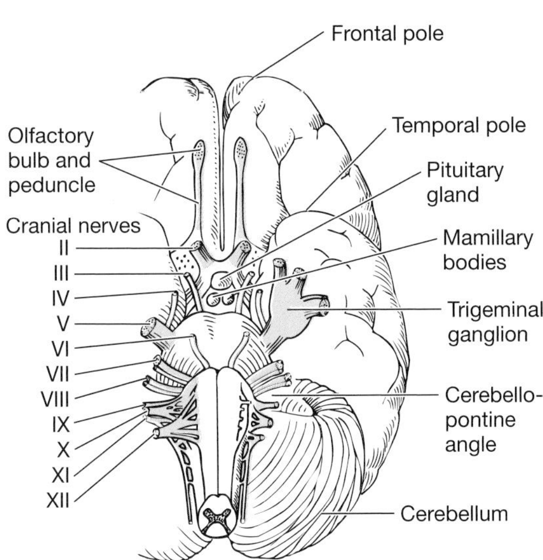

FIGURE 2.17. Ventral view of the brain stem with cranial nerves. (Reproduced, with permission, from Waxman SG. *Clinical Neuroanatomy*, 25th ed. New York: McGraw-Hill, 2003: Figure 8-1.)

Pathway: *Axons from the olfactory bulb* (olfactory stalk) → *anterior olfactory nucleus* → *primary olfactory cortex, entorhinal cortex, amygdala.*
Clinical: Fracture of cribiform plate → anosmia → no taste.

CN II: Optic—Sensory

Component: Special sensory (special afferent).
Function: Visual information from the retina.
Outlet: Optic canal (travels with ophthalmic artery).
Pathway: *Optic nerves* → *optic chiasm* → *optic tracts* → *lateral geniculate nucleus and superior colliculus* → *occiptal cortex* (via the optic radiations).
Clinical: Damage → unilateral blindness when damaged at the nerve.

CN III: Oculomotor—Motor (Figure 2.18)

Component 1: Somatic motor (general somatic efferent).
Function 1: Innervates levator palpebrae superioris, superior rectus, medial rectus, inferior rectus, and inferior oblique muscles (from oculomotor nucleus). See Tables 2.7 and 2.8.
Component 2: Visceral motor (general visceral efferent).
Function 2: Provides parasympathetic supply to constrictor pupillae and ciliary muscles via ciliary ganglion (from Edinger-Westphal nucleus).
Outlet: Superior orbital fissure (travels through the cavernous sinus).
Clinical: Isolated oculomotor nerve palsy.

- Thrombosis in cavernous sinus.
- Aneurysms in posterior cerebral arteries or superior cerebellar arteries.
- Compression caused by tumor, abscess, or trauma leading to herniation → under such conditions, the tentorial notch can displace the cerebral peduncles to the opposite site and compress the oculomotor nerve.
- Ophthalmoplegia (downward, abducted eye due to unopposed action of superior oblique and lateral rectus muscles), ptosis (due to inactivation of levator palpebrae superioris), dilation of pupil (due to decreased tone of the constrictor pupillae), paralysis of accommodation.
- Pupil-sparing CN III palsy: Most likely diabetic neuropathy, atherosclerosis, vasculitis.

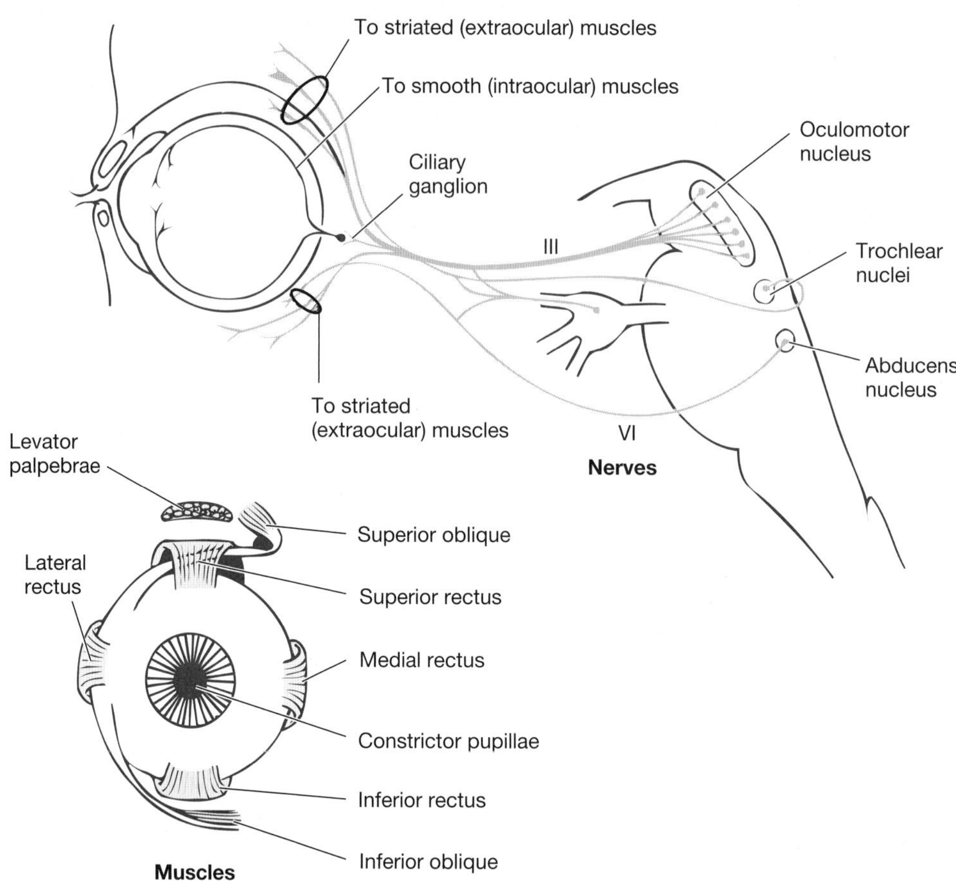

FIGURE 2.18. The oculomotor, trochlear, and abducens nerves; ocular muscles. (Reproduced, with permission, from Waxman SG. *Clinical Neuroanatomy*, 25th ed. New York: McGraw-Hill, 2003: Figure 8-4.)

CN IV: Trochlear—Motor (Figure 2.18)

Component: Somatic motor (general somatic efferent).
Function: Innervates superior oblique muscle.
Outlet: Superior orbital fissure.
Pathway: Trochlear nucleus → crosses within the midbrain → travels through cavernous sinus.
Clinical: Isolated CN IV palsy.

TABLE 2.7. Extraocular Muscles and Their Actions

Muscle	Primary Action	Secondary Action
Lateral rectus	Abduction	None
Medial rectus	Adduction	None
Superior rectus	Elevation	Adduction, intorsion
Inferior rectus	Depression	Adduction, extorsion
Superior oblique	Depression	Intorsion, abduction
Inferior oblique	Elevation	Extorsion, abduction

TABLE 2.8. Deviation Associated with Isolated Extraocular Muscle Weakness

Muscle	Nerve	Deviation of Eyeball	Diplopia Present When Looking	Direction of Image
Lateral rectus	VI	Inward (internal squint)	Toward temple	Vertical
Medial rectus	III	Outward (external squint)	Toward nose	Vertical
Superior rectus	III	Downward and inward	Upward and outward	Oblique
Inferior rectus	III	Upward and inward	Downward and outward	Oblique
Superior oblique	IV	Upward and outward	Downward and inward	Oblique
Inferior oblique	III	Downward and outward	Upward and inward	Oblique

- Etiology includes idiopathic, trauma (40%), microvasculopathy secondary to diabetes, atherosclerosis, or hypertension; can be congenital.
- Paralysis of superior oblique → diplopia, weakness of downward gaze, depression. Patient has difficulty going down stairs. Patients develop a characteristic head tilt, away from affected side to reduce their diplopia.

CN VI: Abducens—Motor (Figure 2.18)

Component: Somatic motor (general somatic efferent).
Function: Innervate lateral rectus.
Outlet: Superior orbital fissure (travels through cavernous sinus).
Clinical: Isolated CN VI palsy.

- Most common due to the long course of the nerve.
- Etiologies include elevated intracranial pressure, aneurysms of posterior inferior cerebellar and basilar arteries or of the internal carotid arteries, tumors, trauma, congenital absence of nerve (Duane syndrome), inflammation/infection (viral), intracranial hypotension.
- Present with binocular horizontal diplopia and esotropia in primary gaze.
- **Tolosa-Hunt syndrome:** A painful ophthalmoplegia caused by nonspecific granulomatous inflammation of the cavernous sinus or superior orbital fissure. Onset is usually a painful ophthalmoplegia with varying degrees of optic and trigeminal nerve involvement. Etiology is unknown and it is considered a diagnosis of exclusion. Treatment is pain relief and prednisone for 7–10 days, then taper. Most patients respond to steroids, but some patients may have incomplete recovery or a recurrence (approximately 30%).

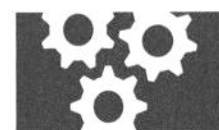

MNEMONIC

LR_6SO_4

Lateral **R**ectus CN **VI** and **S**uperior **O**blique CN **IV**

CN V: Trigeminal—Mixed (Figure 2.19)

Component 1: Branchial motor (special visceral efferent).
Function 1: Innervate muscle of mastication, tensor tympani, tensor palatini, mylohyoid, anterior belly of digastric.
Component 2: General sensory (general somatic afferent).
Function 2: Sensation from face and scalp as far as the top of the head, conjunctiva, bulb of the eye, mucous membranes of paranasal sinuses, nasal and oral cavities including tongue and teeth, part of external aspect of the tympanic membrane, and meninges in anterior middle cranial fossa.
Outlet: Emerges on the midlateral surface of pons as large sensory root and

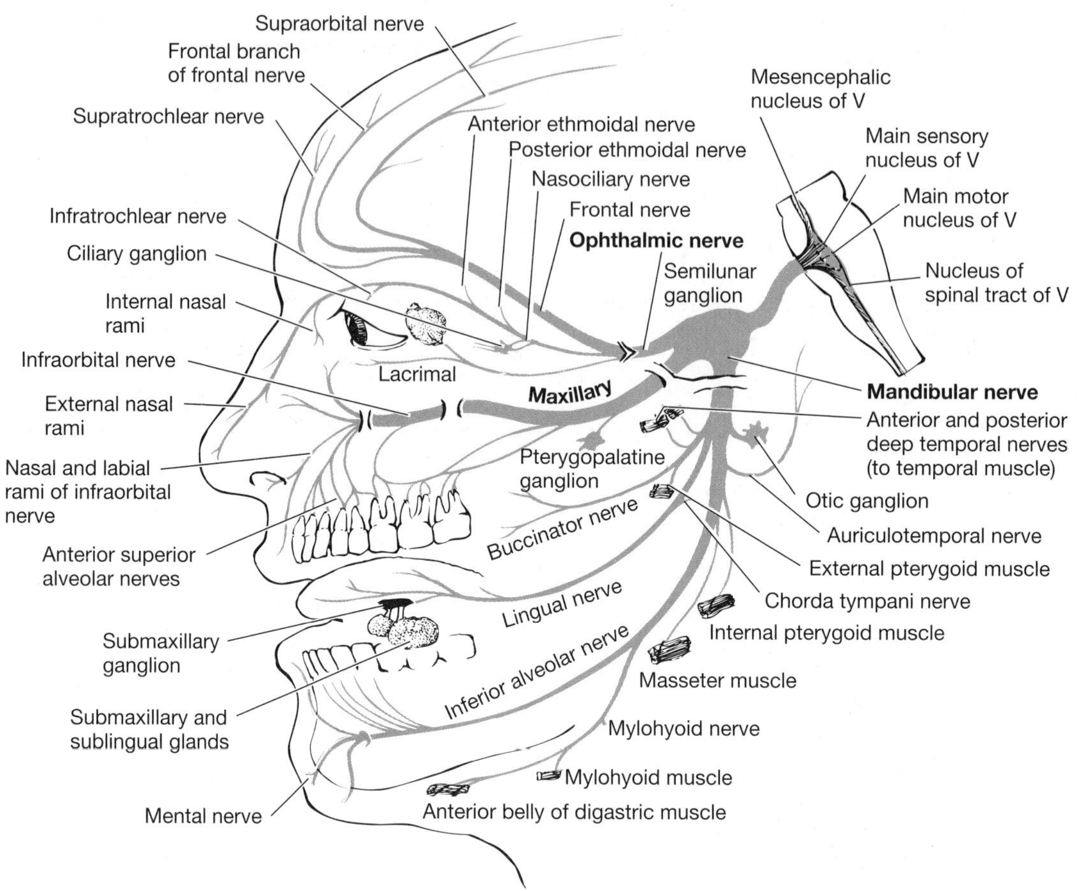

FIGURE 2.19. Trigeminal nerve. (Reproduced, with permission, from Waxman SG. *Clinical Neuroanatomy*, 25th ed. New York: McGraw-Hill, 2003: Figure 8-11.)

smaller motor root. Ophthalmic (V1): superior orbital fissure; maxillary (V2): foramen rotundum; mandibular (V3): foramen ovale.

Clinical: Trigeminal neuralgia → characterized by severe pain in distribution of 1 or more of the branches of the trigeminal. Excruciating paroxysmal pain of short duration can be caused by pressure from a small vessel on the root entry zone of the nerve.

CN VII: Facial—Mixed (Figure 2.20)

Component 1: Branchial motor (special visceral efferent).

Function 1: Innervate stapedius, stylohyoid, posterior belly of digastric muscles, muscles of facial expression, buccinator, platysma, and occipitalis muscle.

Component 2: General sensory (general somatic afferent).

Function 2: Sensation for the skin of the concha of the auricle, a small area of skin behind the ear, and possibly to supplement V3, which supplies the wall of the acoustic meatus and external tympanic membrane.

Component 3: Visceral motor (general visceral efferent).

Function 3: Stimulation of lacrimal, submandibular, and sublingual glands, as well as the mucous membranes of the nose, and hard and soft palate.

Component 4: Special sensory (special afferent).

Function 4: Taste from the anterior two-thirds of tongue and hard and soft palate.

Outlet: Internal acoustic meatus (motor → stylomastoid foramen).

Clinical: Facial nerve palsy: LMN pattern (involves the whole side of the face. If UMN pattern, involves only the lower two-thirds of the face be-

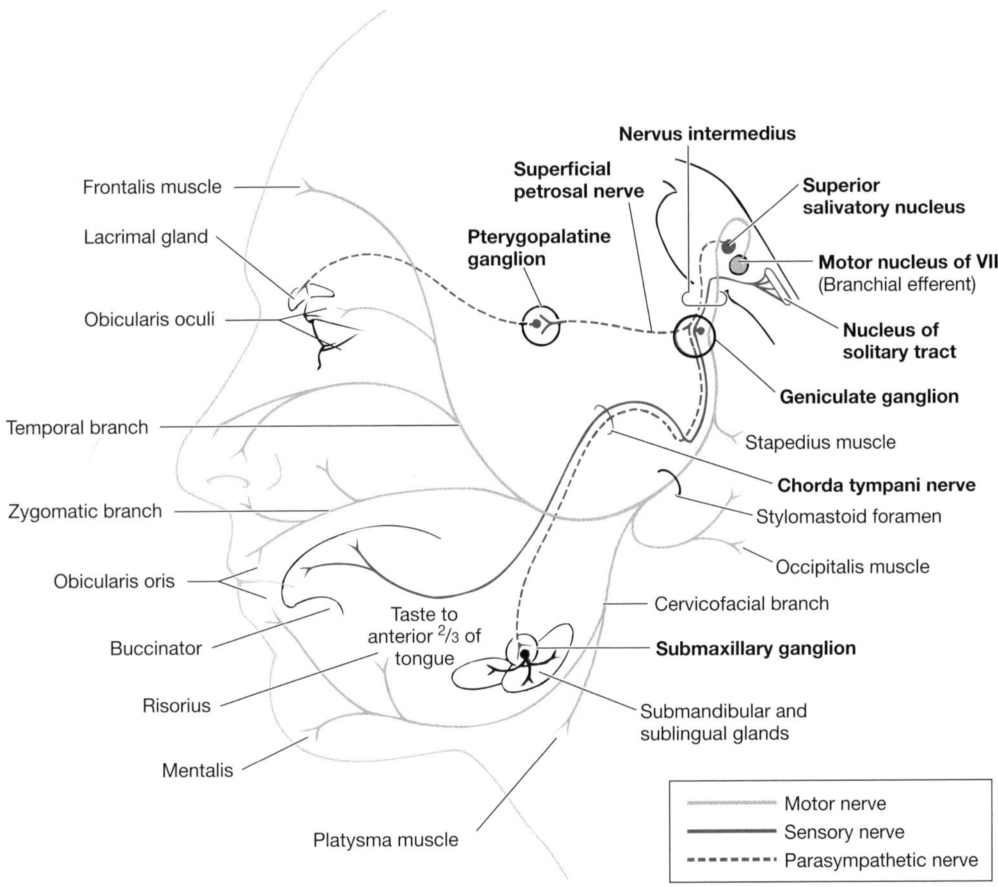

FIGURE 2.20. Facial nerve. (Reproduced, with permission, from Waxman SG. *Clinical Neuroanatomy,* 25th ed. New York: McGraw-Hill, 2003: Figure 8-13.)

cause of bilateral cortical innervation to the upper parts of the face). Loss of taste to anterior two-thirds of tongue; loss of muscles of facial expression.

- Associated with diabetes, herpes viruses, tumors, sarcoidosis, AIDS, Lyme disease.
- If idiopathic, then called Bell palsy.
- Treatment includes 7–10 day course of prednisone +/– acyclovir/valacyclovir.
- Most cases resolve, but there is a risk of facial myokymia → aberrant CN VII regeneration leads to increased tone in the facial muscle.

CN VIII: Vestibulocochlear—Sensory

Component: Special sensory (special afferent).
Function: Auditory information from the cochlea and balance information from the semicircular canals.
Outlet: Internal acoustic meatus.
Clinical: Deafness, dizziness, damage to auditory canal or nerve.

- Vestibular schwannoma (acoustic neuroma): A tumor of Schwann cells that myelinate the CN VIII. Can also cause CN VII palsy.
- Associated with neurofibromatosis type 2.

CN IX: Glossopharyngeal—Mixed

Component 1: Branchial motor (special visceral efferent).
Function 1: Innervate striated muscle, stylopharyngeus muscle.

Component 2: Visceral motor (general visceral efferent).
Function 2: Supplies otic ganglion → parotid gland.
Component 3: Visceral sensory (general sensory afferent).
Function 3: Carries sensation from carotid body and carotid sinus.
Component 4: General sensory (general somatic afferent).
Function 4: Sensation from the posterior one-third of tongue, skin of external ear, internal surface of tympanic membrane.
Component 5: Special sensory (special afferent).
Function 5: Taste from the posterior one-third of tongue.
Outlet: Jugular foramen.
Clinical: Damage to nerve would result in absent gag reflex.

CN X: Vagus—Mixed

Component 1: Branchial motor (special visceral efferent).
Function 1: Innervate striated muscle of pharynx, tongue, and larynx.
Component 2: Visceral motor (general visceral efferent).
Function 2: To smooth muscle and glands of pharynx, larynx, thoracic and abdominal viscera.
Component 3: Visceral sensory (general sensory afferent).
Function 3: From larynx, trachea, esophagus, thoracic and abdominal viscera, stretch receptors in walls of aortic arch, chemoreceptors in aortic bodies in the arch.
Component 4: General sensory (general somatic afferent).
Function 4: Sensation from skin at the back of the ear and in external acoustic meatus, part of the external surface of the tympanic membrane and the pharynx.
Outlet: Jugular foramen.
Clinical: Complete bilateral transection of vagus nerves → **fatal.** Unilateral lesions of vagus → produce widespread dysfunction of the palate, pharynx, and larynx. The soft palate is weak and may be flaccid so that the voice has a nasal twang. Weakness or paralysis of the vocal cord may result in hoarseness. There can be difficulty in swallowing and cardiac arrhythmias may be present.

Damage to the recurrent laryngeal nerve can occur as result of invasion or compression by a tumor or complication of thyroid surgery. It may be accompanied by hoarseness.

CN XI: Accessory—Motor

Component: Branchial motor (special visceral efferent).
Function: Innervate sternocleidomastoid (SCM) and trapezius.
Outlet: Jugular foramen.
Pathway: Has both a cranial and a spinal component.

- Cranial: Nucleus ambiguus → joins the vagus outside of the skull.
- Spinal: Anterior horn motor neurons C1–C6 → ascent as the spinal root of accessory nerve → through jugular foramen → SCM and trapezius.

Clinical: Paralysis of SCM → inability to rotate head to contralateral side. Paralysis of upper portion of trapezius muscle → winglike scapula and inability to shrug ipsilateral shoulder.

CN XII: Hypoglossal—Motor

Component: Somatic motor (general somatic efferent).
Function: Innervates all intrinsic and extrinsic muscles of tongue except palatoglossus.

Outlet: Hypoglossal canal.
Clinical: Tongue deviates toward the side of the lesion.

See Table 2.9 for skull-based cranial nerve syndromes.

Quick Review of Cranial Nerves

See Table 2.10 for a review of cranial nerves and Table 2.11 for important foramina.

BRAIN STEM

General Concepts

- Contains the medulla, pons, and midbrain. Tectum = dorsal. Tegmentum = ventral.
- Lies ventral to cerebellum and is continuous with spinal cord caudally.
- Three major functions:
  1. Conduit functions
  2. Cranial nerve functions
  3. Integrative functions → reticular formation
- In general, the motor nuclei are located in the medial portions of the brain stem and the sensory nuclei are located in the lateral portions of the brain stem.

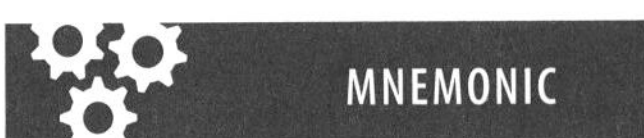

MNEMONIC

Remember **M**otor nuclei are usually **M**edial in the brain stem.

TABLE 2.9. Skull-Based Cranial Nerve Syndromes

Syndrome	CN Involved	Location	Typical Causes	Other Info/Clinical Scenario
Gradenigo	V, VI	Petrous apex	Suppurative otitis media, idiopathic, inflammation	Spread of infection though the skull base can result in Vernet syndrome or prevertebral/parapharyngeal abscess. Pain in V distribution, VI palsy.
Vernet	IX, X, XI	Jugular foramen	Metastatic tumor, schwannoma, meningioma, and glomus tumor	Difficulty in swallowing solids; paralysis of the soft palate with anesthesia of the pharynx; loss of taste in the posterior one-third of the tongue; paralysis of the vocal cords with laryngeal anaesthesia; and paralysis of the SCM and trapezius muscles.
Collet-Sicard	IX, X, XI, XII	Intercondylar space	Mass lesions, usually metastatic	Paralysis of the vocal cords, palate, trapezius muscle, and SCM muscle; it also causes secondary loss of the sense of taste in the back of the tongue, and anesthesia of the larynx, pharynx, and soft palate.
Villaret	IX, X, XI, XII, sympathetics	Retropharyngeal space	Mass lesions, usually metastatic	Weakness of superior constriction of the pharynx with dysphagia for solids; paralysis of soft palate with associated anesthesia of this and of the pharynx; loss of taste in the posterior one-third of the tongue; paralysis of the vocal cord with laryngeal anesthesia; paralysis of the SCM and trapezius; and paralysis of the cervical sympathetic nerves resulting in Horner syndrome.

TABLE 2.10. Cranial Nerve Categories and Functions

Nerves	Categories	Functions
Olfactory (I)	Afferent/sensory	Olfaction; does not make a relay in the brain stem or thalamus.
Optic (II)	Afferent/sensory	Cell bodies in retina that send parallel projections to midbrain and thalamus.
Oculomotor (III)	Efferent/motor	Muscles of eye (medial rectus, superior rectus, inferior rectus, inferior oblique), muscles of eyelids (levator palpabrae—elevation of eyelid), preganglionic parasympathetic projections to ciliary ganglion, sends projections to sphincter muscles to iris (pupil) and lens.
Trochlear (IV)	Efferent/motor	Superior oblique (rotates eye outward and downward).
Trigeminal (V)	Mixed	Afferent: Sensory to front two-thirds of head, anterior two-thirds of tongue, proprioception of the jaw. Efferent: Muscles of mastication, tensor tympani of inner ear.
Abducens (VI)	Efferent/motor	Lateral rectus (moves eye laterally).
Facial (VII)	Mixed	Afferent: Sensory to external ear; taste—anterior two-thirds of tongue. Efferent: Muscles of facial expression, stapedius, preganglionic. Parasympathetic fibers of submandibular, sublingual, and lacrimal glands.
Vestibulocochlear (VIII)	Afferent/sensory	Vestibular and cochlear nuclei: Audition and balance.
Glossopharyngeal (IX)	Mixed	Afferent: Sensory, external ear, pharynx, posterior one-third of tongue, taste from posterior one-third of tongue, carotid sinus, carotid body. Efferent: Muscles of pharynx, preganglionic parasympathetic fibers of parotid salivary glands.
Vagus (X)	Mixed	Afferent: Sensory, external ear, taste from epiglottis, thoracic and abdominal viscera, mucous membranes of larynx and laryngeal pharynx. Efferent: Muscles of larynx and pharynx, thoracic and abdominal viscera.
Accessory (XI)	Efferent/motor	Larynx, trapezius, sternocleidomastoid muscles.
Hypoglossal (XII)	Efferent/motor	Muscles of ipsilateral portion of the tongue.

TABLE 2.11. Important Foramina

Foramina → Structure	Foramen → Structure
Cribriform plate → olfactory nerve bundles	Foramen cecum → vein to superior sagittal sinus
Optic canal → CN II, ophthalmic artery	Hypoglossal canal → CN XII
Superior orbital fissure → CN III, CN IV, CN VI, V1 (ophthalmic nerve)	Foramen spinosum → meningeal branch of V3, middle meningeal artery/vein
Foramen rotundum → V2 (maxillary nerve)	Foramen lacerum → ICA
Foramen ovale → V3 (mandibular nerve), accessory meningeal artery, lesser petrosal nerve	Internal acoustic meatus → CN VII, CN VIII, labyrinthine artery
Jugular foramen → CN IX, CN X, CN XI, sigmoid sinus, posterior meningeal artery	Foramen magnum → spinal roots of CN XI, vertebral arteries

Blood Supply to Brain Stem (Figure 2.21)

- Medial medulla: Caudal → paramedian branches of anterior spinal artery, rostral → paramedian branches of vertebral arteries.
- Lateral medulla: Penetrating branches from vertebral arteries and PICA.
- Medial pons: Paramedian branches of the basilar artery.

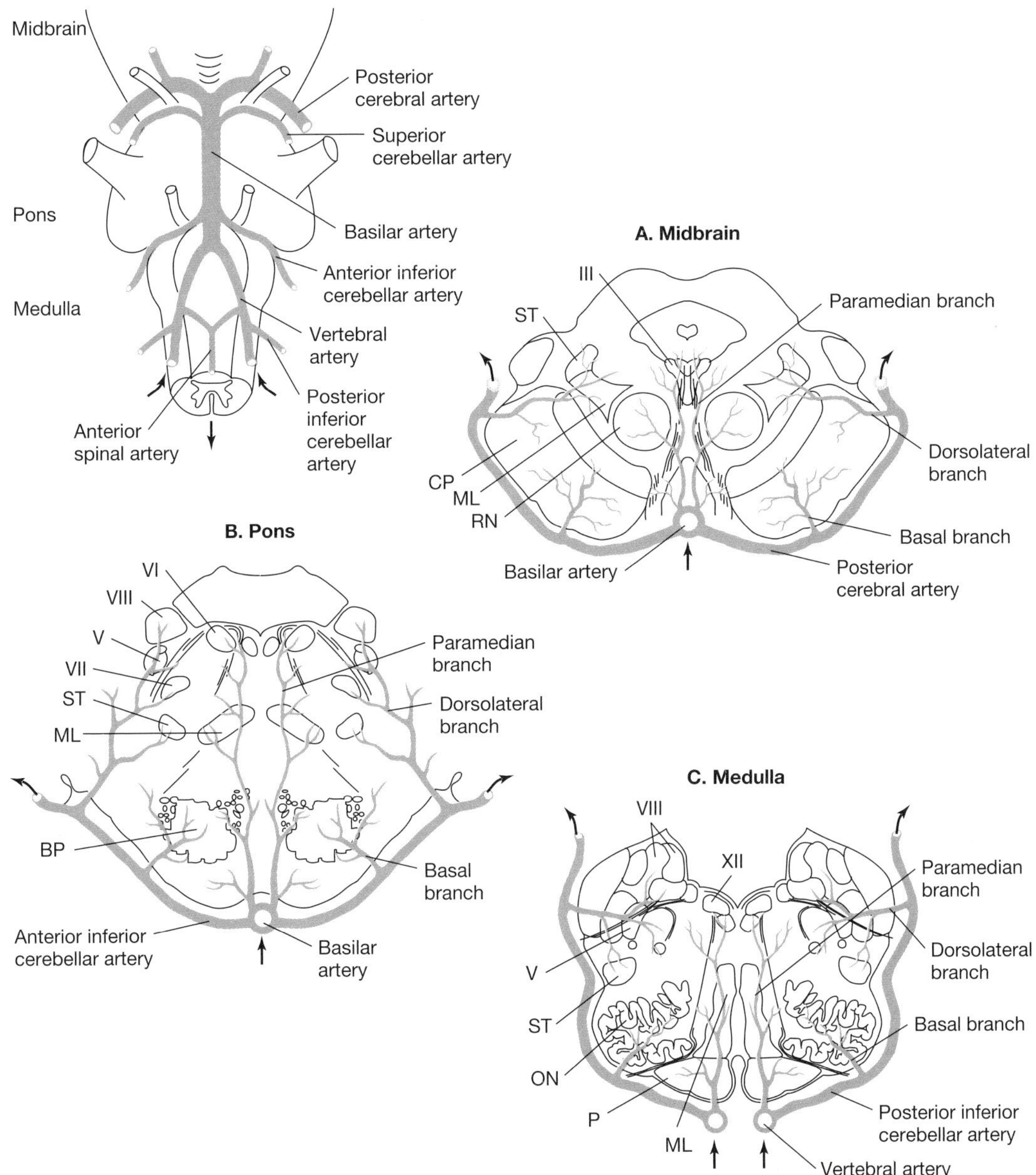

FIGURE 2.21. Arterial supply of the brain stem. (A) Midbrain. The basilar artery gives off paramedian branches that supply the oculomotor (III) nerve nucleus and the red nucleus (RN). A larger branch, the posterior cerebral artery, courses laterally around the midbrain, giving off a basal branch that supplies the cerebral peduncle (CP) and a dorsolateral branch supplying the spinothalamic tract (ST) and medial lemniscus (ML). The posterior cerebral artery continues (upper arrows) to supply the thalamus, occipital lobe, and medial temporal lobe. **(B)** Pons. Paramedian branches of the basilar artery supply the abducens (VI) nucleus and the medial lemniscus (ML). The anterior inferior cerebellar artery gives off a basal branch to the descending motor pathways in the basis pontis (BP) and a dorsolateral branch to the trigeminal (V) nucleus, the vestibular (VIII) nucleus, and the spinothalamic tract (ST), before passing to the cerebellum (upper arrows). **(C)** Medulla. Paramedian branches of the vertebral arteries supply descending motor pathways in the pyramid (P), the medial lemniscus (ML), and the hypoglossal (XII) nucleus. Another vertebral branch, the posterior inferior cerebellar artery, gives off a basal branch to the olivary nuclei (ON) and a dorsolateral branch that supplies the trigeminal (V) nucleus, the vestibular (VIII) nucleus, and the spinothalamic tract (ST), on its way to the cerebellum (upper arrows). (Reproduced, with permission, from Aminoff MJ, Simon RP. *Clinical Neurology*, 6th ed. New York: McGraw-Hill, 2005: Figure 9-12.)

KEY FACT

Internal auditory artery (labyrinthine) supplies the inner ear and is a branch of the AICA.

- Lateral pons: Paramedian branches of basilar artery and AICA.
- Superior dorsolateral pons: Superior cerebellar artery (SCA).
- Midbrain: Penetrating branches of top of basilar artery, proximal PCAs.

Cranial Nerve Nuclei

See Table 2.12 and Figure 2.22.

Other Nuclei and Structures

See Table 2.13 and Figures 2.23 and 2.24.

Important Descending Pathways of Brain Stem

1°, first-order neuron; 2°, secondary order neuron; 3°, third-order neuron; 4°, fourth-order neuron.

TABLE 2.12. Cranial Nerve Nuclei

Cranial Nerve Nuclei	Nerves
Motor	
1. Hypoglossal nucleus: Motor axons to muscles of the tongue (medulla).	XII
2. Spinal accessory nucleus: Motor axons to trapezius and SCM (medulla).	XI
3. Nucleus ambiguus: Muscles of larynx and pharynx (medulla).	IX, X, XI
4. Facial nucleus: Inferior and lateral to abducens nucleus, project superiorly and medially to loop around the abducens nucleus, go ventrolaterally to emerge on the ventrolateral aspect of pons (pons).	VII
5. Abducens nucleus: Lateral rectus, emerge at the caudal border of pons, near midline (pons).	VI
6. Motor nucleus of V: Level of midpons, muscles of mastication (pons).	V
7. Trochlear nucleus: Axons of nucleus decussate and emerge on dorsal surface of caudal midbrain, level of inferior colliculi, supply contralateral superior oblique muscle of eye (midbrain).	IV
8. Oculomotor nucleus: Level of superior colliculi. Extend ventrally and emerge between the cerebral peduncles (midbrain).	III
Preganglionic Parasympathetic	
1. Dorsal motor nucleus of X: Lies lateral to hypoglossal nucleus. Projection to thoracic and abdominal viscera (medulla).	X
2. Inferior salivatory nucleus: Through IX to otic ganglion → parotid gland (medulla).	IX
3. Superior salivatory nucleus: Through VII to submandibular → submandibular and sublingual salivary glands and pterygopalatine ganglia → lacrimal (pons).	VII
4. Edinger-Westphal nucleus: Located along midline, dorsal to oculomotor nuclei, at the level of superior colliculi, axons from this nucleus project through III and synapse in ciliary ganglion → sphincter pupillae and ciliary muscle of the eye (midbrain).	III
Sensory	
1. Nucleus solitarius: Parellels the hypoglossal nucleus, lateral to dorsal motor of X. Sensory from IX and X. Taste from VII, IX, X (medulla).	VII, IX, X
2. Spinal nucleus of V: Continuous with dorsal horn of spinal cord and extends through the medulla to midpons. Receives "Little 3" from two-thirds of head (medulla and pons).	V, VII, IX, X
3. Dorsal and ventral cochlear nuclei: Lie in lateral portion of floor of fourth ventricle, at the pontine-medullary junction. Innervation of spiral ganglion (medulla).	VIII
4. Vestibular nuclei: Medial to cochlear, greater rostrocaudal extent than cochlear. Innervation from vestibular ganglion (medulla).	VIII
5. Principal nucleus of V (main nucleus): Located at the level of midpons and is at the pontine end of spinal nucleus of V. Receives "Big 4" information from face and from outer ear (pons).	V, VII, IX, X
6. Mesencephalic nucleus of V: Posterior pons and anterior midbrain. This nucleus contains the primary sensory cell bodies that project afferents to muscles and joints of jaw, proprioception.	V

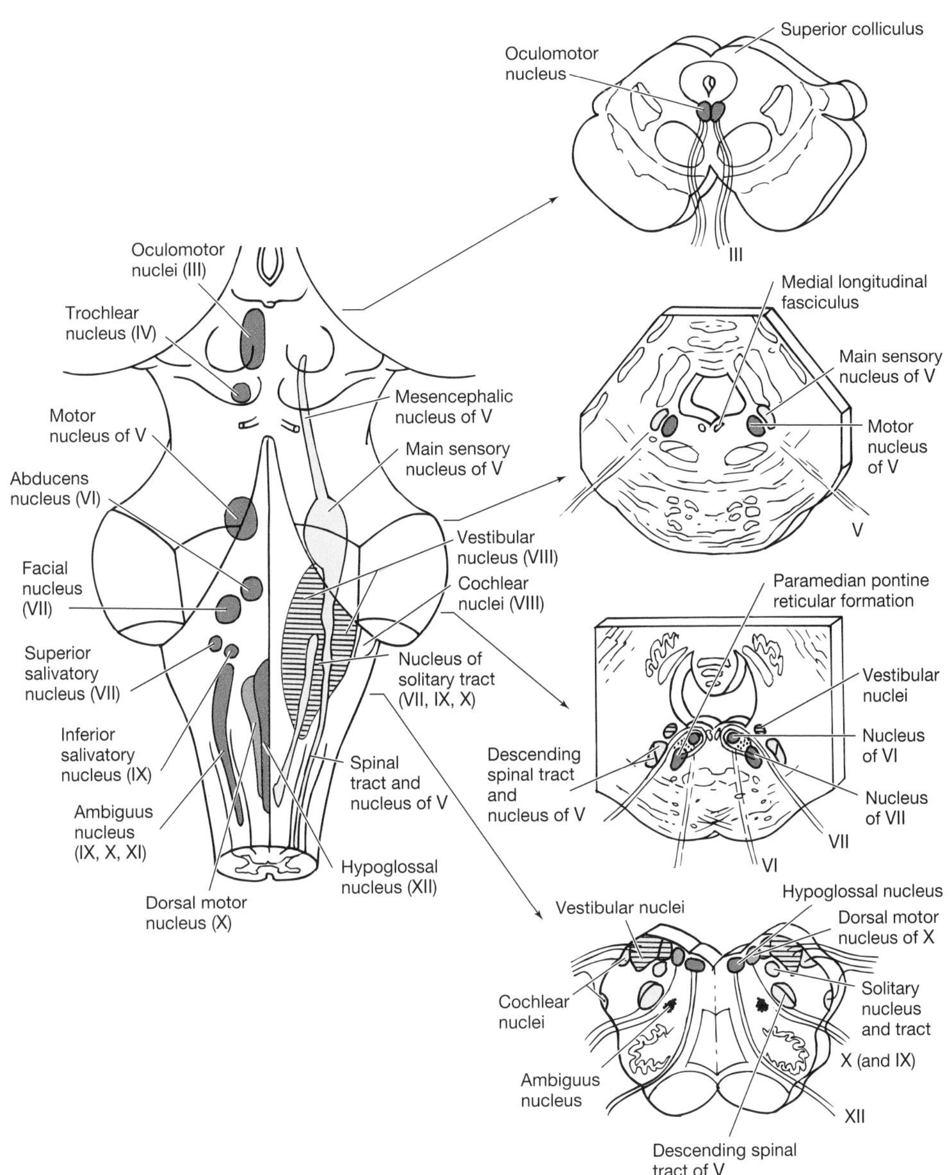

FIGURE 2.22. Cranial nerve nuclei. Left: Dorsal view of the human brain stem with the positions of the cranial nerve nuclei projected on the surface. Motor nuclei are on the left; sensory nuclei are on the right. Right: Transverse sections at the levels indicated by the arrows. (Reproduced, with permission, from Waxman SG. *Clinical Neuroanatomy,* 25th ed. New York: McGraw-Hill, 2003: Figure 7-6.)

Corticospinal Tract

Carry motor information from the cerebral cortex to lower motor neurons.

- 1° (UMN): *Precentral gyrus* → internal capsule (posterior limb) → cerebral peduncles (midbrain) → bundles (pons) → decussate at the caudal end of the medulla at the decussation of pyramids → lateral corticospinal tract and anterior corticospinal tract (do not decussate).
- 2° (LMN): Ventral horn interneurons and alpha motor neurons → muscles.
- Somatotopic organization of this pathway is maintained throughout the entire projection.

TABLE 2.13. Input/Outputs of Specialized Brain Stem Nuclei

Structures	Level	Input	Output	Functions
Lateral (accessory) cuneate nucleus	Medulla	Mechanoreceptors from arms via cuneocerebellar tract.	Ipsilateral cerebellum via inferior cerebellar peduncle (ICP).	Information on limb and joint position in the upper extremities.
Inferior olivary nucleus	Medulla	Red nucleus (via central tegmental tract), cortex, brain stem, and spinal cord.	Cross midline as internal arcuate fibers (olivocerebellar fibers), enter ICP, becomes climbing fibers.	Important relay and integration center. Critical input to the cerebellum involved in Purkinje cell plasticity and motor learning.
Reticular nuclei (rostral: midbrain/ upper pons; caudal: pons/medulla)	All		Goes to thalamus, intralaminar nuclei, hypothalamus, basal forebrain.	Rostral: Maintain alertness. Caudal: Integrate motor, reflex, and autonomic functions.
Caudal raphe nuclei	Caudal pons/ medulla	Inputs from the periaqueductal gray matter.	To cerebellum, medulla, and spinal cord (terminate in the substantia gelantinosa, intermediolateral cell column).	Produce *serotonin;* form part of a central pain-control system, can have excitatory effect on motor neurons.
Area postrema	Medulla		Nucleus solitarius and other centers in the brain stem.	Chemotactic trigger. Lacks a blood-brain barrier thus can detect noxious compounds.
Rostral raphe nuclei	Midbrain/ rostral pons		To hypothalamus basal ganglia, amygdaloid body, hippocampus, and cingulate gyrus.	Produce *serotonin.* VIP in sleep-wake cycle and in affective behavior, food intake, hormone secretion, sexual behavior, thermoregulation, depression.
Pontine nuclei	Pons	Ipsilateral motor and sensory cortex via corticopontine fibers.	Contralateral cerebellar cortex via middle cerebellar peduncle (MCP).	Give rise to the mossy fibers. Function in motor coordination.
Locus ceruleus (means "blue spot")	Pons (near fourth ventricle)			Release *norepinephrine* to nearly all parts of the brain and spinal cord. VIP in sleep-wake cycle and level of alertness.
Superior olivary nuclear complex	Pons	Bilateral ventral cochlear nuclei (via fibers of ventral stria).	To bilateral inferior colliculi (via trapezoid body and lateral lemniscus).	Functions in localizing sounds horizontally in space.
Paramedian pontine reticular formation	Pons	Superior colliculus (via predorsal bundle) and contralateral frontal eye fields (projections cross in midbrain).	To abducens nucleus.	Controls horizontal gaze and sacchades.
Pretectal area	Midbrain	Optic tracts (via extrageniculate pathway in brachium of superior colliculus).	To bilateral Edinger-Westphal nuclei (as posterior commissure).	Mediates pupillary light reflex.

TABLE 2.13. Input/Outputs of Specialized Brain Stem Nuclei *(continued)*

Structures	Level	Input	Output	Functions
Periaqueductal gray	Midbrain	Hypothalamus, amygdala, cortex.	Synapses with caudal raphe nuclei and rostral ventral medulla. Then projects to substantia gelatinosa → release endogenous opioids.	*Enkephalin*-releasing neurons. Inhibits pain transmission. Important in the gate-control theory involving pain modulation.
Substantia nigra pars compacta (dorsal)	Midbrain		To the striatum.	*Dopamine*-containing neurons. Involved in motor control pathways. Lesioned in Parkinson disease.
Substantia nigra pars reticularis (ventral)	Midbrain	Striatum (GABA, substance P—inhibitory) and subthalamic nucleus (glutamate—excitatory).	Inibitory projections to ventrolateral/ventral anterior thalamus. To superior colliculus and reticular formation.	Secretes *GABA.* Inhibitory neurons. Works with globus pallidus internus (GPi) to coordinate movement. Also sends projection to tectospinal (via superior collicullus) and reticulospinal tract (via reticular formation).
Ventral tegmental area	Midbrain	Prefrontal cortex.	To nucleus accumbens, frontal lobes, and other limbic structures.	*Dopamine*-containing neurons. Involved in behavior and reward center. May be affected in schizophrenia.
Red nucleus	Midbrain	Contralateral dentate/interposed nuclei via superior cerebellar peduncle (SCP).	To inferior olivary nucleus (via central tegmental tract) and cervical spinal cord (via rubrospinal tract).	Motor control pathway.
Inferior colliculus	Midbrain	Superior olivary nuclear complex (via lateral lemniscus).	To medial geniculate nucleus (via brachium of the inferior colliculi).	Part of ascending auditory system.
Superior colliculus	Midbrain	Optic tract (bypasses lateral geniculate nucleus as extrageniculate visual pathway), substantia nigra, pars reticularis, prefrontal cortex (Brodmann's area, eight frontal eye fields), inferior parietal lobule.	To pulvinar (part of the extrageniculate visual pathway) to occipital lobe; to cervical cord (via tectospinal tract, crosses in midbrain at dorsal tegmental decussation); paramedian pontine reticular formation.	Generation of saccadic eye movements; eye-head coordination. Involved in reflexive sacchades.
Rostral interstitial nucleus of medial longitudinal fasciculus and interstitial nucleus of Cajal	Midbrain	Prefrontal cortex (Brodmann's area, eight frontal eye fields).	To oculomotor nucleus.	Vertical gaze center. Ventral portion mediates downgaze. Dorsal region (near posterior commissure) mediates upgaze.

G
F
E
D
C
B

A

Nucleus gracilis
Nucleus cuneatus
Dorsal spinocerebellar tract
Spinal nucleus of V
Spinothalamic tract
Ventral horn of C1
Decussation of pyramids

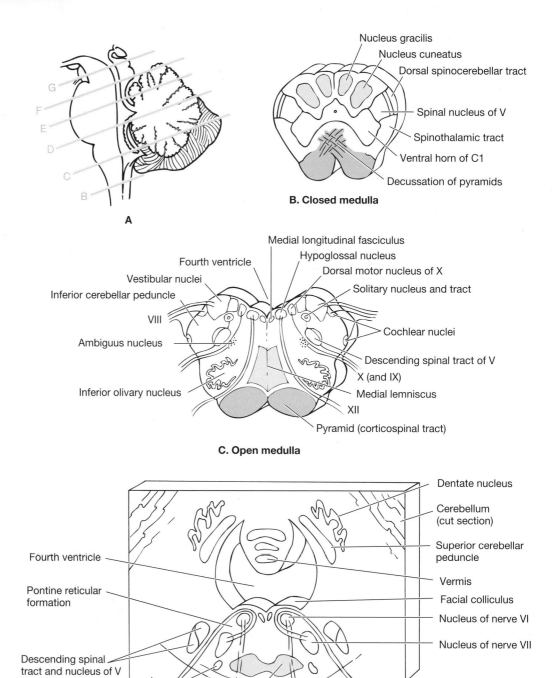

B. Closed medulla

Medial longitudinal fasciculus
Hypoglossal nucleus
Fourth ventricle
Dorsal motor nucleus of X
Vestibular nuclei
Solitary nucleus and tract
Inferior cerebellar peduncle
VIII
Cochlear nuclei
Ambiguus nucleus
Descending spinal tract of V
X (and IX)
Inferior olivary nucleus
Medial lemniscus
XII
Pyramid (corticospinal tract)

C. Open medulla

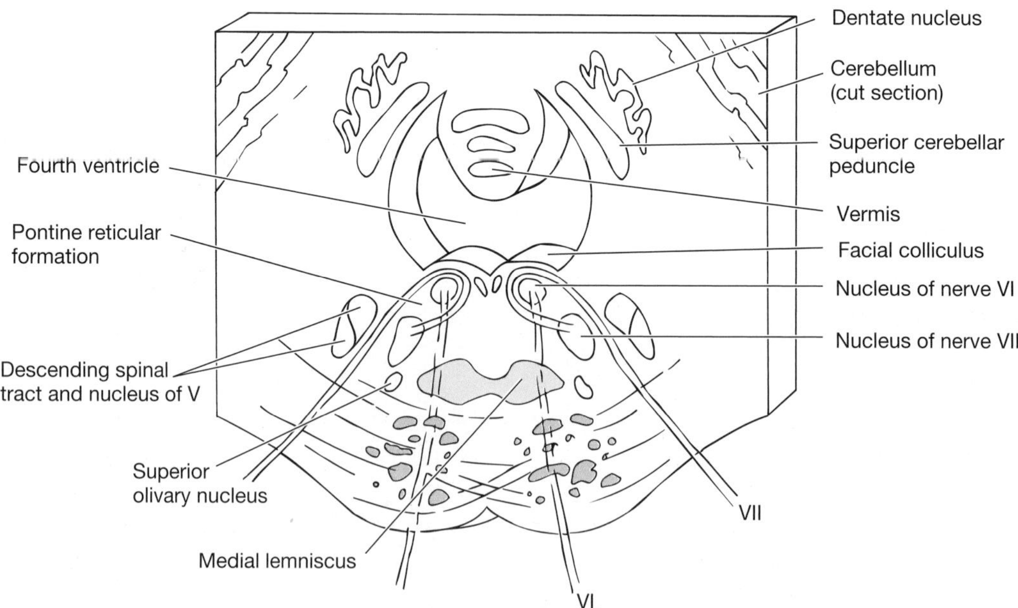

D. Lower pons; level of nerves VI and VII

FIGURE 2.23. Schematic cross-section at various levels of the brain stem. (A) Key to levels of sections. **(B–G)** Schematic transverse sections through the brain stem. The corticospinal tracts and the dorsal column nuclei/medial lemnisci are shaded so that they can be followed as they course through the brain stem. (Reproduced, with permission, from Waxman SG. *Clinical Neuroanatomy*, 25th ed. New York: McGraw-Hill, 2003: Figure 7-7.)

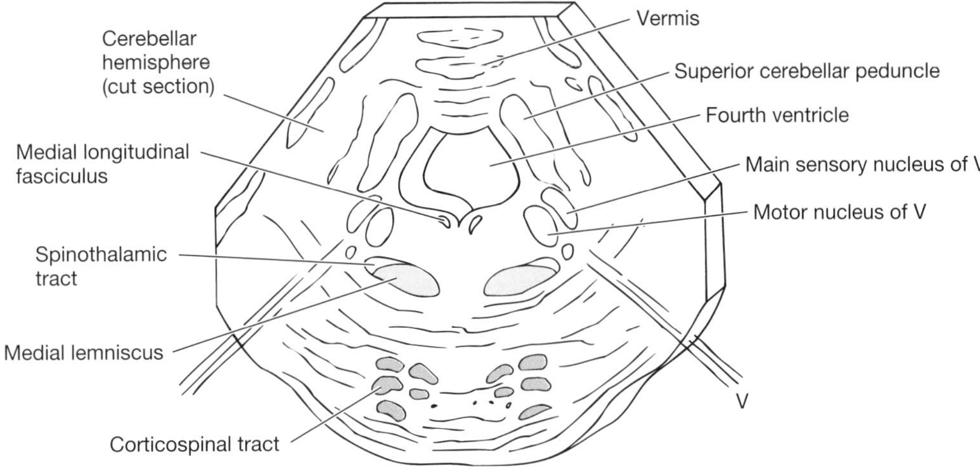

E. Middle pons; level of nerve V

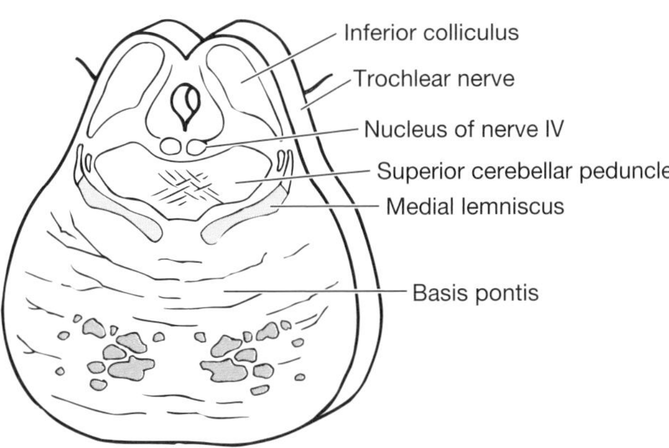

F. Pons/midbrain; level of nucleus VI

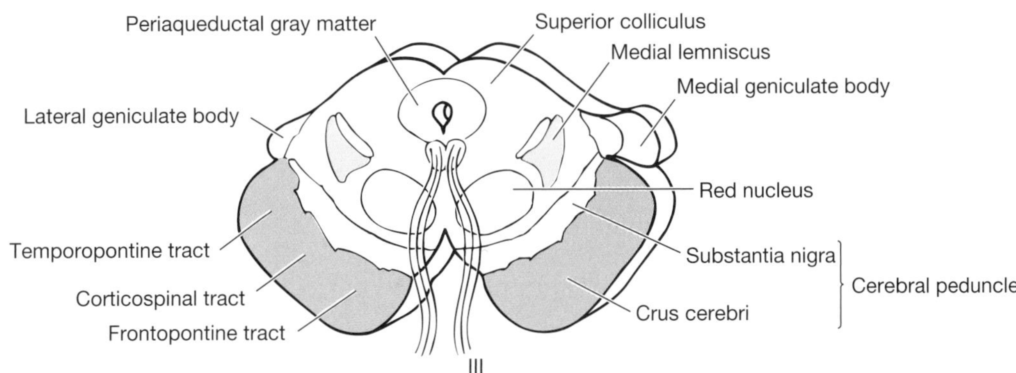

G. Upper midbrain; level of nerve III

FIGURE 2.23. Schematic cross-section at various levels of the brain stem. ***(continued)***

Corticobulbar Tract

Fibers projecting from motor areas of cortex to the cranial nerve nuclei.

- 1° **(UMN)**: *Precentral gyrus* → genu of internal capsule → cerebral peduncles.
- 2° **(LMN)**: *Cranial nerve nuclei* → muscles of face, neck, etc.
- Has ipsilateral and strong contralateral projections to all of the cranial nerve nuclei except for the lower facial nucleus (there is no ipsilateral projection to lower facial nucleus).
- Lesion to corticobulbar tract → UMN paralysis to the contralateral lower face.
- Lesion to facial nerve → LMN paralysis to the ipsilateral face.

Corticopontine Tract

- 1°: *Motor, premotor, somatosensory cortices* → internal capsule cerebral peduncles → base of pons.
- 2°: *Pontine nuclei* → pontocerebellar tracts → cross midline in pontine fibers → middle cerebellar peduncle.

Rubrospinal Tract

Control of movement in the contralateral limbs.

- 1°: Red nucleus → crosses at ventral tegmental decussation.
- 2°: Cervical spinal cord (ventral horn interneurons).

Vestibulospinal Tract

Medial vestibulospinal tract → positioning of head and neck, lateral vestibulospinal tract → balance.

- 1°: Medial/inferior vestibular nuclei → travels crossed and uncrossed in ventral column.
- 2°: Ventral horn interneurons in cervical and upper thoracic cord.
- 1°: Lateral vestibular nuclei → travels uncrossed in ventral column.
- 2°: Ventral horn interneurons in entire cord.

Medial Reticulospinal Tract

Motor function (excitation of flexor and proximal trunk and axial motor neurons).

- 1°: Pontine reticular formation → travels in lateral column → descends uncrossed.
- 2°: Ventral horn interneurons.

Lateral Reticulospinal Tract

Modulation of sensory transmission and spinal reflexes; excitation and inhibition of axial (neck and back) motor neurons.

- 1°: Medullary reticular formation → travels in lateral column → descends crossed and uncrossed.
- 2°: Most of the ventral horn and the basal portion of the dorsal horn.

Tectospinal Tract

Reflex head turning.

- 1°: Superior colliculus → travels in ventral column and crosses in dorsal tegmental decussation.
- 2°: Contralateral ventral horn interneurons in the cervical cord.

Important Ascending Tracts of the Brain Stem

Dorsal Column/Medial Lemniscus

Proprioception, light touch, vibratory sensation, and stereognosis to arms, legs, and trunk.

- 1°: Encapsulated mechanoreceptors → *dorsal root ganglion* → (may synapse in the nucleus proprius of the dorsal horn) → dorsal columns (fasciculus cuneatus and fasciculus gracilis).
- 2°: *Dorsal column nuclei (nucleus gracilis and nucleus cuneatus)*(medulla) → cross as internal arcuate fibers (medulla) → medial lemniscus (located medially in medulla, but it gradually moves laterally through its ascent in the brain stem).
- 3°: *Ventral posterior lateral (VPL) of thalamus* → internal capsule.
- 4°: *Somatosensory cortices (postcentral gyrus).*

Trigeminothalamic Tracts

Sensory pathways for face.

- Proprioception, vibratory sensation, light touch, and stereognosis for face.
  - 1°: Mechanoreceptors → *trigeminal ganglion.*
  - 2°: *Principal nucleus of V* → cross over → ventral trigeminothalamic tract or no cross over → dorsal trigeminothalamic tract.
  - 3°: *Contralateral ventral posterior medial (VPM) or ipsilateral VPM.*
  - 4°: *Somatosensory cortex (postcentral gyrus).*
- Pain, temperature, and crude touch for face.
  - 1°: Trigeminal ganglion.
  - 2°: Spinal nucleus of V → cross over → ventral trigeminothalamic tract.
  - 3°: VPM thalamus.
  - 4°: Somatosensory cortices.
  - **Mesencephalic nucleus of V:** Primary afferents from muscle spindles in the jaw that synapse primarily in the motor nucleus of V. Carries proprioceptive information from the muscles of mastication and are the afferent neurons of jaw jerk reflex.

Anterolateral System

Transmission of pain and temperature sensation and also crude touch.

- Spinothalamic tract:
  - 1°: *Dorsal root ganglion* → Lissauer's tract.
  - 2°: *Marginal zone and substantia gelatinosa* → cross in ventral white commissure → anterolateral system (lower lateral and upper medial).
  - 3°: *VPL of thalamus* → internal capsule.
  - 4°: *Somatosensory cortices.*
- **Spinoreticulothalamic tract:** Synapse in *reticular formation.*

Dorsal Spinocerebellar Tract

- 1°: Mechanoreceptors of legs → *dorsal root ganglion.*
- 2°: *Clarke's nucleus* → dorsal spinocerebellar tract → inferior cerebellar peduncle.
- 3°: *Cerebellar cortex.*

Cuneocerebellar Tract

- 1°: Mechanoreceptors from arms → *dorsal root ganglion.*
- 2°: *Lateral cuneate nucleus* → inferior cerebellar peduncle.
- 3°: *Cerebellar cortex.*

Brain Stem Syndromes/Strokes

Medial (Basal) Medullary Syndrome: Dejerine Syndrome—Alternating Hypoglossal Hemiplegia

- Infarct of paramedian branches of vertebral and anterior spinal arteries.
- Involves the pyramids, part or all of medial lemniscus, and nerve XII.
- Ipsilateral weakness of the tongue.
- Contralateral arm or leg weakness.
- Contralateral decrease in proprioception, vibration, and light touch.

Lateral Medullary Syndrome: Wallenberg Syndrome

- Infarct of PICA or vertebral arteries.
- Involves some or all of the following structures: inferior cerebellar peduncle, vestibular nuclei, fibers or nuclei of nerve IX or X, spinal nucleus and tract of V, spinothalamic tract, and sympathetic pathways.
- Vertigo, nystagmus, nausea, hoarseness, dysphagia.
- Ipsilateral ataxia.
- Ipsilateral decreased taste.
- Ipsilateral Horner syndrome.
- Loss of pain and temperature to contralateral body and ipsilateral face.

Avellis Syndrome

Infarct or damage to the tegmentum of the medulla.

- Involves CN X, spinothalamic tract.
- Ipsilateral weakness of the soft palate and vocal cords.
- Contralateral loss of pain and temperature to the body.

Jackson Syndrome

Infarct of damage to the tegmentum of the medulla.

- Involves CN X, CN XI, CN XII, corticospinal tract, spinothalamic tract.
- Ipsilateral weakness of SCM, trapezius, tongue, soft palate, pharynx, and larynx.
- Contralateral weakness of the body.
- Contralateral loss of pain and temperature to the body.

Locked-in Syndrome

Due to large pontine infarct.

- Large lesions of the basal pons that interrupts the corticobulbar and corticospinal pathways bilaterally, thus interfering with speech, facial expression, and the capacity to activate most muscles.
- Somatosensory system and reticular pathways are spared → patient awake and aware of surroundings.
- Vertical eye movements spared → communicates with eye and eye movements.

AICA Syndrome

Infarct of the lateral caudal pons, caused by blockage of AICA.

- Involves middle cerebellar peduncle (MCP), vestibular nuclei, trigeminal nucleus/tract, spinothalamic tract, descending sympathetic fibers.
- Ipsilateral ataxia, vertigo, nystagmus.
- Loss of pain and temperature to ipsilateral face and contralateral body.
- Ipsilateral Horner syndrome.
- If labyrinthine artery is also blocked, then ipsilateral hearing loss can result.

Superior Cerebellar Artery (SCA) Syndrome

Infarct of dorsolateral rostral pons, caused by blockage of SCA.

- Involves superior cerebellar peduncle (SCP); cerebellum; other lateral structures, which can include vestribular nuclei, dentate nucleus, descending sympathetic fibers, spinothalamic tract, medial lemniscus (lateral portion).
- Primarily leads to ipsilateral ataxia.
- Can include signs and symptoms from other structures.

Medial Pontine Basis and Tegmentum Syndromes

Caused by infarcts of the paramedian branches of the basilar artery. Pontine structures are affected to various degrees depending on the depth of the infarcts.

- **Foville syndrome:** Affects corticospinal and corticobulbar tracts, facial nucleus, and paramedian pontine reticular formation (PPRF); leads to contralateral face, arm, and leg weakness; complete ipsilateral facial weakness; ipsilateral horizontal gaze palsy.
- **Millard-Gubler syndrome:** Affects corticospinal and corticobulbar tracts, tracts of CN VI and CN VII; leads to contralateral face, arm, and leg weakness, complete ipsilateral facial weakness, ipsilateral abducens nerve palsy.
- Foville syndrome and Millard-Gubler syndromes are examples of pontine "wrong-way" eyes syndrome as there is an ipsilateral horizontal gaze palsy or abducens nerve palsy with contralateral weakness. The difference between Foville and Millard-Gubler is that Foville affects PPRF and Millard-Gubler affects the abducens nerve.
- **Pure motor hemiparesis:** Affects corticospinal and corticobulbar tracts; leads to contralateral face, arm, and leg weakness.
- **Ataxic hemiparesis:** Affects corticospinal, corticobulbar, pontine nuclei, pontocerebellar fibers; leads to contralateral face, arm, and leg weakness and contralateral ataxia (sometimes ipsilateral).

Weber Syndrome (Alternating Oculomotor Hemiplegia)

Involves the midbrain basis.

- Infarct of the branches of the PCA and top of basilar artery, can also be caused by tumors.
  - Involves CN III and portions of cerebral peduncles.
  - Ipsilateral CN III palsy and contralateral hemiparesis.

Claude Syndrome

Involves the midbrain tegmentum.

- Infarct of the branches of the PCA and top of basilar artery, can also be due to tumors.
- Involves CN III, red nucleus, SCP.
- Ipsilateral CN III palsy and contralateral ataxia.

Benedikt Syndrome

Involves midbrain basis and tegmentum.

- Infarct of the branches of the PCA; can also be due to tumors or tuberculomas.
  - Involves CN III, red nucleus, corticospinal tract, substantia nigra.
- Ipsilateral CN III palsy with contralateral hemiparesis, ataxia, and tremor and involuntary movments.

Nothnagel Syndrome

Involves midbrain tectum.

- Usually caused by tumor compression.
- Involves CN III (unilateral or bilateral), SCP.
- Paralysis of gaze depending on CN III involvement and cerebellar ataxia.

Parinaud Syndrome

Involves dorsal midbrain.

- Usually caused by pineal tumors or hydrocephalus.
- Interrupts vertical gaze centers.
- Paralysis of upward gaze and accommodation, light-near dissociation.

Other Important Brain Stem Functions and Pathways (Table 2.14)

Medial Longitudinal Fasciculus (MLF)

Fibers involved in coordinated head, neck, and eye movements. Carries fibers that allow conjugate movement of both eyes (Figure 2.24).

- Interconnections of the oculomotor nucleus, trochlear nucleus, abducens nucleus, vestibular nucleus, spinal accessory nucleus, and PPRF.
- For rightward gaze shifts, the lateral rectus of the right eye and the medial rectus of the left eye must be activated together.
- Each abducens nucleus commands a gaze shift to its own side:
  - Motor neurons drive the ipsilateral lateral rectus.
  - Internuclear interneurons send axons in the contralateral MLF, which drive neurons in oculomotor nucleus, which drive the contralateral medial rectus.
  - Vestibular nuclei also connect to this pathway and they are responsible vestibulo-ocular reflex.

TABLE 2.14. Major Ascending and Descending Pathways in the Brain Stem

Ascending	Descending
Medial lemniscus	Corticospinal tract
Spinothalamic tract	Corticonuclear tract
Trigeminal lemniscus	Corticopontine fibers
Lateral lemniscus	Rubrospinal tract
Reticular system fibers	Tectospinal tract
Medial longitudinal fasciculus	Medial longitudinal fasciculus
Inferior cerebellar peduncle	Vestibulospinal tract
Superior cerebellar peduncle	Reticulospinal tract
Secondary vestibulary fibers	Central tegmental tract
Secondary gustatory fibers	Descending tract of nerve V

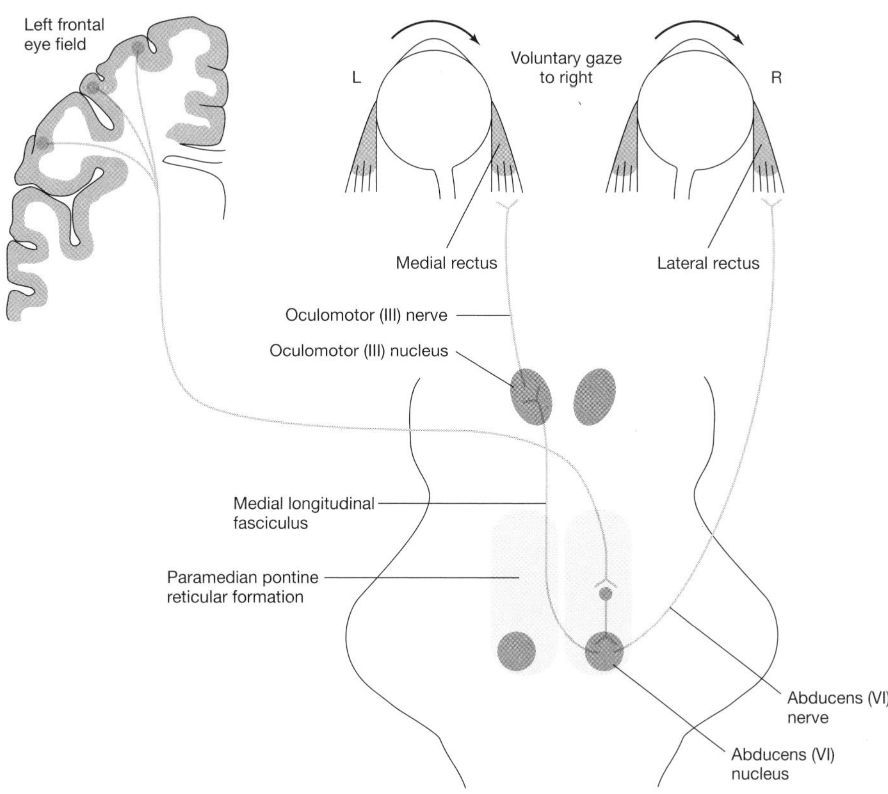

FIGURE 2.24. Neuronal pathways involved in horizontal gaze. (Reproduced, with permission, from Aminoff MJ, Simon RP. *Clinical Neurology*, 6th ed. New York: McGraw-Hill, 2005: Figure 4-6.)

Lesions of MLF/PPRF

1. **Internuclear ophthalmoplegia (INO):** Lesion of MLF. Classically seen in patients with demyelinating diseases such as multiple sclerosis.
   - Side of INO = side of lesion.
   - Impaired eye adduction on the affected side when horizontal gaze is attempted, but eye adduction is normal on convergence.
2. **One-and-a-half syndrome:** Lesion of MLF and adjacent abducens nucleus or PPRF.
   - Ipsilateral eye cannot move at all horizontally, and the contralateral eye loses half of its movements with only preservation of abduction.
3. **Lesion of the PPRF:**
   - Unilateral PPRF lesion leads to a loss of all horizontal rapid eye movements toward the ipsilateral side.

Mollaret Triangle

Connections between the red nucleus, inferior olivary nucleus, and the dentate nucleus of cerebellum.

- Red nucleus to the inferior olivary nucleus (central tegmental tract).
- Inferior olivary nucleus to contralateral dentate (inferior cerebellar peduncle).
- Contralateral dentate to the red nucleus (superior cerebellar peduncle).
- Lesion of central tegmental tract leads to **palatal myoclonus** (associated with hypertrophic olivary degeneration).
- Lesions within other parts of this pathway usually lead to intention tremor.

CEREBELLUM

Controls many aspects of coordination of movement, maintenance of body equilibrium, and movement initiation and planning. Exerts its control over the ipsilateral side of the body. Information is exchanged with the cerebellum via the cerebellar peduncles (see Table 2.15).

External Anatomy (Table 2.15)

Covers most of the posterior surface of the brain stem, forms the "roof" of fourth ventricle.

- Posterolateral fissure: Flocculonodular lobe from posterior lobe.
- Primary fissure: posterior lobe from anterior lobe.
- Anterior and posterior lobes are divided into 3 longitudinal zones:
  - Vermis: Most medial zone.
  - Paravermis: Lies between vermis and hemispheres.
  - Cerebellar hemisphere: Large lateral portions.
- Other structures: Flocculus, tonsils, nodulus, uvula, horizontal fissure.
- There are 10 principal lobules (Figure 2.25).

Functional Anatomy (Figure 2.26)

- **Vestibulocerebellum:** Located in flocculonodular lobe.
  - Input: Vestibular nuclei.
  - Output: Vestibular nuclei.
  - Function: Balance and eye movements, bidirectional communication helps to coordinate eye movements and body equilbrium.
- **Spinocerebellum:** Located in vermis and paravermis of anterior and posterior lobes.
  - Input: Vermis: vestibular nuclei and proprioceptive and sensory inputs from the head and neck. Paravermis: spinal cord (info on limb position from ascending spinocerebellar tracts).
  - Function: Coordinate motor control during motor execution. Vermis: coordinates medial (axial) systems. Paravermis: controls activity of lateral motor system (limb movement during ongoing motor activity).
- **Cerebrocerebellum:** Located in large lateral zone cerebellar hemispheres.
  - Input: Contralateral, pontine nuclei.
  - Output: Motor and premotor cortical areas after stopping in VL thalamus.
  - Function: Involved in motor planning and initiation of movement.

TABLE 2.15. Cerebellar Peduncles

Peduncles	Input	Output
Inferior	1. Afferents from vestibular nuclei 2. Afferents via dorsal spinocerebellar and cuneocerebellar tracts 3. Lateral reticular nucleus 4. Inferior olive nucleus → decussate → internal arcuate fibers	
Middle	Corticopontine fibers → pontine nuclei → decussate (some do not) → enter middle cerebellar peduncle	
Superior		Motor output from cerebellum

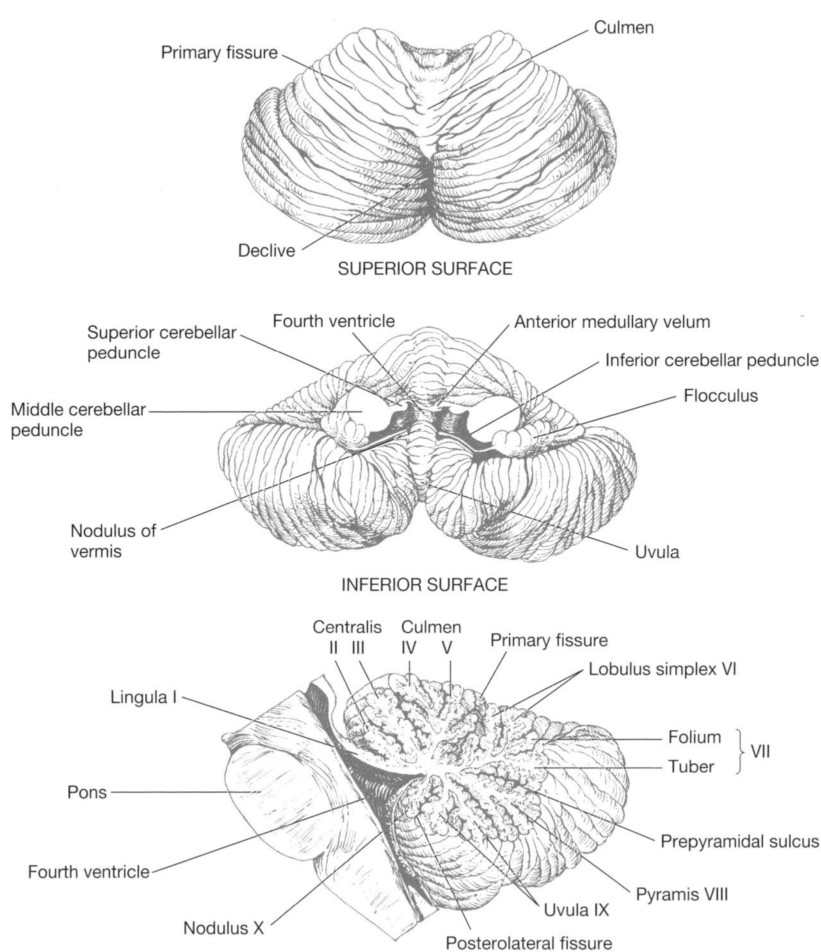

FIGURE 2.25. External anatomy of cerebellum. Superior and inferior views and sagittal section of the human cerebellum. The 10 principal lobules are identified by name and by number (I–X). (Reproduced, with permission, from Ganong WF. *Review of Medical Physiology,* 22nd ed. New York: McGraw-Hill, 2003: 218.)

Microanatomy (Figure 2.27)

Cerebellar cortex consists of 3 layers: Outer molecular layer, Purkinje cell layer, and granular layer (Table 2.16).

- Deep cerebellar nuclei (medial to lateral): Fastigial, globose, embolliform, dentate (Table 2.17).
- Vestibulocerebellum (flocculonodular lobe) doesn't project to a deep nucleus; rather, Purkinje cells send axons directly to vestibular nuclei.

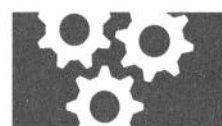
MNEMONIC

Feel Good Each Day
Fastigial
Globose
Embolliform
Dentate

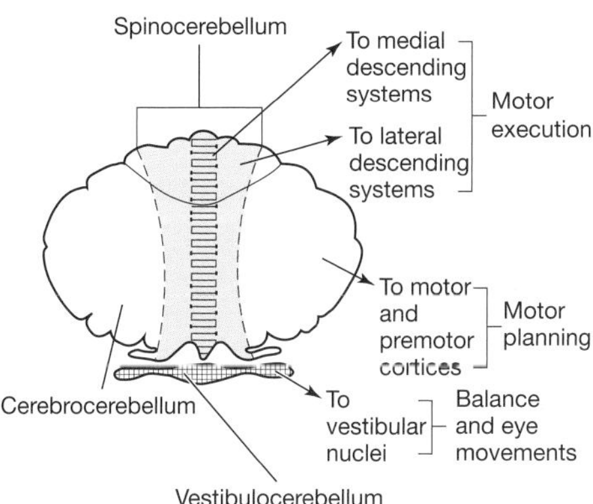

FIGURE 2.26. Functional divisions of the cerebellum. (Reproduced, with permission, from Ganong WF. *Review of Medical Physiology,* 22nd ed. New York: McGraw-Hill, 2003: 221.)

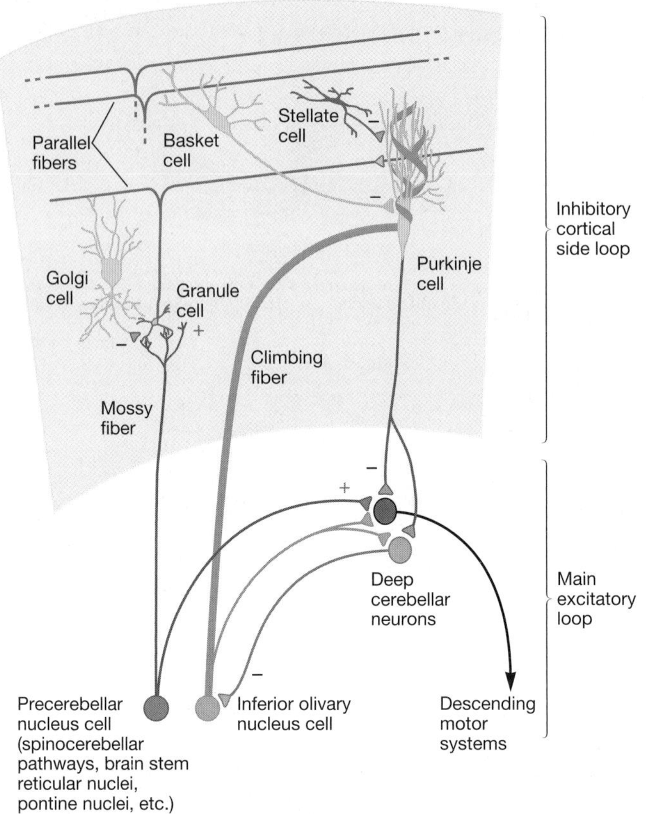

FIGURE 2.27. The physiologic organization of cerebellar circuitry. The main output of the deep cerebellar nuclei is excitatory and is transmitted through mossy and climbing fibers. This "main loop" is modulated by an inhibitory cortical loop, which is effected by Purkinje cell output but indirectly includes the other main cell types through their connections with Purkinje cells. Recurrent pathways between the deep nuclei and cortical cells via mossy and climbing fibers complete the cerebellar servomechanism for motor control. (Reproduced, with permission, from Ropper AH, Brown RH. *Adams and Victor's Principles of Neurology*, 8th ed. New York: McGraw-Hill, 2005: 75.)

TABLE 2.16. Layers of the Cerebellar Cortex

Molecular Layer	Purkinje Cell Layer	Granular Layer
■ Basket cells (receive excitatory inputs from the parallel fibers and project back to Purkinje cells, which they inhibit) ■ Golgi cells (receive excitatory inputs from parallel fibers and from mossy fibers, and project to granule cell, which they inhibit) ■ Stellate cells (excitatory inputs from parellel fibers to give rise to inhibitory to Purkinje)	■ Purkinje cell bodies (inhibitory projections and dendrites that fan out in a single plane) send axons to deep nuclei of cerebellum (can project out of the cerebellar cortex)	■ Granule cell bodies (only excitatory neurons in cerebellar cortex) send axons to molecular layer, then bifurcate and become parallel fibers

TABLE 2.17. **Deep Cerebellar Nuclei**

Dentate	Interposed (Globose + Emboliform)	Fastigial
■ Input: Purkinje cells of cerebrocerebellum ■ Output: Back to motor thalamus	■ Input: From paravermis ■ Output: Red nucleus	■ Input: Vermis ■ Output: Reticular formation

CEREBRUM

Cerebral hemispheres make up the largest portion of the brain (see first section and Figures 2.1 and 2.2).

Microscopic Structure of the Cortex (Figure 2.28)

Neocortex

Six-layered cortex:

- Molecular layer (I): Contains nonspecific afferent fibers that come from within the cortex or from the thalamus:
  - External granular layer (II): A rather dense layer composed of small cells.
  - External pyramidal layer (III): Contains pyramidal cells.
- Internal granular layer (IV): Usually a thin layer with cells similar to those in the external granular layer.
- Internal pyramidal layer (V): Contains, in most areas, pyramidal cells that are fewer in number but larger in size than those in the external pyramidal layer.
- Fusiform (multiform) layer (VI): Consists of irregular fusiform cells whose axons enter the adjacent white matter.

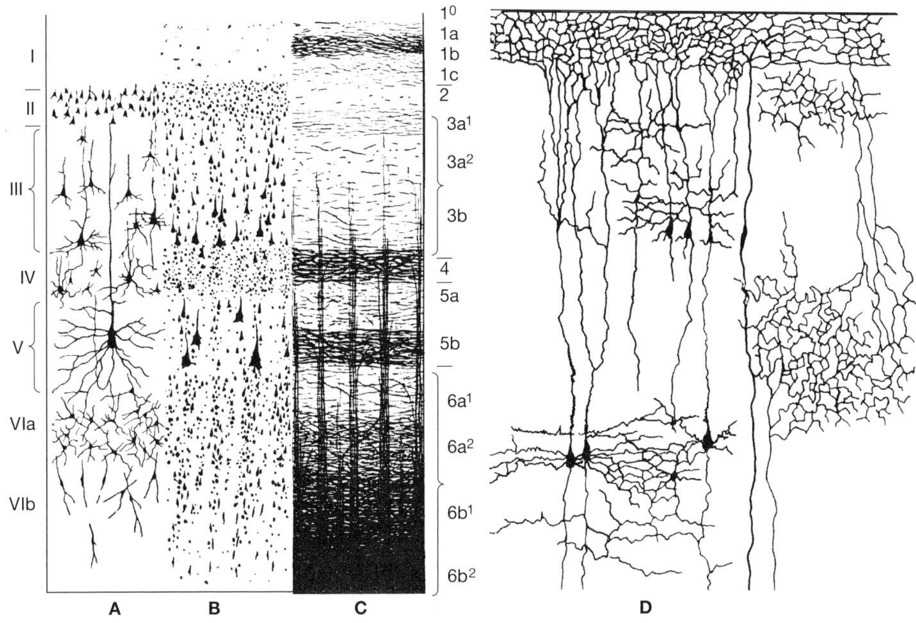

FIGURE 2.28. **Diagram of the structure of the cerebral cortex. (A)** Golgi neuronal stain. **(B)** Nissl cellular stain. **(C)** Weigart myelin stain. **(D)** Neuronal connections. Roman and Arabic numerals indicate the layers of the isocortex (neocortex); 4, external line of Baillarger (line of Gennari in the occipital lobe); 5b, internal line of Baillarger. (A, B, and C reproduced, with permission, from Waxman SG. *Clinical Neuroanatomy*, 25th ed. New York: McGraw-Hill, 2003: Figure 10-10. D reproduced, with permission, from Ganong WG. *Review of Medical Physiology*, 19th ed. Appleton & Lange, 1999.)

Archicortex

Three-layered cortex (also called allocortex):

- Phylogenetically old areas of the limbic system, such as primary olfactory cortex, hippocampus, and the dentate gyrus.
- Mesocortex: 5- to 6-layered cortex, poorly organized.
- Includes inferior and mesial temporal lobes (hippocampal formation).

Brodmann's Areas (Figure 2.29)

Used to designate the cytoarchitecture of different parts of the brain. Now they are used to designate functional anatomy.

Homunculus (Figures 2.30 and 2.31)

Means "little man"; somatotopic organization at the motor and sensory cortices.

Special Systems

Motor System

- Primary motor cortex: Precental gyrus (Brodmann's area 4).
- Premotor area: Lateral surface of Brodmann's area 6.
  - Involved in body posture.
  - Work through reticulospinal, tectospinal, and rubrospinal tracts.
- Supplementary motor area: Medial surface of Brodmann's area 6.
  - Involved in complex movements.
  - Lesion of this area is associated with global akinesia, ideomotor apraxia.

KEY FACT

Lesion at the optic chiasm (in particular a pituitary tumor or mass) can cause a bitemporal hemianopsia.

Somatosensory System

Primary sensory cortex (Brodmann's areas 3, 1, 2).

Visual System (Figure 2.32)

- **Retina:** Detects light and transmits images from the nasal and temporal fields.
- **Optic nerve fibers** from the temporal fields cross at the optic chiasm.
- **Optic tracts:** Nerve fibers past the chiasm.

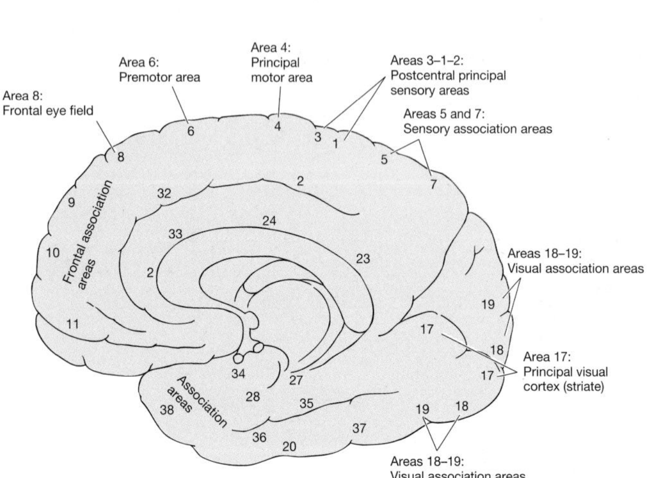

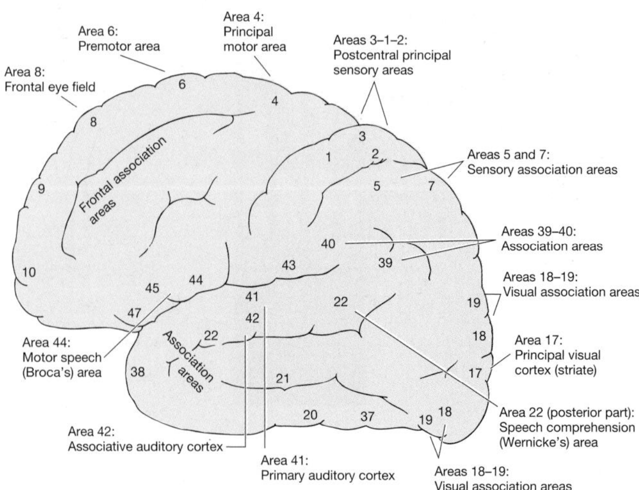

FIGURE 2.29. Medial and lateral aspects of the cerebrum. The cortical areas are shown according to Brodmann with functional localizations.

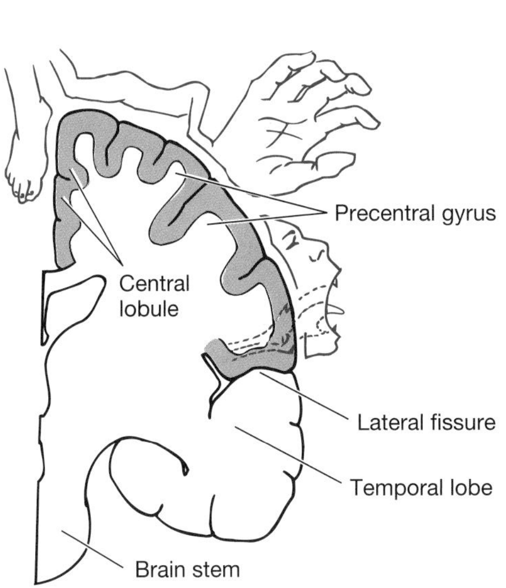

FIGURE 2.30. Motor homunculus. (Reproduced, with permission, from Waxman SG. *Clinical Neurology*, 25th ed. New York: McGraw-Hill, 2003: Figure 10-14.)

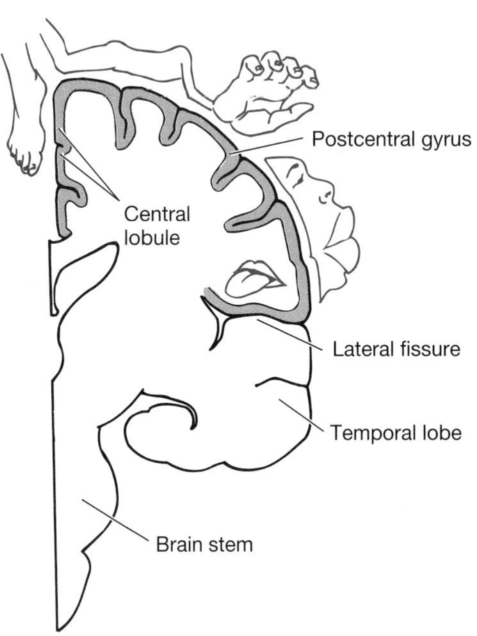

FIGURE 2.31. Sensory homunculus. (Reproduced, with permission, from Waxman SG. *Clinical Neurology*, 25th ed. New York: McGraw-Hill, 2003: Figure 10-15.)

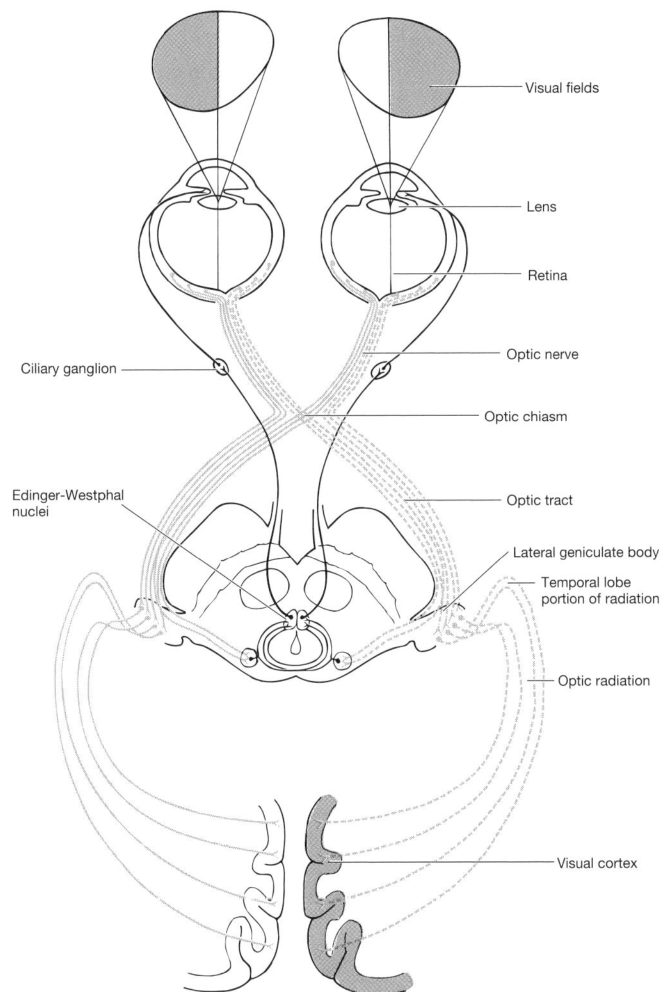

FIGURE 2.32. Visual system. (Reproduced, with permission, from Waxman SG. *Clinical Neurology*, 25th ed. New York: McGraw-Hill, 2003: Figure 15-14.)

- **Lateral geniculate nucleus (LGN):** Posterior thalamic nucleus, receives all info from optic tract except the extrageniculate pathway.
  - Extrageniculate pathway goes straight to the brain stem structures such as the superior colliculus and pretectal area. Therefore, lesion of the LGN spares pupillary function but they can also caused a contralateral homonymous hemianopsia.
  - LGN has 6 separate nuclear layers: Layers 1, 4, 6: receive crossed fibers. Layers 2, 3, 5: receive uncrossed fibers.
- **Optic radiations:**
  - Parietal radiations: From superior retinal quadrants that detect information from the inferior visual fields.
  - Temporal radiations (Meyer loop): From inferior retinal quadrants that detect information from the superior visual fields.
- **Primary visual cortex (Brodmann's area 17):** Occipital lobe.
  - Below the calcarine fissure (lingual gyrus) → superior visual field.
  - Above the calcarine fissure (cuneus) → inferior visual field.
  - Lesion of the occipital lobe leads to a contralateral homonymous hemianopsia that is macula sparing.

KEY FACT

If Wilbrand knee (an anterior deflection of the decussating fibers from the inferior nasal retina) is lesioned, then a superior temporal quadrantanopia contralateral to the lesion will result.

Lesion at optic tract leads to a contralateral homonymous hemianopsia.

Other Lesions Associated with Visual System

- **Anton syndrome:** Bilateral damage to occipital lobes → complete blindness. Patients deny that they are blind. Associated with stroke, posterior reversible leukoencephalopathy, and increased intracranial pressure (leads to compression of PCAs).
- **Balint syndrome:** Bilateral lesions of the lateral occipitoparietal cortex, associated with watershed infarcts. Triad of paralysis of visual fixation, optic ataxia, and simultanagnosia.
- **Prosopagnosia:** Bilateral (or large unilateral) lesion of the ventral occipitotemporal lobes. Leads to an inability to recognize faces.
- **Akinetopsia:** Inability to perceive moving objects, but objects can be recognized once they are stationary. Lesion of the association visual cortex at Brodmann's area 37 (visual area V).

KEY FACT

Lesion of Meyer loop → contralateral superior homonymous quadrantopsia.

Lesion of mesial parietal lobe → contralateral inferior homonymous quadrantopsia.

Auditory System (Figure 2.33)

- **Cochlea and organ of Corti** transmit information to the acoustic portion of CN VIII and then synapse in the cochlear nuclei.
- **Fibers from cochlear nuclei:**
  - Dorsal → cross the pontine tegmentum → contralateral lateral lemniscus.
  - Ventral → synapse bilaterally in superior olivary nucleus complex → bilateral lateral lemnisci.
- **Inferior colliculus:** Receives fibers from the lateral lemniscus.
- **Medial geniculate nucleus:** Receives fibers from the inferior colliculus in the brachium of the inferior colliculus.
- **Primary auditory cortex (Brodmann's area 41):** Receives relay fibers from the medial geniculate nucleus as the auditory radiations.
  - Because the auditory pathway above the cochlear nuclei represents parts of the sound input to both ears, a unilateral lesion in the lateral lemniscus, medial geniculate body, or auditory cortex does not result in marked loss of hearing on the ipsilateral side.

KEY FACT

Crossing fibers from superior olivary nucleus complexes occupy the trapezoid body. The superior olivary nucleus is responsible for localizing sounds horizontally in space.

Vestibular System (Figure 2.34)

Vestibular End Organs

Transmit information by the vestibular portion of CN VIII.

- **Utricle and saccule:** Respond to linear acceleration.
- **Semicircular canal** (superior, lateral, and posterior): Responds to angular acceleration and deceleration.

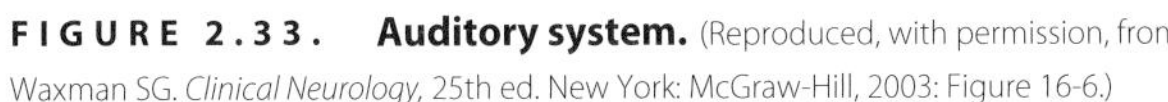

FIGURE 2.33. **Auditory system.** (Reproduced, with permission, from Waxman SG. *Clinical Neurology*, 25th ed. New York: McGraw-Hill, 2003: Figure 16-6.)

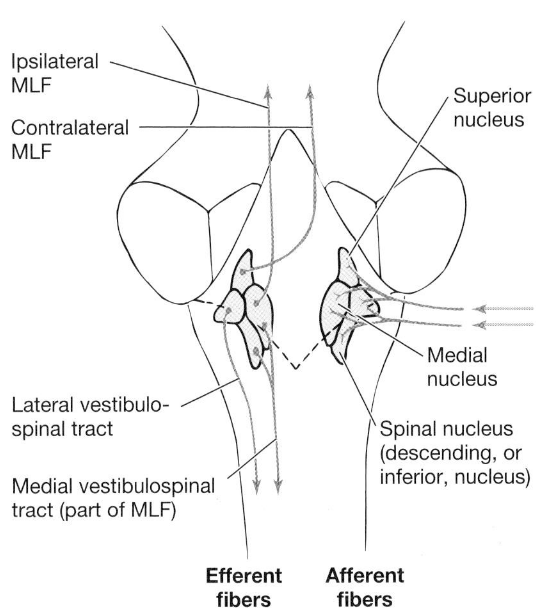

FIGURE 2.34. **Vestibular system.** (Reproduced, with permission, from Waxman SG. *Clinical Neurology*, 25th ed. New York: McGraw-Hill, 2003: Figure 17-2.)

Vestibular Nuclei

Divided into 4 nuclei that receive and transmit separate information.

1. **Superior:**
   - Input: Semicircular canals, flocculonodulus, uvula.
   - Output: Ocular motor nuclei.
2. **Medial:**
   - Input: Semicircular canal, flocculonodulus, uvula.
   - Output: Ocular motor nuclei, cerebellar cortex, medial vestibulospinal tract.
3. **Inferior:**
   - Input: Saccule, fastigial nucleus.
   - Output: Ocular motor nuclei, cerebellar cortex, lateral vestibulospinal tract.
4. **Lateral:**
   - Input: Utricle, anterior vermis, fastigial nucleus.
   - Output: Lateral vestibulospinal tract.

Vestibulospinal Tracts

- Lateral: Goes to entire ipsilateral spinal cord (involved in postural control).
- Medial: Goes to contralateral cervica and thoracic cord (involved in head positioning).

Thalamic/Cortical Representation

Still unclear. May project to parietal lobe and parts of the auditory cortex.

Anton
- bilat occip lobe
- blind but deny

Balint
watershed infarct
Triad:
1) ∅ visual fix
2) optic ataxia
3) simultanagn

Prosopagnosia
bilat ventral occip-temp
∅ recogn. faces

Akinetopsia
assoc. visual cortex
∅ recog "moving" objects (can when stationary)

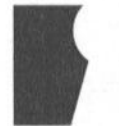

KEY FACT

Olfactory hallucinations: Can be seen in seizures of the mesial temporal lobe or uncus.

Olfactory System

- Cortex components are located near the uncus of the temporal lobes.
- Olfactory bulb → olfactory tracts (medial and lateral olfactory stria).
  - Lateral olfactory stria → pyriform and entorhinal cortex, parts of amygdala.
  - Pyriform cortex → (thalamus) → frontal lobe; this tract is responsible for conscious detection of odors.
  - Medial olfactory stria → anterior olfactory nucleus (which communicates back to the olfactory bulbs) and anterior perforated substance; olfactory reflex reactions.

Gustatory System

Contains sensation of taste from the tongue.

- Taste sensation: Anterior two-thirds of tongue comes from the chorda tympani (branch of CN VII), posterior one-third of tongue comes from CN IX, and palate/epiglottis comes from CN X.
- Taste fibers → nucleus solitarius (in medulla) → ventral posteromedial thalamus → primary gustatory cortex in the opercular and insural regions of the frontal lobes, secondary gustatory cortex in caudolateral orbitofrontal cortex, amygdala, hypothalamus, and basal forebrain.

Limbic System (Figure 2.35)

- Involves emotions, memory, fear, homeostasis, unconscious drives, and olfaction.
  - Hypothalamus: Homeostasis, autonomic/neuroendocrine function.
  - Olfactory cortex: Olfaction.
  - Hippocampal formation: Memory.
  - Amygdala: Fear, emotions.
- Primarily located in medial and ventral portions of the frontal and temporal lobes.
- See Table 2.18 for major limbic pathways.

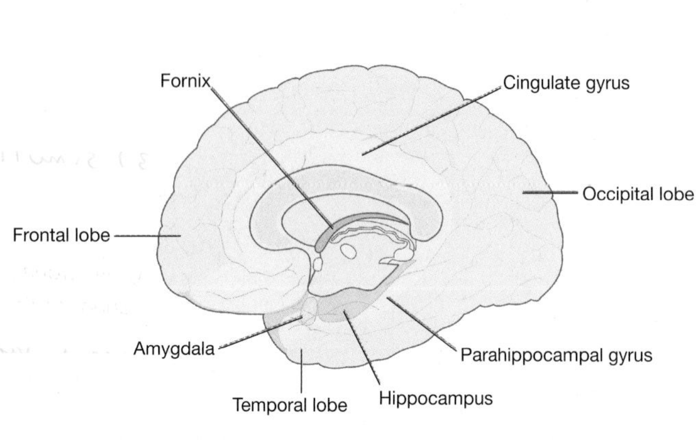

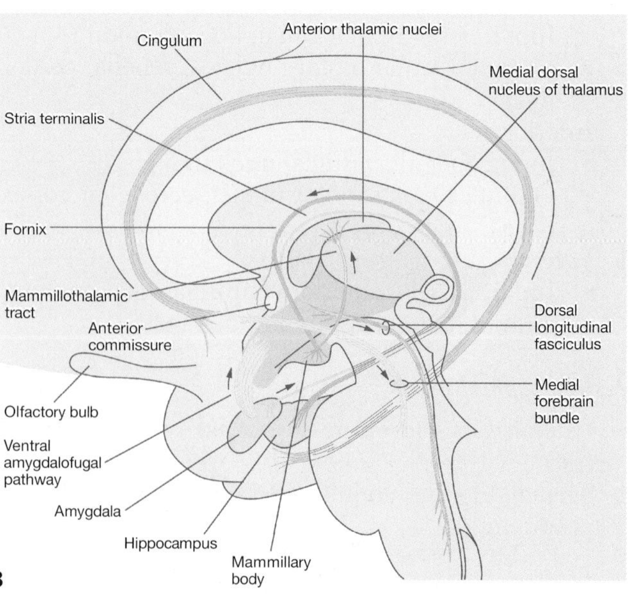

FIGURE 2.35. Sagittal diagram of the limbic system. (A) Surface topography of the limbic system and associated prefrontal cortex. **(B)** Connections of the limbic structures and their relation to the thalamus, hypothalamus, and midbrain tegmentum. The cortical parts of the limbic system, or limbic lobe, are interconnected by a septo-hypothalamic-mesencephalic bundle, ending in the hippocampus, and the fornix, which runs from the hippocampus back to the mamillary bodies, and by tracts from the mamillary bodies to the thalamus and from the thalamus to the cingulate gyrus. The Papez circuit is the internal component of this system. (Reproduced, with permission, from Ropper AH, Brown RH. *Adams & Victor's Principles of Neurology*, 8th ed. New York: McGraw-Hill, 2005: 443.)

TABLE 2.18. Major Limbic Pathways

Pathway	Input	Output
Fornix	Subiculum	Medial and lateral mammillary nuclei; lateral septal nuclei
	Hippocampus	Lateral septal nuclei
	Hippocampal formation	Anterior thalamic nucleus
	Medial septal nucleus	Hippocampal formation
	Nucleus of diagonal band	Hippocampal formation
Mammillothalamic tract	Medial mammillary nucleus	Anterior thalamic nucleus
Cingulum	Cingulate gyrus	Parahippocampal gyrus
Mammillotegmental tract	Mammillary bodies	Brain stem
Stria medullaris	Medial septal nuclei	Habenula
Anterior commissure	Anterior olfactory nucleus	Contralateral anterior olfactory nucleus
	Amygdala	Contralateral amygdala
	Anterior temporal cortex	Contralateral anterior temporal cortex
Stria terminalis	Corticomedial amygdala	Hypothalamus
	Amygdala	Septal nucei
Medial forebrain bundle	Amygdala, other forebrain structures	Brain stem nuclei
	Brain stem nuclei	Amygdala, other forebrain structures
Perforant pathway	Entorhinal cortex	Dentate gyrus granule cells
Alvear pathway	Entorhinal cortex	Hippocampal pyramidal cells

- **Hippocampal formation:** Primary functions in memory.
  - Includes hippocampus, dentate gyrus, and subiculum.
  - Circuitry of the hippocampal formation (Figure 2.36) includes 4 different pyramidal cell sectors at the cornu ammonis (CA). In order they are: CA_1 (closest to subiculum), CA_2, CA_3, CA_4 (within hilus of dentate gyrus).
- Granule cells of the dentate gyrus send axons (mossy fibers) that terminate on pyramidal neurons in the CA_3 region of the hippocampus.
- These neurons, in turn, project to the fornix, which is a major efferent pathway.
- Collateral branches (termed *Schaffer collaterals*) from the CA_3 neurons project to the CA_1 region.

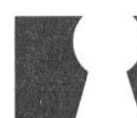

KEY FACT

Sommer sector (CA_1 and CA_2) are prone to ischemic damage in watershed injuries.

THALAMUS/HYPOTHALAMUS

Diencephalon

- **Thalamus:** Relay point between subcortical structures and cerebral cortex and plays a major role in modulating cortical activity, large ovoid gray mass of nuclei that lies between third ventricle and the internal capsule. Short interthalamic adhesion (massa intermedia) that connects the thalami across the narrow third ventricle (see Figure 2.37).
- **Hypothalamus:** Autonomic and regulatory functions (eating, autonomic

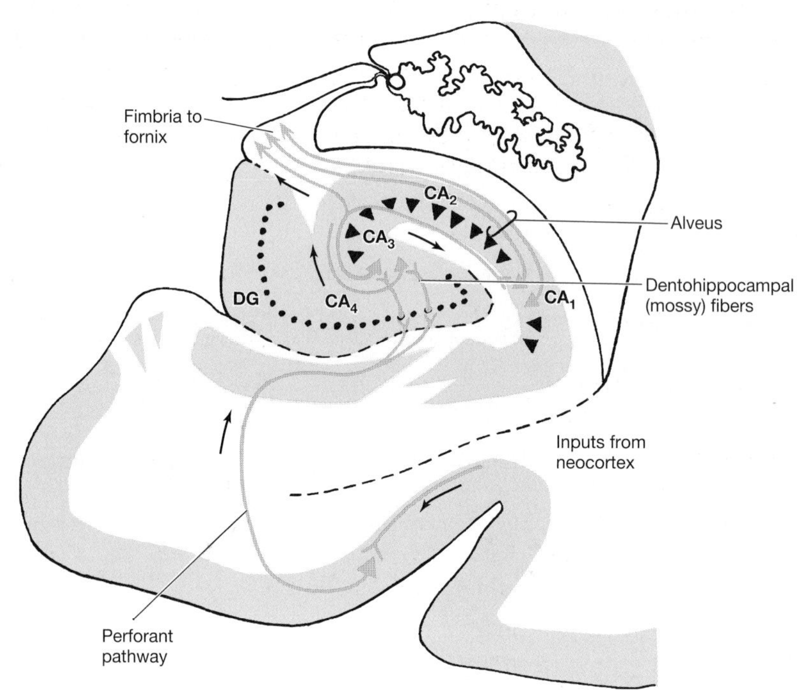

FIGURE 2.36. Hippocampal formation. Schematic illustration of the major connections to, within, and from the hippocampal formation. Dentate granule cells (DG) project to pyramidal neurons in the hippocampus. CA_1 through CA_4 are sectors of the hippocampus. (Reproduced, with permission, from Waxman SG. *Clinical Neurology*, 25th ed. New York: McGraw-Hill, 2003: Figure 19-10.)

body temperature, H_2O balance, hormones, circadian rhythms, expression of emotion).

- **Subthalamus:** Lies between dorsal thalamus and tegmentum, consists of the subthalamic nucleus.
- **Epithalamus:** Consists of habenular trigones, pineal gland, habenular commissure.

Thalamic White Matter

- **Thalamic radiations:** Fiber bundles that emerge from the lateral surface of the thalamus and terminate in cerebral cortex.

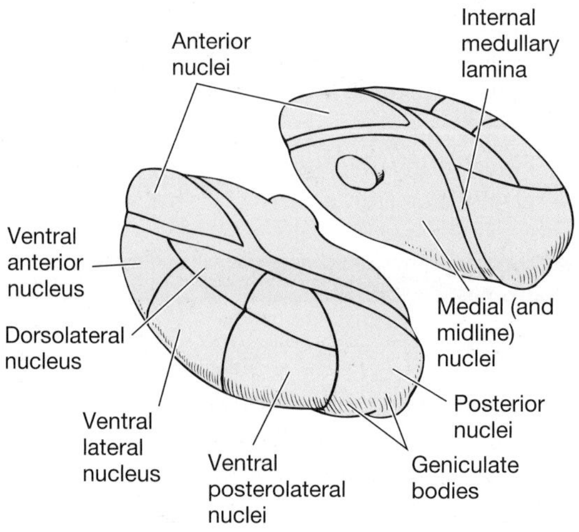

FIGURE 2.37. Diagrams of the thalamus. Oblique lateral and medial views. (Reproduced, with permission, from Waxman SG. *Clinical Neurology*, 25th ed. New York: McGraw-Hill, 2003: Figure 9-3.)

- **External medullary lamina:** Layer of myelinated fibers on the lateral surface of the thalamus close to the internal capsule, separates the thalamic reticular nucleus from the other thalamic nuclei (Table 2.19).
- **Internal medullary lamina:** Vertical sheet of white matter that bifurcates in its anterior portion and divides the gray matter of the thalamus into lateral, medial, and anterior nuclear groups.

Nuclear Groups

Anterior Nuclear Group

- **Anterior nucleus:** Forms anterior tubercle of thalamus, bordered by limbs of internal lamina.
  - Input: Mammillary bodies of hypothalamus via mamillothalamic tract; hippocampus via fornix.
  - Output: To the cingulate gyrus.
  - Role: Memory formation.

Nuclei of the Midline

Lie within the internal medullary lamina.

- **Centromedial (CM) nucleus:**
  - Input: Inhibitory from globus pallidus.
  - Output: Projects to basal ganglia (caudate and putamen).

Medial Nuclear Group

Lie medial to Y band.

- **Dorsomedial (DM) nucleus:** Largest nucleus of medial nuclear group.
  - Input: From olfactory cortex via stria medullaris.
  - Output: To hypothalamus; sends a massive projection to cingulate and orbitofrontal cortex.
  - Role: Emotional behavior.

TABLE 2.19. The Thalamic Nuclei

Type of Nucleus	Thalamic Nucleus
Motor	VA/VL CM
Sensory	VPL VPM LGN MGN
Limbic	A DM
Associational	LD, LP Pulvinar Reticular Intralaminar

LATERAL NUCLEAR GROUP

- **Ventroanterior (VA) nucleus:**
  - Input: From the basal ganglia.
  - Output: To primary motor cortex (area 4) and premotor and supplementary motor cortex (area 6).
  - Role: Faciliates movement.
- **Ventrolateral (VL) nucleus:**
  - Input: From basal ganglia and cerebellum.
  - Output: To primary motor cortex (area 4) and premotor/supplementary motor cortex (area 6).
  - Role: Faciliates movement.
- **Ventroposterolateral (VPL) nucleus:**
  - Input: From ALS and dorsal column/medial lemniscal system.
  - Output: Somatosensory cortices (areas 3, 1, 2).
  - Role: Somatosensory relay nucleus for the body.
- **Ventroposteromedial (VPM) nucleus:**
  - Input: From ventral/dorsal trigeminothalamic tract; from nucleus solitarius.
  - Output: Somatosensory cortices (areas 3, 1, 2); to taste cortex (area 43).
  - Role: Somatosensory relay nucleus for the face; taste relay.
- **Laterodorsal (LD) nucleus:** Sits above VL.
  - Output: Projects to frontal, parietal, and cingulate cortex.
  - Role: Integrates sensory information and emotional behavior.
- **Lateroposterior (LP) nucleus:** Sits above VPL and VPM.
  - Similar connections as LD.

POSTERIOR NUCLEI

- **Lateral geniculate nucleus (LGN):**
  - Input: From the retina.
  - Output: To primary visual cortex (area 17) via the optic radiations (receives a good deal of feedback input from the cortex).
  - Role: Visual relay nucleus.
- **Medial geniculate nucleus (MGN):**
  - Input: From the inferior colliculus via the brachium of inferior colliculus.
  - Output: To auditory cortex (area 41) via auditory radiations.
  - Role: Auditory relay nucleus.
- **Pulvinar:** Caps the back of the thalamus.
  - Input: From parietal and temporal association areas, which include secondary association cortices devoted to vision, somatosensation, and audition, from superior colliculus and primary visual cortex.
  - Output: To parietal and temporal association areas, which include secondary association cortices devoted to vision, somatosensation, and audition.
  - Role: Integration of sensory information and in the modulation of spatial attention.

RETICULAR NUCLEI

Lateral to lateral group of nuclei separated from the rest of the thalamus by the external medullary lamina.

- Only thalamic nucleus that doesn't project to the cerebral cortex.
- Only thalamic nucleus with inhibitory output.

- Sends its output exclusively to other thalamic nuclei (a particular region of the reticular nucleus receives excitatory input from a particular thalamic nucleus and sends inhibitory output back to the same nucleus).
- Role: Regulate flow of information from the thalamus to the cortex, part of the ascending reticular activating system, modulation of arousal and sleep and in the generation of brainwave activity.
- Lesion: Likely site for abnormalities associated with certain epilepsies.

HYPOTHALAMIC NUCLEI

See Table 2.20.

TABLE 2.20. Hypothalamic Nuclei

NUCLEUS	FUNCTION
Lateral Hypothalamus	
Lateral hypothalamic nucleus	Induces eating when stimulated.
	Lesion → anorexia/starvation.
Medial Hypothalamus	
Preoptic region	
Median preoptic nucleus	Regulates release of gonadotropic hormones from adenohypophysis.
Anterior nucleus	Regulates temperature, stimulates parasympathetic system.
	Lesion → hyperthermia.
Lateral preoptic nucleus	γ-aminobutyric acid (GABA) and galanine projections that promote sleep onset.
Supraoptic region	
Supraoptic nucleus	Produces antidiuretic hormone (ADH) and oxytocin.
Paraventricular nucleus	Produces ADH, oxytocin, corticotropin-releasing hormone.
	Lesion → diabetes insipidus.
Suprachiasmatic nucleus	Regulates circadian rhythms, receives direct input from the retina.
Tuberal region	
Ventromedial nucleus	Induces satiety.
	Lesion → hyperphagia.
Arcuate nucleus	Projects to pituitary and influences hormone release from the anterior pituitary. Part of the dopamine system (prolactin-inhibiting factor).
Mammillary region	
Mammillary nucleus	Input from hippocampal formation via fornix. Projects to anterior nucleus of thalamus via mammillothalamic tract.
	Lesion → Wernicke encephalopathy, Korsakoff pychosis.
Dorsomedial nucleus	Involved in behavior control, when stimulated leads to violent behavior in animals.
Posterolateral nucleus	Induces wakefulness via diffuse orexin/hypocretin projections. Projects to cholinergic and monoaminergic neurons in brain stem and lateral preoptic nucleus.
Posterior Hypothalamus	
Posterior hypothalamic nucleus	Involved in thermoregulation.
	Lesion → heat loss and inability to regulate temperature.

INTERNAL CAPSULE/BASAL GANGLIA

Internal Capsule

- Broad band of myelinated fibers that separates some of the basal ganglia from the thalamus and caudate nucleus.
- Consists of anterior limb, posterior limb, and genu.
  - Anterior limb: Separates the putamen and globus pallidus from the caudate nucleus. Contains the following fiber bundles: thalamocortical and corticothalamic fibers that course between lateral thalamic nuclear group and frontal lobe cortex. Tracts, corticopontine tract. Fibers that run transversely from the caudate nucleus to the putamen.
  - Posterior limb: Located between the thalamus and the lentiform nucleus. Contains the following fiber tracts: corticobulbar and corticospinal tracts run in anterior one-half of the posterior limb, with fibers to the face at genu of the internal capsule. Corticorubral fibers from the frontal lobe cortex to the red nucleus accompany the corticospinal tract. Somatosensory fibers from thalamus to the postcentral gyrus of cortex lie in the posterior one-third of the posterior limb. (Face most anteriorly, then arm, and then the leg.)
- There is also an external and extreme capsule.

Basal Ganglia (Figure 2.38)

- Collection of nuclei which participate in control of movement.
  - Input: Descending motor information from the motor/premotor cortex.
  - Output: Stops in motor thalamus (VA/VL) then to motor/premotor cortex (come from GP_i and SN_r).
  - Influence over the movements on the contralateral side of the body.
- Parts of the basal ganglia:
  1. Caudate nucleus.
  2. Lenticular nucleus: Putamen and globus pallidus.

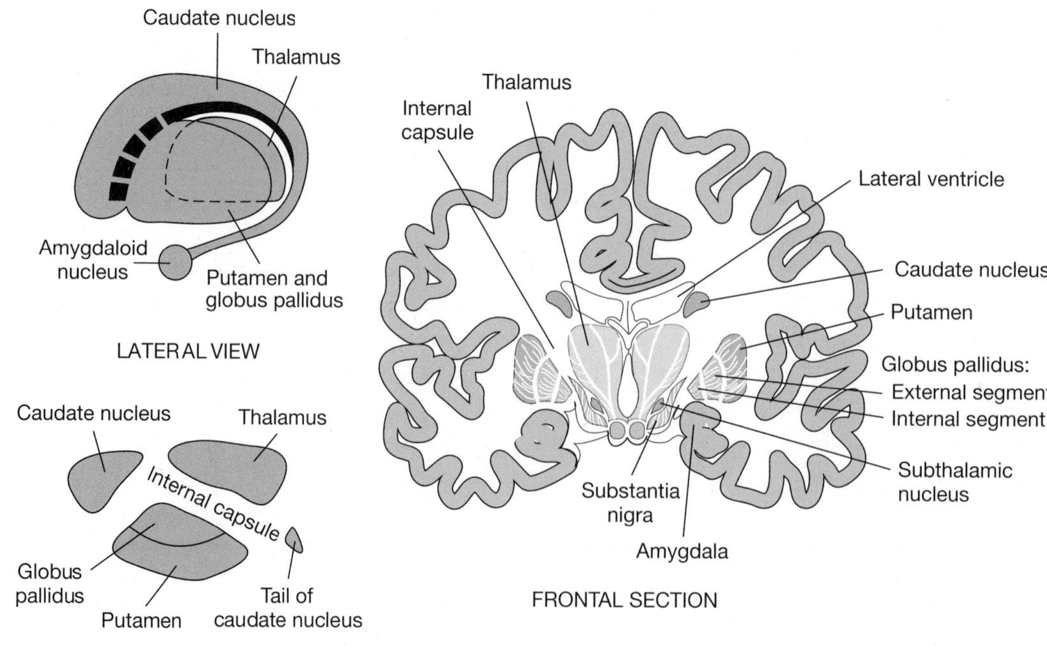

FIGURE 2.38. Basal ganglia. (Reproduced, with permission, from Ganong WF. *Review of Medical Physiology,* 22nd ed. New York: McGraw-Hill, 2003: 213.)

3. Globus pallidus: External and internal.
4. Striatum: Caudate and putamen.
5. Subthalamic nucleus: Junction of midbrain and diencephalon.
6. Amygdala: Involved in the limbic system.
7. Claustrum: Thin layer of gray matter lying between the extreme capsule and external capsule in the brain. Unknown function.

Motor Control Pathways (Figures 2.39 and 2.40)

- **Direct pathway:** Inhibitory outputs from the striatum act to remove the tonic inhibition of GP_i/SN_r output and allow the motor command to be executed (disinhibition).
- **Indirect pathway:** Outputs from the striatum project to GP_e, which in turn inhibits STN. Net effect is to increase the level of inhibition and effectively prevent GP_i/SN_r output and prevent execution of the motor command.

Striatum Projections

- D_2 receptors are mostly found on enkephalin containing striatal neurons, inhibiting the "indirect" pathway.
- D_1 receptors are found on substance P containing striatal neurons that participate in the "direct" pathway.

Peripheral Nervous System

PERIPHERAL NERVE ORGANIZATION

- Lies outside of the brain and spinal cord. Composed of the cranial nerves and 31 pairs of spinal nerves.
- Important nerve groups include cervical plexus, brachial plexus, and lumbosacral plexus.
- In addition to the motor and sensory nerves, there is the autonomic nervous system, which is divided into the sympathetic and parasympathetic systems.

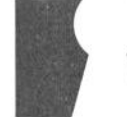

KEY FACT

Cancer cells can infiltrate the perineurium and cause symptoms of neuropathy. This can be seen primarily in patients with skin cancer and often affects the cranial nerves.

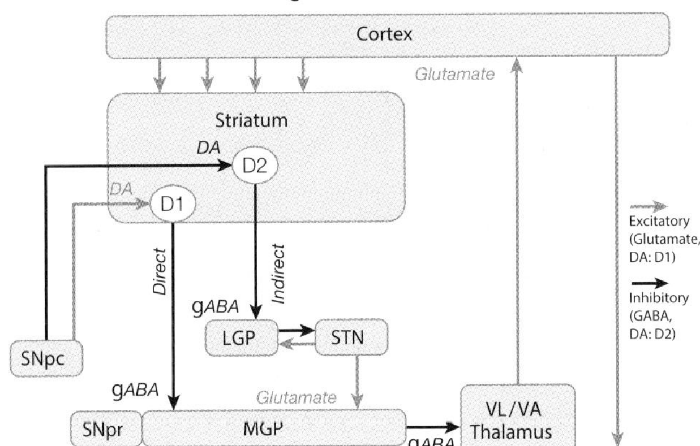

FIGURE 2.39. Functional anatomy of the striatum. Diagram of the main neurotransmitter pathways and their effects in the cortical basal ganglia-thalamic circuits. (Reproduced, with permission, from Ropper AH, Brown RH. *Adams & Victor's Principles of Neurology,* 8th ed. New York: McGraw-Hill, 2005: 592.)

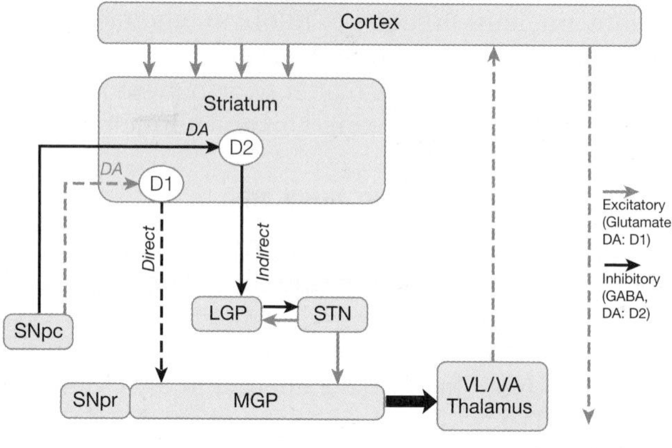

FIGURE 2.40. Functional anatomy and Parkinson disease. Corresponding physiologic state as conceptualized in Parkinson disease, in which hypokinesia is the main finding as a result of reduced dopamine input from the substantia nigra and pars compacta to the striatum via the direct pathway, which results in withdrawal of inhibitory activity of the globus pallidus and, in turn, increased inhibitory drive on the thalamic nuclei, which reduces input to the cortical motor system. (Reproduced, with permission, from Ropper AH, Brown RH. *Adams & Victor's Principles of Neurology*, 8th ed. New York: McGraw-Hill, 2005: 592.)

ANATOMY OF A NERVE

A nerve consists of the nerve fibers plus the connective tissue associated with the nerve (Figure 2.41).

- **Endoneurium:** Connective tissue surrounding 1 nerve fiber.
- **Perineurium:** Connective tissue surrounding 1 nerve fascicle.
- **Epineurium:** Connective tissue surrounding 1 or several nerve fascicles.

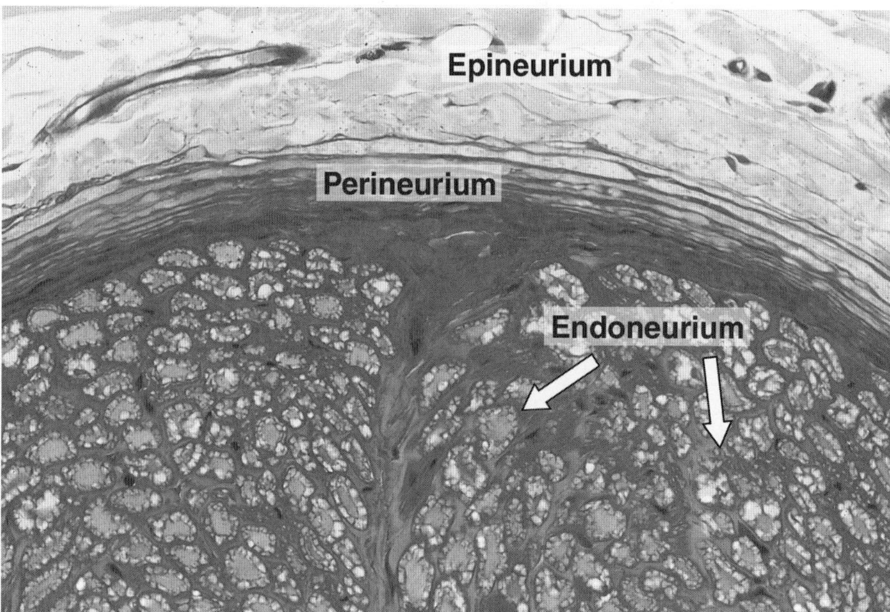

FIGURE 2.41. Peripheral nerve anatomy. (Also see Color Plate.) Cross-section of a thick nerve showing the epineurium, perineurium, and endoneurium. The myelin sheath that envelops each axon was partially removed by the histological technique. PT stain. Medium magnification. (Reproduced, with permission, from Junqueria LC. *Basic Histology Text & Atlas*, 11th ed. New York: McGraw-Hill, 2005: Figure 9-34.)

NERVE FIBER TYPES

See Table 2.21.

MOTOR NEURON WITH AXON

See Figure 2.42.

CERVICAL PLEXUS

- Plexus of the motor roots of C1–C4. Share some innervation with the accessory nerve and hypoglossal nerve.
- Located deep to the sternocleiodomastoid muscle. Because of the deep location, it is rarely subject to injury.
- Provides innervation to the scalenes, lower trapezius, diaphragm, muscles of the neck.
- **Ansa cervicalis** is a loop of nerves that is part of the cervical plexus. Superior root from C1 supplies the superior belly of the omohyoid muscle and the inferior root from C2 and C3 innervate the sternohyoid and sternothyroid muscles.

BRACHIAL PLEXUS (FIGURE 2.43)

- Plexus of the motor and sensory roots from C5 to T1.
- Extends from the cervical roots through the neck below the clavicle and into the axilla. The subclavian artery runs parallel with the trunks, divisions, cords, and branches.
- Roots: 5—C5, C6, C7, C8, and T1.

TABLE 2.21. Nerve Fiber Types

Fiber Type	Function	Fiber Diameter (μm)	Conduction Velocity (m/s)	Spike Duration (ms)	Absolute Refractory Period (ms)
A					
α	Proprioception	12–20	70–120	0.4–0.5	0.4–1
β	Somatic motor				
γ	Touch, pressure, motor	5–12	30–70		
δ	Motor to muscle spindles	3–6	15–30		
	Pain, cold, touch	2–5	12–30		
B	Preganglionic autonomic	< 3	3–15	1.2	1.2
C					
Dorsal root	Pain, temperature, reflex response	0.4–1.2	0.5–2	2	2
Sympathetic	Postganglionic sympathetics	0.3–1.3	0.7–2.3	2	2

Note: A and B fibers are myelinated; C fibers are not myelinated.

Reproduced, with permission, from Ganong WF. *Review of Medical Physiology,* 22nd ed. New York: McGraw-Hill, 2005.

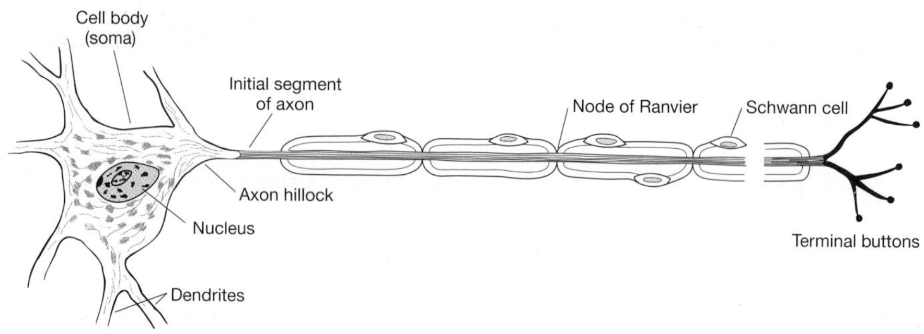

FIGURE 2.42. Motor neuron with axon. (Reproduced, with permission, from Ganong WF. *Review of Medical Physiology*, 22nd ed. New York: McGraw-Hill, 2003: 52.)

- Trunks: 3—superior or upper (C5–C6), middle (C7), and inferior or lower (C8–T1).
- Divisions: 6—anterior and posterior of each trunk.
- Cords: 2—lateral (C5–T1), posterior (C5–C8), and medial (C8–T1).
- Branches: Nerves that emerge from the cords.

KEY FACT

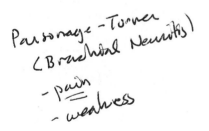

Martin-Gruber anastomosis: Communicating branch from the anterior interosseous nerve to the ulnar nerve in the forearm. It supplies the adductor pollicis, abductor digiti minimi, and first dorsal interosseous muscles. Occurs in 15–30% of the population and it is considered a normal variant.

Brachial Neuritis (Parsonage-Turner Syndrome)

Rare clinical syndrome involving an inflammatory reaction to the nerves in the brachial plexus. Can present with severe pain in the shoulder region, mild fever, and weakness in the muscles of the upper trunk. Weakness usually develops over 2 weeks. Etiologies include viral infection, bacterial infection, trauma, childbirth, vaccinations, rheumatologic illness, surgery. There is a very rare genetic form that is autosomal dominant and localizes to the SEPT9 gene on chromosome 17q. Treatment is usually symptomatic and most patients recover after 2 years.

Nerves of the Brachial Plexus

See Table 2.22.

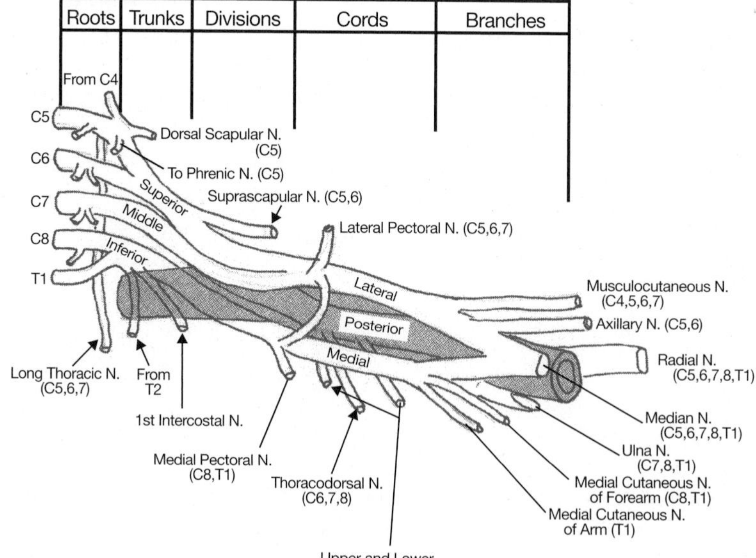

FIGURE 2.43. The brachial plexus. Organization of the roots, trunks, divisions, and cords, as well as root origins of peripheral nerves. (Reproduced, with permission, from Brunicardi FC, Anderson DR, Billiar TR, Dunn DL, Hunter JG, Matthews JB, Poliok RE, Schwartz JT. *Schwartz's Principles of Surgery*, 8th ed. New York: McGraw-Hill, 2005: Figure 43-6.)

TABLE 2.22. **Nerves of the Brachial Plexus**

Nerve	Origin	Spinal Level	Muscles Innervated	Sensory Components
Dorsal scapular	From C5 root	C5	Rhomboids	
Long thoracic	From C5–C7 roots	C5–C7	Serratus anterior	
Suprascapular	From upper trunk	C5, C6	Supraspinatus Infraspinatus	
Nerve to subclavius	From upper trunk	C5, C6	Subclavius	
Lateral pectoral	From lateral cord	C5–C7	Pectoralis major (primarily the clavicular head)	
Lateral antebrachial cutaneous	From lateral cord			Skin of the lateral forearm
Musculocutaneous	From lateral cord	C5–C7	Biceps (C5, C6) Brachialis Coracobrachialis	
Median	From lateral, medial, and posterior cords	C5–T1	Pronator teres (C6, C7) Flexor carpi radialis (C6, C7) Flexor digitorum superficalis (C7–T1) Abductor pollicis brevis (C8, T1) Oppopens pollicis (C8, T1) First lumbrical interosseous (with ulnar) (C8, T1)	Thumb, first and second digits, and one-half of third digit ventolateral part of palm
Anterior interosseous	Deep branch of the median nerve	C7, C8	Flexor pollicis longus Flexor digitorum profundus (I, II) Pronator quadratus	
Medial pectoral	From medial cord	C8, T1	Pectoralis minor Pectoralis major	
Medial antebrachial cutaneous	From medial cord	C8, T1		Skin to the medial forearm
Ulnar	From medial cord	C7–T1	Flexor carpi ulnaris (C7–T1) Flexor digitorum profundus (III, IV) (C7, C8) Abductor digiti minimi (C8, T1) Flexor digit minimi (C8, T1) First dorsal interosseous (C8, T1) Second palmar interosseous (C8, T1) Adductor pollicis (C8, T1)	One-half of the fourth and fifth digits and ventral side of palm
Thoracodorsal	From posterior cord	C6–C8	Latissimus dorsi	
Subscapular	From posterior cord	C5, C6	Teres major Subscapularis	

TABLE 2.22. Nerves of the Brachial Plexus *(continued)*

Nerve	Origin	Spinal Level	Muscles Innervated	Sensory Components
Axillary	From posterior cord	C5, C6	Deltoids Teres minor	Small part of the lateral shoulder
Radial nerve	From posterior cord	C5–T1	Triceps (C6–C8) Brachioradialis (C5, C6) Extensor carpi radialis (C5, C6) Supinator (C6, C7)	Most of the back of the hand, including the web of skin between the thumb and index finger
Posterior interosseous	Branch from the radial nerve	C7, C8	Extensor carpi ulnaris (C7, C8) Extensor digitorum (C7, C8) Abductor pollicis longus (C7, C8) Extensor pollicis longus (C7, C8) Extensor pollicis brevis (C7, C8)	
Posterior antebrachial cutaneous	Branch from the radial nerve			Skin to the dorsal surface of the forearm

Lesions of the Brachial Plexus

Lesions of the Trunk

- **Erb-Duchenne paralysis:** Involves the upper trunk. Occurs during trauma or during traction of the arm at birth. Associated with birth trauma involving maternal obesity and large babies. Called the "waiter's tip" palsy.
  - Roots involved: C5, C6.
  - Nerves affected: Suprascapular nerve, C5 and C6 portions of lateral cord and posterior cord, lateral antebrachial cutaneous nerve.
  - Actions lost: Shoulder abduction, elbow flexion.
  - Arm is internally rotated at shoulder, with an extended elbow and pronated forearm. Deep tendon reflexes at the biceps and brachioradialis are lost.
- **Klumpke paralysis:** Involves the lower trunk. Can occur as a consequence of breech delivery (associated with shoulder dystocia), apical tumors (such as Pancoast tumor), trauma to the shoulder. Often called the "claw hand" palsy.
  - Roots involved: C8, T1.
  - Actions lost: Finger flexion and intrinsic hand movements, weakness of triceps and extensor digitorum communis.
  - Arm is slightly flexed at the elbow and wrist, and the hand appears flaccid and atrophied. There is sensory loss involving the hand and medial forearm.
  - If the T1 root is involved, there can be a Horner syndrome present.
- **Middle trunk lesion:** Very rare. Usually occurs with other lesions of the brachial plexus. Looks similar to a C7 root injury.

Lesions of the Cords

Involved with lesions below the clavicle. This can be seen in trauma such as shoulder dislocation or clavicular fractures.

- Posterior cord: Weakness in upper-extremity extensors and shoulder abduction. Sensory loss over the posterior part of the arm and hand.
- Medial cord: Weakness in most small hand muscles and some loss of finger flexion. Sensory loss over the medial aspect of the forearm.
- Lateral cord: Weakness in upper-extremity flexors (except finger flexion). Sensory loss involves the lateral forearm.

Thoracic Outlet Syndrome

Due to compression of the lower part of the brachial plexus by a cervical rib or band. The subclavian artery and vein can also be compressed. This leads to pain and paresthesias in the medial aspect of forearm and the fourth and fifth digits of the hands. Weakness in the intrinsic hand muscles can be present. Ulnar nerve is primarily affected. Treatment is usually surgical.

LUMBOSACRAL PLEXUS (FIGURE 2.44)

- Plexus of motor and sensory nerves from L1 to S2. It is formed from the lumbar and sacral plexi.
- Travels from the upper lumbar area to the sacrum.
- Lumbar plexus (T12–L4) sits within the psoas muscle and anterior to the vertebral process.
- Sacral plexus (S1–S4) sits between the pelvic fascial layer and piriformis muscle.

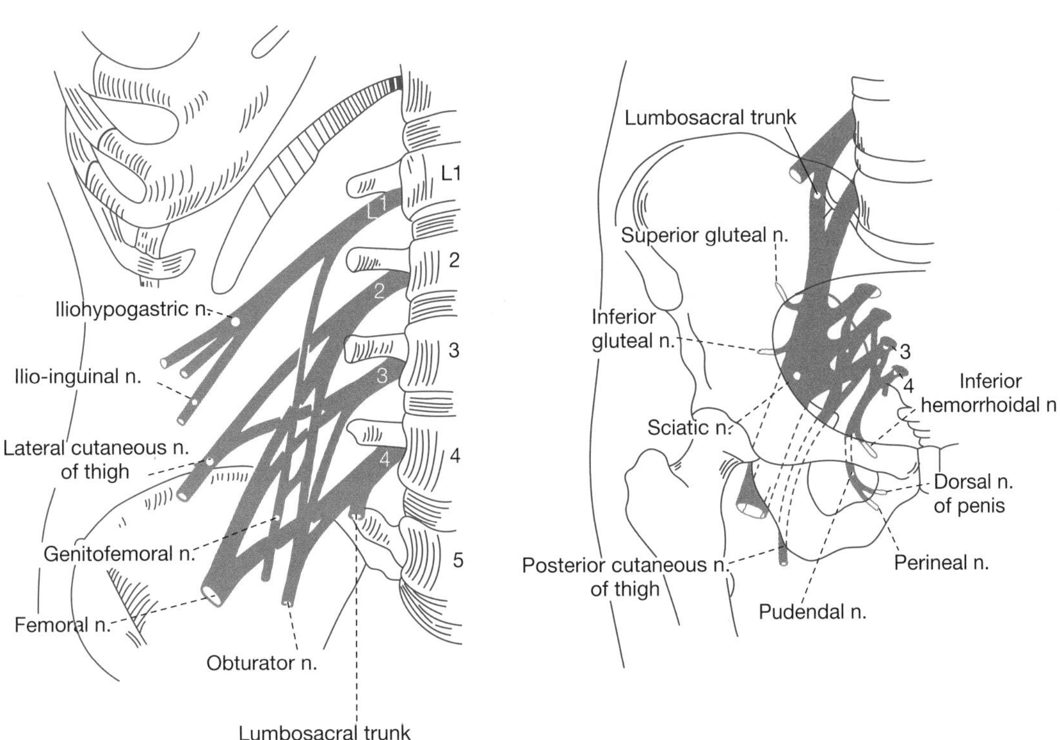

FIGURE 2.44. The lumbosacral plexus. Lumbar plexus (left) and sacral plexus (right). The lumbosacral trunk is the liaison between the lumbar and the sacral plexuses. (Reproduced, with permission, from Ropper AH, Brown RH. *Adams & Victor's Principles of Neurology*, 8th ed. New York: McGraw-Hill, 2005: 1169.)

Lesions of the Lumbosacral Plexus

- Etiologies include tumor involvement via compression or invasion, radiation damage, puerperal and postpartum complications, retroperitoneal pathology including hematomas or abscesses. In contrast to brachial plexus lesions, trauma is not a common cause of damage to the lumbosacral plexus.
- The earliest symptom is usually pain in the distribution of the nerves involved and then weakness is a later finding.
- **Upper plexus lesions:** Primarily involve the lumbar plexus. Weakness would be present in thigh flexion and adduction and leg extension. Sensory loss would be over the anterior thigh and leg.
- **Lower plexus lesions:** Primarily involve the sacral plexus. Weakness would be present in the posterior thigh, leg, and foot. Sensory loss involves the S1 and S2 distribution.

KEY FACT

Pain is usually a presenting factor in lumbosacral plexus injury caused by cancer invasion but not by radiation.

Nerves of the Lumbosacral Plexus

See Tables 2.23 through 2.26.

MERALGIA PARESTHETICA

Syndrome involving pain, burning, numbness, and paresthesias at the anterolateral thigh. Usually due to entrapment of lateral femoral cutaneous nerve. Etiologies include obesity, tight clothing, pregnancy, physical exercise (yoga/pilates positions), diverticulitis, uterine tumors. Treatment is usually risk factor reduction and symptomatic. Surgery can be performed to release the entrapment.

ACCESSORY PERONEAL NERVE

Common anomaly involving a branch from the superficial peroneal nerve that innervates the extensor digitorum brevis in addition to the regular innervation by the deep peroneal nerve. On nerve conduction studies, the compound action potential is larger with stimulation at the knee than at the ankle because the stimulation at the knee is coming from the deep and superficial branches of the peroneal nerve.

DERMATOMES

A dermatome is an area of skin that is mainly supplied by a single spinal nerve (see Figures 2.45 and 2.46). There are 8 cervical nerves, 12 thoracic nerves, 5 lumbar nerves, and 5 sacral nerves. Each of these nerves relays sensation (including pain) from a particular region of skin to the brain.

Along the thorax and abdomen the dermatomes are like a stack of discs forming a human, each supplied by a different spinal nerve. Along the arms and the legs, the pattern is different: the dermatomes run longitudinally along the limbs. Although the general pattern is similar in all people, the precise areas of innervation are as unique to an individual as fingerprints.

A similar area innervated by peripheral nerves is called a peripheral nerve field. Dermatomes are useful in neurology for finding the site of damage to the spine. Viruses that infect spinal nerves such as herpes zoster infections (shingles), can reveal their origin by showing up as a painful dermatomal area.

TABLE 2.23. Nerves of the Lumbosacral Plexus

Nerve	Spinal Level	Muscles Innervated	Sensory Component
Iliohypogastric	T12, L1		Skin over the hypogastric and gluteal regions
Ilioinguinal	L1		Skin over the upper/medial part of thigh; skin covering the root of the penis and scrotum or the mons pubis and labia majora
Lateral femoral cutaneous	L2, L3		Skin over the anterolateral thigh
Genitofemoral	L1, L2	Cremaster	Skin over the upper part of the femoral triangle; skin over the scrotum or the mons pubis and labia majora
Femoral	L1–L4	Iliopsoas (L1–L3) Quadriceps femoris (L2–L4)	Skin over the anteromedial aspect of thigh, knee, and lateral calf
Obturator	L2–L4	Adductor (external obturator, pectineus, adductor longus, adductor brevis, adductor magnus, gracilis)	Skin over the lateral aspect of the thigh
Superior gluteal	L4–S1	Gluteus medius/minimus (L4–S1) Tensor fascia lata	
Inferior gluteal	L5–S2	Gluteus maximus (L5–S2)	
Sciatic	L5-S2	Hamstrings: Semitendinous, semimembranosus, biceps (L5–S2)	Skin over the foot and the postolateral aspect of the calf
Tibial (comes off of sciatic)	L4–S2	Gastrocnemius (S1, S2) Soleus (S1, S2) Tibialis posterior (L4, L5) Flexor digitorum longus, flexor hallucis longus (L5–S2)	
Medial and lateral plantar (comes off of tibial)	S1, S2	Small muscles of the feet (S1, S2)	Soles and toes (medial does medial portion, lateral does lateral portion)
Common peroneal		See deep and superficial portions	Skin over the postolateral aspect of the calf and top of the foot
Deep peroneal	L5, S1	Tibialis anterior Extensor digitorum longus Extensor hallucis longus Extensor digitorum brevis	Skin between the webs of the great toe and second toe
Superficial peroneal	L5, S1	Peroneus longus Peroneus brevis	
Sural (comes off of common peroneal and tibial)			Skin over the lateral aspect of the foot
Calcaneal branch (comes off of distal tibial nerve)			Skin over the sole of the foot

TABLE 2.24. Muscle Fiber Types

Fiber Type	Fiber Diameter	Twitch Speed	Metabolism/Mitochondria	Myoglobin Content	ATPase	NADH
Type I	Small	Slow	Aerobic High	High	pH 9.4 light pH 4.3 dark	Dark
Type II[a]	Large	Fast	Anaerobic Low	Low	pH 9.4 dark pH 4.3 light	Light

[a]Type II is further subdivided into Type IIa and Type IIb. Type IIb are larger and faster than Type IIa fibers. Type IIb are more fatigable than Type IIa.

TABLE 2.25. Upper-Extremity Muscles and Their Associated Actions

Shoulder abduction	Deltoid Supraspinatus	Axillary Suprascapular	**C5,** C6 **C5,** C6
Shoulder adduction	Teres major Latissimus dorsi	Subscapular Thoracodorsal	C5, C6, C7 C6, **C7,** C8
Elbow flexion	Biceps Brachioradialis	Musculocutaneous Radial	C5, C6 C5, **C6**
Elbow extension	Triceps	Radial	C6, **C7,** C8
Pronation	Pronator teres Pronator quadratus	Median Anterior interosseous	C6, C7 C8
Supination	Supinator	Radial	C6, C7
Wrist flexion	Flexor carpi ulnaris Flexor carpi radialis	Ulnar Median	C7, **C8,** T1 C6, C7
Wrist extension	Extensor carpi radialis longus Extensor carpi ulnaris	Radial Posterior interosseous	C5, **C6** **C7,** C8
Proximal thumb flexion	Flexor pollicis brevis	Ulnar Median	C8, **T1** C8, **T1**
Distal thumb flexion	Flexor pollicis longus	Anterior interosseous	C7, **C8**
Thumb abduction	Abductor pollicis brevis	Median	C8, **T1**
	Abductor pollicis longus	Posterior interosseous	**C7,** C8
Thumb extension	Extensor pollicis longus Extensor pollicis brevis	Posterior interosseous Posterior interosseous	**C7,** C8 **C7,** C8
Thumb adduction	Adductor pollicis	Ulnar	C8, **T1**
Thumb opposition	Opponens pollicis	Median	C8, **T1**
Proximal finger flexion	Flexor digitorum superficialis	Median	C7, **C8,** T1
Distal finger flexion	Flexor digitorum profundus I/II Flexor digitorum profundus III/IV	Anterior interosseous Ulnar	C7, **C8** C7, **C8**
Finger extension	Extensor digitorum	Posterior interosseous	**C7,** C8

TABLE 2.26. Lower-Extremity Muscles and Their Associated Actions

Hip adduction	Adductor muscles	Obturator	**L2, L3,** L4
Hip abduction	Gluteus medius and minimus	Superior gluteal	**L4, L5,** S1
Hip flexion	Iliopsoas	Femoral	**L1, L2,** L3
Hip extension	Gluteus maximus	Inferior gluteal	**L5, S1,** S2
Knee flexion	Hamstrings	Sciatic	L5, **S1,** S2
Knee extension	Quadriceps	Femoral	L2, **L3, L4**
Foot plantar flexion	Gastrocnemius Soleus	Tibial Tibial	S1, S2 S1, S2
Foot dorsiflexion	Tibialis anterior	Deep peroneal	**L4,** L5
Foot inversion	Tibialis posterior	Tibial	L4, L5
Foot eversion	Peroneus longus and brevis	Superficial peroneal	L5, S1
Toe flexion	Flexor digitorum longus Flexor hallucis longus	Tibial Tibial	L5, **S1, S2** L5, **S1, S2**
Toe dorsiflexion	Extensor digitorum longus Extensor digitorum brevis	Deep peroneal Deep peroneal	**L5,** S1 **L5,** S1
Great toe dorsiflexion	Extensor hallucis longus	Deep peroneal	**L5,** S1

Autonomic Nervous System

The autonomic nervous system (Figure 2.47) is a special subsection of the nervous system that has both efferent and afferent components that control pupil size, lacrimation, salivation, blood pressure, heart rate, urination, bowel control, and sexual function. It is organized as preganglionic and postganglionic neurons.

- **Sympathetic ("flight or fight" system):** Dilates the pupils, increases heart rate, decreases blood flow to the gastrointestinal (GI) tract, dilates the bronchioles, controls ejaculation.
  - Preganglionic neurons: Intermediolateral cell column from T1–L3 spinal cord segments.
  - Postganglionic neurons: sympathetic chain.
- **Parasympathetic ("rest response"):** Contracts the pupils, decreases heart rate, increases blood flow to the GI tract, stimulates salivary gland secretion, stimulates erection.
  - Preganglionic neurons: Medullary nuclei (dorsal motor nucleus of the vagus, superior salivatory nucleus, inferior salivatory nucleus), midbrain nucleus (Edinger-Westphal nucleus), sacral parasympathetic nucleus from S2–S4 spinal cord segments.
  - Postganglionic neurons: Ganglia close the end organ (ciliary ganglion, pterygopalatine ganglion, submandibular ganglion, otic ganglion, terminal [intramural] ganglia).

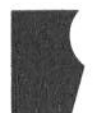

KEY FACT

Patients with parasympathetic dysfunction have poor to no pupillary response to light, but patients with Horner syndrome have a normal pupillary reaction to light.

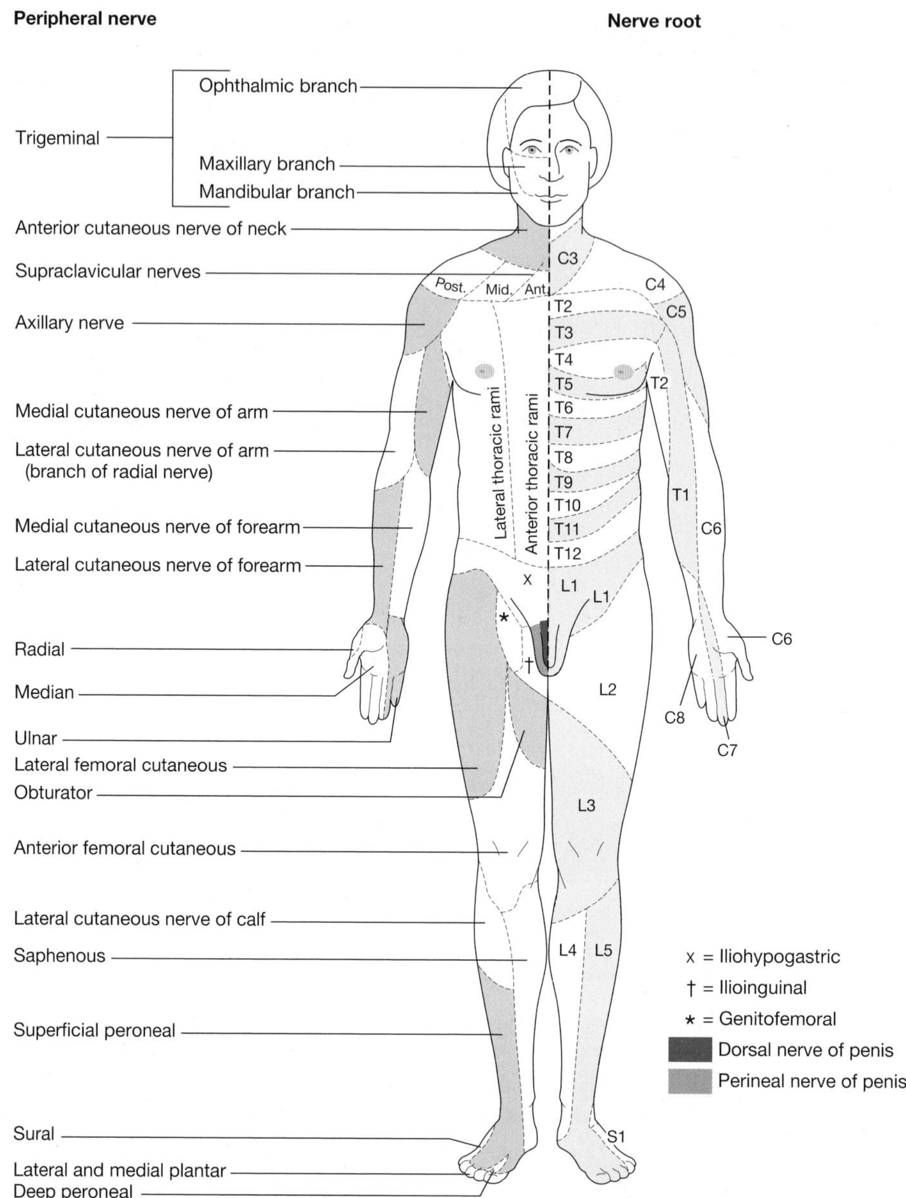

FIGURE 2.45. Dermatomes and cutaneous innervation patterns, anterior view. (Reproduced, with permission, from Aminoff MJ, Simon RP. *Clinical Neurology*, 6th ed. McGraw-Hill, 2005: Figure 6-4A.)

AUTONOMIC DYSREFLEXIA

Disruption of the autonomic reflex arc due to a spinal cord lesion at or above T6. Clinical findings include hypertension; bradycardia; sweating above level of spinal injury; piloerection and cold, clammy skin below level of spinal injury; facial flushing; skin flushing above level of spinal injury; rhinorrhea; nausea; and headache. Attacks are usually precipitated by noxious stimuli below the level of the spinal injury such as urinary tract infections, bladder distention, constipation, or sacral decubitus ulcers. Treatment is blood pressure control and prevention/treatment of noxious stimuli.

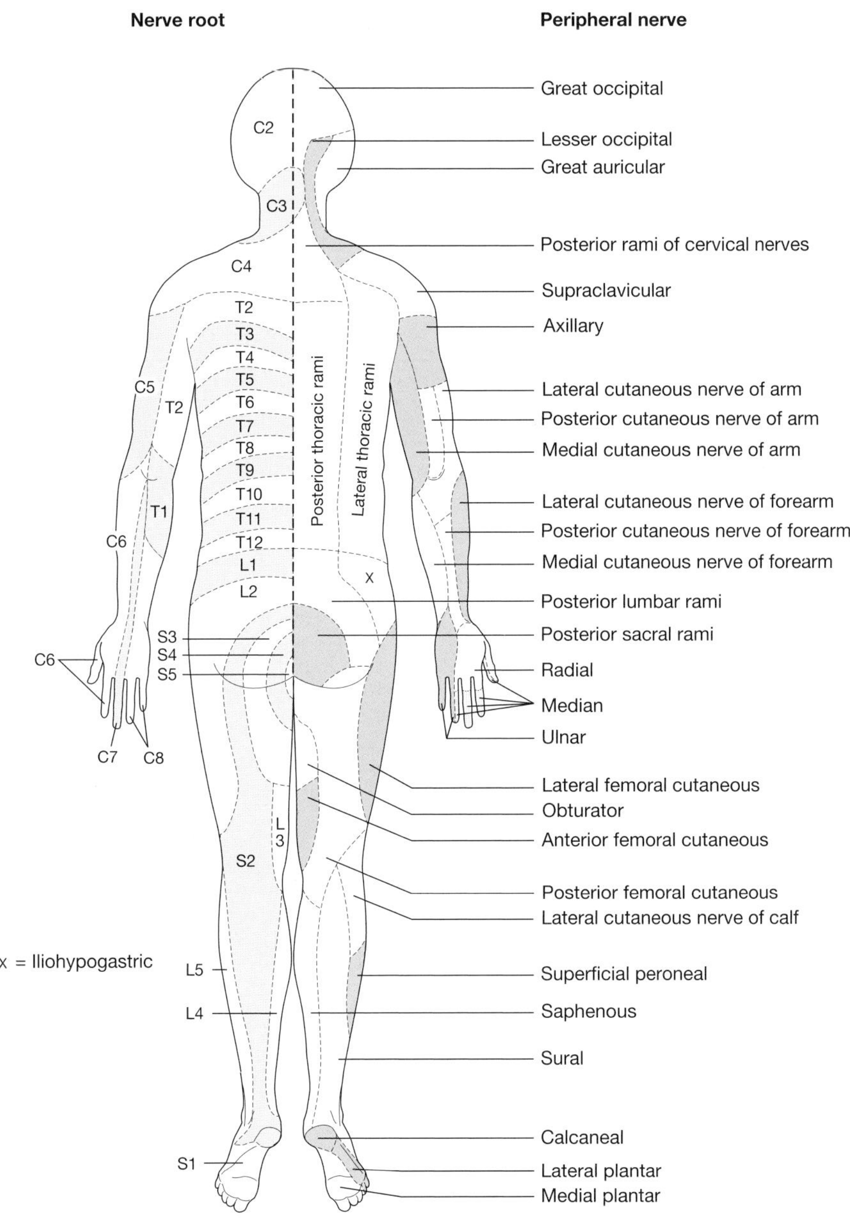

FIGURE 2.46. Dermatomes and cutaneous innervation patterns, posterior view. (Reproduced, with permission, from Aminoff MJ, Simon RP. *Clinical Neurology*, 6th ed. McGraw-Hill, 2005: Figure 6-4B.)

MUSCLE ANATOMY

- Muscle → fascicle → fiber → myofibers (contractile unit) (Figure 2.48).
- **Sarcomere:** Region between the Z-lines.
- Thick filaments: Enriched with myosin, which is connected from the M-line to the Z-disc by titin, and is the A band.
- Thin filaments: Actin filaments, designated by the lighter I-bands.
- H-band and I-band shorten when a contraction occurs, but the length of the thick and thin filaments does not change (Figure 2.49).

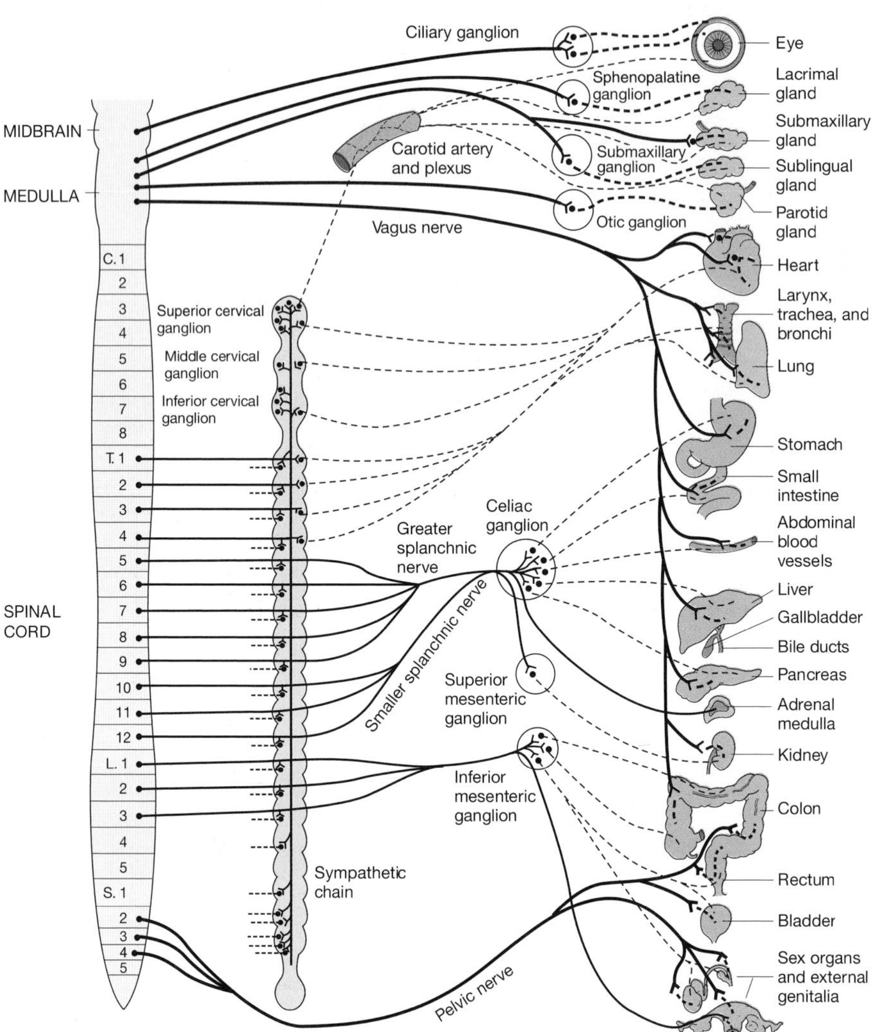

FIGURE 2.47. Autonomic nervous system. (Reproduced, with permission, from Ganong WF. *Review of Medical Physiology*, 22nd ed. New York: McGraw-Hill, 2003: 225.)

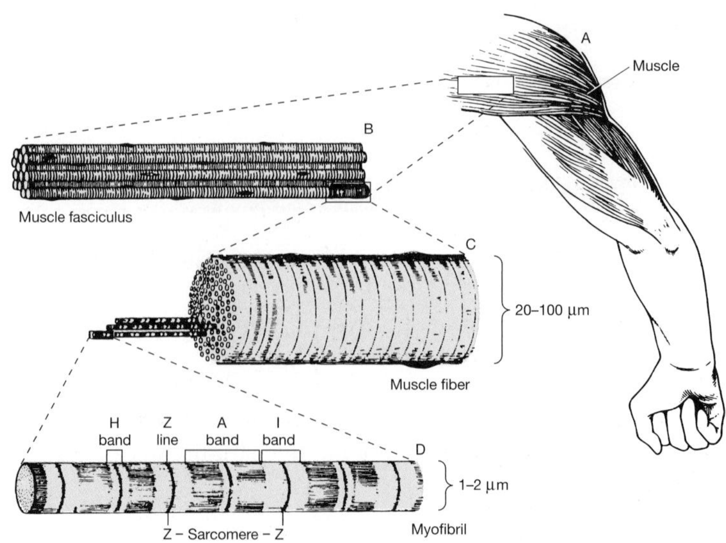

FIGURE 2.48. Organization of skeletal muscle. (A) Extended; **(B)** contracted. (Reproduced, with permission, from Murray RK, Granner DK, Rodwell VW. *Harper's Illustrated Biochemistry*, 27th ed. New York: McGraw-Hill, 2006: 566.)

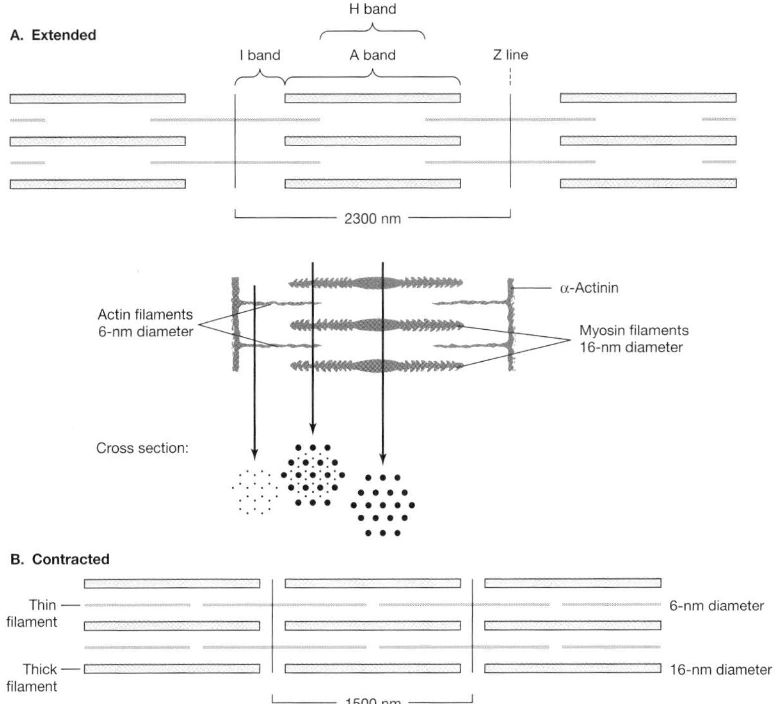

FIGURE 2.49. Arrangement of filaments in striated muscle. (Reproduced, with permission, from Murray RK, Granner DK, Rodwell VW. *Harper's Illustrated Biochemistry*, 27th ed. New York: McGraw-Hill, 2006: 567.)

NOTES

CHAPTER 3

Neuropharmacology

Irfan Qureshi, MD

Principles of Neuropharmacology

ELECTROCHEMICAL GRADIENT

Resting membrane potential is set primarily by permeability of membrane to potassium ions and equals –70 mV. Changes in membrane potential are caused by changes in the relative permeability of these ions via opening or closing of gated ion channels. See Table 3.1.

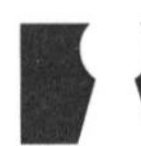

KEY FACT

Channelopathies present with episodic symptoms and often have triggers such as exercise (Table 3.3).

ION CHANNELS

Ion channels (Table 3.2) are transmembrane proteins that form pores in the neuronal membrane. When open, they allow the flow of specific ions down the electrochemical gradient. Channels can be either voltage or ligand gated.

- **Voltage gated:** Open or close as a result of change in membrane voltage. Mostly found at axon hillock, along axon, and at axon terminal.
- **Ligand gated:** Open or close as a result of neurotransmitter binding. Mostly found at dendrites and cell body.

ACTION POTENTIALS

An action potential (AP) is an all-or-none, large-amplitude, brief-duration, and self-propagating membrane depolarization. It results when local stimuli cause an initial depolarization in the neuronal membrane to a threshold value, which is ~15 mV more positive than the resting membrane potential.

- Depolarization is mediated by sodium channel activation with influx of sodium ions into cell.
- Repolarization is mediated by sodium channel inactivation and potassium channel activation resulting in potassium ion efflux out of cell (see Figure 3.1).
- Refractory period is characterized by continued inactivation of sodium channels leading to no APs being generated (absolute refractory) or increased threshold for stimuli to generate AP (relative refractory).

SYNAPTIC TRANSMISSION

- When a propagating AP reaches the presynaptic region:
  - Voltage-dependent calcium channels are activated and calcium ions enter the cell.
  - Vesicle-bound neurotransmitter is released into synapse via exocytosis.

TABLE 3.1. Key Electrolytes Involved in Generating the Membrane Potential

Ion	Intracellular Concentration (mM)	Extracellular Concentration (mM)
Na^+	10	100
K^+	100	5
Cl^-	10	105
Ca^{2+}	2×10^{-4}	4

TABLE 3.2. Toxins Used to Characterize Ion Channels

Channel Types	Mode of Toxin Action	Source
Voltage-gated		
Sodium channels		
Tetrodotoxin (TTX)	Blocks channel from outside	Puffer fish
Batrachotoxin (BTX)	Slows inactivation, shifts activation	Colombian frog
Potassium channels		
Apamin	Blocks "small Ca-activated" K channel	Honeybee
Charybdotoxin	Blocks "big Ca-activated" K channel	Scorpion
Calcium channels		
Omega conotoxin (ω–CTX-GVIA)	Blocks N-type channel	Pacific cone snail
Agatoxin (ω–AGA-IVA)	Blocks P-type channel	Funnel web spider
Ligand-gated		
Nicotinic ACh receptor		
α-Bungarotoxin	Irreversible antagonist	Marine snake
$GABA_A$ receptor		
Picrotoxin	Blocks channel	South Pacific plant
Glycine receptor		
Strychnine	Competitive antagonist	Indian plant
AMPA receptor		
Philanthotoxin	Blocks channel	Wasp

Reproduced, with permission, from Katzung B. *Basic and Clinical Pharmacology,* 11th ed. New York: McGraw-Hill, 2009: Table 21-1.

TABLE 3.3. Examples of Neurological Channelopathies

Category	Disorder	Channel Type	Gene
Ataxias	Episodic ataxia-1	K	*KCNAI*
	Episodic ataxia-2	Ca	*CACNLIAd*
	Spinocerebellar ataxia-6	Ca	*CACNLIAd*
Migraine	Familial hemiplegic migraine	Ca	*CACNLIAd*
Epilepsy	Benign neonaal familial convulsions	K	*KCNQ2, KCNQ3*
	Generalized epilepsy with febrile convulsions plus	Na	*SCNIβ*
Periodic paralysis	Hyperkalemic periodic paralysis	Na	*SCN4A*
	Hypokalemic periodic paralysis	Ca	*CACNLIA3*
Myotonia	Myotonia congenita	C1	*CLCN1*
	Paramyotonia congenita	Na	*SCN4A*
Deafness	Jorvell and Lange-Nielsen syndrome (deafness, prolonged QT interval, and arrythmia)	K	*KCNQ1, KCNE1*
	Autosomal dominant progressive deafness	K	*KCNQ4*

Reproduced, with permission, from Fauci AS, Braunwald E, Kasper DL, et al. (Eds.). *Harrison's Principles of Internal Medicine,* 17th ed. New York: McGraw-Hill, 2008: 2339.

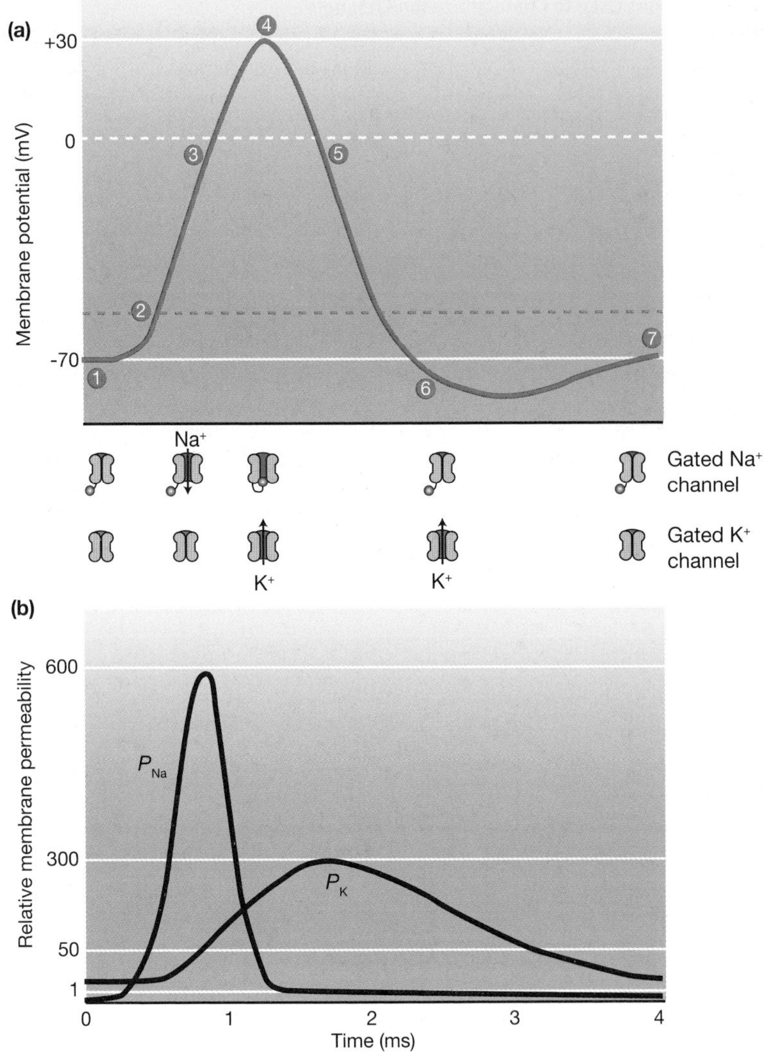

FIGURE 3.1. Action potentials and membrane permeability. The changes in (a) membrane potential (mV) and (b) relative membrane permeabilty (P) to Na^+ and K^+ during an action potential. (Reproduced, with permission, from Widmaier, EP, Raff H, Strang KT. Vander's Human Physiology. McGraw-Hill Education, 2008.)

  - Neurotransmitters bind to postsynaptic receptors.
  - Local synaptic responses ensue that may be excitatory or inhibitory depending on the characteristics of the receptor.
- **Excitatory postsynaptic potentials (EPSPs):** Slightly depolarize postsynaptic membrane and increase likelihood of AP propagation.
- **Inhibitory postsynaptic potentials (IPSPs):** Slightly hyperpolarize postsynaptic membrane and decrease likelihood of AP propagation.

RECEPTORS

Receptors mediate a number of important cellular effects through a variety of mechanisms (Figure 3.2). Major classes of neurotransmitter receptors include:

- **Ionotropic:** Ligand-gated ion channels.
- **Metabotropic:** G protein–coupled receptors that exert actions through second messenger systems, including cyclic adenosine monophosphate (cAMP) and phosphoinositol cascades.

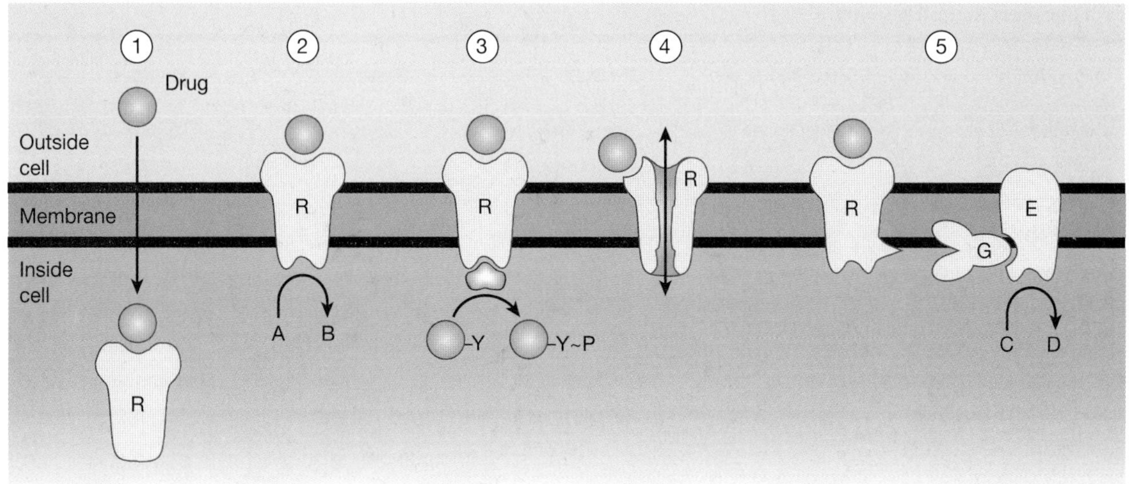

FIGURE 3-2. Receptor signaling mechanisms. Known transmembrane signaling mechanisms: **1:** A lipid-soluble chemical signal crosses the plasma membrane and acts on an intracellular receptor (which may be an enzyme or a regulator of gene transcription); **2:** the signal binds to the extracellular domain of a transmembrane protein, thereby activating an enzymatic activity of its cytoplasmic domain; **3:** the signal binds to the extracellular domain of a transmembrane receptor bound to a separate protein tyrosine kinase, which it activates; **4:** the signal binds to and directly regulates the opening of an ion channel; **5:** the signal binds to a cell-surface receptor linked to an effector enzyme by a G protein. (A, C, substrates; B, D, products; R, receptor; G, G protein; E, effector [enzyme or ion channel]; Y, tyrosine; P, phosphate.) (Reproduced, with permission, from Katzung B. *Basic and Clinical Pharmacology*, 11th ed. New York: McGraw-Hill, 2009: Figure 2-5.)

SYNAPTIC PLASTICITY

- **Long-term potentiation:** Long-term change in amplitude of synaptic response brought about by stimulation. Thought to underlie learning and memory.
- **Long-term depression:** The converse of long-term potentiation. Also thought to underlie learning and memory.

Neurotransmitters

Properties that define neurotransmitters:

- Present in neuron terminals.
- Release with stimulation of neuron.
- When exogenously applied to postsynaptic neurons, evoke same effects as physiologic stimulation of presynaptic neurons.
- Deactivation in synapse by local process such as reuptake or enzymatic breakdown.
- See Table 3.4 for examples of classes of neurotransmitters.

KEY FACT

Dale's principle states that a given neuron secretes the same set of transmitters from all its terminals.

DOPAMINE

Biosynthesis

- Tyrosine $\xrightarrow{\text{tyrosine hydroxylase}}$ DOPA $\xrightarrow{\text{DOPA decarboxylase}}$ Dopamine.
- Tyrosine hydroxylase is rate-limiting enzyme.

Metabolism

Primarily removed from synapse by reuptake into the presynaptic neuron via transporter. Metabolized by catechol-O-methyltransferase (COMT) and monoamine oxidase (MAO). Principal metabolite is homovanillic acid (HVA).

TABLE 3.4. Examples of Classes of Neurotransmitters

Monoamines	Amino Acids	Small Molecule	Purines	Gases	Peptides
Dopamine	*Excitatory*	Acetylcholine	Adenosine triphosphate	Nitric oxide	Opioids
Norepinephrine	Glutamate		Adenosine	Carbon monoxide	Vasopressin
Serotonin	Aspartate				Somatostatin
Histamine	*Inhibitory*				Oxytocin
	γ-Aminobutyric acid				Tachykinins
	Glycine				Cholecystokinin
	Taurine				Neuropeptide Y
	β-Alanine				Neurotensin

Functional Anatomy

Major dopaminergic tracts include:

- **Nigrostriatal tract:** Projects from the substantia nigra to the striatum, comprising the extrapyramidal motor system.
- **Mesolimbic tract:** Projects from the ventral tegmental area to the limbic system including the nucleus accumbens. It plays an important role in cognition and emotion and is implicated in psychosis and substance abuse.
- **Mesocortical tract:** Projects from the ventral tegmental area to the cortex, particularly frontal cortex. It also plays an important role in cognition and emotion and is implicated in psychosis and substance abuse.
- **Tubero-infundibular tract:** Projects from the arcuate nucleus of the hypothalamus to the pituitary. Dopamine secreted in this tract suppresses prolactin release from the anterior pituitary.

Receptors and Pharmacology

Receptors include subtypes D_1–D_5 that are functionally classified into 2 groups. Distribution of D_1 receptors is more widespread. See Table 3.5.

- **Dopaminergic agents** (Table 3.6): Used to treat movement disorders and depression (ie, MAO inhibitors [MAOIs], tricyclics, and buproprion) but also include illicit drugs such as cocaine and amphetamine. Can produce euphoria, nausea, visual hallucinations, psychosis, and hyperkinetic movement disorders.
- **Dopamine antagonists:** Used to treat psychosis. Can produce weight gain, autonomic symptoms (orthostasis, impotence, galactorrhea, etc), parkinsonism, precipitate neuroleptic malignant syndrome, and tardive dyskinesias.

KEY FACT

1-Methyl-4-phenyl-1,2,3,6-tetrahydropyridine (MPTP) is a meperidine analog that is toxic to dopaminergic cells and was responsible for outbreak of parkinsonism in heroin abusers.

NOREPINEPHRINE

Biosynthesis

- Tyrosine $\xrightarrow{\text{tyrosine hydroxylase}}$ DOPA $\xrightarrow{\text{DOPA decarboxylase}}$ Dopamine $\xrightarrow{\text{dopamine β-hydroxylase}}$ Norepinephrine.
- Norepinephrine $\xrightarrow{\text{phenylethanolamine N-methyl-transferase}}$ Epinephrine
- Like dopamine synthesis, tyrosine hydroxylase is the rate-limiting enzyme. Norepiphrine is converted to epinephrine in the adrenal medulla.

Metabolism

Primarily removed by presynaptic reuptake via transporter. Also metabolized by COMT and MAO, and the principal metabolites are vanillylmandelic acid (VMA) and methoxy-hydroxy-phenylglycol (MHPG).

TABLE 3.5. Dopaminergic Receptor Family

Receptor	Agonists[a]	Antagonists[a]	G Protein Coupling	Areas of Localization
D_1	SKF82958*; SKF81297*	SCH23390*; SKF83566; haloperidol	G_s[b]	Neosriatum; cerebral cortex; olfactory tubercle; nucleus accumbens
D_2	Bromocriptine*	Raclopride; sulpiride; haloperidol	$G_{i/o}$[b]	Neostriatum; olfactory tubercle; nucleus accumbens[c]
D_3	Quinpirole*; 7-OH-DPAT	Raclopride	$G_{i/o}$	Nucleus accumbens; islands of Calleja
D_4		Clozapine	$G_{i/o}$	Midbrain; amygdala
D_5	SKF38393	SCH23390	G_s	Hippocampus; hypothalamus

[a] Asterisks indicate selective agonists and antagonists.

[b] G_s: GTP binding stimulator of adenylate cyclase; $G_{i/o}$: GTP binding inhibitor of adenylate cyclase.

[c] D_2 long and D_2 short forms, which differ in the length of the third cytoplasmic loop, have been cloned. Although they are expressed in different brain regions, the functional significance of these splice variants is not known.

Reproduced, with permission, from Nestler E, Hyman S, Malenka R. *Molecular Neuropharmacology: A Foundation for Clinical Neuroscience,* 2nd ed. New York: McGraw-Hill: 2008: Table 8-5.

TABLE 3.6. Select Dopaminergic Agents

Agonists	Bromocriptine Pergolide Pramipexole Ropinirole Apomorphine
Antagonists	*Typical* Metoclopramide Chlorpromazine Haloperidol
	Atypical Risperidone Olanzapine Clozapine Quetiapine
MAO inhibitors	Selegiline Rasagaline
COMT inhibitors	Talcapone Entacapone
Vesicular monoamine transport inhibitors	Reserpine Tetrabenazine
Reuptake inhibitor	Bupropion
Miscellaneous	Amantadine

FUNCTIONAL ANATOMY

- Synthesized principally by the locus ceruleus, which projects diffusely to the cerebral cortex, limbic system, reticular activating system, and spinal cord.
- Neurotransmitter for postganglionic sympathetic neurons, except sweat glands.

RECEPTORS AND PHARMACOLOGY

- **Adrenergic agents:** Used to treat depression (ie, MAOIs, tricyclics, and venlafaxine) but also include illicit drugs such as cocaine and amphetamine. Produce sympathomimetic effects.
- **Adrenergic antagonists:** Used to treat tremor and anxiety (ie, β-blockers for essential tremor).
- See Tables 3.7 through 3.9.

TABLE 3.7. Adrenergic Receptor Family

RECEPTOR	AGONISTS[a]	ANTAGONISTS[a]	G PROTEIN COUPLING	AREAS OF LOCALIZATION IN BRAIN
α_{1A}	A61603* Phenylephrine Methoxamine	Nigulpidine* Prazosin Indoramin	$G_{q/11}$[b]	Cortex Hippocampus
α_{1B}	Phenylephrine Methoxamine	Spiperone* Prazosin Indoramin	$G_{q/11}$	Cortex Brain stem
α_{1D}	Phenylephrine Methoxamine	Prazosin Indoramin	$G_{q/11}$	
α_{2A}	Oxymetazoline*; clonidine	Yohimbine; rauwolscine; prazosin	$G_{i/o}$[b]	Cortex; brain stem; midbrain; spinal cord
α_{2B}	Clonidine	Yohimbine; rauwolscine; prazosin	$G_{i/o}$	Diencephalon
α_{2C}	Clonidine	Yohimbine; rauwolscine; prazosin	$G_{i/o}$	Basal ganglia; cortex; cerebellum; hippocampus
β_1	Isoproterenol; terbutaline*	Alprenolol*; betaxolol*; propranold	G_s[b]	Olfactory nucleus; cortex; cerebellar nuclei; brain stem nuclei; spinal cord
β_2	Procaterol*; zinterol*	Propranolol	G_s	Olfactory bulb; piriform cortex; hippocampus; cerebellar cortex
β_3		Pindolol*; bupranolol*; propranolol	G_s/ $G_{i/o}$	

[a] Asterisks indicate selective agonists and antagonists.

[b] G_s: GTP binding stimulator of adenylate cyclase; $G_{i/o}$: GTP binding inhibitor of adenylate cyclase; $G_{q/11}$: GTP binding stimulator of phospholipase C.

Reproduced, with permission, from Nestler E, Hyman S, Malenka R. *Molecular Neuropharmacology: A Foundation for Clinical Neuroscience,* 2nd ed. New York: McGraw-Hill: 2008: Table 8-5.

TABLE 3.8. Relative Selectivity of Adrenoceptor Agonists

	Relative Receptor Affinities
Alpha agonists	
Phenylephrine, methoxamine	$\alpha_1 > \alpha_2 >>>>> \beta$
Clonidine, methylnorepinephrine	$\alpha_1 > \alpha_2 >>>>> \beta$
Mixed alpha and beta agonists	
Norepinephrine	$\alpha_1 = \alpha_2; \beta_1 >> \beta_2$
Epinephrine	$\alpha_1 = \alpha_2; \beta_1 = \beta_2$
Beta agonists	
Dobutamine	$\beta_1 > \beta_2 >>>> \alpha$
Isoproterenol	$\beta_1 = \beta_2 >>>> \alpha$
Albuterol, terbutaline, metaproterenol, ritodrine	$\beta_2 >> \beta_1 >>>> \alpha$
Dopamine agonists	
Dopamine	$D_1 = D_2 >> \beta >> \alpha$
Fenoldopam	$D_1 >> D_2$

Reproduced, with permission, from Katzung B. *Basic and Clinical Pharmacology,* 11th ed. New York: McGraw-Hill, 2009: Table 9-2.

SEROTONIN

Biosynthesis

- Tryptophan $\xrightarrow{\text{tryptophan hydroxylase}}$ 5-hydroxytryptophan $\xrightarrow{\text{amino acid decarboxylase}}$ 5-hydroxytryptamine (5-HT, serotonin).
- Tryptophan hydroxylase is a rate-limiting enzyme, but tryptophan is a more important rate-limiting reagent.

Metabolism

Mostly synaptic reuptake and also MAO metabolism halt serotonin activity. Major metabolite is 5-hydroxyindoleacetic acid (5-HIAA). Serotonin is also the substrate for melatonin synthesis.

TABLE 3.9. Relative Selectivity of Antagonists for Adrenoceptors

	Receptor Affinity
Alpha antagonists	
Prazosin, terazosin, doxazosin	$\alpha_1 >>> \alpha_2$
Phenoxybenzamine	$\alpha_1 > \alpha_2$
Phentolamine	$\alpha_1 = \alpha_2$
Yohimbine, tolazoline	$\alpha_2 >> \alpha_1$
Mixed antagonists	
Labetalol, carvedilol	$\beta_1 = \beta_2 \geq \alpha_1 > \alpha_2$
Beta antagonists	
Metoprololol, acebutolol, alprenolol, atenolol, betaxolol, celiprolol, esmolol, nebivolol	$\beta_1 >>> \beta_2$
Propranolol, carteolol, penbtolol, pindolol, timolol	$\beta_1 = \beta_2$
Butoxamine	$\beta_2 >>> \beta_1$

Reproduced, with permission, from Katzung B. *Basic and Clinical Pharmacology,* 11th ed. New York: McGraw-Hill, 2009: Table 10-1.

Functional Anatomy

Major serotonergic tracts include:

- Synthesized in the dorsal raphe nuclei, in the dorsal midbrain and pons, which project diffusely to the cerebral cortex, limbic system, striatum, and cerebellum, as well as intracranial blood vessels, including those associated with the trigeminal nerve.
- The caudal raphe nuclei, in the pons and medulla, also synthesize serotonin and project to the spinal cord mediating analgesia.

> **KEY FACT**
>
> Antiemetics, such as ondansetron and metoclopramide, are $5HT_3$ receptor antagonists.

Receptors and Pharmacology

Serotonergic agents: Used for depression and migraine. Can lead to excess serotonergic activity (serotonin syndrome) that is a life-threatening syndrome consisting of mental status change, autonomic hyperactivity and movement disorder difficult to differentiate from neuroleptic malignant syndrome. See Table 3.10.

ACETYLCHOLINE

Biosynthesis

- Acetyl CoA + Choline $\xrightarrow{\text{choline acetyltransferase}}$ ACh.
- The rate-limiting factor is choline.

Metabolism

Synaptic cholinesterases metabolize ACh into acetyl CoA and choline.

Functional Anatomy

- Synthesized in basal forebrain nuclei, such as the nucleus basalis of Meynert, which project to the olfactory bulb cortex, hippocampus, amygdala, and cortical association areas.
- Neurotransmitter of the neuromuscular junction.
- Neurotransmitter of the autonomic nervous system, except most postganglionic sympathetic neurons (which use norepinephrine).

Receptors and Pharmacology (Table 3.11)

- **Anticholinergics:** Used to treat movement disorders but can produce cognitive impairment. Side effects can include accommodation paresis, drowsiness, dry mouth, difficulty urinating, constipation, and, in severe cases, tachycardia, hypertension, hyperthermia, and delirium.
- **Acetylcholinesterase inhibitors:** Used to treat myasthenia gravis and Alzheimer disease. Include reversible inhibitors, such as pyridostigmine and physostigmine, as well as irreversible inhibitors, such as organophosphates and nerve gas. Can cause cholinergic crisis characterized by sweating, salivation, bronchial secretions, and miosis, as well as flaccid paralysis and respiratory failure.

> **KEY FACT**
>
> Postganglionic sympathetic neurons innervating sweat glands use acetylcholine.

HISTAMINE

Biosynthesis

Histidine $\xrightarrow{\text{histidine decarboxylase}}$ histamine.

Metabolism

Degraded by histamine methyltransferase.

TABLE 3.10. Serotonergic Receptor Family

Receptor[a]	Agonists	Antagonists	G Protein	Localization
5 HT_{1A}	8-OH-DPAT; buspirone, gepirone	WAY 100135	$G_{i/o}$[b]	Hippocampus; septum; amgdala; dorsal raphe; cortex
5 HT_{1B}	Sumatriptan and related triptans		$G_{i/o}$	Substantia nigra; basal ganglia
5 HT_{1D}	Sumatriptan and related triptans	GR 127935	$G_{i/o}$	Substantia nigra; striatum nucleus; accumbens; hippocampus
5 HT_{1E}			$G_{i/o}$	
5 HT_{1F}			$G_{i/o}$	Dorsal raphe; hippocampus; cortex
5 HT_{2A}	DMT and related psychedelics[c]	Ketanserin; cinanserin; MDL900239	$G_{q/11}$[b]	Cortex; olfactory tubercle; claustrum
5 HT_{2B}	DMT		$G_{q/11}$	Not located in brain
5 HT_{2C}	DMT; MCPP	Mesulergine; fluoxetine	$G_{q/11}$	Basal ganglia; choroid plexus; substantia nigra
5 HT_3		Ondanseron; granistetron	Ligand-gated channel	Spinal cord; cortex; hippocampus; brain stem nuclei
5 HT_4	Metoclopramide	GR 113808	G_s[b]	Hippocampus; nucleus accumbens; striatum substantia nigra
5 HT_{5A}		Methiothepin	G_s	Cortex; hippocampus; cerebellum
5 HT_{5B}		Methiothepin	Unknown	Habenula; hippocampal CA1
5 HT_6		Methiothepin; clozapine; amitriptyline	G_s	Striatum; olfactory tubercle; cortex; hippocampus
5 HT_7		Methiothepin; clozapine; amitriptyline	G_s	Hypothalamus; thalamus; cortex; suprachiasmatic nucleus

[a] The nomenclature of 5-HT receptors is extremely complicated because so many subtypes have been cloned. Some require further characterization before definitive classifications may be made. Represented in the table is the nomenclature recently approved by the International Union of Pharmacology Classification of Receptors Subcommittee on 5-HT Receptors.

[b] G_s: GTP binding stimulator of adenylate cyclase; $G_{i/o}$: GTP binding inhibitor of adenylate cyclase; $G_{q/11}$: GTP binding stimulator of phospholipase C.

[c] Other examples include lysergic acid (LSD), psilocybin, and mescaline.

DMT, N,N-dimethylamine; MCPP, metachlorophenylpiperazine.

Reproduced, with permission, from Nestler E, Hyman S, Malenka R. *Molecular Neuropharmacology: A Foundation for Clinical Neuroscience*, 2nd ed. New York: McGraw-Hill: 2008: Table 9-3.

Functional Anatomy

Produced in the tuberomammillary nucleus of the hypothalamus, which projects throughout the CNS, particularly into cortex and limbic system. Regulates arousal, body temperature, and vascular dynamics.

Receptors and Pharmacology

See Table 3.12.

TABLE 3.11. Major Autonomic Receptor Types, Cholinoceptors

Agonists	Antagonists
α-Latrotoxin	*Nicotinic*
	Curare derivatives
Nicotinic	Succinylcholine
Nicotine	Botulinum toxin
	α-Bungarotoxin
Muscarinic	
Muscarine	*Muscarinic*
Bethanecol	Atropine
Pilocarpine	Scopolamine
	Tricyclic antidepressants

Reproduced, with permission, from Katzung B. *Basic and Clinical Pharmacology*, 11th ed. New York: McGraw-Hill, 2009: Figure 6-2.

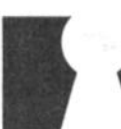

KEY FACT

Effects of tetanus and strychnine are mediated by blocking glycine.

γ-AMINOBUTYRIC ACID (GABA)

Major inhibitory neurotransmitter in the CNS, along with glycine (which is also inhibitory and found in the brain stem and spinal cord).

Biosynthesis

- Glutamate $\xrightarrow{\text{glutamate decarboxylase}}$ GABA.
- Requires vitamin B_6 (pyridoxine) cofactor.

Metabolism

GABA activity in the synapse is halted by synaptic reuptake and enzymatic deactivation.

Functional Anatomy

Widely distributed within the CNS. Mediates the inhibitory actions of local interneurons in the brain.

TABLE 3-12. Histamine Receptor Family

Receptor	Agonists	Antagonists	G Protein	Localization
H_1		Mepyramine[a]; triprolidine; diphenhydramine; dimenhydrinate	$G_{q/11}$[b]	Cortex; hippocampus; nucleus accumbens; thalamus
H_2	Dimaprit[a]	Ranitidine[a]; cimetidine[a]	G_s[b]	Basal ganglia; hippocampus; amygdala; cortex
H_3	R-α-methylhistamine[a]; imetit[a]	Thioperamide[a]	$G_{i/o}$[b]	Basal ganglia; hippocampus; cortex

[a] Selective agonists or antagonists.

[b] G_s: GTP binding stimulator of adenylate cyclase; $G_{i/o}$: GTP binding inhibitor of adenylate cyclase; $G_{q/11}$: GTP binding stimulator of phospholipase C.

Reproduced, with permission, from Nestler E, Hyman S, Malenka R. *Molecular Neuropharmacology: A Foundation for Clinical Neuroscience,* 2nd ed. New York: McGraw-Hill: 2008: Table 9-8.

RECEPTORS AND PHARMACOLOGY (TABLE 3.13)

- $GABA_A$ receptor has binding sites for:
  - Benzodiazepines: Increase Cl^- channel opening frequency.
  - Barbiturates: Increase Cl^- channel opening duration.

TABLE 3.13. GABA Receptors

IONOTROPIC $GABA_A$ RECEPTOR	METABOTROPIC $GABA_B$ RECEPTOR
Gene Families	
α_1–a_6	$GABA_BR_{1a}$
β_1–β_4	$GABA_BR_{1b}$
γ_1–γ_2	
δ	$GABA_BR_2$
p1–p3	
ε	
π	
Agents that Bind to the GABA Site	
Agonists	**Antagonists**
GABA	L-Baclofen
Isoguvacine	CGP27492
Muscimol	
THIP	
Piperidine 4-sulphonic acid	
Antagonists	**Antagonists**
Bicuculline	2-OH-s-saclofen
	CGP35348
	CGP55845
	CGP64213
Agents that Bind to the Benzodiazepine Site	
Agonists	**Antagonists**
Flunitrazepam	Flumazenil
Zolpidem	AK93426
Abecarnil	
Inverse agonists	
DMCM	
Ro194603	
Antagonists that Bind to Other Sites	
Picrotoxin	
Zn^{2+}	

Reproduced, with permission, from Nestler E, Hyman S, Malenka R. *Molecular Neuropharmacology: A Foundation for Clinical Neuroscience,* 2nd ed. New York: McGraw-Hill: 2008: Table 7-3.

- Picrotoxin site.
- Steroid site.
- GABA.
- $GABA_B$ receptor:
  - Agonist: Baclofen
  - Antagonist: Phaclofen
- **GABA-ergic agents:** Used as muscle relaxants, sedatives, and antiepileptics. For example, tiagabine is a GABA reuptake inhibitor, vigabatrin inhibits GABA-transaminase activity, and topiramate enhances GABA receptor activity.
- **γ-hydroxybutyrate (GHB):** GABA analog. Also known as sodium oxybate and used to treat narcolepsy with cataplexy. Illicit use as "date rape drug."
- **GABA receptor antagonists:** Flumazenil is used to treat benzodiazepine overdose.

GLUTAMATE

Major excitatory neurotransmitter in the brain, while asparate plays this role in the spinal cord.

Biosynthesis

Glutamine $\xrightarrow{\text{glutaminase}}$ Glutamate.

Metabolism

Reuptake into presynaptic neurons terminates glutamate activity.

Functional Anatomy

Distributed widely throughout the CNS.

Receptors and Pharmacology (Table 3.14)

- *N*-methyl-*D*-aspartate (NMDA) receptor is a ligand- and voltage-gated calcium channel with binding sites for:
  - Glutamate: Increase.
  - Glycine: Increase.
  - Polyamine (phencyclidine and ketamine): Voltage-dependent increase.
  - Magnesium: Voltage-dependent decrease.
  - Zinc: Voltage-independent decrease.
- **Glutamate analogs:** Domoic acid causes seizures.
- **Glutamate excitotoxicity:** Excessive NMDA activity can lead to neuronal death and has been implicated in the pathophysiology of many neuropsychiatric conditions including stroke and neurodegenerative disease.
- **Glutamate receptor antagonists:** Used to treat epilepsy (ie, lamotrigine and gabapentin). Also:
  - **Memantine:** Noncompetitive NMDA receptor antagonist that prevents excitotoxicity by inhibiting prolonged influx of calcium. Used for treatment of moderate to severe Alzheimer disease.
  - **Riluzole:** NMDA receptor antagonist that prolongs survival in amyotrophic lateral sclerosis (ALS).

KEY FACT

Autoantibodies to glutamate receptor GluR3 are associated with Rasmussen encephalitis.

Rasmussen encephalitis = GluR3 ab

NITRIC OXIDE (NO)

Neurological functions include regulating cerebral blood flow and facilitating penile erections.

TABLE 3.14. Glutamate Receptors

Functional Gene	Families Classes	Agonists	Antagonists
	Ionotropic		
AMPA	G1uR1	Glutamate	CNQX
	G1uR2	AMPA	NBQX
	G1uR3	Kainate	
GYK153655	G1uR4	(S)-5-fluorowillardine	
Kainate	G1uR5	Glutamate	CNQX
	G1uR6	Kainate	
LY294486	G1uR7	ATPA	
	KA1		
	KA2		
NMDA	NR1	Glutamate	D-AP5, D-APV
	NR2A	Aspartate	2R-CPPene
	NR2B	NMDA	MK-801
	NR2C	Ketamine	
	NR2D	Phencyclidine	
	Metabotropic		
Group I	mG1uR1 1S,	3R-ACPD	AIDA
	mG1uR5 DHPG		CBPG
Group II	mG1uR2 1S,	3R-ACPD	EGLU
	mG1uR3 DCG-IV		PCCG-4
			APDC
Group III	mGluR4 l-AP4	3R-ACPD	MAP4
	mGluR6 1S,		MPPG
	mGluR7		
	mGluR8		

Reproduced, with permission, from Nestler E, Hyman S, Malenka R. *Molecular Neuropharmacology: A Foundation for Clinical Neuroscience*, 2nd ed. New York: McGraw-Hill: 2008: Table 5-1.

Biosynthesis

Arginine + Oxygen $\xrightarrow{\text{nitric oxide synthase}}$ Nitric oxide + Citrulline

Receptors and Pharmacology

NO diffuses directly into cells and does not require specific receptors. NO activity leads to production of cyclic guanosine monophosphate (cGMP).

KEY FACT

Capsaicin mediates analgesia by depleting substance P.

OTHER NEUROPEPTIDES

- Most neuropeptides are derived from precursor molecules and are released along with other neurotransmitters to modulate their function (Table 3.15).
- Hypocretins (orexins): Synthesized in the hypothalamus. Play a role in the sleep-wake cycle and are deficient in narcolepsy.

BRIEF SUMMARY OF NEUROTRANSMITTER PHARMACOLOGY

See Table 3.16.

Key Neurotransmitter-Disease Correlations

EPILEPSY

Pyridoxine deficiency: Characterized by decreased GABA synthesis and seizures that resolve with intravenous pyridoxine administration.

HEADACHE

Migraine: Treated with ergot derivatives and triptans that are agonists of 5-HT_{1D} receptors.

TABLE 3.15. Neuropeptide Cotransmission

Dopamine	Cholecystokinin (CCK) Neurotensin
Norepinephrine	Neuropeptide Y Somatostatin Enkephalin
Serotonin	Substance P Thyrotropin-releasing hormone Enkephalin
Acetylcholine	Vasoactive intestinal polypeptide Substance P
GABA	Somatostatin CCK Substance P Enkephalin Dynorphin
Vasopressin	CCK Dynorphin
Oxytocin	Enkephalin

TABLE 3.16. Summary of Neurotransmitter Pharmacology in the Central Nervous System

Transmitter	Anatomy	Receptor Subtypes and Preferred Agonists	Receptor Antagonists	Mechanisms
Acetylcholine	Cell bodies at all levels; long and short connections	Muscarinic (M_1): muscarine	Pirenzepine, atropine	Excitatory: ↓ in K^+ conductance; ↑ IP_3, DAG
		Muscarine (M_2): muscarin, bethanechol	Atropine, methoctramine	Inhibitory: ↑ K^+ conductance; ↓ cAMP
	Motoneuron-Renshaw cell synapse	Nicotinic: nicotine	Dihydro-β-erythroidine, α-bungarotoxin	Excitatory: ↑ cation conductance
Dopamine	Cell bodies at all levels; short medium, and long connections	D_1	Phenothiazines	Inhibitory(?): ↑ cAMP
		D_2: bromocriptine	Phenothiazines, butyrophenones	Inhibitory (presynaptic): ↓ Ca^{2+}; Inhibitory (postsynaptic): ↑ in K^+ conductance, ↓ cAMP
GABA	Supraspinal and spinal interneurons involved in pre- and postsynaptic inhibition	$GABA_A$: muscimol	Bicuculline, picrotoxin	Inhibitory: ↑ Cl^- conductance
		$GABA_B$: baclofen	2-OH saclofen	Inhibitory (presynaptic): ↓ Ca^{2+} conductance; Inhibitory (postsynaptic): ↑ K^+ conductance
Glutamate	Relay neurons at all levels and some interneurons	N-Methyl-D-aspartate (NMDA): NMDA	2-Amino-5-phosphonovalerate, dizocilpine	Excitatory: ↑ cation conductance, particularly Ca^{2+}
		AMPA: AMPA	CNQX	Excitatory: ↑ cation conductance
		Kainate: kainic acid, domoic acid		
		Metaboropic: ACPD, quisqualate	MCPG	Inhibitory (presynaptic): ↓ Ca^{2+} conductance ↓ cAMP; Excitatory: ↓ K^+ conductance; ↑ IP_3, DAG
Glycine	Spinal interneurons and some brain stem interneurons	Taurine, β-alanine	Strychnine	Inhibitory: ↑ Cl^- conductance
5-Hydroxytryptamine (serotonin)	Cell bodies in midbrain and pons project to all levels	$5\text{-}HT_{1A}$: LSD	Metergoline, spiperone	Inhibitory: ↑ in K^+ conductance, ↓ cAMP
		$5\text{-}HT_{2A}$: LSD	Ketanserin	Excitatory: ↓ K^+ conductance, ↑ IP_3, DAG
		$5\text{-}HT_3$: 2-methyl-5-HT	Ondansetron	Excitatory: ↑ cation conductance
		$5\text{-}HT_{4A}$		Excitatory: ↓ K^+ conductance

TABLE 3.16. Summary of Neurotransmitter Pharmacology in the Central Nervous System *(continued)*

TRANSMITTER	ANATOMY	RECEPTOR SUBTYPES AND PREFERRED AGONISTS	RECEPTOR ANTAGONISTS	MECHANISMS
Norepinephrine	Cell bodies in pons and brain stem project to all levels	α_1: phenylephrine	Prazosin	Excitatory: ↓ K^+ conductance, ↑ IP_3, DAG
		α_2: clonidine	Yohimbine	Inhibitory (presynaptic): ↓ Ca^{2+} conductance; Inhibitory (postsynaptic): ↑ K^+ conductance, ↓ cAMP
		β_1: isoproterenol, dobutamine	Atenolol, practolol	Excitatory: ↓ K^+ conductance, ↑ cAMP
		β_2: albuterol	Butoxamine	Inhibitory: may involve ↑ in electrogenic sodium pump; ↑ cAMP
Histamine	Cells in ventral posterior hypothalamus	H_1: 2(*m*-fluorophenyl)-histamine	Mepyramine	Excitatory: ↓ K^+ conductance; ↑ IP_3, DAG
		H_2: dimaprit	Ranitidine	Excitatory: ↓ K^+ conductance, ↑ cAMP
		H_3: *R*-α-methyl-histamine	Thioperamide	Inhibitory autoreceptors
Opioid peptides	Cell bodies at all levels; long and short connections	Mu: bendorphin	Naloxone	Inhibitory (presynaptic): ↓ Ca^{2+} conductance, ↑ cAMP
		Delta: enkephalin	Naloxone	Inhibitory (postsynaptic): ↑ K^+ conductance, ↓ cAMP
		Kappa: dynorphin	Naloxone	
Tachykinins	Primary sensory neurons, cell bodies at all levels; long and short connections	NK1: Substance P methylester, aprepitant	Aprepitant	Excitatory: ↓ K^+ conductance; ↑ IP_3, DAG
		NK2		
		NK3		
Endocannabinoids	Widely distributed	CB1: Anandamide, 2-arachidonylglycerol	Rimonabant	Inhibitory (presynaptic): ↓ Ca^{2+} conductance, ↓ cAMP

Note: Many other central transmitters have been identified (see text).

ACPD, *trans*-1-amino-cyclopentyl-1,3-dicarboxylate; AMPA, DL-α-mino-3-hydroxy-5-methylisoxazole-4-propionate; cAMP, cyclic adenosine monophosphate; CQNX, 6-cyano-7-nitroquinoxaline-2,3-dione; DAG, diacylglycerol; IP_3, inositol trisphosphate; LSD, lysergic acid diethylamide; MCPG, α-methyl-4-carboxyphenylglycine.

Reproduced, with permission, from Katzung B. *Basic and Clinical Pharmacology,* 11th ed. New York: McGraw-Hill, 2009: Table 21-2.

MOVEMENT DISORDERS

- **Dopamine responsive dystonia (Segawa syndrome):** Characterized by striatal dopamine deficiency, secondary to tyrosine hydroxylase deficiency, therefore L-dopa effectively treats symptoms.

- **Essential tremor:** Treated with β-blockers and phenobarbital.
- **Medication-induced parkinsonism:** Induced by antagonists of basal ganglia D_2 receptors.
- **Neuroleptic malignant syndrome:** Precipitated by withdrawal of dopaminergic medication or receptor blockade.
- **Parkinson disease:** Characterized by degeneration of substantia nigra pars compacta; therefore, pharmacotherapy consists of supplying exogenous L-dopa and dopamine receptor agonists while inhibiting metabolism with agents such as carbidopa, which inhibits DOPA decarboxylase; entacapone, which inhibits COMT; and selegiline, which inhibits MAO-B.
- **Restless leg syndrome:** Treated with dopamine agonists like ropinirole and pramipexole.
- **Stiff-person syndrome:** Autoimmune disorder or paraneoplastic characterized by glutamic acid decarboxylase antibodies (anti-GAD; or anti-ampiphysin) antibodies leading to decreased GABA activity. Symptoms include muscle stiffness and spasms triggered by minimal stimuli.
- **Tardive dyskinesias:** Result from increased sensitivity of postsynaptic dopamine receptors because of previous dopamine receptor antagonism.

NEUROPSYCHIATRIC DISORDERS

- **Alzheimer disease:** Associated with cholinergic deficit, so can be treated with long-acting cholinesterase inhibitors. Also associated with glutamate excitotoxicity, so can be treated with NMDA receptor antagonists.
- **Addiction:** Drugs that increase dopaminergic activity in the nucleus accumbens possess addiction potential. Agents used to reduce addiction-related craving (ie, bupropion) provide compensatory dopamine increase.
- **Depression:** Associated with low catecholamine activity, especially low concentrations of cerebrospinal fluid serotonin metabolites (ie, HIAA). Treatments include MAOIs, tricyclics, selective serotonin reuptake inhibitors (SSRIs), selective dopamine reuptake inhibitors (SDRIs—bupropion), and serotonin and norepinephrine reuptake inhibitors (SNRIs—venlafaxine). See Table 3.17 for pharmacologic differences among several antidepressants.
- **Lesch-Nyhan disease:** Striatal dopamine pathways are implicated in the neurological deficits, such as choreoathetoid dyskinesia and dystonia, that are symptoms of this disease, which is caused by **hypoxanthine-guanine phosphoribosyl transferase** (HGPRT) deficiency with X-linked recessive inheritance.
- **Schizophrenia:** Excessive mesolimbic dopaminergic activity is implicated in pathophysiology; therefore, treatment includes dopamine receptor antagonists. See Table 3.18 for antipsychotic drugs.
- **Tourette syndrome:** Symptoms are associated with hypersensitivity of D_2 receptors in the caudate.

NEUROMUSCULAR TRANSMISSION DISORDERS

- **Botulism:** Caused by impairment of acetylcholine (ACh) release from presynaptic neurons because of botulinum toxin leading to severe weakness.
- **Congenital myasthenic syndromes:** Heterogenous disorders caused by mutations in neuromuscular junction components (Table 3.19).
- **Lambert-Eaton myasthenic syndrome (LEMS):** Paraneoplastic disorder with antibodies against presynaptic calcium channels that inhibit release of ACh and cause weakness.

TABLE 3.17. Pharmacologic Differences Among Several Antidepressants

ANTIDEPRESSANT	ACH M	α_1	H_1	5-HT_2	NET	SERT
Amitriptyline	+++	+++	++	0/+	+	++
Amoxapine	+	++	+	+++	++	+
Bupropion	0	0	0	0	0/+	0
Citalopram, escitalopram	0	0	0		0	+++
Clomipramine						
Desipramine	+	++	+	+	++	+++
Doxepin	+	+	+	0/+	+++	+
Fluoxetine	++	+++	+++	0/+	+	+
Fluvoxamine	0	0	0	0/+	0	+++
Imipramine	0	0	0	0	0	+++
Maprotiline	++	+	+	0/+	+	++
Mirtazapine	+	+	++	0/+	++	0
Nefazodone	0	0	+++	+	+	0
Nortriptyline	0	+	0	++	0/+	+
Paroxetine	+	+	+	+	++	+
	+	0	0	0	+	+++
Protriptyline	+++	+	+	+	+++	+
Sertraline	0	0	0	0	0	+++
Trazodone	0	++	0/+	++	0	+
Trimipramine	++	++	+++	0/+	0	0
Venlafaxine	0	0	0	0	+	++

ACh M, acetylcholine muscarinic receptor; α_1, alpha$_1$-adrenoceptor; H_1, histamine$_1$ receptor; 5-HT_2, serotonin 5-HT_2 receptor; NET, norepinephrine transporter; SERT, serotonin transporter. 0/+, minimal affinity; +, mild affinity; + +, moderate affinity; + + +, high affinity.

Reproduced, with permission, from Katzung B. *Basic and Clinical Pharmacology,* 11th ed. New York: McGraw-Hill, 2009: Table 30-2.

TABLE 3-18. Antipsychotic Drugs: Relation of Chemical Structure to Potency and Toxicities

CHEMICAL CLASS	DRUG	D_2/5-HT_{2A} RATIO[a]	CLINICAL POTENCY	EXRAPRAMIDAL TOXICITY	SEDATIVE ACTION	HYPOTENSIVE ACTIONS
Phenothiazines						
Aliphatic	Chlorpromazine	High	Low	Medium	High	High
Piperazine	Fluphenazine	High	High	High	Low	Very Low
Thioxanthene	Thiothixene	Very High	High	Medium	Medium	Medium
Butyrophenone	Haloperidol	Medium	High	Very High	Low	Very Low
Dibenzodiazepine	Clozapine	Very Low	Medium	Very Low	Low	Medium
Benzisoxazole	Risperidone	Very Low	High	Low[b]	Low	Low
Thienobenzodiazepine	Olanzapine	Low	High	Very Low	Medium	Low
Dibenzothiazepine	Quetiapine	Low	Low	Very Low	Medium	Low to Medium
						Very Low
Dihydroindolone	Ziprasidone	Low	Medium	Very Low	Low	Low
Dihydrocarbostyril	Aripiprazole	Medium	High	Very Low	Very Low	

[a] Ratio of affinity for D_2 receptors to affinity for 5-HT_{2A} receptors.

[b] At dosages below 8 mg/d.

Reproduced, with permission, from Katzung B. *Basic and Clinical Pharmacology,* 11th ed. New York: McGraw-Hill, 2009: Table 29-1.

TABLE 3.19. The Congenital Myasthenic Syndromes

Type	Clinical Features	Electrophysiology	Genetics	End-Plate Effects	Treatment
Slow channel	Most common; weak forearm extensors; onset 2d to 3d decade; variable severity	Repetitive muscle response on nerve stimulation; prolonged channel opening and MEPP duration	Autosomal dominant; α, β, ∊ AChR mutations	Excitotoxic end-plate myopathy; decreased AChRs; postsynaptic damage	Quinidine: decreases end-plate damage; made worse by anti-AChE
Low-affinity fast channel	Onset early; moderately sever; ptosis, EOM involvement; weakness and fatigue	Brief and infrequent channel openings; opposite of slow channel syndrome	Autosomal recessive; may be heteroallelic	Normal end-plate structure	3,4-DAP; anti-AChE
Severe AChR deficiencies	Early onset variable severity; fatigue; typical MG features	Decremental respose to repetitive nerve stimulation; decreased MEPP amplitudes	Autosomal recessive; ∊ mutations most common; may different mustations	Increased length of end plates; variable synaptic folds	Anti-AChE; ?3,4-DAP
AChE deficiency	Early onset; variable severity; scoliosis; may have normal EOM, absent pupillary responses	Decremental response to repetitive nerve stimulation	Mutant gene for AChE's collagen anchor	Small nerve terminals; degenerated junctional folds	Worse with anti-AChE drugs

Abbreviations: AChR, acetylcholine receptor, AChE, acetylcholinesterase; EOM, extraocular muscles; MEPP, miniature end-plate potential; 3,4-DAP, 3-4-Diaminopyridine.

Reproduced, with permission, from Fauci AS, Braunwald E, Kasper DL, et al. (Eds). *Harrison's Principles of Internal Medicine,* 16th ed. New York: McGraw-Hill, 2006: Table 366-2.

- **Myasthenia gravis:** Autoimmune disease frequently associated with antibodies against postsynaptic ACh receptors or muscle-specific kinase (MuSK), often presenting with weakness of extraocular and bulbar muscles. Treated with cholinesterase inhibitors that decrease breakdown of ACh in the synapse.
- **Tick paralysis:** Also due to presynaptic ACh release blockade.

OTHER

- **Hypertension:** Patients taking MAOIs can develop hypertension with consumption of tyramine found in cheese, sausage, pickled fish, and yeast supplements.
- **Pheochromocytoma:** Symptoms are due to excess norepinephrine and epinephrine activity and include hypertension, tachycardia, anxiety, and headache.
- **Pituitary adenoma:** Dopamine agonists decrease prolactin production and reduce size in prolactin-secreting tumors. ↘ DA as tx

Drugs of Abuse

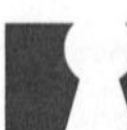

KEY FACT

The brain's reward circuit includes projections from the ventral tegmental area of the midbrain to the nucleus accumbens and other forebrain structures.

Drugs of abuse are rewarding and reinforcing through actions on dopamine and other neurotransmitter systems.

PSYCHOSTIMULANTS

Pharmacology

Cocaine blocks reuptake of monoamines (dopamine [DA] > norepinephrine [NE]), leading to increased synaptic concentrations and receptor activation. Amphetamines principally provoke presynaptic monoamine release (DA > NE) but also block reuptake. Half-lives are typically longer than cocaine, from 6 to 12 hours, so effects are also longer lasting.

Signs and Symptoms

Intoxication initially produces euphoria with heightened feelings of sexual, physical, and mental power as well as appetite suppression, hypervigilance, paranoia, and hallucinations. Signs include tachycardia, hypertension, and pupillary dilation. Sleep time is reduced with suppression of rapid eye movement (REM) sleep. Involuntary movements commonly include chorea, tremor, dystonia, and stereotypies.

Overdose

Can manifest with delirium, psychosis, arrhythmia, vasospasm, myocardial infarction, stroke, or seizure.

Withdrawal

Symptoms include hyperphagia, anhedonia, depression, dysphoria, and sleep disturbances.

Treatment

Symptomatic treatment with antipsychotics, sedatives, antidepressants, and, for severe hypertension, α-blocker antihypertensives (eg, phentolamine).

Clinical Notes

- Cocaine can be injected locally for local anesthesia because it blocks peripheral nerve impulses.
- Amphetamine can treat attention-deficit hyperactivity disorder (ADHD) and narcolepsy.
- Testing with topical cocaine can differentiate Horner syndrome, in which the pupil does not dilate, from physiologic anisocoria; hydroxyamphetamine can differentiate central and preganglionic from postganglionic lesions.

3,4-METHYLENEDIOXYMETHAMPHETAMINE (MDMA, ECSTASY)

Pharmacology

Chemically related to amphetamine. Causes transporter-dependent serotonin efflux into synapse through amphetamine-like effect on serotonin reuptake transporter.

SIGNS AND SYMPTOMS

Acts as psychostimulant and weak psychedelic. Produces feelings of enhanced emotional warmth, sensation, and energy. Signs include chills, teeth clenching, muscle cramping, and blurred vision.

OVERDOSE

Hypertension, encephalopathy, and seizures.

WITHDRAWAL

Anxiety, paranoia, panic attacks, and depression.

TREATMENT

Symptomatic.

MDMA is toxic to serotonergic neurons and can cause cognitive impairment.

OPIOIDS

PHARMACOLOGY

See Table 3.20.

SIGNS AND SYMPTOMS

Opioids cause euphoria in addition to relieving pain and reducing anxiety. Side effects can include sedation, nausea, vomiting, and constipation.

OVERDOSE

Coma, miosis, and respiratory depression.

WITHDRAWAL

Not life threatening. Dysphoria, increased pain sensitivity, insomnia, diarrhea, and autonomic hyperactivity.

TREATMENT

- Receptor antagonists (eg, naloxone) displace opioids from their receptors, reversing the effects of overdose and may even induce withdrawal symptoms.

TABLE 3.20. Opioid Receptor Subtypes, Their Functions, and Their Endogenous Peptide Affinities

RECEPTOR SUBTYPE	FUNCTIONS	ENDOGENOUS OPIOID PEPTIDE AFFINITY
μ (mu)	Supraspinal and spinal analgesia; sedation; inhibition of respiration; slowed gastrointestinal transit; modulatin of hormone and neurotransmitter release	Endorphins > enkephalins > dynorphins
δ (delta)	Supraspinal and spinal analgesia; modulatin of hormone and neurotransmitter release	Enkephalins > endorphins and dynorphins
κ (kappa)	Supraspinal and spinal analgesia; psychotommetic effects; slowed gastrointestinal transit	Dynorphins > > endorphins and enkephalins

Reproduced, with permission, from Katzung B. *Basic and Clinical Pharmacology,* 11th ed. New York: McGraw-Hill, 2009: Table 31-1.

KEY FACT

Phenytoin and carbamazepine induce methadone metabolism, causing opioid withdrawal in patients on methadone maintainence.

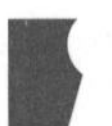

KEY FACT

Ketamine is chemically related to PCP and is also an NMDA receptor antagonist.

- Clonidine can treat autonomic symptoms of opioid withdrawal. Long-acting opioids like methadone, as well as buprenorphine, a receptor agonist-antagonist, can also be used to treat withdrawal.

PHENCYCLIDINE (PCP)

Pharmacology

PCP is a noncompetitive NMDA receptor antagonists that prevents glutamate-induced calcium influx.

Signs and Symptoms

Acts as dissociative anesthetic. Produces euphoria, ataxia, and nystagmus at lower doses and emotional withdrawal, thought disorders, delusions, and hallucinations at higher doses.

Overdose

Can be characterized by rigidity leading to rhabdomyolysis, horizontal and vertical nystagmus, stereotypies, seizures, psychosis, catatonia, and violence.

Treatment

Includes sedation and symptomatic management (ie, muscle relaxants to prevent rhabdomyolysis).

CANNABINOIDS

Pharmacology

The most commonly abused drug in the United States is marijuana, which contains the potent cannabinoid tetrahydrocannabinol (THC), which binds to cannabinoid receptors located in cerebral cortex, basal ganglia, and cerebellum.

Signs and Symptoms

Produces euphoria, altered perceptions, and impaired judgment as well as hunger and conjunctival injection. Long-term use can lead to disturbance of memory, executive function, and psychomotor speed.

Overdose

Causes severe anxiety or psychosis that includes hallucinations and delusions.

Withdrawal

Irritability, restlessness, sleep disturbance, and nausea.

Treatment

Anxiolytics and antipsychotics, if necessary.

NICOTINE

Pharmacology

Agonist of nicotinic ACh receptors that increases catecholamines and mesolimbic dopamine.

Signs and Symptoms

Mild euphoria, increased alertness, muscle relaxation, nausea, and increased psychomotor activity.

Withdrawal

Anxiety, restlessness, tremulousness, increased appetite, and craving.

Treatment

Smoking cessation can be achieved by employing alternate nicotine delivery systems to alleviate withdrawal symptoms, including gum and transdermal patches. Bupropion can also help treat withdrawal symptoms, like craving, by increasing mesolimbic system dopamine.

BRIEF SUMMARY OF DRUGS OF ABUSE

See Table 3.21.

TABLE 3.21. Acute Pharmacologic Actions of Drugs of Abuse

Drug	Action
Opiates/opioid receptors	Agonist at μ, δ, and κ
Cocaine	Inhibits monoamine reptake transporters
Amphetamine release	Stimulates monoamine
Ethanol	Facilitates $GABA_A$ receptor function and inhibits NMDA glutamate receptor function
Nicotine	Agonist at nicotinic acetylcholine receptors
Cannabinoids	Agonist at cannabinoid (CB_1 and CB_2) receptors
Hallucinogens	Partial agonist at $5HT_{2A}$ serotonin receptors
Phencyclidine (PCP)	Antagonist at NMDA glutamate receptors

Reproduced, with permission, from Nestler E, Hyman S, Malenka R. *Molecular Neuropharmacology: A Foundation for Clinical Neuroscience*, 2nd ed. New York: McGraw-Hill: 2008: Table 16-1.

NOTES

CHAPTER 4

Neuroimmunology

Maria K. Houtchens, MD, MMSCI

Multiple Sclerosis (MS)

A 53-year-old man presents with 6 months of gradually worsening leg weakness, spasticity, and hyperreflexia. His exam also reveals mild appendicular ataxia. MRI reveals more than 10 nonenhancing T2 hyperintensities in subcortical white matter, brain stem, and cerebellum, as well as spinal cord atrophy.

What alternatives to MS should be considered? Infections (eg, Lyme disease, syphilis), inflammatory (eg, CNS vasculitis), others (eg, CNS lymphoma). See Table 4.1. Serological testing, CSF analysis, and MRI characteristics should be used to exclude MS mimics.

What is this patient's likely diagnosis? Primary progressive MS (PPMS).

T-cell-mediated autoimmune central nervous system (CNS) disease triggered by unknown exogenous agents such as viruses or bacteria, in genetically susceptible subjects.

Epidemiology

- Most common neurologic disease among young adults.
- Incidence is highest from ages 20 to 40, but can start in childhood or after age 50.
- Female-to-male ratio: 7:3.
- Prevalence decreases with proximity to equator.
- US prevalence: 500,000+.
- In the United States there are 8,500–10,000 new cases per year.
- Genetic risk:
  - General population: 0.1%.
  - If 1 parent or first-degree relative is affected: 4%.
  - If both parents are affected: 20%.
- Associated with major histocompatibility complex II (MHC-II) and certain DR2 haplotypes.

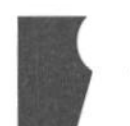

KEY FACT

MS is associated with MHC-II and 3 specific alleles in DR2 haplotype.

Signs and Symptoms

- Constellation depends on location of lesion(s) within brain, spinal cord, and optic nerves. Initially, attacks of inflammation and CNS dysfunction are usually followed by full recovery, but over time, deficits may persist. Attacks typically worsen over several days, plateau, and then improve over days to weeks. Most common symptoms include:
  - Visual/oculomotor disturbances (49%).
  - Leg paresis/leg paresthesias (42%).
  - Cerebellar ataxia (24%).
  - Cognitive impairment (4%).
- Other symptoms include:
  - Lhermitte phenomenon: Electrical paresthesias induced by neck flexion.
  - Uthoff phenomenon: Worsening symptoms/signs with increased body temperature (showering, exercising).
  - Neuropathic pain.
  - Fatigue.
  - Depression.

Pathology/Pathophysiology

- Historically considered a disease of white matter, but recent data suggest additional neurodegeneration and primary involvement of gray matter. Viruses may be implicated in pathogenesis of MS:

- Epstein-Barr virus (EBV) and human herpesvirus 6 (HHV-6) are most consistently and recently implicated.
- Other possibilities include measles, rubella, mumps, coronavirus, parainfluenza, herpes simplex virus type 1 (HSV-1), vaccinia, and human T-lymphotropic virus type 1 (HTLV-1).

- Inflammation is characterized by an **immunologic cascade:**
  - Activation of CD4+ autoreactive T cells in peripheral immune system.
  - Migration of Th1 cells into CNS.
  - Reactivation in-situ by myelin antigen.
  - Activation of B cells and macrophages and secretion of proinflammatory cytokines and antibodies.
  - Typical pathology: Inflammation, demyelination, axonal disruption/loss, atrophy/neurodegeneration.
- **Gross external pathology:** Usually normal, though may see atrophy and widening of sulci with enlargement of lateral and third ventricles. Spinal cord may be slightly shrunken with thickened pia and arachnoid.
- **Gross sections:** "MS plaques"—numerous small, irregular, discolorations (gray in *old* lesions, pink in *acute* lesions), predominantly in periventricular white matter. Superolateral angle of the body of the lateral ventricle is often affected. Optic nerves may look shrunken.
- **Microscopic:** There are 4 patterns of immunohistopathology in MS lesions: a macrophage/T-cell inflammatory type, an antibody-dependent/complement-driven type, an oligodendroglial/myelin-associated glycoprotein-directed inflammatory type, and a degenerative type (lack of perivascular demyelination and absence of remyelination). Usually, one type predominates in an individual patient.
  - Myelin stains show sharply demarcated circumscribed lesions devoid of myelin.
  - Within lesions: Destruction, swelling or fragmentation of myelin sheaths, proliferation of glial cells, variable axonal destruction (new and old plaques).
  - Early/acute lesion (days to weeks): Marked hypercellularity, macrophage infiltration, astrocytosis, perivenular inflammation with plasma cells and lymphocytes, disintegration of myelin.
  - Active/nonacute lesion (weeks to months): Lipid-laden phagocytes, inflammatory response minimal at the center of lesions but prominent at edges of lesion with increased numbers of macrophages, lymphocytes, plasma cells.
  - Chronic inactive plaque (months to years): Prominent demyelination (severe loss of oligodendrocytes), gliosis, hypocellularity, no myelin degradation products.
  - Remyelinating plaques may result from differentiation of precursor cells common to type II astrocytes and oligodendrocytes; uniform areas of aberrant and incomplete myelination (shadow plaques).
- **Electron microscopy:**
  - Widening of outer myelin lamellae.
  - Splitting/vacuolization of myelin sheaths.
  - Vesicular dissolution of myelin.
  - Myelin sheath fragmentation, ball and ovoid formation.
  - Thinning of myelin sheaths.
  - Macrophage-associated pinocytosis and peeling of myelin sheaths.
- **Immunohistochemistry of MS plaques:**
  - Decrease in lipid and protein component of normal myelin.
  - Decrease in staining for myelin basic protein (MBP) and myelin-associated glycoprotein (MAG).

KEY FACT

The pathologic hallmarks of MS are demyelination and inflammation, predominantly perivenular. Severe or advanced disease also involves axonal disruption and cortical atrophy/neurodegeneration. Lesions can be present in the cortex and in basal ganglia.

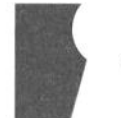

KEY FACT

Viruses that may be implicated in pathogenesis of MS: **EBV, HHV6** (most consistently and recently implicated), measles, rubella, mumps, coronavirus, parainfluenza, HSV-1, vaccinia, HTLV-1.

KEY FACT

MRI fluid-attenuated inversion recovery (FLAIR) suppresses CSF T2 signal for better lesion identification. In early MS, FLAIR is more predictive than other MRI sequences of subsequent disease course.

KEY FACT

MRI measures of gray matter atrophy and whole brain atrophy correlate best with disease progression, disability scores, and MS-related cognitive impairment.

Diagnostic Criteria

- Must exclude alternatives (Table 4.1) and have at least:
  - One clinical attack with objective evidence of neurologic disease *plus*
  - Second attack by magnetic resonance imaging (MRI) criteria, positive spinal fluid findings, *or* abnormal evoked potentials.
- "Revised McDonald criteria" are 87% sensitive at 1 year and 85% specific at 3 years for diagnosis of MS (Table 4.2).
- **What is an attack?**
  - New or recurrent neurological disturbance of kind seen in MS.
  - Subjective report or objective observation.
  - At least 24 hours' duration in absence of fever or infection.
  - Excludes pseudoattacks, single paroxysmal symptoms (multiple episodes of paroxysmal symptoms occurring over 24 hours or more are acceptable as evidence).
  - Some historical events with symptoms and pattern typical for MS can provide reasonable evidence of previous demyelinating event(s), even in the absence of objective findings.
- **Determining time between attacks:** 30 days between onset of event 1 and onset of event 2.
- **MRI criteria:** Dissemination in space.
- **What provides evidence for dissemination in space (DIS)?**
  - ≥ 1 T2 lesion in at least 2 out of 4 areas of the CNS: periventricular, juxtacortical, infratentorial, or spinal cord.
  - Gadolinium enhancement of lesions is not required for DIS.
  - If a subject has a brain stem or spinal cord syndrome, the symptomatic lesions are excluded and do not contribute to lesion.
  - **Dissemination in time.**
- **What provides MRI evidence of dissemination in time (DIT)?**
  - A new T2 and/or gadolinium-enhancing lesion(s) on follow-up MRI, with reference to a baseline scan, irrespective of the timing of the baseline MRI *or*
  - Simultaneous presence of asymptomatic gadolinium-enhancing and nonenhancing lesions at any time.
- **Differential diagnosis** is broad because of the many potential manifestations of MS (see Table 4.1).
- Cerebrospinal fluid (CSF) analysis:
  - CSF pleocytosis: Occasional, mild (≤ 25 cells/mm^3).
  - Protein: Normal to modestly elevated, almost always < 100 mg/L.
  - Oligoclonal bands (OCBs): 50–60% of clinically isolated syndrome (CIS), 95% of clinically definite MS (CDMS). Can have OCBs in

TABLE 4.1. MS Mimics

Infection	**Metabolic**
Lyme disease	Vitamin B$_{12}$ and E deficiency
Neurosyphilis	**Other**
Progressive multifocal leukoencephalopathy, HIV, HTLV-1	Cerebral autosomal dominant arteriopathy with subcortical infarcts and leukoencephalopathy (CADASIL), other rare familial diseases
Inflammatory/Autoimmune	
Systemic lupus erythematosus	CNS lymphoma
Sjogren syndrome	Cervical spondylosis
Other CNS vasculitis	Motor neuron disease
Sarcoidosis	Hereditary leukodystrophies
Behçet disease	Cerebrovascular disease
Acute disseminated encephalomyelitis	

TABLE 4.2. Revised McDonald Criteria for MS Diagnosis (2010)

Clinical (Attack)	Lesions	Additional Criteria to Make Diagnosis
2 or more	Objective clinical evidence of 2 or more lesions or objective clinical evidence of 1 lesion with reasonable historical evidence of a prior attack	None. Clinical evidence alone will suffice; additional evidence desirable but must be consistent with MS
2 or more	Objective clinical evidence of 1 lesion	Dissemination in space, demonstrated by ■ 1 T2 lesion in at least 2 MS typical CNS regions (periventricular, juxtacortical, infratorial, spinal cord); OR ■ Await further clinical attack implicating a different CNS site
1	Objective clinical evidence of 2 or more lesions	Dissemination in time, demonstrated by simultaneous asymptomatic contrast-enhancing and nonenhancing lesions at any time; OR ■ A new T2 and/or contrast-enhancing lesion(s) on follow-up MRI, irrespective of its timing; OR ■ Await a second clinical attack
1	Objective clinical evidence of 1 lesion	Dissemination in space, demonstrated by ■ 1 T2 lesion in at least 2 MS typical CNS regions (periventricular, juxtacortical, infratentorial, spinal cord); OR ■ Await further clinical attack implicating a different CNS site AND Dissemination in time, demonstrated by ■ Simultaneous asymptomatic contrast-enhancing and nonenhancing lesions at any time; OR ■ A new T2 and/or contrast-enhancing lesion(s) on follow-up MIR, irrespective of its timing; OR ■ Await a second clinical attack
0	Progression from the onset	One year of disease progression (retrospective or prospective) AND at least 2 out of 3 criteria: ■ Dissemination in space in the brain based on 1 T2 lesion in periventricular, juxtacortical or infratentorial regions; ■ Dissemination in space in the spinal cord based on 2 T2 lesions; OR ■ Positive CSF

other conditions (eg, HIV, Lyme disease, neurosarcoidosis, subacute sclerosing panencephalitis, neurosyphilis).

- Increased immunoglobulin G (IgG) synthesis (3.3 mg/day in 90% of patients).
- High IgG index (≥ 0.7 in 90% of patients).
- MBP: Usually < 1 ng/mL, but increases to 4 ng/mL in 80% of acute relapses.

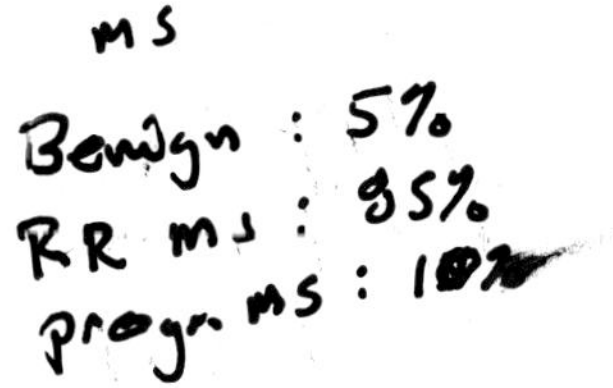

Classification by Disease Course (Figure 4.1)

- Benign MS: 5% of all patients.
- Relapsing-remitting (RRMS): 85% at initial diagnosis.
- Primary progressive (PPMS): 10–20% at initial diagnosis.

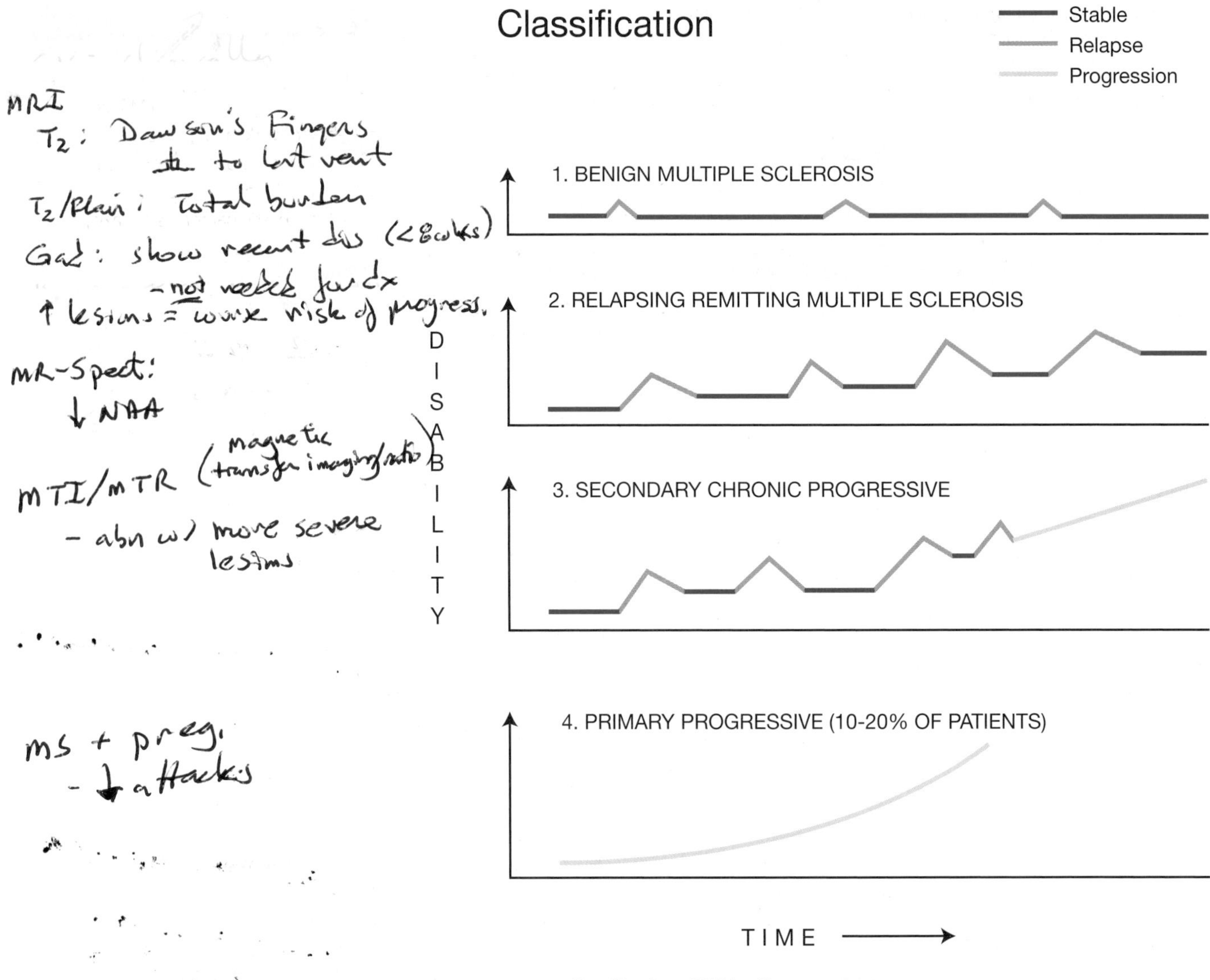

FIGURE 4.1. Classification of MS by disease course.

- Secondary progressive (SPMS): 60% of RRMS becomes SPMS after 15 years.
- **Favorable prognostic indicators:**
  - Younger age of onset.
  - Female sex.
  - Monosymptomatic onset.
  - Sensory rather than motor symptoms at onset.
  - Few T2/FLAIR lesions on original MRI.
  - Long interval between first and second attacks.
  - Low attack frequency in the first 2 years.
  - Full recovery of function after the first attack.
- **MRI findings in MS:**
  - Dawson fingers: T2 hyperintensities arranged perpendicular to the plane of lateral ventricles. Reflect demyelination and perivenular inflammation.
  - T2/FLAIR hyperintensities: Reflect total disease burden, including reversible and irreversible pathology.
  - T1 gadolinium enhancement: Inflammation, blood-brain barrier disruption, and recent disease activity (< 8 weeks) with new lesion formation.

KEY FACT

Benign MS: No or minimal neurologic disability after 10–15 years: 5% of all patients.

Malignant MS: Neurologic disability requiring ambulation assistance after ≤ 5 years—5–7% of all patients.

KEY FACT

There is no consistent evidence that pregnancy worsens clinical outcome for women with MS. MS patients have decreased number of relapses in pregnancy and are at a higher risk for having MS attack for up to 6 months after delivery.

- T1 hypointensities ("black holes"): Reflect severe tissue pathology, axonal loss, and clinical disability.
- Global and focal cerebral atrophy measures in brain and spinal cord: Correlate with axonal loss, neuronal loss, physical and cognitive impairment.
- N-acetyl aspartate (NAA) levels (measured with MR spectroscopy): Marker of neuronal and axonal metabolism. NAA decreased in MS lesions and in normal-appearing white matter in brains of MS patients.
- Magnetization transfer imaging or ratio (MTI/MTR): Abnormal with more severe lesions with tissue destruction; can be abnormal despite normal routine sequences.
- Functional MRI (fMRI): Measures critical circuitry involved in response to injury, activation, loss of function, and recovery of function in MS.

KEY FACT

Fifty to 70% of patients with MS are not able to work in prior occupation 10–15 years after disease onset. Causes of disability: Cognitive and memory disorders, spastic paraparesis, ataxia, sphincter dysfunction.

TREATMENT

- Disease-modifying therapy: Aim to alter natural course of the disease and maximize the quality of life by decreasing:
  - Frequency of relapses.
  - New brain and spinal cord lesions (overall and active).
  - Progression of brain atrophy.
  - Disability progression—physical and cognitive.
- Immunomodulatory agents (IMAs) also known as disease modifying drugs (DMDs) are used continuously before, during, and between relapses. Immunosuppressive agents are used for acute treatment of severe relapses and occasionally for long-term management of severe or progressive disease. IMAs decrease annual relapse rate by ~30% injectable (interferons [IFNs], injectable glatiramer acetate and oral teriflunomide),40–50% (oral fingolimod and dimethyl fumarate), and ~60% (intravenous natalizumab). They decrease the rate of new MRI lesions by 90% (natalizumab) and by 40–80% (glatiramer acetate, IFNs, and oral agents respectively, depending on trial data). May decrease disability progression over typical trial duration (1–3 years), but long-term benefits aren't known.
  - **IFNs used in MS:** Recombinant proteins IFN-β_{1b} (Betaseron) and 2 formulations of IFN-β_{1a} (Avonex and Rebif). Do not cross the blood-brain barrier (BBB)—effects occur in the periphery (eg, lymphoid organs.) Possible mechanisms of action: antiproliferative effect, blocks T-cell activation, apoptosis of autoreactive T cells, IFN-γ antagonism, cytokine shifts (increase in interleukin [IL]-10, decrease in IL-12 production), antiviral effect.
  - **Glatiramer acetate (Copaxone)** is a polypeptide mixture with peripheral and CNS effects. It may work by blocking autoimmune T cells, inducing anergy, inducing anti-inflammatory Th2 cells, bystander suppression.
  - **Natalizumab** (Tysabri) is a recombinant monoclonal antibody that selectively inhibits 4-α_1 integrin receptor on lymphocytes in the periphery (not CNS). Prevents binding to vascular cell adhesion molecule (VCAM)-1 on endothelium. Decreases lymphocyte migration across the BBB.
  - Fingolimod hydrochloride (Gilenya) is an oral once-daily tablet used for treatment of relapsing forms of MS. In vivo, it is metabolized to the active metabolite fingolimod phosphate, which is a sphingosine 1-receptor modulator. The exact mechanism of action of fingolimod in patients with MS is unknown; however, it may work by reducing lymphocyte migration to the CNS.
  - Dimethyl fumarate (Tecfidera) is a twice-daily oral agent that is an in vitro nicotinic acid receptor agonist and an in vivo activator of the nu-

clear factor (erythroid-derived 2)-like 2 (Nrf2) pathway that is involved in the cellular response to oxidative stress. It is used for treatment of relapsing forms of MS.
  - Teriflunomide (Aubagio) is the primary active metabolite of leflunomide, is an immunomodulatory agent with anti-inflammatory properties. It inhibits dihydroorotate dehydrogenase, which is a mitochondrial enzyme involved in de novo pyrimidine synthesis. Although the exact mechanism of action in multiple sclerosis is unknown, it may involve a reduction in activated lymphocytes in the CNS. It is a once daily oral formulation.
- Side effects of IMAs include:
  - **IFNs:** Injection site reactions, flulike symptoms, neutropenia, liver function test elevation, formation of interferon-specific antibodies (partially inactivate effects of the drugs).
  - **Glatiramer acetate:** Injection site reactions, postinjection reaction (chest pain, facial erythema, tachypnea), fat necrosis at sites of prolonged injections.
  - **Natalizumab:** Infusion reaction, opportunistic infections—sometimes fatal (progressive multifocal leukoencephalopathy, disseminated varicella-zoster virus), antibody formation.
  - **Fingolimod:** Cardiac arrythmia/bradicardia (first dose to be administered at the doctor's office with ECG monitoring), macular edema, neutropenia, LFT elevation, increased risk of infections.
  - **Dimethyl fumarate:** Neutropenia, facial flushing, gastrointestinal distress.
  - **Teriflunomide:** LFTs elevations (monthly monitoring for the first 6 months of treatment), hair loss, pregnancy category X, increased risk of infections.
- Immunosuppressive therapies:
  - **Mitoxantrone:** Used in severe RRMS or SPMS (only FDA-approved agent for SPMS). Antineoplastic medicine with cardiac toxicity, 1% risk of leukemia, and standard chemotherapeutic side effects. Reduced relapse rate, MRI lesions and disability progression (trials 2 years' duration).
  - **Cyclophosphamide:** Positive anecdotal data for disease stabilization in SPMS or severe RRMS. Off label.
  - **Other agents** used "off label" in SPMS or in combination treatments of severe RRMS: azathioprine, methotrexate, mycophenolate mofetil, intravenous immunoglobulin (IVIG), monthly intravenous steroid infusions, rituximab, and alemtuzamab.

KEY FACT

Mitoxantrone is the only FDA-approved agent for treatment of secondary progressive multiple sclerosis. It is seldom used due to delayed adverse events, especially lymphoid malignancies and cardiac dysfunction. All other agents are used "off label."

Clinically Isolated Syndrome (CIS)

A 26-year-old woman developed mild left leg weakness and numbness that worsened over several days, plateaued, then resolved fully after several weeks. MRI reveals only a single nonenhancing T2 hyperintense lesion in the subcortical white matter of the right hemisphere. Does this patient have MS?

No, this should be considered a clinically isolated syndrome (CIS).

What is her likelihood of conversion to clinically definite MS (CDMS)? About 1 in 3 (see Table 4.3). Should she be treated with immunomodulatory agents (IMAs)?

IMAs reduce the rate of conversion to CDMS, and are an option for patients at high risk of developing CDMS. This patient's risk is probably not high enough to warrant IMAs.

MS often presents for the first time with a clinically isolated syndrome (CIS) such as optic neuritis (ON), an acute brain stem syndrome, or transverse myelitis (TM). Not all patients with CIS develop CDMS. IMAs have been shown to decrease rate of conversion to CDMS, and may be offered to CIS patients at high risk for developing MS (see Table 4.3).

Optic Neuritis

Acute-subacute inflammation of the optic nerve with visual loss.

KEY FACT

The number of MRI lesions suggestive of inflammatory disease at the time of CIS correlates with future development of CDMS.

Symptoms

- Acute/subacute unilateral decrease or loss of vision.
- Central vision most affected.
- Color vision impaired.
- Orbital pain with eye movement common.

Exam

- Reduced visual acuity on the affected side.
- Relative afferent papillary defect (RAPD)—ipsilateral pupil: Brisk consensual response to light in the unaffected eye, but poor response to direct light.
- Inflamed optic nerve head.
- Red color desaturation.
- Enlarged blind spot/central scotoma.

Differential Diagnosis

- Retinal or macular disease.
- Compressive or infiltrative optic neuropathy.
- Granulomatous (sarcoidosis).
- Tumors (lymphoma, glioma, melanoma, metastatic foci).
- Infectious (fungal).
- Mitochondrial disease.
- Ischemic optic neuropathy.
- Vasculitis.

Additional Tests

- Visual evoked responses: Prolonged P100 latency.
- Visual field defect on Goldmann Visual Field test.
- Color vision defect on Ishihara Color Plates test.
- Post-gadolinium T1 enhancement in optic nerve.

Treatment

- Intravenous methylprednisolone 1 g/day × 3–5 days: Speeds visual recovery but does not improve eventual outcome. Decreases rate of second clinical event. Data from optic neuritis treatment trial.

TABLE 4.3. Risk of CIS Conversion to CDMS Based on MRI Lesions

Number of MRI lesions	0	1	≥ 2
Risk of CDMS	11%	33%	≥ 85%

- Rx of CIS with IFN-α_{1a} shown in one large study to reduce conversion rate to CDMS by 50%.

Transverse Myelitis

A 22-year-old man develops numbness and paresthesias beginning in his feet, ascending over several days to the level of his umbilicus. This was soon accompanied by weakness and spasticity in the legs, and he is now having constipation. When he urinates, he has incomplete bladder emptying. What studies should be performed?

MRI of the thoracic and cervical spinal cord. CSF analysis including oligoclonal bands. Viral PCR (eg, CMV, VZV, HSV, EBV) should be considered, especially if there is CSF pleocytosis. Serum testing for HTLV-1, HIV, Lyme, syphilis, and forms of vasculitis.

MRI reveals an enhancing T2 hyperintensity of the spinal cord from T7 to T9. What is the likely diagnosis, and how should he be treated? Transverse myelitis. IV corticosteroids can be considered, though there is no clear evidence of efficacy.

Acute/subacute inflammation of the spinal cord. Usually limited to ≤ 3 vertebral segments and occupies less than two-thirds of cross-sectional cord diameter.

Symptoms

- Ascending numbness and paresthesias in the legs.
- Sensory symptoms involving the trunk and the perineum.
- Difficulty with or loss of bladder and/or bowel control.
- Leg weakness.
- Sensory and/or motor symptoms involving the arms (< 20%).
- Back pain.

Exam

- Decreased sensation to various modalities in the legs and/or the arms.
- Spinal sensory level.
- Paraparesis.
- Loss of sensation in the perineum.
- Increased deep tendon reflexes (DTRs), Babinski responses, increased muscle tone.
- DTRs may be depressed and muscles may be flaccid acutely.

Differential Diagnosis

- Idiopathic autoimmune transverse myelitis.
- Acute disseminated encephalomyelitis (postinfectious or postvaccination).
- Viral myelitis.
- MS.
- Vasculitis from systemic autoimmune disease.
- Spinal cord infarction.
- Spinal cord compression.
- Paraneoplastic myelopathy (especially anti-Hu antibodies, also associated with sensory neuronopathy, seen mostly in small cell lung cancer, rarely in neuroblastoma and prostate cancer).
- Other infections (eg, Lyme disease, syphilis).
- HTLV-1.

Additional Tests

- MRI T2 spinal cord hyperintensity.
- MRI post-gadolinium T1 enhancement.
- Abnormal somatosensory evoked potentials.
- Mild CSF lymphocytic pleocytosis and elevated protein.

Treatment

- IV methylprednisolone 1 g/day × 3–5 days (no clear published evidence of efficacy but done frequently and is considered the standard of care if motor involvement).
- Other options:
  - Immunomodulating medicines (see below).
  - Anti-inflammatory medicines.
  - Immunosuppressant medicines.
  - Symptomatic therapy.

Variants of MS

NEUROMYELITIS OPTICA (DEVIC DISEASE)

Severe acute myelitis (usually cervical) and bilateral optic neuritis. Usually monophasic. Common in Africa and Asia, rarer in North America.

- Usually spans > 3 spinal segments, often involves swelling of the spinal cord.
- Pathology: Extensive demyelination, cavitating necrosis, acute axonal injury, loss of oligodendrocytes. Plaques: CD3+, CD8+, macrophages, granulocytes, eosinophils, perivascular immunoglobulin M deposition.
- IgG anti-NMO antibodies in > 73%; may predict recurrence.
- Oligoclonal bands present in 85% of patients.
- Brain MRI may show few T2 hyperintense lesions.
- CSF may show pleocytosis with 50 or more lymphocytes or neutrophils.
- Monophasic or relapsing course.
- Immunosupression (eg, corticosteroids, plasma exchange, azathioprine, micophenolate) partially effective in nonrandomized trials.

BALÓ CONCENTRIC SCLEROSIS

Rare variant of multiple sclerosis. Characterized by alternating bands of demyelinated and myelinated white matter in concentric rings or irregular stripes. Lesions may be multiple or mixed with other, more typical MS plaques. Often a feature of aggressive disease but can occur in chronic MS.

MARBURG VARIANT

Severe, sometimes monophasic, form of MS leading to advanced disability or death within a period of weeks to months. No consistently successful treatment. MRI: extensive, diffuse, confluent cerebral involvement giving the appearance of "MS cerebritis" or large solitary expanding lesion (tumefactive MS). High-dose steroids are usually ineffective. Improvement with aggressive chemotherapy regimens has been described.

Acute Disseminated Encephalomyelitis (ADEM)

- Monophasic, or polyphasic acute, demyelinating inflammatory illness, typically following upper respiratory infection (50–75%) or vaccination. More common in children. First symptoms 7–14 days postinfection, most hospitalized within a week.
- Various forms of ADEM:
  - Bickerstaff brain stem encephalitis.
  - Postinfectious transverse myelitis.
  - Bilateral optic neuritis (following chickenpox).
  - Acute hemorrhagic leukoencephalitis (aka, acute hemorrhagic encephalopathy or Weston-Hurst syndrome). Always preceded by respiratory infection, often *Mycoplasma*.

SIGNS AND SYMPTOMS

- Children > adults: Prolonged fever, headache, imbalance/gait instability, dysphagia/dysarthria, diplopia.
- Adults > children: Limb paresthesias and weakness.
- **General clinical features:**
  - First clinical attack of inflammatory or demyelinating disease in the CNS.
  - Acute or subacute onset.
  - Affects multifocal areas of the CNS.
  - Polysymptomatic presentation.
  - Must include encephalopathy: Acute behavioral change such as confusion or irritability and/or alteration in consciousness ranging from somnolence or coma.
  - Attack should be followed by improvement on clinical and/or neuroradiologic (MRI) measures.
  - Sequelae may include residual deficits.
  - No other etiologies can explain the event.
  - ADEM relapses (with new or fluctuating symptoms, signs or MRI findings) occurring within 3 months of the inciting ADEM episode are considered part of the same acute event. In addition, ADEM relapses that occur during a steroid taper or within 4 weeks of completing a steroid taper are considered part of the initial inciting ADEM episode.
- **Lesion characteristics on MRI FLAIR and T2 weighted images:**
  - Large (> 1–2 cm in size) multifocal, hyperintense, bilateral, asymmetric lesions in the supratentorial or infratentorial white matter. Rarely, brain MRI shows a single large (≥ 1–2 cm) lesion predominantly affecting white matter.
  - Gray matter, especially basal ganglia and thalamus, may be involved.
  - Spinal cord MRI may show confluent intramedullary lesion(s) with variable enhancement, in addition to the abnormalities on brain MRI.
  - No radiologic evidence of previous destructive white matter changes.
- **Suspect ADEM when:**
  - Close temporal relation to infection or vaccination.
  - MRI shows > 50% involvement of white matter; may also involve deep gray.
  - When enhancement present in majority of lesions.
  - Biopsy discouraged, but sometimes done for tumefactive/solitary lesions to exclude alternatives. ADEM shows perivascular infiltration macrophages and T cells; in very early stages, polymorphonuclear granulocytes; and demyelination restricted to perivascular area (unlike MS).

KEY FACT

Encephalopathy is a required feature for the diagnosis of ADEM, but is not a typical feature of multiple sclerosis. In addition, a cerebrospinal fluid pleocytosis ≥ 50 white blood cells/mm can be observed in ADEM, whereas this finding is highly atypical for multiple sclerosis.

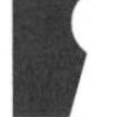

KEY FACT

Strict diagnostic criteria for ADEM are not established. Controlled treatment trials in ADEM have not been done.

Differential Diagnosis

- Viral, bacterial, or parasitic meningoencephalitis. (Herpes simplex encephalitis is a frequent clinical mimic.)
- Other vasculitic/autoimmune conditions:
  - Initial presentation of antiphospholipid antibody syndrome.
  - Primary CNS angiitis.
  - Systemic lupus erythematosus (SLE)-related vasculitis.
  - Neurosarcoidosis.
  - Behçet disease.
  - Primary or metastatic CNS neoplastic disease.
  - Mitochondrial leukoencephalopathy.

Treatment and Prognosis

- Variable success with:
  - IV corticosteroids
  - Oral immunosuppressants
  - Plasmapheresis
  - IVIG
  - Cytotoxic chemotherapy
- Full recovery in > 70%.
- Ten to 20% mild-moderate disability.
- Five percent mortality.
- Sudden severe polysymptomatic onset implies worse prognosis.

Isolated CNS Vasculitis (Granulomatous Angiitis of the Brain)

- Characteristic histologic lesions: Granulomatous lesions with multinucleated giant cells in small or large cerebral blood vessels.
- May involve spinal cord, or spinal cord disease may occur in isolation (spinal cord arteritis).
- Some association with herpes zoster ophthalmicus.
- Clinical course: Subacute progressive encephalopathy, dementia, headache, followed by mental obtundation.
- CSF pleocytosis (> 500 cells per HPF), elevated CSF protein (> 100 mg/dL).
- Cerebral angiography shows beading of the arteries.
- Brain and meningeal biopsy essential for diagnosis.
- Usually fatal within months to several years.
- Cytotoxic chemotherapy can be tried.

Eales Disease

Retinal perivasculitis characterized by inflammation and possible blockage of retinal blood vessels, abnormal growth of new blood vessels, and recurrent retinal and vitreal hemorrhages.

- Adult males, 20–35.
- Avascular regions in the retina, with microaneurysms, dilation of capillary channels, tortuosity of neighboring vessels, and spontaneous chorioretinal scars.
- Variable visual acuity, no known treatment.

NOTES

CHAPTER 5

Neurodegenerative Disorders

Saurav Das, MBBS
Adam Fleisher, MD, MAS
Michael S. Rafii, MD, PhD

Dementias

The National Institute on Aging–Alzheimer's Association (NIA-AA) core clinical criteria for diagnosis of all causes of dementia:

- Dementia is diagnosed when there are cognitive or behavioral (neuropsychiatric) symptoms that:
  - Interfere with the ability to function at work or at usual activities;
  - Represent a decline from previous levels of functioning and performing; and
  - Are not explained by delirium or major psychiatric disorder.
- Cognitive impairment is detected and diagnosed through a combination of (a) history taking from the patient and a knowledgeable informant and (b) an objective cognitive assessment—either a "bedside" mental status examination or neuropsychological testing.
  - Neuropsychological testing should be performed when the routine history and bedside mental state examination cannot provide a confident diagnosis.
  - The cognitive or behavioral impairment involves a minimum of 2 of the following domains:
    1. Impaired ability to acquire and remember new information. Symptoms include repetitive questions or conversations, misplacing personal belongings, forgetting events or appointments, getting lost on a familiar route.
    2. Impaired reasoning and handling of complex tasks, poor judgment. Symptoms include poor understanding of safety risks, inability to manage finances, poor decision-making ability, and inability to plan complex or sequential activities.
    3. Impaired visuospatial abilities. Symptoms include inability to recognize faces or common objects or to find objects in direct view despite good acuity, inability to operate simple implements, or orient clothing to body.
    4. Impaired language functions (speaking, reading, writing). Symptoms include difficulty thinking of common words while speaking, hesitations; speech, spelling, and writing errors.
    5. Changes in personality, behavior or comportment. Symptoms include uncharacteristic mood fluctuations such as agitation, impaired motivation, initiative, apathy, loss of drive, social withdrawal, decreased interest in previous activities, loss of empathy, compulsive or obsessive behaviors, and socially unacceptable behaviors.

ALZHEIMER DISEASE (AD)

Mrs. A, a 72-year-old woman, comes to the clinic complaining of increasing forgetfulness. She is accompanied by her husband, who is 77 years old and worked as an engineer. They live in their own house and have a son who works in Chicago and visits them occasionally. Mrs. A's husband states that she has been struggling with her memory for the past few months. She worked as a schoolteacher most of her life and used to be an outgoing person. However, she faces a profound word-finding difficulty now. The previous week, she got lost in the parking lot and had to call a friend to help her drive home. She has made frequent mistakes in paying the bills online. Mrs. A was always fond of cooking. However, they got really worried when they found that she left the kitchen stove turned on the night before. Mrs. A's husband feels that it was she who was the more careful of the two and such a behavior was very uncharacteristic of her. Therefore, they decided to see a doctor.

She slipped and fell down in the bathroom last week, hurting her knee, and has a slight limp on the left side. Mrs. A has a good level of hygiene. She takes a shower every day on her own and takes their dog for a walk. She has an insight to her memory problems. She occasionally gets frustrated in the course of conversation when she is unable to recall the correct word, but she is not depressed.

Mrs. A has a past history of hypertension, hyperlipidemia, coronary vascular disease, a cardiac stent, and osteoarthritis. Her current medications include simvastatin, atenolol, a baby aspirin, and analgesics. She has no known drug allergies. She does not smoke cigarettes or consume alcohol.

Differential diagnosis includes Alzheimer disease, dementia with Lewy bodies, frontotemporal dementia, vascular dementias, dementias from infection, a metabolic disorder such as hypothyroidism, B_{12} deficiency, neoplasms such as brain tumors, drugs and toxins such as effects of alcohol, repeated head trauma, normal pressure hydrocephalus, and pseudodementia. Additionally, dementia can be seen in late stages of Parkinson disease as well.

However, given her age, presentation, risk factors, and the prevalence of these diseases, the differentials can be narrowed to Alzheimer disease or vascular dementia. A brain imaging is done to rule out a cerebrovascular pathology. Management of Alzheimer disease is directed toward symptomatic relief. The patient can be started on acetylcholinesterase inhibitors such as donepezil. It is known to slow the progression of cognitive decline. If during the follow-up visits, a single-drug therapy is found inadequate, adding a new drug like memantine (NMDA receptor antagonist) should be considered.

Also, it is interesting to note the difference in patterns of memory loss in Mrs. A and her husband. It is also the difference between normal aging and pathological dementia.

Background

Alzheimer disease is the most common dementia in the United States. The prevalence is increasing due to an aging population. It is the sixth leading cause of death in the United States, and the fifth leading cause of death over the age of 65.

- Prevalence: > 5.4 million cases in the United States. This figure includes 5.2 million people aged 65 and older, and 200,000 individuals under the age of 65 have younger-onset Alzheimer disease.
- Incidence: The estimated annual incidence of Alzheimer disease appears to increase dramatically with age, from approximately 53 new cases per 1000 people age 65–74, to 170 new cases per 1000 people age 75–84, to 231 new cases per 1000 people over age 85.
- The US NIA-AA and International Working Group (IWG) have both contributed criteria for the diagnosis of AD that better define clinical phenotypes; and integrate biomarkers into the diagnostic process, covering the full staging of the disease.
- The National Institute on Aging–Alzheimer's Association (NIA-AA) classifies progression of AD into 3 stages:
  1. Preclinical stages
  2. Mild cognitive impairment
  3. Dementia due to AD

It also defines both core-clinical criteria (Figure 5.1) as well as research criteria incorporating biomarkers (Figure 5.2) to diagnose each of the above 3 stages.[1]

IWG criteria proposed in 2007 has now been refined to IWG-2 criteria in 2014. On the basis of these refinements, the diagnosis of AD can be simpli-

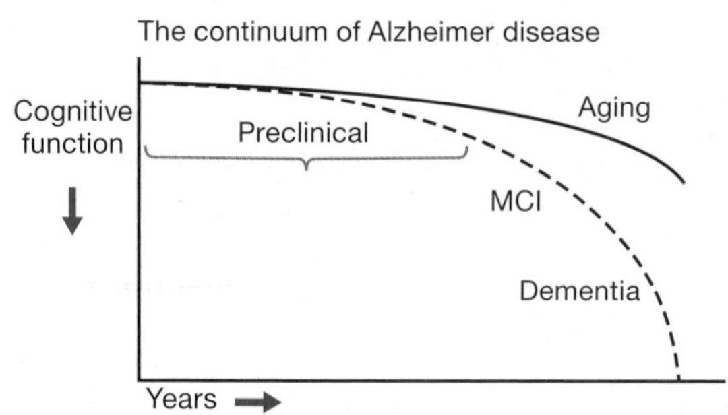

FIGURE 5.1. Clinical trajectory of Alzheimer disease (AD). Preclinical AD includes (a) presymptomatic autosomal dominant mutation carriers, (b) asymptomatic biomarker positive individuals at risk for progression to MCI due to AD and AD dementia, (c) biomarker positive individuals who have demonstrated subtle decline from their own baseline that exceeds the decline expected with typical aging, but would not meet the criteria for MCI.

fied, requiring the presence of an appropriate clinical AD phenotype (typical or atypical) and a pathophysiological biomarker consistent with AD pathology (such as decreased A-beta 1-42 and increased T Tau and P Tau in CSF; increased tracer retention on amyloid PET).

The current guidelines, therefore, define the criteria for the diagnosis of the following:

(a) Typical AD (amnestic syndrome of hippocampal type).
(b) Atypical forms of AD (posterior cortical atrophy, lopogenic variant, frontal variant, Down syndrome variant).
(c) Mixed AD (both clinical and biomarker evidence of AD + clinical and biomarker evidence of mixed pathology, eg, previous history of stroke or MRI evidence of vascular lesions in the brain; extrapyramidal signs, hallucinations, or abnormal dopamine transporter PET scan).
(d) Preclinical stages of AD:
    (i) Asymptomatic at risk = Absence of clinical phenotype, typical or atypical + in-vivo evidence of AD pathology.
    (ii) Presymptomatic = Absence of clinical phenotype, typical or atypical + proven autosomal dominant mutations including PSEN1, PSEN2, or APP, or other proven genes, including trisomy 21.

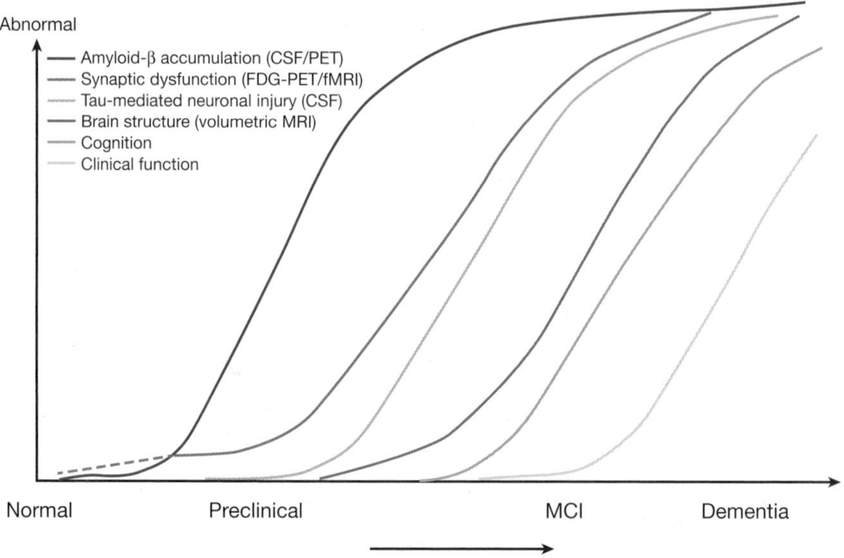

FIGURE 5.2. Biomarker trajectories for different stages of AD.

Atypical AD

It is diagnosed in the presence of *in vivo* evidence of AD pathology along with the presence of any of the following symptoms

1. Posterior variant
   (a) Occipito-temporal
   Visuoperceptive impairment: Impaired identification of objects, symbols, words and faces.
   (b) Biparietal
   Visuospatial function impairment: Symptoms of Gerstaman syndrome, Balint syndrome, limb apraxia, and neglect.
2. Lopogenic variant
   Single word retreival and sentence repitition problems with a spared semantic, syntactic, and motor speech.
3. Frontal variant
   Primary apathy and behavioral disinhibition.
4. Down syndrome variant.

Preclinical Stages of AD

The NIA-AA defines the diagnostic criteria encompassing biomarker, epidemiological, and neuropsychological evidence to define the preclinical phase of AD (Table 5.1). However, these recommendations are solely intended for research purposes and do not have any clinical implications.

MILD COGNITIVE IMPAIRMENT (MCI)

Background

- MCI is a neurodegenerative disorder that represents an incipient stage of dementia.
- It does not represent an extreme of normal aging.
- Early detection is the key to delaying progression to dementia.
  - Prevalence: 12–15% among nondemented subjects over the age of 65 years.
  - Incidence: 1% per year.

Classification

The criteria for "mild cognitive impairment (MCI) due to Alzheimer disease" as outlined in the NIA-AA diagnostic guidelines:

- Clinical diagnosis criteria[2]:
  1. Concern regarding a change in cognition (obtained from patient/informant/clinician).

TABLE 5.1. Stages of Preclinical AD

Stage	Description	Aβ (PET or CSF)	Markers of Neuronal Injury (tau, FDG, sMRI)	Evidence of Subtle Cognitive Change
Stage1	Asymptomatic cerebral amyloidosis	Positive	Negative	Negative
Stage 2	Asymptomatic amyloidosis + "downstream" neurodegeneration	Positive	Positive	Negative
Stage 3	Amyloidosis + neuronal injury + subtle cognitive/behavioral decline	Positive	Positive	Positive

AD, Alzheimer disease; Aβ, amyloid beta; PET, positron emission tomography; CSF, cerebrospinal fluid; FDG, fluorodeoxyglucose (18F); sMRI, structural magnetic resonance imaging.

2. Impairment in 1 or more cognitive domains (memory/executive function/attention/ language/visuospatial skills).
3. Preservation of independence in functional abilities.
4. Not demented (the impairment should be so mild that the patient has no evidence of significant social or occupational functioning).

Table 5.2 summarizes the NIA-AA research diagnosis criteria for classifying MCI.

- Original Petersen criteria:
  - Memory complaint, preferably qualified by an informant.
  - Memory impairment for age and education.
  - Preserved general cognitive function.
  - Intact activities of daily living.
  - Not demented.
- MCI subtypes and revised criteria (Figure 5.3): There must be a decline in cognitive function with preservation of most activities of daily living, but not meeting criteria for dementia.[3]
  - Amnestic MCI
  - Nonamnestic MCI

Pathophysiology

Patients with MCI often have similar pathology to those with AD; this is more likely in those with amnestic MCI. Patients with amnestic MCI typically have pathologic changes intermediate between normal and AD. Pathology in amnestic MCI usually consists of:

- Medial temporal lobe atrophy.
- Medial temporal lobe intracellular neurofibrillary tangles consisting of phosphorylated tau protein.
- Sparse diffuse extracellular neocortical beta amyloid plaques.

Investigations

- MCI patients typically progress to dementia at a rate of 10–15% per year.
- Severity of symptoms predicts rate of progression to dementia. Those with greater memory impairment or multiple-domain MCI progress to dementia more rapidly. Those with multiple-domain MCI also have worse overall survival rates.
- Hippocampal atrophy on MRI predicts progression to dementia. Ventricular and whole brain rates of change also predict conversion.

TABLE 5.2. NIA-AA Research Diagnosis Criteria for Classifying MCI

Diagnostic Category	Biomarker Probability of AD Etiology	Aβ (PET or CSF)	Neuronal Injury (tau, FDG, sMRI)
MCI–core clinical criteria	Uninformative	Conflicting/indeterminant/ untested	Conflicting/indeterminant/ untested
MCI due to AD—intermediate likelihood	Intermediate	Positive Untested	Untested
MCI due to AD—high likelihood	Highest	Positive	Positive
MCI—unlikely due to AD	Lowest	Negative	Negative

AD, Alzheimer disease; Aβ, amyloid beta; PET, positron emission tomography; CSF, cerebrospinal fluid; FDG, fluorodeoxyglucose (18F); sMRI, structural magnetic resonance imaging.

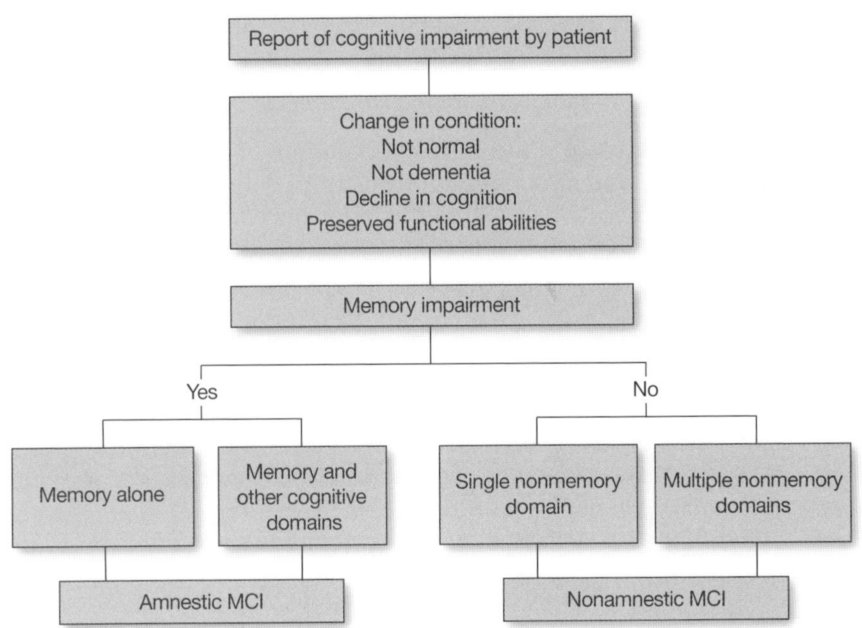

FIGURE 5.3. Amnestic versus nonamnestic MCI.

- The presence of 1 or more *APOE4* alleles predicts faster conversion to AD, although testing is currently not recommended.
- A combination of elevated cerebrospinal fluid (CSF) tau and low amyloid beta levels predicts more rapid progression to AD.
- FDG-PET (**2-deoxy-2[F-18]fluoro-D-glucose positron emission tomography**) hypometabolism in the parietal and temporal lobes likely predict progression to AD.
- Amyloid imaging shows AD-like patterns of uptake in some patients with MCI. It has been shown to distinguish normal from MCI and AD.
- The American Academy of Neurology recommends the following for all dementia evaluations:
  - Noncontrasted brain CT or MRI.
  - Screening for depression.
  - Testing for B_{12}/folate and thyroid deficiencies.
  - Screening for syphilis in high-risk populations only.

Treatment

- There are no FDA-approved treatments for MCI.
- Donepezil slows progression to AD for up to 18 months, and up to 24 months in those with the *APOE4* gene, but is not currently a recommended treatment.
- Vitamin E is not effective in slowing progression to AD.
- Rivastigmine, galantamine, and rofecoxib did not slow progression in clinical trials.
- No vitamins, supplements, or behavioral modifications have been shown to be effective in the treatment of MCI.

DEMENTIA DUE TO ALZHEIMER DISEASE (AD)

- NIA-AA criteria for the classification of dementia due to AD[4]:
  1. Probable AD dementia.
  2. Possible AD dementia.
  3. Probable or possible AD dementia with evidence of AD pathophysiological process.

- Core clinical criteria: Probable AD dementia is diagnosed when the patient:
  1. Meets criteria for all-cause dementia and, in addition, has following characteristics:
     (a) Insidious onset.
     (b) Clear-cut history of worsening of cognition by report or observation.
     (c) The initial and most prominent cognitive deficits are evident on history and examination in 1 of the following categories:
       - Amnestic presentation.
       - Nonamnestic presentations (including language, visuospatial presentation, or executive dysfunction).
     (d) The diagnosis of probable AD should *not* be applied when there is an evidence of:
       - Substantial concomitant cerebrovascular disease.
       - Core feature of dementia with Lewy bodies (DLB), other than dementia itself.
       - Prominent features of behavioral variant of FTD.
       - Prominent features of semantic variant primary progressive aphasia or nonfluent/agrammatic variant primary progressive aphasia.
       - Another concurrent, active neurological disease, or a non-neurological medical comorbidity or use of medication that could have a substantial effect on cognition.
- Possible AD dementia is diagnosed in either of the following circumstances:
  1. Atypical course: In terms of the nature of cognitive deficits for AD dementia, but either has a sudden onset of cognitive impairment or demonstrates insufficient historical detail or objective cognitive documentation of progressive decline, or
  2. Etiologically mixed presentation: Meets all core criteria for AD dementia but has evidence of concomitant cerebrovascular disease, DLB, another neurological disease or non-neurological medical comorbidity, or medication use that could have a substantial effect on cognition.
- Table 5.3 summarizes the NIA-AA research diagnostic criteria for AD dementia.

Pathophysiology

- **Cerebral atrophy:**
  - Begins in the entorhinal cortex and hippocampus.
  - Atrophy increases and spreads globally over time.
  - Typically spares the occipital lobe until late stages.
- **Histology:**
  - Global loss of neurons and synaptic connections.
  - Amyloid plaque deposition: The amyloid precursor protein (APP) is a transmembrane protein spliced by beta and gamma secretase to produce Aβ1-40 and Aβ1-42. Amyloid plaques are extracellular protein deposits made of up beta amyloid (Aβ) fragments consisting of Aβ1-40 and Aβ1-42. Aβ1-42 is the primary constituent of the amyloid plaque core. Diffuse plaques: Thought to be benign and often found in normal elderly. Compact plaques: Associated with neuritic changes caused by toxic effects to dendrites and axons. Cerebral amyloid angiopathy: Amyloid often deposits in blood vessels, increasing risk for hemorrhages in AD patients. Primary constituent is Aβ1-42.
- **Neurofibrillary tangles:**
  - Intracellular deposits starting in neurons in the entorhinal cortex and hippocampus, later spreading more globally.
  - Consist of paired helical filaments composed of hyperphosphorylated tau proteins.
- **Genetics:**
  - *APOE* Σ4: A lipid transport gene product found to significantly ↑ risk

TABLE 5.3. AD Dementia Research Diagnostic Criteria (Including Biomarkers)

Diagnostic Category	Biomarker Probability of AD Etiology	Aβ (PET or CSF)	Neuronal Injury (CSF tau, FDG-PET, sMRI)
Probable AD dementia			
Based on clinical criteria	Uninformative	Unavailable, conflicting, or indeterminate	Unavailable conflicting, or indeterminate
With 3 levels of evidence of AD pathophysiological process	Intermediate Intermediate High	Unavailable or indeterminate Positive Positive	Positive
Possible AD dementia (atypical clinical presentation)			
Based on clinical criteria	Uninformative	Unavailable, conflicting, or indeterminate	Unavailable, conflicting, or indeterminate
With evidence of AD pathophysiological process	High but does not rule out second etiology	Positive	Positive
Dementia unlikely due to AD	Lowest	Negative	Negative

AD, Alzheimer disease; Aβ, amyloid beta; PET, positron emission tomography; CSF, cerebrospinal fluid; FDG, fluorodeoxyglucose (18F); sMRI, structural magnetic resonance imaging.

of late-onset Alzheimer disease. This is by far the gene with the strongest association with sporadic late-onset AD. Fifteen percent of the population carries this allele. With 1 copy of *APOE* Σ4, there is a 50% chance of having AD by the mid to late 70s. With 2 copies of *APOE* Σ4, there is a 50% chance of having AD by the mid to late 60s. *APOE* Σ2 allele is protective against AD.

- Familial Alzheimer disease (FAD): Autosomal dominant inheritance. Typically early onset, late 30s to 60s. APP: Located on chromosome 21. Mutations cause FAD with onset at ages 40–60s. People with Down syndrome develop Alzheimer-type dementia typically by age 30–40. Presinilin 1 on chromosome 14. Involved in the gamma secretase complex. Mutations cause FAD with onset typically before age 40. Presinilin 2 on chromosome 1. Involved in the gamma secretase complex. Mutations cause FAD with onset typically before age 40. This mutation is quite rare compared to mutations in presinilin 1 and APP.

Risk Factors

- Age: At age 65, 1–2% of the population has AD; by age 85, 35–50% of people have AD.
- Head trauma: History of significant head trauma increases risk of AD.
- Education: Lower education predisposes to onset of AD.
- Sex: Controversial evidence shows women may be at slightly ↑ risk. Many feel this is an artifact of the fact that women typically live longer than men.

Investigations

- AAN guidelines for dementia workup:
  1. Structural neuroimaging using a computed tomography/magnetic resonance (CT/MR) scan is appropriate in initial evaluation.

2. Screening for depression, B_{12} deficiency, and hypothyroidism should be performed as a part of routine workup for all dementia.
3. Screening for syphilis in patients with dementia is *not* justified unless clinical suspicion for neurosyphilis is present.
4. The CSF 14-3-3 protein is useful for confirming or rejecting the diagnosis of Creutzfeldt-Jakob disease (CJD).

- FDG-PET scan is approved by Medicare to differentiate AD from frontotemporal dementia.
- Amyloid PET is approved to rule out fibrillar amyloid plaques associated with AD.
- CSF levels of Aβ and tau can be useful if clinical diagnosis is uncertain.
- If indicated by history or examination, sedimentation rate, hemoglobin A_{1C}, heavy metal screen, HIV testing can be done.

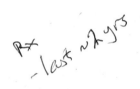

Treatment

Current approved therapies include (1) acetylcholinesterase inhibitors (including donepezil, rivastigmine, and galantamine) and (2) the NMDA receptor antagonist memantine.

- These drugs have demonstrated improvement above the baseline only in some patients; however, they delay the decline in most patients. Most patients benefit by slowed or halted decline for 1–2 years after treatment initiation.
- Acetylcholinesterase inhibitors: Increase acetylcholine levels in the basal forebrain and medial temporal lobe structures. These drugs are approved for mild to moderate AD. However, Aricept is approved for severe AD as well.
- Memantine: Inhibits glutamate at the NMDA receptor for neuroprotection. Indicated as add-on treatment to acetylcholinesterase inhibitors in moderate to severe AD.

The mechanism of action, indications, and the initial and maximum dose of administration for these drugs is summarized in Table 5.4.[5]

The common side effects associated with acetylcholinesterase inhibitors are broadly gastrointestinal, including nausea, vomiting, diarrhea, weight loss, loss of appetite, and muscle weakness. Side effects associated with memantine include dizziness, headache, constipation, and confusion.

TABLE 5.4. Treatment Recommendations for AD

Mechanism of Action		Cholinesterase Inhibitors		NMDA Receptor Antagonist
Drug	**Donepezil**	**Galantamine**	**Rivastigmine**	**Memantine**
Indication	Mild-moderate AD; severe AD	Mild-moderate AD	Mild-moderate AD	Moderate-severe AD
Initial dose	Tablet: 5 mg qd	Tablet/oral solution: 4 mg bid XR capsule: 8 mg qd	Capsule/oral solution: 1.5 mg bid Patch: 4.6 mg qd	Tablet/oral solution: 5 mg qd
Maximal dose	Tablet: 10 mg qd 23 mg (mod-sev)	Tablet/oral solution: 12 mg bid XR capsule: 16 or 24 mg qd	Capsule/oral solution: 6 mg bid Patch: 9.5 mg qd or 13.3 mg	Tablet/oral solution: 10 mg bid 28 mg XR qd

XR, extended release; MOA, mechanism of action; NMDA, *N*-methyl-D-aspartate.

DEMENTIA WITH LEWY BODIES

Dementia with Lewy bodies (DLB) is the second most common neurodegenerative dementia after Alzheimer disease. DLB is a diagnosis that now encompasses dementias that have combined AD pathology with Lewy bodies (Lewy body variant of AD [LBV]), and those with pure Lewy body pathology (pure diffuse Lewy body disease [pDLBD]). It does not include those with Parkinson disease that later develop dementia, Parkinson disease with dementia (PDD), although there is reason to believe that PDD and pDLBD may be the same disease with different presentations. In fact, they are quite difficult to distinguish clinically and pathologically in moderate to severe dementia.

Classification

- Central features (essential): Dementia with progressive cognitive decline of sufficient magnitude to interfere with social or occupational function. Memory impairment may not necessarily occur early but usually develops with progression. Deficits on tests of attention, executive function, and visuospatial ability may be present.
- Core features (2 or more = probable DLB, 1 = possible DLB):
  - Fluctuating cognition—pronounced variation in attention and alertness.
  - Recurrent visual hallucinations, typically wellformed and detailed.
  - Spontaneous parkinsonism.
- Suggested features (1 core + 1 suggestive = probable DLB; 0 core + 1 or more suggestive = possible DLB):
  - Rapid eye movement (REM) sleep behavior disorder.
  - Severe neuroleptic sensitivity.
  - Single-photon emission computed tomography (SPECT) or PET imaging showing low dopamine transporter activity in basal ganglia.
- Supportive features:
  - Repeated falls and syncope.
  - Transient, unexplained loss of consciousness.
  - Autonomic dysfunction.
  - Other types of hallucinations.
  - Systematized delusions.
  - Depression.
  - Relatively preserved medial temporal lobe structures on CT/MRI.
  - Low uptake on SPECT diffusion scan with ↓ occipital activation.
  - Low uptake on meta-iodo-benzyl-guanidine (MIBG) myocardial scintigraphy.
  - Prominent slow wave activity on electroencephalogram (EEG), with temporal lobe transient sharp waves.
- A diagnosis of DLB is less likely:
  - In the presence of stroke evident as focal neurologic signs or on brain imaging.
  - In the presence of other physical illness or brain disorder that can account in part or in total for the clinical picture.
  - If parkinsonism only appears first at a stage of severe dementia.
- Temporal sequence of symptoms:
  - DLB is diagnosed when dementia precedes or is concurrent with parkinsonism.
  - Parkinson disease dementia (PD-D) and Parkinson disease mild cognitive impairment (PD-MCI) should be used to describe dementia and MCI that occurs in the context of well-established Parkinson disease. The Movement Disorder Society Task Force has proposed a 2-level diagnostic criteria for PD-D and PD-MCI. For research studies that distinguish between DLB and PD-D, the 1-year rule that dementia

should begin no later than 1 year after onset of parkinsonism for a diagnosis of DLB is recommended. However, presence of 1 of the behavioral symptoms, including apathy, depressed or anxious mood, hallucinations, delusions, and excessive daytime sleepiness, supports the diagnosis of PD-D.

- Parkinsonism may be more subtle in DLB than in primary Parkinson disease.
  - Predominance of axial signs including gait difficulty and postural instability.
  - Tremor is less common.
- Age of onset is typically between 60 and 90 years.
- Slightly more common among men.
- LBV progresses more rapidly than AD, whereas pDLBD tends to progress more slowly than AD.
- Severe sensitivity to neuroleptic drugs is common. This may cause worsening psychosis or sedation.

Pathophysiology

- Lewy bodies are found in limbic and cortical regions in about 20% of patients with dementia, and restricted to the amygdalae in 20–30%.
- AD pathology often coexists with Lewy body pathology.
- Neocortical Lewy bodies consist of intracytoplasmic eosinophilic inclusions:
  - α-synuclein is the primary protein that makes up the Lewy body.
  - Lewy bodies stain with ubiquitin and anti-α-synuclein antibodies.
  - Usually located in cortical layers V and VI.
  - Most commonly found in the cingulated cortex, amygdala, and insular and frontal cortices, a distribution that correlates with mesolimbic dompaminergic projections.
  - Degeneration of the cholinergic projections result from interruption of basal forebrain neurons.

Investigations

- Primarily relies on the history and exam to meet the criteria outlined above.
- History for a caretaker is essential, as those with early dementia often have little insight or memory for the symptoms of their disease.
- MRI or CT should be used to rule out focal structural pathologies and vascular disease which may contribute to the clinical picture.
- Fluorodopa PET scanning or SPECT tracers with beta-citalopram can show low striatal dopamine transporter activity compared to AD.
- Fluordeoxyglucose PET and standard SPECT scanning have demonstrated hypometabolism in the occipital lobes, and may be suggestive of DLB or PDD.
- MIBG imaging of the heart has demonstrated ↓ sympathetic innervation in subjects with DLB but is not widely used for this clinical purpose.

Treatment

Few evidence-based treatments are available given the wide range of pathologies in DLB. In addition, there are no known disease-modifying drugs for DLB. Following are some basic guidelines:

- Many DLB patients also have AD pathology. Similar treatments for DLB are recommended for management of dementia symptoms.
- Patients with DLB are less likely to show a good response to levodopa

compared to PD or PDD. But these drugs should be tried to treat disabling parkinsonian symptoms.

- DLB patients tend to be very sensitive to side effects of CNS-active drugs. Therefore, start low and titrate slowly.
- Targeted therapy:
  - Cognitive impairment: Acetylcholinesterase inhibitors (AChEIs): Donepezil, rivastigmine, galantamine. Memantine as add-on therapy for moderate to severe dementia.
  - Hallucinations (these treatments may worsen parkinsonism): Risperidone, olanzapine, aripiprazole.
  - Insomnia: Trazodone, chloral hydrate.
  - Depression: Selective serotonin reuptake inhibitors (SSRIs).
  - Motor impairment: Levodopa/carbidopa: Risk of hallucinations, anxiety, agitation, and somnolence. Dopamine agonists: Avoid these medications due to significantly higher risk of hallucinations in DLB patients.

FRONTOTEMPORAL LOBAR DEMENTIA (FTLD)

- FTLD accounts for up to 20% of degenerative dementias.
- Prevalence: 15 per 100,000 persons between the ages of 45 and 64.
- It may be more common than AD in people younger than 60 years old.

Classification

- Commonly presents between ages 45 and 65, with 40% having a positive family history.
- Three phenotypic variants:
  - **Frontal/Behavioral variant of frontotemporal dementia (bvFTD/fvFTD):** 56% of all FTLD. Male predominance: 2:1. Earliest age of onset with a mean of 58 years at diagnosis. Most rapidly progressive (3.4 years from diagnosis to death). Twenty percent are autosomal dominant inheritance. Associated with amyotrophic lateral sclerosis (FTD with motor neuron disease: FTD-MND). Fifteen percent of patients with FTD develop ALS. Either ubiquitin or tau inclusion postmortem. Table 5.5 summarizes the Revised International Consensus Criteria for diagnosis of bvFTD.
  - **Semantic dementia (SD):** < 20% of FTLD. Similar age of onset to FTD. Slowest rate of progression (5.2 years from diagnosis to death). Most cases are sporadic without clear pattern of inheritability. Predominantly have ubiquitin staining inclusions postmortem.
    - Behavioral symptoms: Emotional withdrawal, depression, mental rigidity, compulsions.
    - Cognitive symptoms: Semantic knowledge breakdown: Poor naming, word recall, and word recognition. Long-term memory loss. Agnosia for faces and objects.
    - Neurologic symptoms: Late neurologic findings with atypical parkinsonism.
  - **Progressive nonfluent aphasia (NFA):** 25% of FTLD. Moderate progression (4.3 years from diagnosis to death). Less than 20% with genetic inheritance patterns. Associated with corticobasal degeneration (CBD) and progressive supranuclear palsy (PSP). Nearly all have tau inclusions on pathology.
    - Behavioral symptoms: Typically manifest late in disease. Normal insight and awareness. Social withdrawal, depression.
    - Cognitive symptoms: Changes in verbal fluency and pronunciation, word finding difficulties, agrammatism, and phonemic paraphasias.

TABLE 5.5. Revised International Criteria for bvFTD

I. Neurodegenerative disease

The following symptom must be present to meet criteria for bvFTD:

- A. Shows progressive deterioration of behavior and/or cognition by observation or history (as provided by a knowledgeable informant).

II. Possible bvFTD

Three of the following behavioral/cognitive symptoms (A–F) must be present to meet criteria. Ascertainment requires that symptoms be persistent or recurrent, rather than single or rare events.

- A. Early[a] behavioral disinhibition (one of the following symptoms [A.1–A.3] must be present):
  - A.1. Socially inappropriate behavior
  - A.2. Loss of manners or decorum
  - A.3. Impulsive, rash, or careless actions
- B. Early apathy or inertia (one of the following symptoms [B.1–B.2] must be present):
  - B.1. Apathy
  - B.2. Inertia
- C. Early loss of sympathy or empathy (one of the following symptoms [C.1–C.2] must be present):
  - C.1. Diminished response to other people's needs and feelings
  - C.2. Diminished social interest, interrelatedness, or personal warmth
- D. Early perseverative, stereotyped, or compulsive/ritualistic behavior (one of the following symptoms [D.1–D.3] must be present):
  - D.1. Simple repetitive movements
  - D.2. Complex, compulsive, or ritualistic behaviors
  - D.3. Stereotypy of speech
- E. Hyperorality and dietary changes (one of the following symptoms [E.1–E.3] must be present):
  - E.1. Altered food preferences
  - E.2. Binge eating, increased consumption of alcohol or cigarettes
  - E.3. Oral exploration or consumption of inedible objects
- F. Neuropsychological profile: Executive/generation deficits with relative sparing of memory and visuospatial functions (all of the following symptoms [F.1–F.3] must be present):
  - F.1. Deficits in executive tasks
  - F.2. Relative sparing of episodic memory
  - F.3. Relative sparing of visuospatial skills

III. Probable bvFTD

All of the following symptoms (A–C) must be present to meet criteria.

- A. Meets criteria for possible bvFTD
- B. Exhibits significant functional decline (by caregiver report or as evidenced by Clinical Dementia Rating Scale or Functional Activities Questionnaire scores)
- C. Imaging results consistent with bvFTD (one of the following [C.1–C.2] must be present):
  - C.1. Frontal and/or anterior temporal atrophy on MRI or CT
  - C.2. Frontal and/or anterior temporal hypoperfusion or hypometabolism on PET or SPECT

IV. Behavioral variant FTD with definite FTLD pathology

Criterion A and either criterion B or C must be present to meet criteria.

- A. Meets criteria for possible or probable bvFTD
- B. Histopathological evidence of FTLD on biopsy or at postmortem
- C. Presence of a known pathogenic mutation

V. Exclusionary criteria for bvFTD

Criteria A and B must be answered negatively for any bvFTD diagnosis. Criterion C can be positive for possible bvFTD but must be negative for probable bvFTD.

- A. Pattern of deficits is better accounted for by other nondegenerative nervous system or medical disorders
- B. Behavioral disturbance is better accounted for by other nondegenerative nervous system or medical disorders
- C. Biomarkers strongly indicative of Alzheimer disease or other neurodegenerative process

[a]As a general guideline, "early" refers to symptom presentation within the first 3 years.

bvFTD, behavioral variant FTD.

May have stuttering, impaired repetition, apraxia of speech. May develop impaired executive function and working memory.
- Neurologic symptoms: Supranuclear gaze problems, axial rigidity, alien limb, and focal dystonias.

PATHOPHYSIOLOGY

- Degeneration begins in the frontal and anterior temporal lobes.
- **Atrophy:**
  - FTD: Symmetric frontal and temporal lobe atrophy, with frontal more than temporal.
  - SD: Often asymmetric left frontal and temporal lobe atrophy, with temporal more than frontal, insula, amygdalae, and anterior hippocampus.
  - NFA: Asymmetric left frontal, insular, anterior parietal, and superior temporal cortices, with prominent the left perisylvian atrophy.
- A simple algorithm for bedside clinical assessment and syndromic diagnosis of progressive aphasias is summarized in Table 5.6.
- **Microscopic findings:**
  - Only a minority of patients will have classic "Pick's" pattern of pathology at autopsy.
  - Pick bodies: Tau protein deposits within ballooned neurons (Pick cells). Often found in amygdalae and hippocampus, paralimbic structures, ventral temporal cortex, and sometimes in the anterior frontal and dorsal temporal lobes.
  - Many FTLD patients have diffuse tau staining rather than distinct Pick bodies in the cortex of affected regions.
  - Some cases of FTLD show non-tau pathology, with ubiquitin staining neuronal changes. A protein called TAR-DNA-binding protein 43 (TDP-43) has been discovered to account for some ubiquitin staining in FTD patients. Loss of myelin and axons is seen in involved areas.
  - Loss of large pyramidal cells in cortical layer III and sometimes V. Loss of small pyramidal and nonpyramidal cells of layer II.
- **FTD-MND:**
  - Loss of large pyramidal cells, microvacuolation, and mild gliosis.
  - Substantia nigra is pale, with reactive fibrous astrocytosis.
  - Tau-negative, ubiquitin-positive inclusions in the frotal cortex and hippocampus (dentate gyrus).
  - Hypoglossal nucleus atrophy.

TABLE 5.6. Progressive Aphasias

TYPES[a]	BEDSIDE CLINICAL TEST
Progressive nonfluent aphasia	■ Effortful dysarthric speech ■ Expressive agrammatism Terse telegraphic phrasing with error in tense or function words
Logopenic progressive aphasia	Impaired phrase repetition (disproportionate to repetition of single polysyllabic words)
Semantic dementia	Impaired word comprehension Select a nominated item from an array or supply a definition
Atypical primary progressive aphasia	Pure anomia, disorders affecting language pathways other than speech, or pure dysprosody

[a]These diagnoses of the primary aphasias are made only after brain imaging to rule out the possibility of a nondegenerative brain lesion (eg, tumor).

- **Genetics:**
  - FTD has a substantial genetic component, with an autosomal dominant inheritance pattern or identifiable disease-causing mutations in around 10–20% of the patients who have some family history in a higher proportion.[6]
  - Most familial cases of FTD have mutations in the microtubule associated protein tau (**MAPT**), progranulin (**GRN**) genes, or the recently identified hexanucleotide repeat expansion in the **C9ORF72** gene. Less often, mutations in the gene encoding valosin containing protein (**VCP**) cause FTD in association with inclusion body myositis and Paget disease of bone.

Investigations

Rule out reversible dementias:

- Complete blood count.
- Chemistry panel.
- Vitamin B_{12}, folic acid levels.
- Thyroid function tests.
- CSF levels of Aβ and tau can be useful if clinical diagnosis is uncertain.
- If indicated by history or examination: sedimentation rate, hemoglobin A_{1C}, heavy metal screen, HIV testing, RPR for syphilis if in a high-risk population, CSF level of 1-4-3-3 protein to support diagnosis of Creutzfeldt-Jakob disease.
- Imaging:
  - CT or MRI for structure lesions and significant vascular disease and demonstrate atrophy patterns discussed above.
  - PET scan is approved by Medicare to differentiate AD from FTD. Frontal and temporal hypometabolism can be seen.
  - PET using amyloid-binding ligands is under development, which may result in methods for differentiating AD from FTLD.

Treatment

- There are no known effective treatments for FTLD.
- Acetylcholine esterase inhibitors are not indicated.
- SSRIs may improve compulsive behaviors and carbohydrate cravings.
- Atypical antipsychotics can improve aggressive and delusional behaviors.
- Avoid typical antipsychotics due to exacerbation of parkinsonism.
- Trazodone has shown benefit in behavioral management.

VASCULAR DEMENTIA

- Vascular dementia (VaD) is the second most common contributor to dementia after AD.
- Mixed dementia with AD and VaD is common.
- Lifetime risk of VaD is greater than AD.
- Twenty-five to 32% of people meet criteria for dementia 3 months after a stroke.
- Stroke increases risk of dementia by 2- to 4-fold.
- Age adjusted incidence rate: 14.6 per 1000 person-years (vs 19.2 per 1000 person-years for AD).
- Two times more common in African-Americans compared to whites.
- Mortality rate in VaD is likely higher than AD.
- Cognitive decline tends to be slower than AD.

Classification

The American Heart Association (AHA)/American Stroke Association (ASA) classifies vascular cognitive impairment into the following diagnoses:

1. Vascular mild cognitive impairment (VaMCI)
   - VaMCI
   - Possible VaMCI
   - Probable VaMCI
   - Unstable MCI
2. Vascular dementia (VaD)
   - VaD
   - Possible VaD
   - Probable VaD

A diagnosis of VaMCI is made only in patients who are not in delirium, are free of alcohol or any other substance abuse/dependence, and are free of any type of substance at least in the past 3 months.[7]

The diagnostic criteria for vascular cognitive impairment are summarized in Table 5.7.

- Hachinski criteria (1975):
  - Score of ≥ 7 suggests multi-infarct dementia.
  - Score of 5–6 suggests mixed AD/VaD.
  - Score ≤ 4 suggests nonvascular dementia.
  - Two points each: Abrupt onset cognitive symptoms, history of stroke, focal neurological signs, focal neurological symptoms.
  - One point each: Stepwise progression, nocturnal confusion, preservation of personality, depression, somatic complaints, emotional incontinence, hypertension, atherosclerosis.
- NINDS-AIREN (National Institute of Neurological Disorders and Stroke and Association Internationale pour la Recherché et l'Enseignement en Neurosciences, 1993): Used most often in clinical trials.
  - Probable VaD: Memory loss plus impairment in 2 other cognitive domains; focal signs on neurologic exam; imaging findings of vascular brain injury; and onset of dementia within 3 months after a recognized stroke or abrupt deterioration in cognitive function or fluctuating, stepwise progression of cognitive deficits.
  - Possible VaD: Imaging findings, temporal relationship, abrupt onset, or stepwise/fluctuating course.
- DSM-IV-TR (1994):
  - Memory loss sufficient to interfere with everyday function.
  - No clouding of consciousness.
  - Stepwise deteriorating course and "patch" distribution of deficits.
  - Focal neurologic signs and symptoms.
  - Evidence from the history, physical examination, or laboratory tests of cerebrovascular disease that is judged to be etiologically related to the disturbance.

Pathophysiology

- There are no consensus criteria for the pathological diagnosis of VaD.
- About 20% of elderly have silent infarcts that can → slow, subtle cognitive decline.
- Worsening of white matter hyperintensities correlates with decline in cognition and processing speed.
- Autopsy studies suggest a diagnosis of VaD should include:
  - Cortical infarcts in at least 3 areas of the parietal, frontal, or temporal lobes.
  - Excluding infarcts in the primary and secondary visual cortex.

TABLE 5.7. Vascular Cognitive Impairment

1. The term *VCI* characterizes all forms of cognitive deficits from VaD to MCI of vascular origin.
2. These criteria cannot be used for subjects who have an active diagnosis of drug or alcohol abuse/dependence. Subjects must be free of any type of substance for at least 3 months.
3. These criteria cannot be used for subjects with delirium.

Dementia

1. The diagnosis of dementia should be based on a decline in cognitive function from a prior baseline and a deficit in performance in ≥ 2 cognitive domains that are of sufficient severity to affect the subject's activities of daily living.
2. The diagnosis of dementia must be based on cognitive testing, and a minimum of 4 cognitive domains should be assessed: executive/attention, memory, language, and visuospatial functions.
3. The deficits in activities of daily living are independent of the motor/sensory sequelae of the vascular event.

Probable VaD

1. There is cognitive impairment and imaging evidence of cerebrovascular disease and
   a. There is a clear temporal relationship between a vascular event (eg, clinical stroke) and onset of cognitive deficits, or
   b. There is a clear relationship in the severity and pattern of cognitive impairment and the presence of diffuse, subcortical cerebrovascular disease pathology (eg, as in CADASIL).

Possible VaD

There is cognitive impairment and imaging evidence of cerebrovascular disease but

1. There is no clear relationship (temporal, severity, or cognitive pattern) between the vascular disease (eg, silent infarcts, subcortical small-vessel disease) and the cognitive impairment.
2. There is insufficient information for the diagnosis of VaD (eg, clinical symptoms suggest the presence of vascular disease, but no CT/MRI studies are available).
3. Severity of aphasia precludes proper cognitive assessment. However, patients with documented evidence of normal cognitive function (eg, annual cognitive evaluations) before the clinical event that caused aphasia *could* be classified as having probable VaD.
4. There is evidence of other neurodegenerative diseases or conditions in addition to cerebrovascular disease that may affect cognition, such as
   a. A history of other neurodegenerative disorders (eg, Parkinson disease, progressive supranuclear palsy, dementia with Lewy bodies);
   b. The presence of Alzheimer disease biology is confirmed by biomarkers (eg, PET, CSF, amyloid ligands) or genetic studies (eg, *PS1* mutation); or
   c. A history of active cancer or psychiatric or metabolic disorders that may affect cognitive function.

VaMCI

1. VaMCI includes the 4 subtypes proposed for the classification of MCI: amnestic, amnestic plus other domains, nonamnestic single domain, and nonamnestic multiple domain.
2. The classification of VaMCI must be based on cognitive testing, and a minimum of 4 cognitive domains should be assessed: executive/attention, memory, language, and visuospatial functions. The classification should be based on an assumption of decline in cognitive function from a prior baseline and impairment in at least 1 cognitive domain.
3. Instrumental activities of daily living could be normal or mildly impaired, independent of the presence of motor/sensory symptoms.

Probable VaMCI

1. There is cognitive impairment and imaging evidence of cerebrovascular disease and
   a. There is a clear temporal relationship between a vascular event (eg, clinical stroke) and onset of cognitive deficits, or
   b. There is a clear relationship in the severity and pattern of cognitive impairment and the presence of diffuse, subcortical cerebrovascular disease pathology (eg, as ain CADASIL).
2. There is no history of gradually progressive cognitive deficits before or after the stroke that suggests the presence of a nonvascular neurodegenerative disorder.

Possible VaMCI

There is cognitive impairment and imaging evidence of cerebrovascular disease but

1. There is no clear relationship (temporal, severity, or cognitive pattern) between the vascular disease (eg, silent infarcts, subcortical small-vessel disease) and onset of cognitive deficits.
2. There is insufficient information for the diagnosis of VaMCI (eg, clinical symptoms suggest the presence of vascular disease, but no CT/MRI studies are available).
3. Severity of aphasia precludes proper cognitive assessment. However, patients with documented evidence of normal cognitive function (eg, annual cognitive evaluations) before the clinical event that caused aphasia could be classified as having probable VaMCI.
4. There is evidence of other neurodegenerative diseases or conditions in addition to cerebrovascular disease that may affect cognition, such as
   a. A history of other neurodegenerative disorders (eg, Parkinson disease, progressive supranuclear palsy, dementia with Lewy bodies);
   b. The presence of Alzheimer disease biology is confirmed by biomarkers (eg, PET, CSF, amyloid ligands) or genetic studies (eg, *PS1* mutation); or
   c. A history of active cancer or psychiatric or metabolic disorders that may affect cognitive function.

Unstable VaMCI

Subjects with the diagnosis of probable or possible VaMCI whose symptoms revert to normal should be classified as having "unstable VaMCI."

VCI indicates vascular cognitive impairment; VaD, vascular dementia; MCI, mild cognitive impairment; CADASIL, cerebral autosomal dominant arteriopathy with subcortical infarcts and leukoencephalopathy; CT/MRI, computed tomography/magnetic resonance imaging; PET, positron emission tomography; CSF, cerebrospinal fluid; VaMCI, vascular mild cognitive impairment.

- Subcortical vascular dementia:
  - Isolated infarcts confined to subcortical regions are usually not sufficient to cause clinical dementia.
  - However, multiple small infarcts in the deep white matter can cause dementia (Binswager syndrome): Presents with severe confluent white matter changes with slowly progressive decline in cognition, urinary incontinence, and gait problems; thought to be caused by chronic white matter hypoperfusion.
  - Rare, strategically placed single, symptomatic, subcortical infarcts can cause dementia: Anterior or dorsomedial thalamus; genu of the internal capsule; head of the caudate; history of global cerebral hypoxic event at the time of stroke increases the risk of dementia.

INVESTIGATIONS

- Clinical evaluation should be the same as a standard dementia workup.
  - Rule out reversible dementias: Complete blood count; chemistry panel; vitamin B_{12}, folic acid levels; thyroid function tests; CT or MRI for structure lesions and significant vascular disease; CSF levels of Aβ and tau can be useful if clinical diagnosis is uncertain. If indicated by history or examination: sedimentation rate, hemoglobin A_{1C}, heavy metal screen, HIV testing, RPR for syphilis if in a high-risk population, CSF level of 1-4-3-3 protein to support diagnosis of Creutzfeldt-Jakob disease.
- There is no good evidence that *APOE* Σ4 is associated with VaD.
- Cognitive deficits present in a more varied fashion than Alzheimer disease. Memory, attention, executive function, language, visuospatial abilities, and learning may all be impacted in various degrees.
- Most common cognitive deficits include slowness of processing, poor mental flexibility, and working memory as opposed to short-term memory as seen in early AD.
- As a quick screen at the bedside, clinicians can focus on the following cognitive tests:
  - MMSE.
  - Letter fluency—number of "F" words in a minute (normal is > 12).
- Affective disorders should also be screened for.
- Cognitive symptoms based on cortical infarct territory:
  - Middle cerebral artery: Aphasia, neglect.
  - Anterior cerebral artery: Apathy, abulia, akinetic mutism.
  - Posterior cerebral artery: Amnesia, anomia, agnosia.
  - Subcortical infarcts and deep white matter infarcts: Interrupt fronto-subcortical networks, bradyphrenia, gait problems, executive dysfunction.

TREATMENT

Mainstay of management is stroke prevention:

- Blood pressure control: Most important modifying risk factor to reduce progression.
- Cholesterol lowering.
- Diabetic screening and management.
- Mediterannean diet and physical exercise.
- Smoking cessation.
- Aspirin or other antiplatelet agent.
- Among achetylcholine esterase inhibitors, donepezil can be useful for cognitive enhancement in patients of VaD, and galantamine is shown to benefit patients with mixed VaD and AD. The benefits of memantine and rivastigmine are not well established in VaD.

- Depression is often responsive to SSRIs.
- Cautious use of atypical antipsychotics for can be useful, but added extra-pyramidal symptoms can ↑ fall rates and should be monitored carefully.

NORMAL PRESSURE HYDROCEPHALUS (NPH)

An 80-year-old man presents to the clinic with a 6-week history of difficulty walking and worsening problems with memory. The patient's wife reports that he developed these problems approximately 2 months ago. The patient's wife says that he has great difficulty getting up from a chair and that once he gets up, he starts to shuffle slowly, as if it were a "frozen walking." She notes that he is quite unsteady even while standing still. The patient's memory problems are insidious in onset and gradually progressive. He had a major word-finding difficulty to start with and has progressed to a level where he is unable to perform his daily chores now. They started most prominently around the same time as the walking problem, 6 weeks ago. The patient is a known hypertensive and is on Lasix for that. He has no other significant past history. On review of systems, the patient's wife says that he developed urinary incontinence 1 month prior and has had frequent episodes every day. He has never had any such problem in the past nor has he been treated for a prostrate problem. He was first seen by his primary doctor and referred to a neurologist for further examination and evaluation. A CT scan of the brain demonstrates moderate ventriculomegaly in the setting of mild diffuse cortical atrophy.

The differential diagnosis here includes normal pressure hydrocephalus, Alzheimer disease, Parkinson disease, and vascular dementia. Benign prostratic hyperplasia is a common diagnosis in the elderly presenting with urinary incontinence. In our patient, the CT scan is most consistent with normal pressure hydrocephalus. Additionally, the workup should include a lumbar puncture with an opening pressure to evaluate for the presence of hydrocephalus. The upper limit of normal opening pressure is 180 mm of water.

The triad of dementia, gait apraxia, and urinary incontinence are classic for normal pressure hydrocephalus. The presence of pyramidal signs is a frequent finding on neurological examination. This patient's history, physical findings, and response to removal of CSF are in favor of the diagnosis. A large-volume lumbar puncture, withdrawing 30–50 cc of CSF, is often therapeutic. In this patient, if there is a response including improvement in his symptoms, then he may be a candidate for a ventriculoperitoneal shunt.

- Approximately 175,000 persons in the United States have NPH.
- Diagnosis should be considered based on clinical findings and imaging results.
- All the cardinal features of NPH are also common in the elderly in general, with multiple causes. This makes diagnosis of NPH challenging.

Classification

- It is important to evaluate the patient's general clinical health for surgical candidacy.
- Alcohol abuse worsens prognosis.
- If nonobstructive hydrocephalus is caused by previous subarachnoid hemorrhage, meningitis, prior brain surgery, or head injury, it will likely respond better to surgical shunting.

- Large head size may indicate congenital hydrocephalus that has become symptomatic later in life. Ten to 20% of elderly with hydrocephalus may have congenital hydrocephalus.
- Cardinal features: There are no consensus diagnoses established.
  - Gait difficulty: Typical "glue foot" or "magnetic gait" with difficulty initiating movement; however, there is no festination as seen in parkinsonism. If gait abnormality began first or at the same time as dementia, then the chance for improvement with surgical shunting is better.
  - Cognitive decline: If present for > 2 years, a response to surgery is unlikely. Characterized by psychomotor slowing, memory impairment, and executive functioning difficulty. Compared to AD, NPH scores better on orientation and delayed recall. Impaired, compared to AD, on attention and concentration measured by digit span, arithmetic, block design, and symbol/digit matching from the Wechler Memory Scale and Adult Intelligence Scale.
  - Urinary incontinence: Enlarged ventricles.
- Differential diagnosis:
  - Combinations of dementias, gait problems, and ventriculomegaly: Cervical spondylosis, arthritis, peripheral neuropathy, antipsychotic use, neurodegenerative dementia (AD, DLB, FTLD).
  - Cerebral vascular disease: Vascular dementia; strokes without dementia causing gait abnormalities or vestibular dysfunction; Binswanger disease with dementia, gait difficulty, and urinary incontinence.
  - Parkinson disease with dementia and ventriculomegaly.
  - Multiple systems atrophy, progressive supranuclear palsy, or corticobasal degeneration.

Pathophysiology (Figure 5.4)

- Normal ventricular enlargement can begin prior to age 60.
- Less than half of biopsies show arachnoid fibrosis.
- Typically, cortical biopsies show normal parenchyma.
- Close to one-third show AD pathology or vascular disease, consistent with the prevalence of these diseases in general elderly populations.
- Deep white matter hyperintensities are sometimes seen, but not likely associated to hydrocephalus directly. It is more likely that white matter disease is related to the effects of hypertension, which is increased in NPH patients. White matter hyperintensities are often associated with underlying gliosis, axonopathy, demyelination or vacuolization, but not necessarily infarctions.

Investigations

- Evaluate factors that could aggravate hydrocephalus:
  - Hypertension
  - Recent head injury
  - Sleep apnea
  - Congestive heart failure
  - Obesity
- Evaluate for causes of gait disturbance:
  - Arthritis
  - Cervical myelopathy
  - Visual impairment
  - Lumbar stenosis
  - Radiculopathy
  - Peripheral neuropathy
- Evaluate for other causes of dementia: AD, VaD

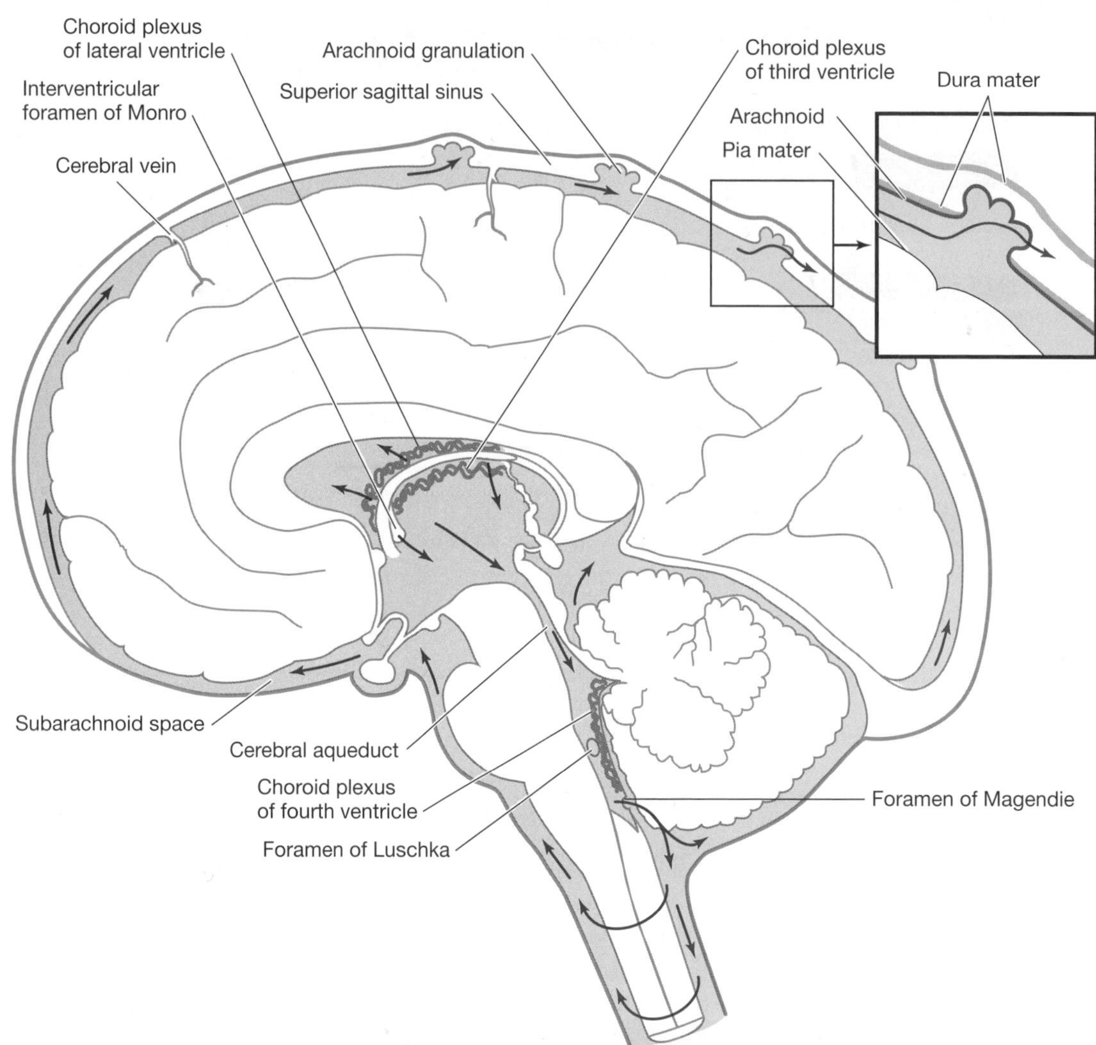

FIGURE 5.4. CSF flow in the brain. CSF is produced by the choroid plexus, which consists of specialized secretory tissue located within the cerebral ventricles. It flows from the lateral and third ventricles through the cerebral aqueduct and fourth ventricle and exits the ventricular system through 2 laterally situated foramina of Luschka and a single, medially located foramen of Magendie. CSF then enters and circulates through the subarachnoid space surrounding the brain and spinal cord. It is ultimately absorbed through arachnoid granulations into the venous circulation. (Reproduced, with permission, from Aminoff MJ, Greenberg, DA, Simon RP. *Clinical Neurology*, 6th ed. New York: McGraw-Hill, 2005: 405.)

- Examination:
  - Head circumference: If > 59 cm in men or 57.5 cm in women, suspect congenital hydrocephalus.
  - Evaluate for signs of other disease: Parkinsonism, predominant memory problems (AD, DLB), behavioral problems (FTD), focal neurologic signs (stroke, neuropathy).
  - Cognitive evaluation: Detailed neurocognitive testing can often distinguish AD from NPH patterns of cognitive deficits.
- Neuroimaging:
  - MRI is superior to CT, with the ability to better evaluate for aqueduct stenosis, cerebellar tonsil herniation, and brain stem infarcts. MRI can also be used to measure medial temporal lobe structures more accurately to differentiate NPH from AD.
  - Characteristic MRI findings (Figure 5.5): Ventriculomegaly: Evans ratio of > .31. Evans ratio is the ratio of the maximum width of the frontal horns of the lateral ventricles divided by the diameter of the skull measured from the 2 sides of the inner table at the same level. Relative

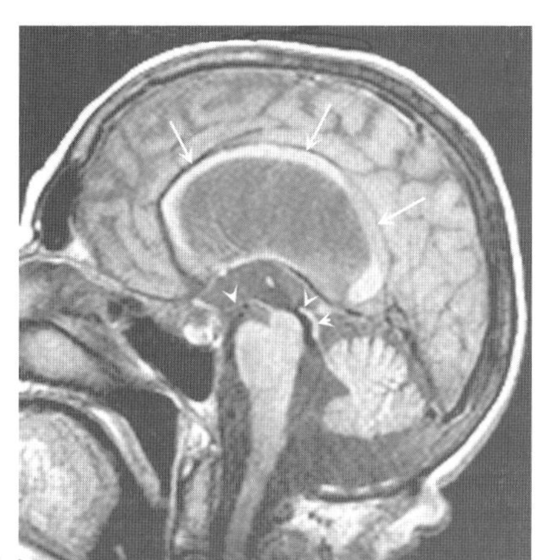
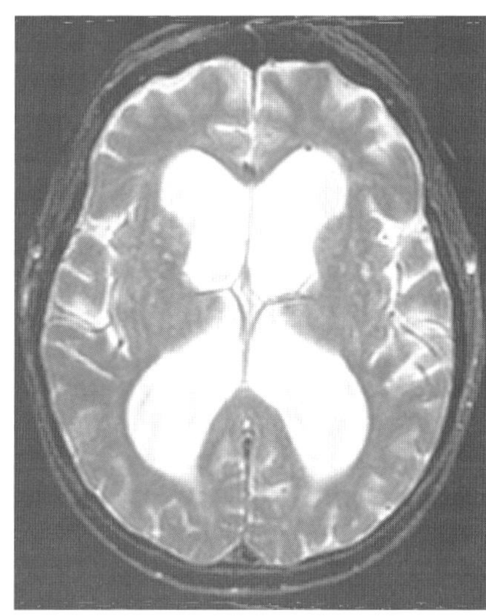

FIGURE 5.5. Normal pressure hydrocephalus. A: Sagittal T1-weighted MR image demonstrates dilatation of the lateral ventricle and stretching of the corpus callosum (arrows), depression of the floor of the third ventricle (single arrowhead), and enlargement of the aqueduct (double arrowheads). Note the diffuse dilatation of the lateral, third, and fourth ventricles with a patent aqueduct, typical of communicating hydrocephalus. **B:** Axial T2-weighted MR images demonstrate dilatation of the lateral ventricles without generalized cortical atrophy. This patient underwent successful ventriculoperitoneal shunting. (Reproduced, with permission, from Kasper DL, Braunwald E, Fauci AS, et al. *Harrison's Principles of Internal Medicine*, 16th ed. New York: McGraw-Hill, 2004: 1143.)

lack of global atrophy. Presence of global atrophy or disproportionate medial temporal lobe atrophy does not exclude NPH; however, it may implicate comorbid AD. "Thinning" or elevation of the corpus callosum. Distention of the third ventricle. Dilated aqueduct of Sylvius is often seen. Look for structural causes associated with congenital hydrocephalus: Arnold Chiari malformations, lack of white matter abnormalities, aqueductal stenosis. Temporal horn enlargement can be seen in both NPH and AD: Measurements of CSF flow with techniques such as cine MRI, have not proven to be strong predictors of surgical outcome. Cisternography showing presence of radioisotope in the ventricles 48–72 hours after lumbar injection has not proven to be a consistent predictor of good surgical outcome.

- Large-volume CSF drainage from lumbar puncture:
  - Gait improvement after drainage of 30–50 cc of CSF indicates good surgical candidacy for ventriculoperitoneal shunting.
  - High specificity but low sensitivity.
- Prolonged CSF drainage and pressure monitoring by lumbar catheterization:
  - CSF drainage of about 10 cc per hour over 2–3 days with repeated gait and cognitive testing.
  - Pressure monitoring can be done to evaluate for transient B-waves, implicating transient spikes in CSF pressure. Adding this to clinical evaluation does not clearly improve prediction of shunt success.
  - Sensitivity 50–100% for successful response to shunting.
  - Specificity 60–100%.
  - Positive predictive value 80–100%.
  - Higher–risk procedure than drainage by lumbar puncture. Risks include meningitis, nerve root irritation, subdural hemorrhage if drainage occurs too fast.
  - Should be performed only at a center with experience placing and managing CSF drains.

- CSF infusion testing:
  - Infusion of fluid by lumbar puncture needle to assess resistance levels.
  - Resistance at ≥ 18 mm Hg/mL/min predicts good shunting response.

Treatment

- The only treatment for NPH is ventriculoperitoneal shunting.
- There is an ↑ prevalence of systemic hypertension in those with NPH. The causal relationships between hypertension and NPH are unknown. Nonetheless, hypertension should be evaluated for and treated in all patients with NPH.
- Improvement can be assessed by objective measures of gait change, activities of daily living (such as the Katz index or the Rankin scale).
- Ventriculoperitoneal shunting:
  - Sustained improvement can be seen in gait at 3 years postsurgery in about 75% of cases.
  - Cognitive improvement seen in up to 80% at 3 years.
  - Improved urinary incontinence seen in over 80% at 3 years.
  - Predictive factors:
    1. Favoring postshunt improvement: Gait disturbance preceding cognitive problems; mild cognitive deficits; short duration of cognitive deficits; clinical improvement after lumbar drainage; CSF flow resistance of ≥ 18 mm Hg/mL/min during CSF infusion test; presence of B waves ≥ 50% of time during continuous lumbar CSF monitoring.
    2. Not favoring postshunt improvement: Moderate to severe cognitive impairment; dementia for > 2 years; cognitive impairment preceding gait disturbance; presence of aphasia; history of alcohol abuse; MRI showing significant white matter involvement or diffuse cerebral atrophy.
  - Known shunting complications: Risks of general anesthesia; acute intracerebral hemorrhage; infection of shunt; subdural hygroma or hematoma; seizures; shunt malfunctions; headaches; hearing loss; tinnitus; oculomotor palsies; damage to intra-abdominal organs.

OTHER DEMENTIAS

- There are many less common causes of dementia, many of which are treatable (Table 5.8).
- Atypical dementia presentations such as rapid onset, early presentation, or unusual neurological features should raise the suspicion of less common causes of dementia.
- Certain risk populations warrant further workup for uncommon dementia. These may include family history or risky sexual practices, for example.
- The American Academy of Neurology recommends routine testing only during initial dementia evaluations for 3 common causes of cognitive impairment. Although cognitive impairment in these disorders is rare, the disorders are quite common and treatable.
  - Vitamin B_{12} deficiency
  - Hypothyroidism
  - Depression
- Each less common cause of dementia requires specific evaluations and management, which should be guided by clinical suspicion and based on a thorough history and exam.

TABLE 5.8. Less Common Causes of Dementia

Vitamin deficiencies
- Thiamine (B_1): Wernicke encephalopathy[a]
- B_{12} (pernicious anemia)[a]
- Nicotinic acid (pellagra)[a]

Endocrine and other organ failure
- Hypothyroidism[a]
- Adrenal insufficiency and Cushing syndrome[a]
- Hypo- and hyperparathyroidism[a]
- Renal failure[a]
- Liver failure[a]
- Pulmonary failure[a]

Chronic infections
- HIV
- Neurosyphilis[a]
- Papovavirus (progressive multifocal leukoencephalopathy)
- Prion (Creutzfeldt-Jakob and Gerstmann-Sträussler-Scheinker diseases)
- Tuberculosis, fungal, and protozoal[a]
- Sarcoidosis[a]
- Whipple disease[a]

Head trauma and diffuse brain damage
- Dementia pugilistica
- Chronic subdural hematoma[a]
- Postanoxia
- Postencephalitis
- Normal pressure hydrocephalus[a]

Neoplastic
- Primary brain tumor[a]
- Metastatic brain tumor[a]
- Paraneoplastic limbic encephalitis

Toxic disorders
- Drug, medication, and narcotic poisoning[a]
- Heavy metal intoxication[a]
- Dialysis dementia (aluminum)
- Organic toxins

Psychiatric
- Depression (pseudodementia)[a]
- Schizophrenia[a]
- Conversion reaction[a]

Degenerative disorders
- Huntington disease
- Progressive supranuclear palsy
- Corticobasal degeneration
- Multiple systems atrophy
- Hereditary ataxias (some forms)
- Motor neuron disease (amyotrophic lateral sclerosis [ALS])
- Multiple sclerosis
- Adult Down syndrome with Alzheimer
- ALS-Parkinson-dementia complex of Guam

Miscellaneous
- Vasculitis[a]
- Cerebral autosomal dominant arteriopathy with subcortical infarcts and leukoencephalopathy (CADASIL)
- Acute intermittent porphyria[a]
- Recurrent nonconvulsive seizures[a]

Additional conditions in children or adolescents
- Hallervorden-Spatz disease
- Subacute sclerosing panencephalitis
- Metabolic disorders (eg, Wilson and Leigh diseases, leukodystrophies, lipid storage diseases, mitochondrial mutations)

[a] Potentially reversible.

Adapted, with permission, from Fauci AS, Braunwald E, Kasper DL, et al. *Harrison's Principles of Internal Medicine,* 16th ed. New York: McGraw-Hill, 2007: 1254.

PARKINSON DISEASE

A 58-year-old right-handed man presents with a tremor in his right hand. Over the past year, the patient has noticed a worsening tremor in his right hand. His tremor is most noticeable when he is walking or watching television. It gets worse when he is at a restaurant and eating. It is not relieved by alcohol and disappears when he is playing tennis and golf. He has a history of hypertension and has had an appendectomy. Medications include metoprolol 50 mg twice a day. He has no known drug allergies.

The patient most likely has a diagnosis of idiopathic Parkinson disease with the cardinal findings of tremor, bradykinesia, rigidity, loss of postural reflexes, and freezing phenomena. Freezing postural instability and bradykinesia are grouped as negative phenomena, and are more disabling than the tremor and rigidity, which are positive phenomena. Unfortunately, the negative symptoms do not respond well to treatment. Masked facies, micrographia, ↓ glabellar reflex, stooped posture, ↓ arm swing, and difficulties with pivot turns are all associated features of the disease, sometimes beginning asymmetrically or unilaterally; however, as the disease progressed, the motor symptoms worsened and often became resistant to treatment. Autonomic symptoms may appear, involving constipation and orthostasis, and cognitive ineffective symptoms such as depression may also develop.

The first test to order would be an MRI to rule out structural findings, such as a mass that might → similar symptoms. In addition, the MRI would help rule out vascular parkinsonism, which occurs with strokes in the basal ganglia.

- Most frequent neurodegenerative movement disorder.
- Prevalence of 1–3% in people older than 55.
- Slight male predominance.
- Pathologic feature is Lewy bodies in the substantia nigra.
- Majority of cases are sporadic, but more than 10% of cases are familial, with an autosomal dominant inheritance as in the rare cases with α-synuclein mutations, or autosomal recessive as in cases with parkin gene or DJ-1 gene mutations in juvenile parkinsonism.
- Diagnosis of PD is based on clinical criteria. In addition to motor syndrome, PD patients present different nonmotor manifestations, including:
  - Neuropsychiatric disturbances
  - Autonomic dysfunction
  - Abnormalities in olfactory perception
  - Sensory symptoms
  - Sleep disorders
- **Motor syndrome:** Cardinal clinical features of PD include:
  - Bradykinesia
  - Rigidity
  - Resting tremor
  - Gait
  - Postural reflex abnormalities
- **Nonmotor syndrome:** Disturbances of cognition and emotion are common. The most frequent neuropsychiatric symptoms are:
  - Depression
  - Visual hallucinations
  - Anxiety
- In PD patients, prevalence of dementia has been estimated as 25–30%. Dementia is "subcortical" type.
- Sexual dysfunction due to both loss of libido and impotence, and urinary symptoms such as urgency, frequency, and incontinence of urine are also common complaints.
- In late stages of the disease, PD may cause complications such as choking, pneumonia, and falls that can → death.

Treatment

- **Carbidopa/levodopa:**
  - Most widely used form of treatment is L-dopa, which is transformed into dopamine in the dopaminergic neurons by L-aromatic amino acid decarboxylase (often known by its former name dopa-decarboxylase).
  - Only 1–5% of L-dopa enters the dopaminergic neurons. The remaining L-dopa is often metabolized to dopamine elsewhere, causing a wide variety of side effects.

  - Carbidopa and benserazide are dopa decarboxylase inhibitors. They help to prevent the metabolism of L-dopa before it reaches the dopaminergic neurons and are generally given as combination preparations of carbidopa/levodopa (eg, Sinemet, Parcopa).
- **Catechol-O-methyl transferase (COMT) inhibitors:** Tolcapone inhibits the COMT enzyme, thereby prolonging the effects of L-dopa, and so has been used to complement L-dopa. However, due to its possible side effects such as liver failure, its availability is limited.
- **Dopamine agonists:**
  - The dopamine agonists bromocriptine, pergolide, pramipexole, ropinirole, cabergoline, apomorphine, and lisuride are moderately effective.
  - These have their own side effects, including those listed above in addition to somnolence, hallucinations, and/or insomnia.
  - Several forms of dopamine agonism have been linked with a markedly ↑ risk of problem gambling and hypersexuality.
  - Dopamine agonists initially act by stimulating some of the dopamine receptors.
- **Symptomatic therapy:**
  - Levodopa, coupled with a peripheral decarboxylase inhibitor (PDI), remains the standard of symptomatic treatment for PD. It provides the greatest antiparkinsonian benefit with the fewest adverse effects in the short term.
  - Dopamine agonists provide symptomatic benefit comparable to levodopa/PDI in early disease but lack sufficient efficacy to control signs and symptoms by themselves in later disease.
  - Dopamine agonists cause more sleepiness, hallucinations, and edema than levodopa.
  - Prospective, double-blind studies have demonstrated that initial treatment with a dopamine agonist, to which levodopa can be added as necessary, causes fewer motor fluctuations and dyskinesias than levodopa alone.
- **Monoamine oxidase-B (MAO-B) inhibitors:**
  - Selegiline and rasagiline reduce the symptoms by inhibiting (MAO-B), which inhibits the breakdown of dopamine secreted by the dopaminergic neurons.
  - Metabolites of selegiline include L-amphetamine and L-methamphetamine (not to be confused with the more notorious and potent dextrorotary isomers).
  - Unlike other nonselective MAO inhibitors, tyramine-containing foods do not cause a hypertensive crisis.
- **Surgery and deep brain stimulation.**
- **Deep brain stimulation (DBS):**
  - FDA-approved treatment for PD.
  - Consists of an electrical lead being implanted into the targeted brain structure (thalamus, GPi, STN).
  - Lead is connected to an implantable pulse generator (IPG) implanted in the subclavicular region of the chest cavity.
  - Lead and IPG are connected by extension wire that is tunneled down the neck under the skin.
  - DBS provides monopolar or bipolar electrical stimulation to the targeted brain area.
  - Stimulation amplitude, frequency, and pulse width adjusted to control symptoms and eliminate adverse events.
  - Patient controls stimulator off using a handheld magnet.
  - Mechanism of action is resetting abnormal firing patterns.
  - The response from DBS is only as good as the patient's best on-time with the exception of tremor, which may have greater improvement than with medication.

Ataxias

FRIEDREICH ATAXIA

- Friedreich ataxia is a progressive disorder with significant morbidity.
- Loss of ambulation typically occurs 15 years after disease onset.
- More than 95% of patients are wheelchair bound by age 45 years.
- Cardinal features include progressive limb and gait ataxia, dysarthria, loss of joint position and vibration senses, absent tendon reflexes in the legs, and extensor plantar responses.
- Onset of Friedreich ataxia is early in life, with gait ataxia being the usual presenting symptom, and lower extremities are affected equally.
- Some patients may have hemiataxia initially before the symptoms become generalized.
- Gait ataxia manifests as progressively slow and clumsy walking, which often begins after normal walking has developed. The ataxia may be associated with difficulty standing and running.
- The gait ataxia is of both a sensory and a cerebellar type.
- The cerebellar features of gait ataxia in Friedreich ataxia include a wide-based gait with constant shifting of position to maintain balance. Sitting and standing are associated with titubation.
- The sensory ataxia resulting from a loss of joint position sense contributes to the wide-based stance and gait but a steppage gait also is present, characterized by uneven and irregular striking of the floor by the bottom of the feet.
- As the disease progresses, ataxia affects the trunk, legs, and arms. As the arms become grossly ataxic, both action and intention tremors may develop. Titubation of the trunk may appear.
- Facial, buccal, and arm muscles may become tremulous and occasionally display choreiform movements.

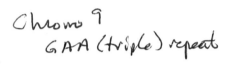

Pathophysiology

- "Dying back phenomenon" of axons, beginning in the periphery with ultimate loss of neurons and a secondary gliosis.
- The primary sites of these changes are the spinal cord and spinal roots.
- This results in loss of large, myelinated axons in peripheral nerves, which increases with age and disease duration.
- Unmyelinated fibers in sensory roots and peripheral sensory nerves are spared.
- The posterior columns and corticospinal, ventral, and lateral spinocerebellar tracts all show demyelination and depletion of large, myelinated nerve fibers to differing extents.
- The corticospinal tracts are relatively spared down to the level of the cervicomedullary junction, below which they are severely degenerated and become progressively more severe moving down the spinal cord.
- This explains the common finding of bilateral extensor plantar responses and weakness late in the disease.

Investigations

The cardinal features of Friedreich ataxia are as follows:

- Progressive limb and gait ataxia develops before the age of 30 years.
- Lower extremity tendon reflexes are absent.
- Evidence of axonal sensory neuropathy is noted.
- Dysarthria, areflexia, motor weakness of the lower extremities, extensor plantar responses, and distal loss of joint position and vibration senses are not found in all patients within the first 5 years, but are eventually universal.

- Foot deformity, scoliosis, diabetes mellitus, and cardiac involvement are other common characteristics. Clinical evidence of ventricular hypertrophy, systolic ejection murmurs, and third or fourth heart sounds may be noted.
- Genetic test to verify the GAA repeat expansion on chromosome 9.

TREATMENT

None.

SPINOCEREBELLAR ATAXIAS

- Spinocerebellar ataxia (SCA) is one of a group of genetic disorders characterized by slowly progressive incoordination of gait and often associated with poor coordination of hands, speech, and eye movements. Frequently, atrophy of the cerebellum occurs. See Table 5.9 for genetic and clinical features of hereditary spinocerebellar ataxias.
- As with other forms of ataxia, SCA results in unsteady and clumsy motion of the body due to a failure of the fine coordination of muscle movements, along with other symptoms.
- The symptoms of the condition vary with the specific type (there are several), and with the individual patient. Generally, a person with ataxia retains full mental capacity but may progressively lose physical control.

Dystonias

- Dystonia consists of sustained or repetitive involuntary muscle contractions, frequently causing twisting movements with abnormal postures.
- Dystonia can range from minor contractions in an individual muscle group to severe and disabling involvement of multiple muscle groups.
- The frequency is estimated at 300,000 cases in the United States but is likely greater since many cases are not recognized.
- Dystonia is often initially brought out by voluntary movements (action dystonia) and can later become sustained and extend to other body regions.

PRIMARY TORSION DYSTONIA

- Idiopathic torsion dystonia (ITD), or Oppenheim dystonia, is predominantly a childhood-onset form of dystonia with an autosomal dominant pattern of inheritance that primarily affects Ashkenazi Jewish families.
  - Typically begins in a foot or arm and can progress to involve the other limbs as well as the head and neck.
  - In severe cases, patients can suffer disabling postural deformities. Severity can vary even within a family, with some affected relatives having mild dystonia that may not even have been appreciated.
- Dopa-responsive dystonia (DRD) or the Segawa variant (DYT5) is a dominantly inherited form of childhood-onset dystonia due to a mutation in the gene that encodes for guanosine triphosphate (GTP) cyclohydrolase I, the rate-limiting enzyme for the synthesis of tetrahydrobiopterin.
  - DRD typically presents in early childhood (1–12 years) and is characterized by foot dystonia that interferes with walking. Patients often experience diurnal fluctuations, with worsening of gait as the day progresses and improvement with sleep.
  - DRD is typified by an excellent and sustained response to small doses of levodopa. Some patients may present with parkinsonian features but

TABLE 5.9. Genetic and Clinical Features of Hereditary Spinocerebellar Ataxias

Disease	Gene	Protein	Gene Defect	Syndrome
Autosomal recessive				
Friedreich ataxia	*FRDA1*	Frataxin	GAA_n[a]	Childhood onset, ataxia, dysarthria, pyramidal signs, neuropathy, scoliosis, cardiomyopathy, diabetes
Autosomal dominant				
SCA1	*SCA1*	Ataxin-1	CAG_n	ADCA I[b]
SCA2	*SCA2*	Ataxin-2	CAG_n	ADCA I
SCA3/MJD	*SCA3*	Ataxin-3	CAG_n	ADCA I
SCA4	*SCA4*	Unknown	Unknown	ADCA I
SCA5	*SCA5*	Unknown	Unknown	ADCA III
SCA6	*CACNL1A 4*	Ca channel P/Q-type voltage-gated calcium channel, 1A- subunit	CAG_n	ADCA III
SCA7	*SCA7*	Ataxin-7	CAG_n	ADCA II
SCA8	*SCA8*	Unknown	CTG_n	ADCA I
SCA10	*SCA10*	Ataxin-10	$ATTCT_n$	ADCA III
SCA11	*SCA11*	Unknown	Unknown	ADCA III
SCA12	*PPP2R2B*	PPase2 Protein phosphatase 2, regulatory subunit B, isoform	CAG_n	ADCA I
SCA13	*SCA13*	Unknown	Unknown	Childhood onset, ataxia, and mental retardation
SCA14	*PRKCG*	PKC	Missense	ADCA III
SCA15	*SCA15*	Unknown	Unknown	ADCA III
SCA16	*SCA16*	Unknown	Unknown	ADCA III
SCA17	*TBP*	TATA-binding protein	CAG_n	ADCA I
SCA18	*SCA18*	Unknown	Unknown	Ataxia, muscle atrophy, sensory deficit
SCA19	*SCA19*	Unknown	Unknown	Ataxia, mild cognitive defect
SCA20	*SCA20*	Unknown	Unknown	Ataxia, dysphonia, palatal tremor
SCA21	*SCA21*	Unknown	Unknown	Ataxia, extrapyramidal signs
SCA22	*SCA22*	Unknown	Unknown	ADCA III
SCA23	*SCA23*	Unknown	Unknown	Ataxia, tremor, dyskinesia
SCA + tremor	*FGF14*	Fibroblast growth factor-14	Missense	ADCA I
SCA25	*SCA25*	Unknown	Unknown	Ataxia, sensory neuropathy

MJD, Machado-Joseph disease (same as SCA3); PKC, protein kinase C, gamma subunit; SCA, spinocerebellar ataxia.

[a] XYZ_n, expanded XYZ trinucleotide repeat; $VWXYZ_n$, expanded VWXYZ pentanucleotide repeat.

[b] ADCA I includes ataxia, dysarthria, pyramidal signs, extrapyramidal signs, ophthalmoplegia, and dementia; ADCA II includes ataxia, dysarthria, and pigmentary maculopathy; ADCA III includes ataxia, dysarthria, and sometimes mild pyramidal signs.

Adapted, with permission, from Aminoff MJ, Greenberg, DA, Simon RP. *Clinical Neurology,* 7th ed. New York: McGraw-Hill, 2009: 234.

can be differentiated from juvenile PD by normal striatal fluorodopa uptake on PET and the absence of levodopa-induced dyskinesias.

- DRD patients may occasionally present with spasticity, ↑ reflexes, and Babinski responses and be misdiagnosed as cerebral palsy.

- Focal dystonias: These are the most common forms of dystonia. They typically present in the fourth to sixth decades and affect women more than men. The major types are:

- Blepharospasm: Dystonic contractions of the eyelids with ↑ blinking that can interfere with reading, watching TV, and driving.
- Oromandibular dystonia (OMD): Contractions of muscles of the lower face, lips, tongue, and jaw (opening or closing). Meige syndrome is a combination of OMD and blepharospasm that predominantly affects women over the age of 60 years.
- Spasmodic dysphonia: Dystonic contractions of the vocal cords during phonation, causing impaired speech. Most cases affect the adductor muscles and cause speech to have a choking or strained quality. Less commonly, the abductors are affected, → speech with a breathy or whispering quality.
- Cervical dystonia: Dystonic contractions of neck muscles, causing the head to deviate to one side (torticollis), in a forward direction (anterocollis), or in a backward direction (retrocollis). Muscle contractions can be painful and associated with dystonic tremor and a secondary cervical radiculopathy.
- Limb dystonias: These can be present in either arms or legs and are often brought out by task-specific activities such as handwriting (writer's cramp), playing a musical instrument (musician's cramp), or putting in golf (the yips).
- Focal dystonias can extend to involve other body regions (~30% of cases) and are frequently misdiagnosed as psychiatric or orthopedic problems. Their cause is not known, but genetic factors, autoimmunity, and repeated trauma have been implicated.

HUNTINGTON DISEASE (HD)

HD is a genetic, autosomal dominant, neurodegenerative disorder characterized clinically by disorders of movement, progressive dementia, and psychiatric and/or behavioral disturbance.

Pathophysiology

HD is associated with an excessive sequence of CAG repeats in the *IT15* gene located on arm 4p; researchers are looking into which chromosome contains that gene. The *HD* gene codes for a protein called huntingtin. This protein is found in neurons throughout the brain; its normal function is unknown. Possibly, the abnormal huntingtin protein undergoes proteolysis and is then transported to the nucleus, where it undergoes aggregation.

Investigations

- The first symptoms typically are choreic movements or psychiatric disorders, whereas global cognitive decline generally becomes obvious later and eventually expresses itself as a triad of disordered movement, cognitive decline, and psychiatric disturbance.
- Psychiatric symptoms are prominent in patients with HD, as follows: Symptoms range from personality alterations to mood disorders, aggressiveness, hypersexuality or impotence, alcoholism, and psychosis, including schizophrenia.
- Early motor symptoms often include dystonic posturing and rigidity, but these changes give way to prominent choreiform activity in most affected adults.
- Frequent, irregular, and sudden jerks and movements of any of the limbs or trunk occur.
- Grimacing, grunting, and poor articulation of speech may be prominent.
- DNA repeat expansion:
  - This study forms the basis of a diagnostic blood test for the *HD* gene. Direct gene testing via polymerase chain reaction can identify the *HD* gene and carrier states.

- In addition to being a sensitive indicator of the inheritance of HD, CAG expansion is also highly specific because it is not observed in other neuropsychiatric disorders with which HD frequently is confused.
- MRI: In fully developed cases, these studies show cerebral atrophy, especially of the caudate and putamen, to a degree that is almost specific to the disease.

TREATMENT

Cholinesterase inhibitors for cognitive issues, antidepressants for mood disorders, and antipsychotics for behavioral issues.

ESSENTIAL TREMOR (ET)

A 48-year-old, right-handed man presents with a fluctuating tremor in his right hand, which he has noticed becoming worse over the past 2 years. He first noticed it when trying to sign a legal document 2 years ago. Over the past year he has noticed it daily, and now has difficulty holding a cup of water up to his mouth without any spilling. It is present at rest. He used to be an excellent orator; however, his speech has become tremulous during the past few lectures that he has given. His past medical history is unremarkable; he has had no surgeries, is taking no medications, and has no known drug allergies.

The patient most likely has essential tremor given his physical examination findings, including bilaterality, the duration of his tremor, and now the appearance of an episodic vocal tremor. He has not been taking any drugs associated with action tremors. He does have a positive family history of tremors, and the tremors are occurring even in a private setting when he is not nervous. Patients with essential tremor respond well to primidone, propranolol, or diazepam. The patient should avoid caffeine and nervousness. A diagnostic clue to essential tremor is that patients often report several hours of relief after ingesting low doses of alcohol. Differential diagnosis includes Parkinson disease and vascular parkinsonism.

First test to order would be an MRI to rule out structural findings, such as a mass that might → similar symptoms. In addition, the MRI would help rule out vascular parkinsonism, which occurs with strokes in the basal ganglia.

- The most common movement disorder.
- Tremor usually begins in 1 upper extremity and soon affects the other. ET rarely extends from the upper extremity to the ipsilateral leg.
- A mild degree of asymmetry is not unusual.
- In about 30% of cases, tremor involves the cranial musculature; the head is involved most frequently, followed by voice, jaw, and face.
- Tremor may be intermittent initially, emerging only during periods of emotional activation. Over time, the tremor becomes persistent.
- At any point of time the frequency of tremor is relatively fixed, but amplitude is highly variable depending on the state of emotional activation. Tremor amplitude is worsened by caffeine, emotion, hunger, fatigue, and temperature extremes. The baseline tremor amplitude slowly increases over several years.
- A degree of voluntary control is typical, and the tremor may be suppressed by skilled manual tasks.
- The tremor resolves during sleep.

- Alcohol intake temporarily reduces tremor amplitude in an estimated 50–70% of cases.
- A family history of ET is noted in 50–60% of cases.

Pathophysiology

ET is familial in at least 50–70% of cases. Transmission is autosomal dominant, with incomplete penetrance. Some cases are sporadic with unknown etiology.

Investigations

- No biological markers exist for ET.
- If the family history and examination findings are indicative of ET, no laboratory or imaging studies are required.
- If the family history and examination findings are not indicative of ET, laboratory and imaging studies should be considered.
- Laboratory investigations include standard electrolyte panel, thyroid function tests, BUN, creatinine, liver function tests, and serum ceruloplasmin (for Wilson disease).

Treatment

- Primidone and propranolol are the cornerstones of maintenance medical therapy for ET. The mechanism of action of propranolol is related to peripheral $beta_2$-receptor antagonism. The mechanism of action is unknown. Active metabolites are phenylethylmalonamide (PEMA) and phenobarbital. PEMA has no effect on tremor, and phenobarbital has only modest effect on tremor.
- Provide good benefit in reducing tremor amplitude in approximately 75% of patients.

PARKINSON-PLUS SYNDROMES

Clues suggestive of Parkinson-plus syndromes include the following:

- Lack of response to levodopa/carbidopa (Sinemet) or dopamine agonists in the early stages of the disease.
- Early onset of dementia.
- Early onset of postural instability.
- Early onset of hallucinations or psychosis with low doses of levodopa/carbidopa or dopamine agonists.
- Ocular signs, such as impaired vertical gaze, blinking on saccade, square-wave jerks, nystagmus, blepharospasm, and apraxia of eyelid opening or closure.
- Pyramidal tract signs not explained by previous stroke or spinal cord lesions.
- Autonomic symptoms such as postural hypotension and incontinence early in the course of the disease.
- Prominent motor apraxia.
- Alien-limb phenomenon.
- Marked symmetry of signs in early stages of the disease.
- Truncal symptoms more prominent than appendicular symptoms.
- Absence of structural etiology such as NPH.
- **Multiple system atrophy**—4 overlapping syndromes:
  - **Olivopontocerebellar atrophy:** Parkinsonism, pyramidal signs, and cerebellar signs. Due to degeneration of neurons in cerebellum, pons, inferior olives, and substantia nigra.

  - **Striatonigral degeneration:** Parkinsonism and pyramidal signs due to degeneration of neurons in caudate and putamen. Refractory to L-dopa.
  - **Shy-Drager:** Parkinsonism and dysautonomia. Orthostatic hypotension, impotence, and urinary incontinence/retention. Due to degeneration of preganglionic sympathetic neurons.
  - **Cortical basal ganglionic degeneration (CBGD):** Characterized by frontoparietal cortical atrophy in addition to degeneration within the extrapyramidal system.
- The disease tends to occur in those aged 60–80 years, with a mean age of onset of 63 years. CBGD is a rare syndrome with an estimated incidence of 0.02–0.92 per 100,000 population per year. Symptoms on long-term follow-up include focal or asymmetric rigidity, bradykinesia, postural and action tremor, and marked dystonia. These problems usually arise predominantly in 1 upper extremity. Limb apraxia may become a serious problem, with independent movements occasionally as severe as an "alien limb."
- **Progressive supranuclear palsy:** Supranuclear gaze palsy. ↓ balance with recurrent falls, dysphagia, dysarthria, pseudobulbar palsy.

REFERENCES

1. Jack CR Jr, Albert MS, Knopman DS, et al. Introduction to the recommendations from the National Institute on Aging–Alzheimer's Association workgroups on diagnostic guidelines for Alzheimer's disease. *Alzheimers Dement.* 2011;7(3):257–262.
2. Albert MS, DeKosky ST, Dickson D, et al. The diagnosis of mild cognitive impairment due to Alzheimer's disease: recommendations from the National Institute on Aging–Alzheimer's Association workgroups on diagnostic guidelines for Alzheimer's disease. *Alzheimers Dement.* 2011;7(3):270–279.
3. Petersen RC. Mild cognitive impairment. *N Engl J Med.* 2011;364:2227–2234.
4. McKhann GM, Knopman DS, Chertkow H, et al. The diagnosis of dementia due to Alzheimer's disease: Recommendations from the National Institute on Aging–Alzheimer's Association workgroups on diagnostic guidelines for Alzheimer's disease. *Alzheimers Dement.* 2011;7(3):263–269.
5. National Institute on Aging. Alzheimer's disease medications. November 2008. NIH Publication No. 08-3431. Available at: http://www.nia.nih.gov/Alzheimers/Publications/medicationsfs.htm. Accessed May 1, 2014.
6. Warren JD, Rohrer JD, Rossor MN. Frontotemporal dementia. *BMJ.* 2013;347:f4827. doi: 10.1136/bmj.f4827.
7. Gorelick PB, Scuteri A, Black SE, et al. Vascular contributions to cognitive impairment and dementia: a statement for healthcare professionals from the American Heart Association/American Stroke Association. *Stroke.* 2011, July 21 [online].

CHAPTER 6

Headache and Pain

David W. Chen, MD

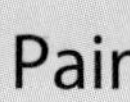

Pain

Pain can be classified as nociceptive (due to disease or damage to non-neural tissues) or neuropathic (due to disease or dysfunction of neural tissues). Table 6.1 summarizes medications for pain.

DEFINITIONS

- Analgesia: Absence of pain from noxious stimuli.
- Anesthesia: Absence of all sensation.
- Allodynia: Pain caused by non-noxious stimuli.
- Hyperalgesia: ↑ sensitivity to noxious stimuli.
- Hypesthesia: ↓ sensitivity to stimuli.
- Paresthesia: Abnormal sensation, spontaneous or evoked.
- Dyesthesia: Unpleasant, abnormal sensation, spontaneous or evoked.

NOCICEPTIVE PAIN

- Pain caused by damage to non-neural tissues from inflammation, injury, irritation, or infection. Common sites include skin, muscles, bone, ligament, viscera.
- Mediated by small, thinly myelinated A-delta and unmyelinated C nerve fibers. Prostaglandins, histamine, bradykinin, substance P.
- Responds to opioids or nonsteroidal anti-inflammatories (NSAIDs).

NEUROPATHIC PAIN

- Pain caused by primary peripheral nervous system (PNS) or central nervous system (CNS) insult.
- Can be continuous or paroxysmal (commonly "burning," "electric," "tingling," "shooting").
- Congenital insensitivity to pain identified as a mutation of nerve growth factor (NGF) tyrosine kinase A receptor. The following are examples of specific neuropathic pain syndromes.

POSTHERPETIC NEURALGIA (PHN)

- Ten to 15% of patients with shingles have dermatomal pain (including V1–3) persisting ≥ 3 months later.
- Hypesthesia and/or hyperalgesia.
- Corneal hypesthesia can lead to corneal scarring and visual loss with herpes zoster ophthalmicus (V1).
- ↑ risk in elderly and immunocompromised.
- Antiviral treatment within 72 hours of varicella-zoster virus (VZV) reactivation may reduce likelihood of PHN.

TABLE 6.1. Summary of Pain Medications

Class/Drug	Notes
Tricyclic antidepressants	Anticholinergic side effects.
Amitriptyline	Mixed NE/5-HT reuptake inhibition. Tertiary amine (more side effect potential).
Imipramine	Mixed NE/5-HT reuptake inhibition; also histamine antagonist. Tertiary amine.
Nortriptyline	NE > 5-HT reuptake inhibition. Secondary amine.
Desipramine	May be activating. Secondary amine.
Atypical antidepressants	
Venlafaxine	SNRI. 5-HT > NE >> DA. Withdrawal hypertension.
Duloxetine	SNRI. Gastrointestinal side effects: Nausea, anorexia. FDA indicated for use in painful diabetic neuropathy, fibromyalgia, MDD, GAD.
Bupropion	DA and NE reuptake inhibition. Lowers seizure threshold.
Anticonvulsants	
Valproic acid[a]	↑ availability of GABA. Monitor LFTs. Category D: Avoid in pregnancy/childbearing age. Weight gain, alopecia, tremor.
Carbamazepine	Na channel. Can cause hyponatremia. Rarely associated with aplastic anemia.
Oxcarbazepine	Na channel. Can cause hyponatremia.
Gabapentin	α-2(δ) Ca^{++} channel. Extremity edema.
Pregabalin	α-2(δ) Ca^{++} channel. FDA indicated for use in painful diabetic neuropathy, fibromyalgia, PHN, epilepsy.
Topiramate[a]	Mixed Ca^{++}, Na^{+}. Paresthesias, nephrolithiasis, weight loss, cognitive impairment. Rare narrow angle glaucoma.
Lamotrigine	Na^{+} channel. Rash and Stevens-Johnson syndrome—titrate slowly. Major interaction with valproate and enzyme-inducing meds.
Muscle relaxants	
Baclofen	GABA-B agonist.
Benzodiazepines	GABA-A agonist.
Tizanidine	Central alpha-2-adrenergic agonist, less hypotension.
Alpha agonist	
Clonidine	Transdermal and PO, hypotension.
NMDA antagonists	Adjuvant to opioids to help avoid tolerance.
Memantine	
Ketamine	IV and SC. Hallucinations.
Opioid analgesics	Tolerance, respiratory depression. No dosage ceiling.
Morphine	
Fentanyl	IV, transdermal.
Hydromorphone	
Meperidine	Can lower seizure threshold; avoid long-term, IM or IV.
Oxycodone	
Codeine	Less potent than other opioids, PO.
Methadone	Weak NMDA receptor activity. Appropriate in renal disease.
Tramadol	Weak mu receptor, NE and 5-HT.

TABLE 6.1. Summary of Pain Medications *(continued)*

CLASS/DRUG	NOTES
NSAIDs	Gastropathy, hepatic metabolism—renal excretion, can cause renal insufficiency.
Aspirin	Salicylic acid. Strong cyclooxygenase inhibition.
Ibuprofen	= Propionic acid.
Indomethacin	= Acetic acid.
Ketorolac	IV, IM, PO. 5 days max, monitor renal function.
Celecoxib	COX-2 inhibitor. Cardiovascular thrombotic events. Contraindicated in sulfonamide hypersensitivity.
Other	
Acetaminophen	Hepatotoxicity.
Capsaicin	Binds TRPV1—heat activated Ca^{++} channel; depletes substance P. Topical.

[a] FDA indication for migraine.

COX-2, cyclooxygenase-2; DA, dopamine; GABA, gamma-aminobutyric acid; GAD, generalized anxiety disorder; 5-HT, 5-hydroxytryptamine; LFTs, liver function tests; MDD, major depressive disorder; NE, norepinephrine; NSAIDs, nonsteroidal anti-inflammatory drugs; PHN, postherpetic neuralgia; SNRI, serotonin and norepinephrine reuptake inhibitor; TRPV1, transient receptor potential vanilloid 1.

TRIGEMINAL NEURALGIA (TIC DOULOUREUX)

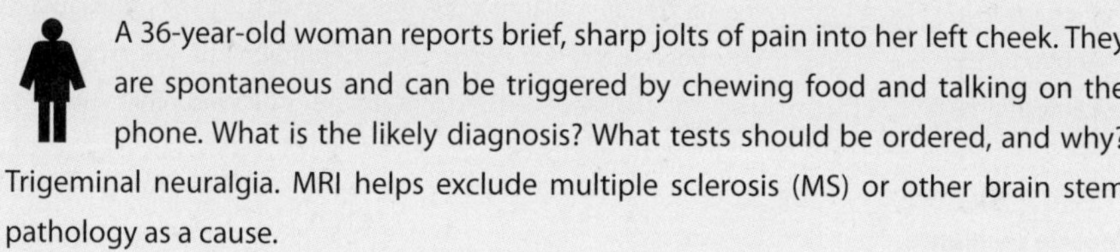
A 36-year-old woman reports brief, sharp jolts of pain into her left cheek. They are spontaneous and can be triggered by chewing food and talking on the phone. What is the likely diagnosis? What tests should be ordered, and why?

Trigeminal neuralgia. MRI helps exclude multiple sclerosis (MS) or other brain stem pathology as a cause.

- Sudden, brief attacks of severe pain in trigeminal distribution (V2 > V3 > V1). Characteristically shooting, lancinating, or "lightning-like."
- Spontaneous or triggered (eg, chewing, talking, smiling, drinking cold or hot fluids, brushing teeth, or touching the face, so called "trigger zone").
- Facial grimace or spasm common.
- No neurological deficits.
- Often idiopathic. Exclude compression of trigeminal nerve by a vascular loop, multiple sclerosis in young patients, Lyme disease, diabetes, pontine tumor.
- **Treatment:**
  - Carbamazepine and oxcarbazepine, other anticonvulsants, and clonazepam
  - Other neuropathic pain medications
- **Surgical:** Decompression of vascular loop, radiofrequency ablation of trigeminal ganglion.

COMPLEX REGIONAL PAIN SYNDROME (CRPS)

- Continuous, severe, disabling regional neuropathic pain out of proportion to recognizable pathology, associated with regional autonomic dysfunction.
- Symptoms: Edema, skin discoloration, altered temperature and sweating, allodynia, and hyperalgesia.
- Formerly called reflex sympathetic dystrophy (RSD); also called causalgia.

- Spontaneous (type I) or after nerve injury (type II).
- Most common after limb injury or limb immobilization.

ERYTHROMELALGIA

- Paroxysmal erythema and severe burning pain, especially in lower extremities. Can be triggered by warming the limb.
- Nerve fiber hypoexcitability → microvascular alterations (ie, blockage).
- Associated with autosomal dominant mutations in voltage-gated Na channel (NaV 1.7) alpha-subunit encoding gene *SCN9A*.
- Can be associated with mercury poisoning, mushroom poisoning (specific Japanese and French species), small-fiber neuropathy, hypercholesterolemia, heat exposure, alcohol, and caffeine.

Headache

Pain caused by disorders that affect pain-sensitive structures (meninges, blood vessels, nerves, muscles) of head and neck:

- CN V mediates sensation from the face, mucous membranes of sinuses and nasal cavity.
- Meninges and vessels of anterior and middle cranial fossa, venous sinuses innervated by trigeminal V1.
- Posterior fossa innervated by upper cervical dorsal roots.
- Nociceptive fibers synapse in trigeminal nucleus caudalis (substantia gelatinosa from C1 to C3; see Figure 6.1). Second-order neurons cross and join spinothalamic tract.

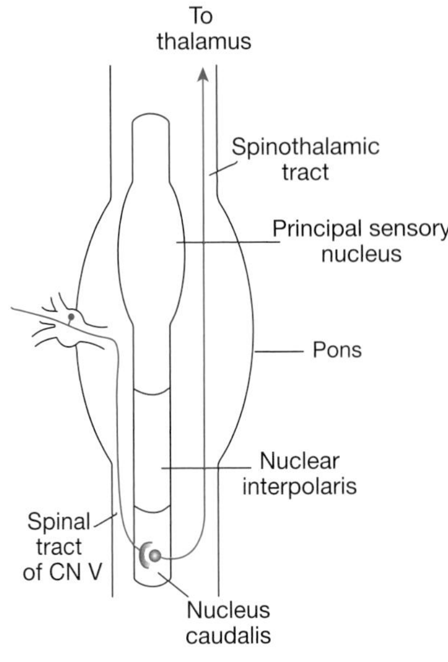

FIGURE 6.1. Trigeminal pain pathways.

PRIMARY HEADACHE

- Primary headaches are caused by intrinsic, often genetic, dysfunction of the nervous system resulting in ↑ vulnerability to headache.
- Categories include migraine, tension-type headache, cluster headache and trigeminal autonomic cephalalgias, and short-lasting headache disorders, such as hypnic or exertional headaches.

Migraine

- More than five headaches lasting 4–72 hours, with at least two of the following: unilateral, pulsating, moderate to severe intensity (inhibiting daily activities), aggravation with routine physical activity; and at least one of the following: nausea and/or vomiting, photophobia, phonophobia.
- With aura (~20%): > 5 and < 60 minutes of reversible visual scotoma, unilateral sensory symptoms, or dysphasic speech. Usually precedes headache, but can develop during.
- Familial hemiplegic migraine (FHM): Migraine with aura causing reversible motor weakness. Rare. Highly penetrant autosomal dominant inheritance. Symptoms include hemiplegia, sensory deficit, seizure, confusion or coma, transient or permanent cerebellar ataxia, nystagmus, or dysarthria.
  - FHM 1: Mutation of *CACNA1A* gene (chromosome 19) coding for voltage-gated P/Q calcium channel. Same gene mutation as spinocerebellar ataxia type 6.
  - FHM 2: Mutation of *ATP1A2* gene (chromosome 1) encoding abnormal Na^+/K^+ ATPase.

    - FHM 3: Mutation of *SCN1A* gene (chromosome 2) coding for neuron voltage-gated sodium channel.
- Status migrainosus: > 72-hour refractory headache. Treat with IV fluids, corticosteroids, IV NSAIDs, metoclopramide, triptans or dihydroergotamine, magnesium.
- Migraine variants: Ophthalmoplegic migraine, basilar-type (Bickerstaff syndrome), acephalgic. In children, cyclic vomiting syndrome and abdominal migraine.
- **Treatment:**
    - Prophylaxis: Beta blockers, calcium channel blockers, valproate, topiramate, tricyclic antidepressants (TCAs).
    - Abortive: NSAIDs, triptans (5-hydroxytryptophan [5-HT] 1B/D), dihydroergotamine and ergotamine, butalbital, corticosteroids, antiemetics.

Tension-Type Headache

- Bilateral, mild to moderate nonpulsatile headache, not aggravated by routine physical activity, without nausea, lasting 30 minutes to 7 days.
- "Tight band around the head."
- Can have photophobia or phonophobia, but not both, and no visual aura. Can overlap with migraine; can become chronic.
- **Treatment:** NSAIDs.

Cluster Headache

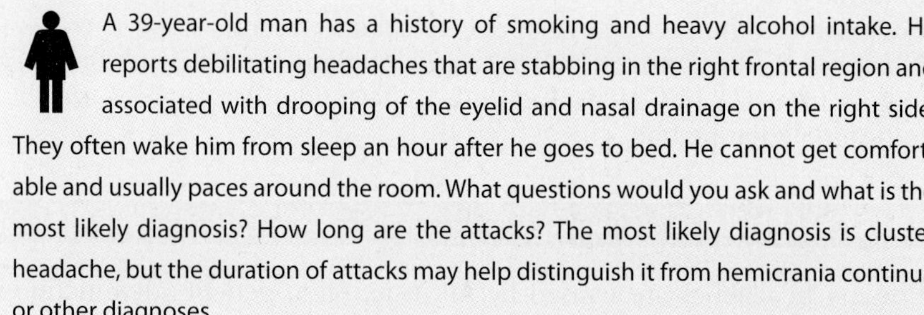

A 39-year-old man has a history of smoking and heavy alcohol intake. He reports debilitating headaches that are stabbing in the right frontal region and associated with drooping of the eyelid and nasal drainage on the right side. They often wake him from sleep an hour after he goes to bed. He cannot get comfortable and usually paces around the room. What questions would you ask and what is the most likely diagnosis? How long are the attacks? The most likely diagnosis is cluster headache, but the duration of attacks may help distinguish it from hemicrania continua or other diagnoses.

- Severe, unilateral periorbital headache, accompanied by lacrimation, rhinorrhea/nasal congestion, miosis, ptosis, eyelid edema, or conjunctival injection.
- Cycles lasting weeks to months, 1–3 attacks/day, each lasting 15–180 minutes. Can wake from sleep, often same time each night.
- Associated with smoking, excessive alcohol intake, rugged facial features, blue or hazel eyes.
- See Table 6.2 for comparison with migraine.
- **Treatment:** 100% oxygen, prednisone, sumatriptan (SC), oral zolmitriptan, injection dihydroergotamine and ergotamine, lidocaine nasal drops, and octreotide in patients with cardiac disease.
- **Prevention:** Calcium channel blockers, lithium, divalproex sodium, steroids.

Trigeminal Autonomic Cephalalgias

- Trigeminal neuralgia: Discussed earlier, under Neuropathic Pain.
- Hemicranias:
    - Hemicrania continua: Steady and continuous with superimposed episodic severe attacks, unilateral headache with autonomic features of cluster headache as well as migraine features.

TABLE 6.2. Comparison of Migraine and Cluster Headache

FEATURE	MIGRAINE	CLUSTER
Location	Unilateral/bilateral	Always unilateral periorbital +/– occipital referral
Pain quality	Throbbing, pulsating	Stabbing, boring, burning
Typical age of onset	10–50	20 or older
Gender	Female > male	Male > female
Time of day	Any time	Can be same time of day, often P.M.
Frequency	1–10 per month	1–3 per day
Duration	4–72 hr	30–180 min
Aura	Sometimes present	Uncommon
Nausea/Vomiting	Often	Almost never
Miosis	Never	50% of the time
Ptosis	Rare	30% of the time
Rhinorrhea	Sometimes	70% of the time
Lacrimation	Rare	Frequent
Blurred vision	Frequent	Infrequent
Behavior	Lying still, dark room	Pacing, manic, difficult to get comfortable
Family history	80%	Rare

  - Chronic and episodic paroxysmal hemicrania (PH): Attacks last 2–45 minutes (shorter duration than cluster), from 5 to 40 times a day. Female predominance.
- SUNCT syndrome (short-lasting unilateral neuralgiform pain with conjunctival injection and tearing): Attacks last 5–250 seconds, typically about five attacks/hour (up to 30/hour), typically men over 50.
- **Treatment:** Indomethacin for PH and lamotrigine for SUNCT.

SECONDARY HEADACHE

- Headaches associated with another disorder known to cause headache.
- Most important is to distinguish from primary headache and exclude treatable or serious causes.
- Clues that suggest secondary headache and should prompt imaging are found in Table 6.3.
- Over 300 conditions are described as causing secondary headache. Some common/important causes follow.

TABLE 6.3. Indications for Imaging in Headache

Headache features
"First or worst" headache
Subacute headache with increasing frequency or severity
New daily persistent headache
Chronic daily headache
Side-locked (headache always on same side)
Not responding to usual treatment
Demographics
History of malignancy or immune compromise
New onset after age 50
Associated signs and symptoms
Abnormal neurological exam with focal deficit (aside from migraine with aura)
Meningeal signs (stiff neck, nausea, fever)
Postural headache
New seizures
Impaired cognition or personality change

Adapted, with permission, from Evans RW, ed. *Diagnostic Testing in Neurology*. Philadelphia: WB Saunders, 1999: 2.

Idiopathic Intracranial Hypertension (Pseudotumor Cerebri)

- Idiopathic headache syndrome, probably caused by combination of ↑ production/↓ reabsorption of cerebrospinal fluid (CSF).
- Peak incidence 20–30 years old.
- Women >> men, obese.
- Associated with some medications (vitamin A, oral contraceptives, tetracycline, corticosteroids).
- Possibly related to narrowing of transverse dural sinus → ↓ CSF reabsorption.

Diagnosis

- CSF pressure > 25 cm H_2O.
- No focal signs other than possible CN VI palsy.
- Normal CSF profile.
- Normal or small ventricles, no mass on CT/MRI.

Symptoms

- Diffuse headache (~95%).
- Transient visual obscurations.
- Pulsatile tinnitus.
- Papilledema and eventual visual loss (peripheral visual loss followed by central).
- Diplopia (due to CN VI palsy).

Treatment

- Mild: Carbonic anhydrase inhibitors.
- Short-term corticosteroids.
- CSF shunt or serial lumbar punctures.
- Severe, with visual loss: Optic nerve sheath fenestration.

Intracranial Hypotension

Postural headache (worse upright) due to low CSF pressure. Usually caused by CSF leak; can be spontaneous, often caused by trivial events, such as severe coughing, leaking diverticulum around spinal nerve root, after spinal anesthesia, lumbar puncture, or spine surgery.

Symptoms

- Worsened by Valsalva.
- Causes orthostatic dizziness, nausea, vomiting, tinnitus and hearing loss.

Imaging

- Subdural hygroma, diffuse meningeal thickening and enhancement.
- CT myelography or radioisotope cisternography can diagnose location of leak.

Treatment

- Bedrest.
- Caffeine.
- Epidural blood patch, epidural saline infusion, or surgical dural repair.

Giant Cell Arteritis

A 72-year-old woman reports 2 months of insidious onset of generalized fatigue, 10-pound weight loss, and headache. Headache is bilateral, moderate in intensity, and described as dull. It is present all the time. She also describes a transient episode of visual disturbance, lasting 15 minutes, where it appeared as if a curtain came down over the right eye. What test should be ordered and what is the most likely diagnosis? ESR, temporal artery biopsy (to exclude temporal arteritis).

- Subacute granulomatous inflammation of medium-sized vessels of head, most frequently the temporal branch of the external carotid artery.
- Unilateral or bilateral, malaise, myalgia, arthralgia, weight loss, fever, jaw claudication, transient monocular blindness, anemia.
- Thrombosis may occur in severely affected arteries, resulting in stroke.
- Women > men, average age about 70 years old.
- Erythrocyte sedimentation rate (ESR) usually > 100 mm/hour (range 29–144 mm/hour), but can be normal or only slightly above normal.
- **Treatment:** Corticosteroids +/– steroid-sparing immunomodulators.

Other Causes of Secondary Headache

A 32-year-old woman reports history of severe left frontal throbbing headaches with associated nausea, photophobia, and phonophobia. These have occurred episodically, especially around her menses. Now she has a continuous headache that is at the vertex of her head. She has the same nausea, photophobia, and phonophobia as usual. She has no other medical history, and her only medication is an oral contraceptive. What test should be ordered and what is the likely diagnosis? MRV or CTV (to look for venous sinus thrombosis).

See Table 6.4.

TABLE 6.4. Other Causes of Secondary Headache

Cause	Notes
Subarachnoid hemorrhage	First or worst headache, CT for acute diagnosis, LP for xanthochromia and RBCs.
Carotid or vertebral dissection	Can be spontaneous, but especially post trauma, partial Horner syndrome, T1-weighted MRI with fat saturation.
Reversible vasoconstriction syndrome	Thunderclap headache, seizures, reversible multifocal arterial narrowing, associated with serotonergic drugs, postpartum.
Venous sinus thrombosis	Can mimic migraine, "empty delta sign" on contrast CT, hypercoagulable state (eg, pregnancy, oral contraceptive use, malignancy).
Pituitary apoplexy	Acute infarction or hemorrhage of pituitary, visual field cut or ophthalmoplegia, associated with pregnancy.
Meningitis/encephalitis	Fever, confusion, photophobia, meningismus (Kernig and Brudzinski signs); if immunocompromised, rule out *Cryptococcus*.
Leptomeningeal disease	Can be lymphomatous or from metastasis, involvement of cranial nerves.
Cerebral autosomal dominant arteriopathy with subcortical infarcts and leukoencephalopathy (CADASIL)	Vascular smooth muscle deterioration, notch 3 mutation (chromosome 19), migraines, transient ischemic attacks, and early dementia.
Metabolic disorders	Hypothyroidism, renal failure, hypercalcemia, anemia.

CHAPTER 7

Neuro-oncology

Jan Drappatz, MD

Primary Central Nervous System (CNS) Tumors

Primary brain tumors arise from the brain or related structures. See Table 7.1 for a guide to classification.

- Only 1 in 10 brain tumors is primary.
- An estimated 70,000 new cases of primary brain tumors were diagnosed in 2013; 25,000 malignant and 45,000 nonmalignant (*Central Brain Tumor Registry of the United States*).
- The most common benign primary brain tumors are meningiomas and the most common malignant tumors are gliomas. Each represent 30% of all primary brain tumors.
- Most common glioma subtype is glioblastoma = WHO grade 4 glioma (50% of all gliomas). Other subtypes including anaplastic astrocytomas (WHO grade III) and lower grade gliomas (WHO grade I and II) are less common.
- Pituitary adenomas are the third most common brain tumor (15% of all primary brain tumors, usually benign).
- All other primary brain tumors are much less common.
- Primary brain tumors have a slight male predominance.
- Peaks of incidence in childhood (gliomas, medulloblastoma/PNET) and older adulthood (Glioblastoma, meningioma).

KEY FACT

Metastatic brain tumors are 10 times more common than primary malignant brain tumors and therefore the most common brain tumor overall.

Symptoms

- Nonspecific, related to increased intracranial pressure:
  - Headache
  - Nausea
  - Vomiting
- Specific symptoms are referable to the particular location of the tumor:
  - Seizures common (including as a presenting symptom) in ~25% of patients with high-grade gliomas and 50% of patients with low-grade tumors.
  - High-grade gliomas and oligodendrogliomas can present with stroke-like symptoms due to intracerebral hemorrhage.

KEY FACT

Low-grade tumors are more epileptogenic than high-grade tumors and metastases.

Exam

Lateralizing signs, including hemiparesis, aphasia, and visual field deficits present in ~50%. Papilledema in 10%.

Differential Diagnosis

Infection (abscess, encephalitis), demyelinating disease, arteriovenous malformations, stroke.

Diagnosis

MRI +/– contrast should be the first test obtained in a patient with signs or symptoms suggestive of an intracranial mass.

- High-grade gliomas and metastases appear as contrast-enhancing intra-axial mass lesions (Figure 7.1) surrounded by edema.
- Low-grade gliomas are typically nonenhancing (exception: pilocytic astrocytoma) and diffusely infiltrative.
- Low-grade gliomas best appreciated with T2/FLAIR (Figure 7.2).
- Benign tumors that homogenously enhance include meningiomas, pilocytic astrocytomas, hemangioblastomas, acoustic neuromas and schwannomas.

TABLE 7.1. Simplified Brain Tumor Classification (with WHO grades I–IV)

Glial tumors	Astrocytic
	■ Circumscribed (I):
	  ■ Pilocytic astrocytoma
	  ■ Pleomorphic xanthoastrocytoma (PXA)
	  ■ Subependymal giant cell astrocytoma (SEGA)
	■ Diffuse astrocytoma:
	  ■ Low grade astrocytoma (II)
	  ■ Anaplastic astrocytoma (III)
	  ■ Glioblastoma (IV)
	Oligodendroglial
	■ Oligodendroglioma (II)
	■ Anaplastic oligodendroglioma (III)
	Mixed
	■ Oligoastrocytoma (II)
	■ Anaplastic oligoastrocytoma (III)

Ependymal tumors	Myxopapillary ependymoma (I) Ependymoma (II) Anaplastic ependymoma (III)
Pineal region tumors	Pineocytoma Pineal tumors of intermediate differentiation Pineal parenchymal tumors (II) Pineoblastoma (IV)
Sellar region tumors	Pituitary adenoma Craniopharyngioma (I)
Germ cell tumors (no WHO grade)	Germinoma Embryonal carcinoma Yolk sac tumor (endodermal sinus tumor) Choriocarcinoma Teratoma Mixed germ cell tumor
Meningeal tumors	Benign meningioma (I) Atypical, clear cell, choroid meningioma (II) Rhabdoid, papillary, or anaplastic (malignant) meningioma (III) Hemangiopericytoma (II-III)
Embryonal tumors	Medulloblastoma (IV) Supratentorial primitive neuroectodermal tumor (PNET) (IV) Atypical teratoid/rhabdoid tumor (IV)
Neuronal tumors	Dysembryoplastic neuroepithelial tumor (DNET) (I) Ganglioglioma (I–II) Central neurocytoma (II)
Choroid plexus tumors	Papilloma (II) Carcinoma (III)
Other	Hemangioblastoma (I)

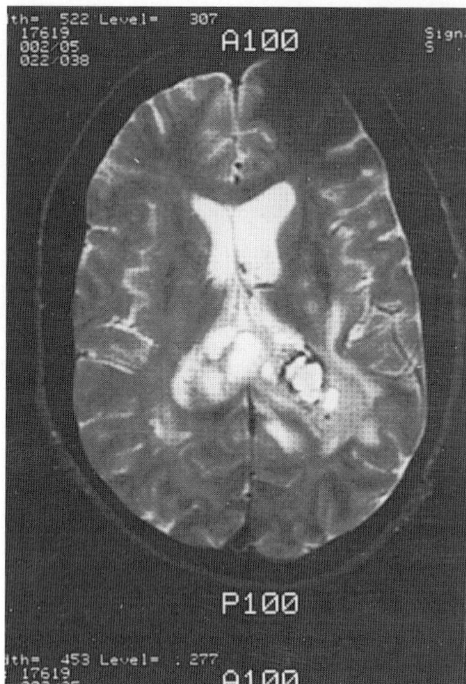

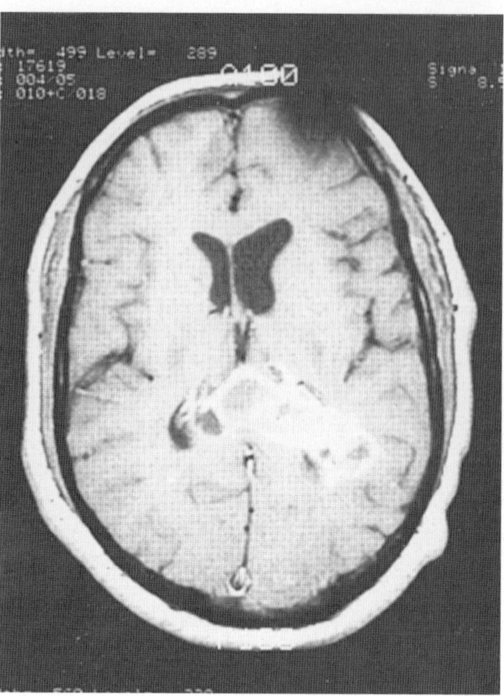

FIGURE 7.1. Glioblastoma multiforme (GBM). T1 gadolinium–enhanced MRI sequence: Heterogeneously enhancing lesion with nonenhancing cystic core reflecting central necrosis. (Reproduced, with permission, from Kantarjian HM, Wolff RA, Koller CA. *MD Anderson Manual of Medical Oncology.* New York: McGraw-Hill, 2006: Fig. 31-2.)

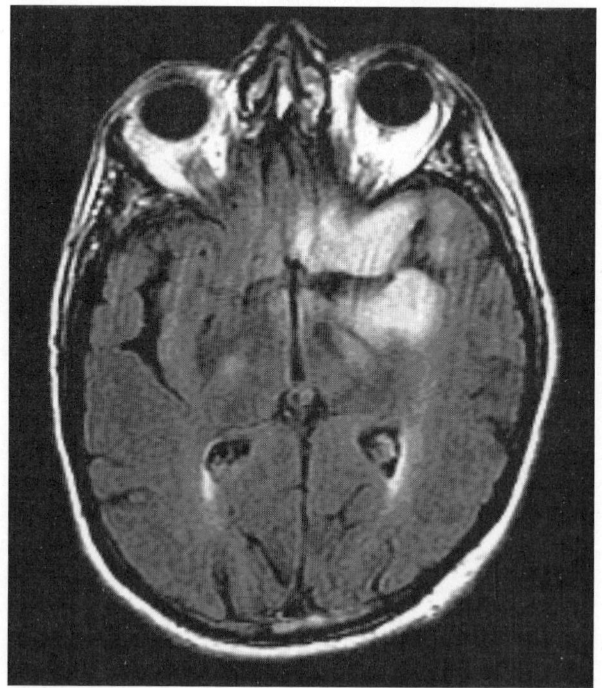

FIGURE 7.2. Low-grade glioma. FLAIR MRI demonstrating T2 hyperintensity. Gadolinium enhancement usually absent. Indistinct margins reflect diffuse infiltration of brain parenchyma. (Reproduced, with permission, from Kantarjian HM, Wolff RA, Koller CA. *MD Anderson Manual of Medical Oncology.* New York: McGraw-Hill, 2006: Fig. 30-3.)

Treatment

- Supportive therapy
  - Corticosteroids: Relief of headache and improvement of lateralizing signs within 24 hours. Dexamethasone first choice—start at 16 mg/d, adjust to minimum dose necessary.
  - Anticonvulsants: Stop prophylactic antiepileptic drugs (AEDs) after the immediate perioperative period; several prospective studies have failed to show efficacy in patients who did not present with seizures.
- Definitive treatment depends on tumor type. Can include:
  - Surgery
  - Radiotherapy
  - Chemotherapy
  - Alternating electric field therapy

Complications

- Thromboembolism in patients with high-grade gliomas and meningiomas (up to 30% of patients).
- Seizures.
- Infection (immunosuppression due to chemotherapy and steroids, especially *Pneumocystis jiroveci* pneumonia).
- Radiation-induced necrosis → cerebral edema, focal neurological symptoms.
- Intracranial hemorrhage.
- Complications of surgery.

KEY FACT

Any spontaneous intracranial hemorrhage can harbor an underlying neoplasm and requires follow-up imaging with gadolinium-enhanced MRI once the blood has resolved.

NEUROEPITHELIAL TUMORS

Astrocytic Tumors

Arise from astrocytic glial cells and stain for glial fibrillary acidic protein (GFAP). Classified as either circumscribed or diffuse.

Circumscribed Astrocytomas

- All are benign (WHO grade I); curable if completely resected and more common in children.
- Radiation and chemotherapy unnecessary if resectable.
- Three different subtypes:
- **Pilocytic astrocytoma:** Cerebellum, optic nerve, hypothalamus, and brain stem. Imaging: Cyst with enhancing mural nodule. Pathology: Rosenthal, eosinophilic granular bodies fibers (Table 7.2).
- **Pleomorphic xanthoastrocytoma (PXA):** Cortical. Pathology: eosinophilic granular bodies, high grade of pleomorphism.
- **Subependymal giant cell astrocytoma (SEGA):** Intraventricular location, associated with tuberous sclerosis, often presents with CSF obstruction.

Diffuse Astrocytomas

- Infiltrate brain parenchyma and tend to undergo anaplastic progression over time.
- The most malignant region determines grading ("low grade" = WHO grade II; "high grade" = WHO grades III and IV.) Grade depends on four main features: nuclear atypia, mitoses, microvascular proliferation, and necrosis.
- Mitoses are required to make it a grade III tumor.
- If either of the last two features is present, the tumor is WHO grade IV tumor—by definition, **glioblastoma.**

TABLE 7.2. Pathologic Eponyms

Rosenthal fibers (magenta intracytoplasmatic elongated inclusions):	**Eosinophilic granular bodies (EGBs):**
■ Pilocytic astrocytoma ■ Surrounding slow-growing tumors such as craniopharyngioma, hemangioblastoma, and pineal cysts ("reactive Rosenthal fibers") ■ Also seen in Alexander disease (see leukodystrophies)	■ Pilocytic astrocytoma ■ Pleomorphic xanthoastrocytoma ■ Ganglioglioma
True rosettes (with lumen):	**Pseudorosettes (without lumen):**
■ Flexner-Wintersteiner rosettes: Retinoblastomas and other primitive neuroectodermal tumors (PNETs)	■ Homer Wright rosettes: Neuroblastoma, medulloblastoma, and other PNETs and pinecytoma ■ In ependymomas

- **Low-grade astrocytoma:**
  - Often referred to simply as "low-grade glioma."
  - **Pathology:** Increased cellularity (Figure 7.3).
  - **Treatment:** Radiotherapy (RT) and chemotherapy. In resected, asymptomatic tumors in younger patients RTcan be withheld. No survival benefit of early RT, but delays time to neurologic progression. Larger tumors (> 4 cm), tumors in older patients (> 40 y) and tumors producing focal symptoms require immediate treatment as time to progression is usually short. There is additional benefit of upfront chemotherapy in this setting. Progressive tumors after RT can be treated with chemotherapy (procarbazine, lomustine [CCNU], and vincristine [PCV] or temozolomide). *Note:* Gemistocytic subtype has worse prognosis and is treated more aggressively.
  - Mean survival: 36–48 months.
- **Anaplastic astrocytoma:**
  - **Pathology:** Increased cellularity and mitoses.
  - **Treatment:** RT and chemotherapy (temozolomide or PCV).
  - **Prognosis:** Median survival 18–24 months. Presence of IDH 1 or 2 mutations confers a better prognosis.
- **Glioblastoma:**
  - Two major pathways lead to glioblastoma multiforme (GBM): Primary

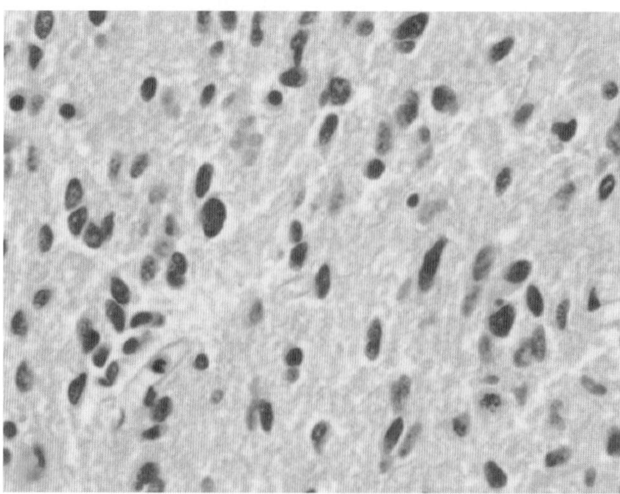

FIGURE 7.3. Low-grade glioma, WHO-grade II (x 400). (Also see Color Plate.) Diffuse infiltration of the brain parenchyma by neoplastic glial cells. (Reproduced, with permission, from Kantarjian HM, Wolff RA, Koller CA. *MD Anderson Manual of Medical Oncology*. New York: McGraw-Hill, 2006: Fig. 30-12.)

de novo: epidermal growth factor receptor (EGFR) amplification, p16 gene deletion, phosphatase and tensin homolog (PTEN) mutation, older patients. Secondary, arising from anaplastic progression of lower-grade tumors (associated with p53 mutation): Younger patients.

- **Pathology** (Figure 7.4): Either necrosis with surrounding tumor cell pseudopalisading or endothelial proliferation in a glial tumor.
- **Treatment:** RT (area of tumor plus 2-cm margin) with concurrent temozolomide, followed by 6–12 months of temozolomide. Bevacizumab (a VEGF targeted monoclonal antibody), and radiosurgery at recurrence. Alternating electric field therapy may also offer benefit.
- **Prognosis:** Median survival 12 months. Some patients have a methylated (∴inactive) DNA repair enzyme (MGMT [O6-methylguanine-**DNA** methyltransferase]) and survive longer when treated with temozolomide (DNA-damaging alkylating agent). Tumors with IDH mutations have a better prognosis similar to WHO grade III tumors.
- **Special cases:**
  - **Gliomatosis cerebri**: Diffuse infiltration of multiple lobes or contralateral hemispheres without dominant mass. Treatment includes chemotherapy (temozolomide) and/or radiation.
  - **Brain stem glioma:** Often slow growing; produces a variable clinical picture, depending on location in the brain stem. Initial manifestation frequently cranial nerve palsy, followed by long tract signs: hemiparesis, unilateral ataxia, and hemisensory symptoms. Slowly progressive over several years unless anaplastic transformation occurs. **Treatment:** Radiation and/or temozolomide. Exophytic tumors have better prognosis than diffusely infiltrating tumors.

Oligodendroglial Tumors

WHO classification includes two grades: low grade (grade II) and anaplastic (grade III).

Pathology

- Uniform "fried egg" cells with clear cytoplasm (perinuclear halos) (Figure 7.5). Mixed oligodendroglial and astrocytic tumors also exist.
- Most oligodendroglial tumors have loss of heterozygosity for chromosomes 1p and 19q. Response to chemotherapy better in patients with 1p and 19q loss.

Prognosis: Best prognosis of all malignant brain tumors. Median survival > 10 years even for anaplastic tumors (with 1p deletion present).

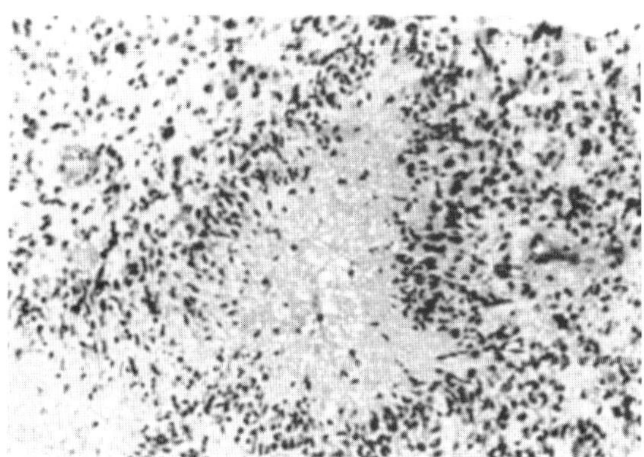

FIGURE 7.4. Glioblastoma.
Areas of necrosis surrounded by palisading neoplastic astrocytes. (Reproduced, with permission, from Chandrasoma P, Taylor CR. *Concise Pathology*, 3rd ed. New York: McGraw-Hill, 1997: Fig. 65-4.)

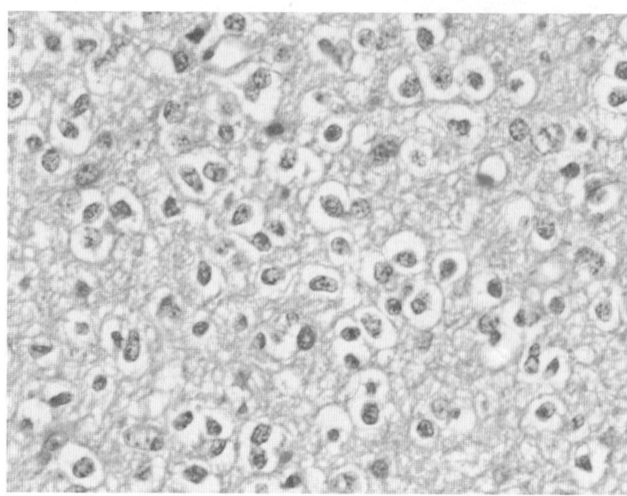

FIGURE 7.5. Oligodendroglioma (x400). (Also see Color Plate.) Characteristic "fried-egg" appearance due to clearing of the cytoplasm around the nuclei. (Reproduced, with permission, from Kantarjian HM, Wolff RA, Koller CA. *MD Anderson Manual of Medical Oncology*. New York: McGraw-Hill, 2006: Fig. 30-14.)

KEY FACT

In adults and adolescents, 75% of ependymomas arise within the spinal canal. Ependymomas are the most common primary spinal cord tumor.

KEY FACT

Intracranial ependymomas are most common in infants and usually involve the 4th ventricle.

Treatment: Adjuvant therapy can usually be deferred for low-grade oligodendrogliomas (unless symptomatic, large and unresectable). Anaplastic tumors are treated with chemotherapy (PCV or temozolomide) and/or radiation.

Ependymomas and Subependymomas

Tumors arise from ependymal cells (lining of ventricle), but a large percentage of ependymomas arise within the brain parenchyma without ventricular communication. Most common in posterior fossa and spinal cord. WHO classification includes three grades:

- Subependymomas and myxopapillary ependymomas (I)
- Ependymomas (II)
- Anaplastic ependymomas (III)

Symptoms/Exam

- Depend on location; often present with increased intracranial pressure. Other symptoms include vomiting, difficulty in swallowing, paresthesias of the extremities, abdominal pain, vertigo, and pain with neck flexion.
- Subependymomas arise from the ventricular lining and cause symptoms only when obstructing cerebrospinal fluid (CSF) flow or involving the spinal cord.
- Myxopapillary ependymomas usually involve the cauda equina only (as with paraganglioma). Myxopapillary tumors of the filum terminal cause bilateral sciatic or anterior thigh pain, sphincter difficulty and upper motor neuron signs.

Imaging

- Intracranial tumors are often heterogeneous and enhance slightly.
- Spinal tumors usually are more homogenous and enhance brightly.

Pathology

- Perivascular pseudorosettes.
- Ependymomas can involve the ventricular system, brain parenchyma, and spinal cord.

Treatment

Curable by complete resection. In anaplastic tumors, which have a higher chance to recur, surgery is followed by radiation. The extent of resection is the most important predictor of outcome.

Complications

Ependymomas have a tendency to spread through the CSF.

Neuronal and Neuroglial Tumors

All benign except neuroblastoma.

Neuronal Tumors

- Gangliocytoma and dysplastic gangliocytoma (Lhermitte-Duclos disease):
  - Hamartomatous cerebellar lesion with mature ganglion cells. (Hamartomatous: borderline between malformation and neoplasm.)
  - Associated with Cowden syndrome and mutation in the PTEN tumor suppressor gene.
- Central neurocytoma: Intraventricular location.
- Paraganglioma: Cauda equina or just filum terminale.
- Cerebral neuroblastoma (can also be classified as PNET—see section on PNET for details).

Mixed Neuroglial Tumors (Mixture of Astrocytic and Neuronal Cells)

- Ganglioglioma:
  - **MRI:** Cyst with enhancing mural nodule.
  - **Pathology:** Eosinophilic granular bodies.
  - **Treatment:** Resection whenever possible.
- Dysembryoplastic neuroepitelial tumor (DNET):
  - Benign cortical nodules.
  - Common cause of seizures in children.

Symptoms/Exam

- Depend on the location of the tumor, often presents with seizures.
- Focal neurological deficits are uncommon.
- Central neurocytoma presents with symptoms of increased intracranial pressure due to hydrocephalus.
- Lhermitte-Duclos disease presents with cerebellar symptoms for a number of years prior to establishing the diagnosis, and hydrocephalus is common.

Diagnosis

- MRI → biopsy.
- Gangliogliomas have a characteristic cyst with enhancing mural nodule.
- Neurocytomas are usually large, nonenhancing lesions arising from the ventricle.
- Synaptophysin is a marker of neuronal differentiation, and immunohistochemistry can aid diagnosis.

Treatment

- Resection of benign lesions is curative.
- Treatment of cerebral neuroblastoma involves resection, radiation, and chemotherapy.

Complications

- Gangliogliomas are not always completely resectable. They can also progress to higher-grade lesions.
- Cerebral neuroblastoma has a tendency to disseminate within the CNS.

KEY FACT

Over half (55%) of all childhood brain tumors arise in the posterior fossa. Children under 5 years of age have the greatest incidence of brain tumors.

Embryonal Tumors

- Referred to as primitive neuroectodermal tumors (PNETs) because of resemblance to primitive neuroectodermal elements.
- All are aggressive, mitotically active, highly malignant tumors.
- All can disseminate throughout the CNS and metastasize outside of the CNS, especially to bone (need for staging scans of brain, spine, and CSF).
- All are typically childhood tumors but occasionally occur in adults.
- All embryonal tumors are treated with resection, radiation, and chemotherapy, and are curable in the majority of patients.

Infratentorial PNET (Medulloblastoma)

Cerebellar tumor with peak incidence in childhood (midline location), occasionally in middle-aged adults (lateral hemisphere).

Pathology

Small blue cells (large nucleus, very little cytoplasm) with Homer Wright rosettes.

Signs and Symptoms

Due to obstructive hydrocephalus: Lethargy, vomiting, morning headache, stumbling gait, frequent falls, diplopia, papilledema, and occasionally sixth nerve palsies. Papilledema is usually present.

Diagnosis

MRI (Figure 7.6), followed by resection that is as complete as possible.

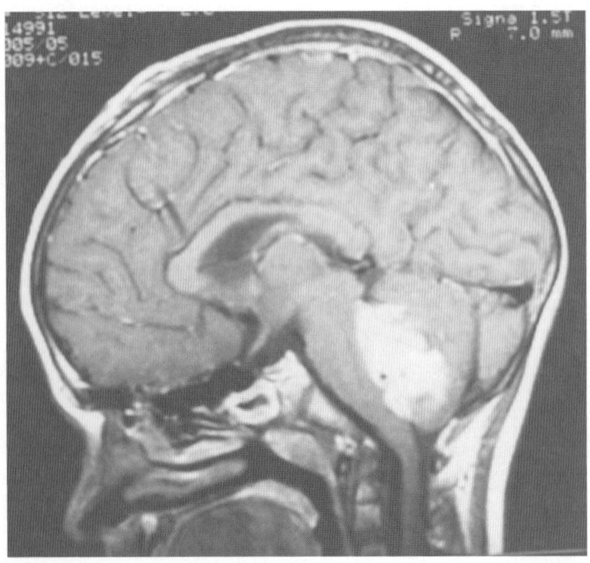

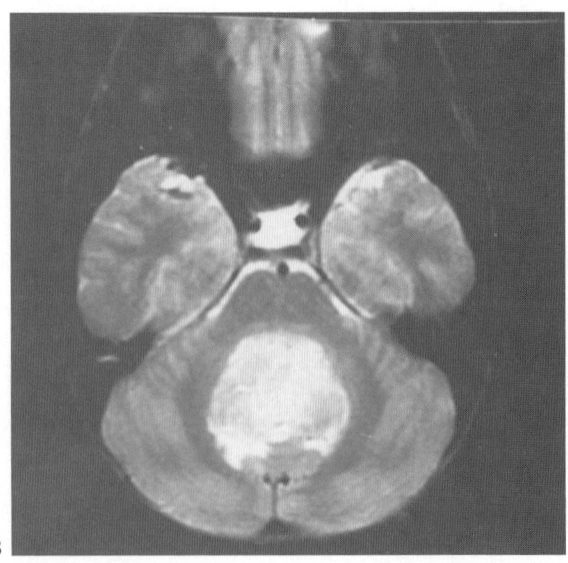

FIGURE 7.6. Medulloblastoma. MRI in the sagittal (A) and axial (B) planes, illustrating involvement of the cerebellar vermis and obliteration of the fourth ventricle. (Reproduced, with permission, from Ropper AH, Brown RH. *Adams and Victor's Principles of Neurology*, 8th ed. New York: McGraw-Hill, 2005: 567.)

Treatment

Resection, multiagent chemotherapy, and either radiation of posterior fossa (in low-risk patients with complete resection and no evidence of CSF spread) or craniospinal irradiation (in patients with presumed disseminated disease). Curable in the majority of patients.

Supratentorial PNET

Histologically similar to medulloblastoma, but referred to simply as PNET when supratentorial. A few special subtypes also exist:

- Pineoblastoma: PNET arising from pineal gland; see under Pineal Region Tumors.
- Cerebral neuroblastoma—not to be confused with peripheral neuroblastoma arising from the sympathetic chain and adrenal medulla, often associated with opsoclonus and myoclonus characterized by an unsteady, trembling gait, myoclonus (brief, shock-like muscle spasms), and opsoclonus (irregular, rapid eye movements) [see also under neuronal tumors].
- Familial retinoblastoma: Often bilateral, associated with osteosarcoma and soft tissue sarcoma.
- Esthesioneuroblastoma, arising from olfactory epithelium.
- Retinoblastoma: PNET of the retina.

Signs and Symptoms

Most frequent presenting sign: leukocoria, a white pupillary reflex.

Diagnosis

Dilated indirect ophthalmoscopic examination.

Pathology

Requires inactivation of the tumor suppressor Rb gene; half AD (13q deletion). Half sporadic. Flexner-Wintersteiner rosettes (in contrast to Homer Wright rosettes which are also seen, these are true rosettes).

Treatment

Include enucleation (only in patients with poor visual prognosis), radiation therapy, and chemotherapy.

Complications

All patients with retinoblastoma should undergo molecular genetic testing. Patients who have germline mutations should be referred to a genetic specialist for testing of parents and siblings. Patients with genetic disease must be carefully monitored for contralateral disease and other cancers.

Atypical Teratoid/Rhabdoid Tumor (ATRT)

Contain elements similar to PNETs (small blue cells) plus intermixed rhabdoid cells (eccentric nucleus, pink cytoplasm). Seventy-five percent occur in the cerebellum. Presentation and imaging findings are similar to medulloblastomas and PNETs. Highly malignant, very poor survival in infants.

PINEAL REGION TUMORS

In descending order of frequency:

- Germinomas
- Pineal parenchymal tumors
- Astrocytomas
- Other germ cell tumors (see below)
- Meningiomas
- Metastases

SYMPTOMS/EXAM

Clinical presentations:

- Endocrine (precocious puberty or amenorrhea).
- Obstructive hydrocephalus due to compression of sylvian aqueduct.
- Parinaud syndrome (vertical gaze palsy, convergence-retraction nystagmus, and light-near dissociation).

DIAGNOSIS

MRI, followed by biopsy or resection. Occasionally CSF markers (alpha-fetoprotein, placental alkaline phosphatase [PLAP], human chorionic gonadotropin [hCG]) can be helpful.

TREATMENT

In all pineal region tumors, as much resection as possible. Less important in germinomas, which are very sensitive to radiation.

Pineal Parenchymal Tumors

- Pineocytoma (benign): Treated with resection only.
- Pineal tumor of intermediate differentiation: Variable clinical behavior; often treated with resection, megavoltage radiotherapy (XRT), and chemotherapy.
- Pineoblastoma (see PNET): Aggressive multiagent chemotherapy and XRT (if disseminated, craniospinal XRT).

Germ Cell Tumors

- Germinomas: Most common. Typically in young adults. Often involves suprasellar area. Stains for placental alkaline phosphatase. High cure rate with radiation alone.
- Embryonal carcinoma.
- Choriocarcinoma (hCG positive).
- Endodermal sinus tumor = yolk sac tumor (alpha-fetoprotein positive).
- Teratomas (mature and immature).
- Mixed germ cell tumors (containing elements of all of the above).

MENINGEAL AND NERVE SHEATH TUMORS

Arise from the meninges and nerve sheaths; neurologic symptoms depend on location.

Meningioma

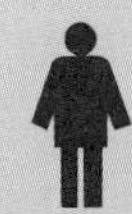

A 76-year-old woman presents with a new-onset single seizure. An MRI reveals a 1-cm extra-axial homogenously enhancing mass with a "dural tail" in the left temporal lobe. There is no T2 hyperintensity in the brain parenchyma. What is her diagnosis, and how should she be managed?

The tumor is most likely a meningioma, and can be followed with serial imaging. Given her advanced age, and the expected slow growth rate, surgery can usually be deferred.

- Most common benign brain tumor, arises from arachnoid cells.
- Peak incidence in older adults.
- Female predilection.
- Prior radiation is a risk factor.
- Most common over the cerebral convexities, but can be adjacent to brain stem, spinal canal, optic nerve, and choroid plexus.

Symptoms/Exam

Depend on location; headaches, occasionally seizures.

Diagnosis

- Homogenously gadolinium enhancing extra-axial lesion (Figure 7.7).
- Majority are benign but can grow and cause neurological dysfunction.
- Nine histologic subtypes; four are more aggressive—"2CPR":
  - Clear cell (atypical, grade II)
  - Chordoid (atypical, grade II)
  - Papillary (anaplastic, grade III)
  - Rhabdoid (anaplastic, grade III)
- Other subtypes can also progress to atypia or anaplasia.

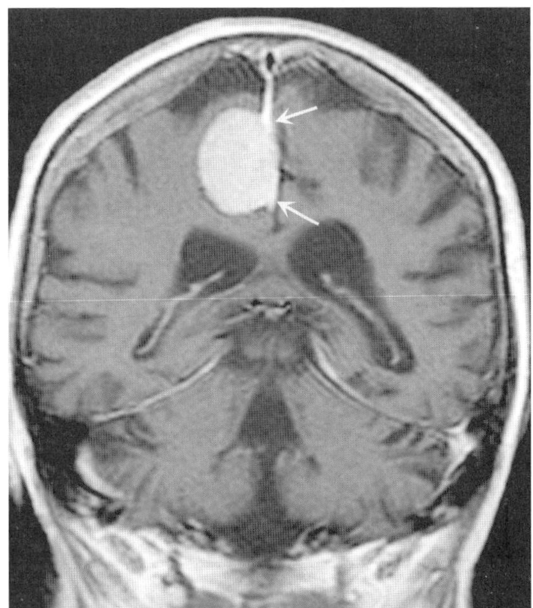

FIGURE 7.7. Meningioma. Coronal postcontrast T1-weighted MR image demonstrates an enhancing extra-axial mass arising from the falx cerebri (*arrows*). There is a "dural tail" of contrast enhancement extending superiorly along the intrahemispheric septum. (Reproduced, with permission, from Kasper DL, Braunwald E, Fauci AS, et al. *Harrison's Principles of Internal Medicine*, 16th ed. New York: McGraw-Hill, 2004: 2456.)

KEY FACT

Differential diagnosis of dural based mass lesion:

- Meningioma
- Hemangiopericytoma
- Dural metastasis (mostly breast, occasionally prostate)

Treatment

- Resection.
- XRT only in anaplastic tumors or incompletely resected atypical tumors.
- Recurrence: XRT.

Hemangiopericytoma

- Very vascular with typical branching vascular pattern ("staghorn pattern"). Higher recurrence and metastasis rates than meningiomas.
- **Treatment:** Resection, followed by radiotherapy.

Schwannoma

- Arise from Schwann cells of cranial nerves and spinal roots, most commonly CN VIII (vestibular schwannoma, a.k.a. acoustic neuroma).
- Eighty to 90% of posterior fossa lesions are schwannomas.
- Bilateral vestibular schwannomas are associated with neurofibromatosis type 2 (NF2) due to a mutation in the NF2 gene on chromosome 22.

KEY FACT

Vestibular schwannoma ("acoustic neuroma") accounts for 80–90% of posterior fossa lesions. Bilateral vestibular schwannomas are associated with neurofibromatosis type 2 (NF2) due to a mutation in the NF2 gene on chromosome 22.

Pathology

- Dense cellular **(Antoni A)** regions, and areas with loose stroma and fewer cells.
- Organized linear palisades of nuclei are called **Verocay bodies.**
- Vast majority are benign.

Symptoms/Exam

- Cranial nerve dysfunction, and occasionally cerebellar compression.
- Acoustic nerve (hearing loss) is involved in almost all cases, followed by the vestibular (dysequilibrium), trigeminal (facial sensory disturbance), and facial nerve (facial weakness).

Diagnosis

Hearing test demonstrates asymmetric sensorineural hearing loss. Imaging reveals tumor arising from the cerebellopontine angle (CPA) (Figure 7.8).

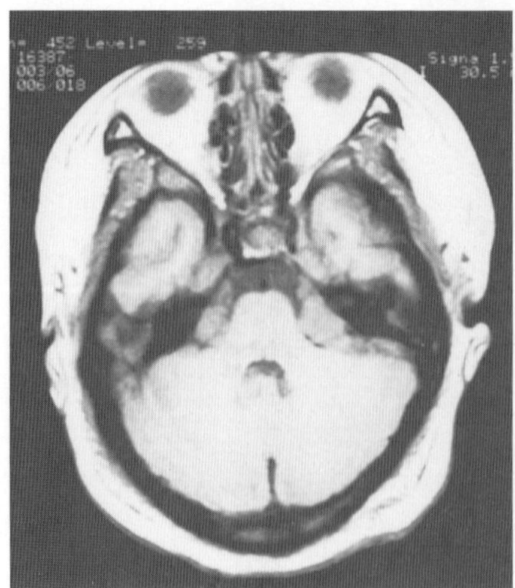

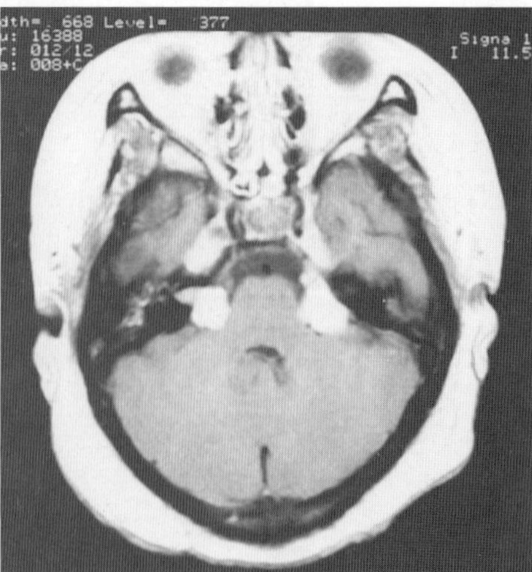

FIGURE 7.8. Bilateral acoustic schwannomas in neurofibromatosis type 2. Axial T1 weighted MRI, without (*left*) and with (*right*) enhancement. (Reproduced, with permission, from Ropper AH, Brown RH. *Adams and Victor's Principles of Neurology*, 8th ed. New York: McGraw-Hill, 2005: 572.)

TREATMENT

- Resection.
- Tumors arise eccentrically and displace axons, usually making nerve-sparing surgery possible.
- Radiosurgery is sometimes preferred with increased surgical risk or bilateral vestibular schwannoma.

Neurofibroma and Malignant Peripheral Nerve Sheath Tumor (MPNST)

Summarized in Table 7.3. Arise from a mixture of Schwann cells and fibroblastic cells on peripheral nerves and spinal roots. Cause enlargement of the nerve.

PATHOLOGY

- Axons embedded in Schwann cells.
- Sporadic or associated with neurofibromatosis type 1 (NF-1).
- Usually benign but progression to MPNST can occur.

SYMPTOMS/EXAM

Depend upon location. Large tumors can cause spinal cord compression → myelopathy. Foraminal neurofibromas commonly cause radicular pain and sensory changes. Typically worse at night and in the morning; better during the day.

DIAGNOSIS

Enhance diffusely with contrast on MRI.

TABLE 7.3. Neurofibromatosis

	NF-1	NF-2
Chromosome	17, autosominal dominant	22, autosominal dominant
Associated tumors	**"NO"** ■ **N**eurofibromas (spinal root, peripheral nerve and skin) ■ **O**ptic gliomas (benign), incidence 15% Other tumors mentioned under NF2 can rarely also occur	**"MISMEG"** ■ **M**ultiple **I**nherited **S**chwannomas ■ **M**eningiomas ■ **E**pendymomas ■ Rarely **G**liomas Neurofibromas are rare in NF2
Symptoms/exam findings	■ Cutaneous neurofibromas ■ Café au lait spots ■ Axillary and inguinal freckling ■ Lisch nodules (iris)	■ Hearing loss ■ Cataracts at young age ■ NB: Skin findings are uncommon
Age at diagnosis	Children	Younger adults (< 40)
Incidence	1:3000	1:30,000–40,000
Treatment principles	**"Watch and wait"** Neurofibromas: Surgery only for symptoms Optic gliomas: Surgery and XRT only for aggressive growth	Surgery or radiation to tumors

TREATMENT

Function-sparing surgical resection. In patients with NF-1 and multiple tumors, only symptomatic tumors should be surgically addressed. Prognosis is good for neurofibromas, poor for MPNSTs.

PRIMARY CENTRAL NERVOUS SYSTEM LYMPHOMA (PCNSL)

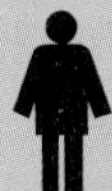

A 43-year-old HIV-positive man (owner of a pet cat) presents with lethargy, headache, and left-sided weakness. MRI reveals enhancing lesions in the right thalamus and left frontal lobe. What tests do you perform?

CSF for cytology, flow cytometry, Epstein-Barr virus polymerase chain reaction (EBV-PCR), and *Toxoplasma* serology. The main differential for multiple enhancing lesions in an immunocompromised host is toxoplasmosis versus PCNSL. Even if no definitive diagnosis can be established with noninvasive measures, patients are often treated with an empiric regimen for toxoplasmosis. (In this case, *Toxoplasma* serology was negative; the patient underwent biopsy, which revealed PCNSL).

Most common in immunosuppressed patients (PCNSL is an AIDS-defining condition) but also seen in immunocompetent older patients.

PATHOLOGY

Perivascular cuffing by malignant lymphocytes and diffuse brain infiltration by malignant lymphocytes. Vast majority are B-cell lymphomas (CD-20 positive); T-cell lymphomas are very rare.

SIGNS AND SYMPTOMS

Progressive focal neurological symptoms; sometimes seizure.

DIAGNOSIS

- Can present as solitary or multifocal enhancing lesion on CT or MRI.
- PCNSLs are very sensitive to steroids! When PCNSL is in the differential, avoid steroids until after diagnostic procedure.
- Staging exam includes neuro-ophthalmologic evaluation (because of high rate of concurrent ocular lymphoma); imaging of entire neuraxis, chest, abdomen, and pelvis (to rule out systemic involvement); and CSF cytology and flow cytometry.

TREATMENT

- Potentially curable.
- High-dose methotrexate-based chemotherapy regimens.
- XRT best deferred initially, especially in elderly patients.
- Most will remit with methotrexate, although remission often is not durable.
- High dose chemotherapy with autologous stem cell transplantation for selected patients.

COMPLICATIONS

Methotrexate or radiation can cause leukoencephalopathy.

SELLAR REGION TUMORS

A number of tumor types can arise in the sellar region. Large masses can cause focal neurological dysfunction. Endocrine dysfunction can be caused by both secreting and nonsecreting tumors.

- MRI is the single best imaging procedure for most sellar masses.
- Masses physically separate from the pituitary gland are usually not pituitary adenomas.

Symptoms

- Headache is common.
- Larger lesions (eg, macroadenomas or other tumors > 1 cm) can compress the optic chiasm, CN III, IV, V, or VI.
- Large, nonsecreting tumors can cause endocrine symptoms, including:
  - Hyperprolactinemia (compression of pituitary stalk interrupts dopamine's inhibition of prolactin production). Causes galactorrhea and amenorrhea in women; gynecomastia in men but often asymptomatic.
  - Hypopituitarism (especially growth retardation in children, sexual dysfunction in adolescents/adults).
- Pituitary microadenomas (< 1 cm) often secrete hormones:
  - Prolactin (most common) → hyperprolactinemia.
  - Growth hormone (GH) → acromegaly.
  - Adrenocorticotropic hormone (ACTH) → Cushing disease.

Differential Diagnosis

- Pituitary adenoma.
- Craniopharyngioma.
- Meningioma.
- Metastatic tumor.
- Optic glioma.
- Aneurysm.
- Arachnoid cyst.
- Rathke cleft cyst (often incidental, arising from remnants of the pharyngeal pouch).
- Lymphocytic hypophysitis (autoimmune).

Pituitary Tumors

Pathology

- Reticulin stain shows loss of lobular pattern. Classification based on immunostaining for various hormones (eg, prolactin, ACTH, GH).
- Multiple endocrine neoplasia (MEN-l) is associated with familial pituitary adenomas (in addition to parathyroid and pancreas tumors).

Exam

Most common finding with macroadenomas: Bitemporal hemianopsia due to central compression of the optic chiasm.

Diagnosis

- Serum prolactin concentration > 200 ng/mL suggests prolactinoma.
- If acromegaly is present, serum insulin-like growth factor (IGF)-I should be measured.
- Elevated 24-hour urine cortisol excretion and high ACTH concentration indicate an ACTH-secreting adenoma.

COMPLICATIONS

Acute expansion of a pituitary adenoma from infarction or hemorrhage (pituitary apoplexy) is a surgical emergency (symptoms: headache, visual symptoms, nausea).

TREATMENT

- Hyperprolactinemia: Can be controlled with dopamine agonist (eg, bromocriptine). Surgery rarely necessary.
- Microadenomas secreting GH (acromegaly) or ACTH (Cushing disease) require surgery.
- Macroadenomas (> 1 cm), require surgery. Occasionally, prolactinomas can go unnoticed in men and present as macroadenoma.

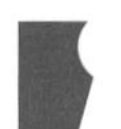

KEY FACT

MEN-1 is associated with familial pituitary adenomas (in addition to parathyroid and pancreas tumors).

Craniopharyngioma

- Extra-axial, slow-growing tumor involving the sella and suprasellar space (occasionally third ventricle). Derived from elements of Rathke cleft.
- Craniopharyngiomas are cystic tumors arising from Rathke cleft, are filled with fluid resembling crank-case oil, and can compress the chiasm.

EXAM

Endocrine dysfunction and visual field cut (most common bitemporal hemianopsia).

DIAGNOSIS

MRI demonstrates cystic suprasellar mass with enhancement of solid components (Figure 7.9).

TREATMENT

Resection followed by radiation therapy. Incompletely resected tumors have worse prognosis.

COMPLICATIONS

Surgery is high risk (vision loss, hypothalamic injury, etc). Many patients develop postoperative diabetes insipidus.

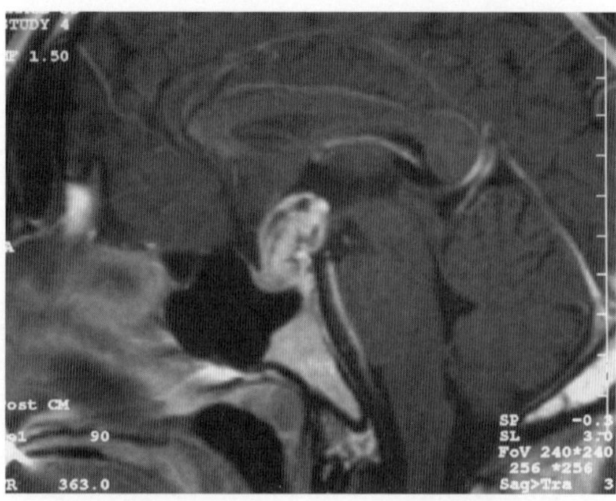

FIGURE 7.9. Suprasellar craniopharyngioma (sagittal MRI). (Reproduced, with permission, from Riordan-Eva P, Whitcher JP. *Vaughan & Asbury's General Ophthalmology,* 16th ed. New York: McGraw-Hill, 2003: 283.)

CHOROID PLEXUS TUMORS

Three types:

- Choroid plexus (CP) papilloma (benign, in children and young adults, immunopositive for transthyretin).
- CP carcinoma.
- CP meningioma.
- Metastatic lesions (in adults, more common than all of the above).

Symptoms

Headache, often due to hydrocephalus.

Exam

Usually nonfocal.

Imaging

MRI reveals an intraventricular mass. Papillomas are often calcified and enhance. Can be difficult to distinguish from ependymomas.

Treatment

Surgery, occasionally shunt required. Papillomas do not recur after complete resection.

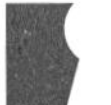

KEY FACT

Intraventricular Tumors

- Intraventricular meningioma
- Central neurocytoma
- Subependymal giant cell astrocytoma (SEGA)
- Supependymoma
- Ependymoma
- Choroid plexus papilloma

HEMANGIOBLASTOMA

- Arise in cerebellum or spinal cord.
- Most common in children and young adults.
- Pathology: Highly vascular tumor.
- Sporadic or associated with Von Hippel–Lindau syndrome (autosomal dominant). (See Table 7.4 for summary of tumor syndromes associated with brain tumors.)

Symptoms

- Depends upon tumor location, and often includes cerebellar ataxia.
- Patients with spinal hemangioblastomas frequently present with pain.
- Can also present with catastrophic neurologic symptoms due to hemorrhage.

Exam

Often cerebellar dysfunction.

Diagnosis

MRI: Cyst with enhancing mural nodule (Figure 7.10).

Treatment

Resection. If unresectable, radiosurgery can be considered.

Complications

Tumors are very vascular and can bleed.

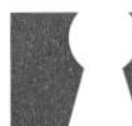

KEY FACT

Tumors with Cyst and Enhancing Mural Nodule

- Hemangioblastoma
- Ganglioglioma
- Pilocytic astrocytoma

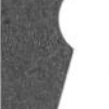

KEY FACT

Tumors associated with Von Hippel–Lindau: Hemangioblastoma, renal cell carcinoma, pheochromocytoma.

TABLE 7.4. Cancer Syndromes Associated with Nervous System Tumors

Tuberous sclerosis	■ Autosominal dominant ■ Cortical tubers (hamartomas) ■ Subependymal giant cell astrocytoma ■ Renal angiomyolipoma ■ Subungual fibroma ■ Adenoma sebaceum of face
Von Hippel–Lindau syndrome	■ Autosominal dominant ■ Cerebellar and spinal cord hemangioblastomas ■ Renal cell carcinoma ■ Pheochromocytoma ■ Retinal angiomas
Li-Fraumeni syndrome	■ Autosominal dominant, p-53 mutation ■ Sarcomas ■ Breast cancer ■ Astrocytomas
Cowden syndrome	■ Autosominal dominant, phosphatase and tensin homolog (PTEN) mutation ■ Dysplastic gangliocytoma of cerebellum (Lhermitte-Duclos) ■ Colon polyps ■ Breast cancer ■ Thyroid cancer
Turcot syndrome	■ Colorectal tumors ■ Gliomas ■ Medulloblastomas

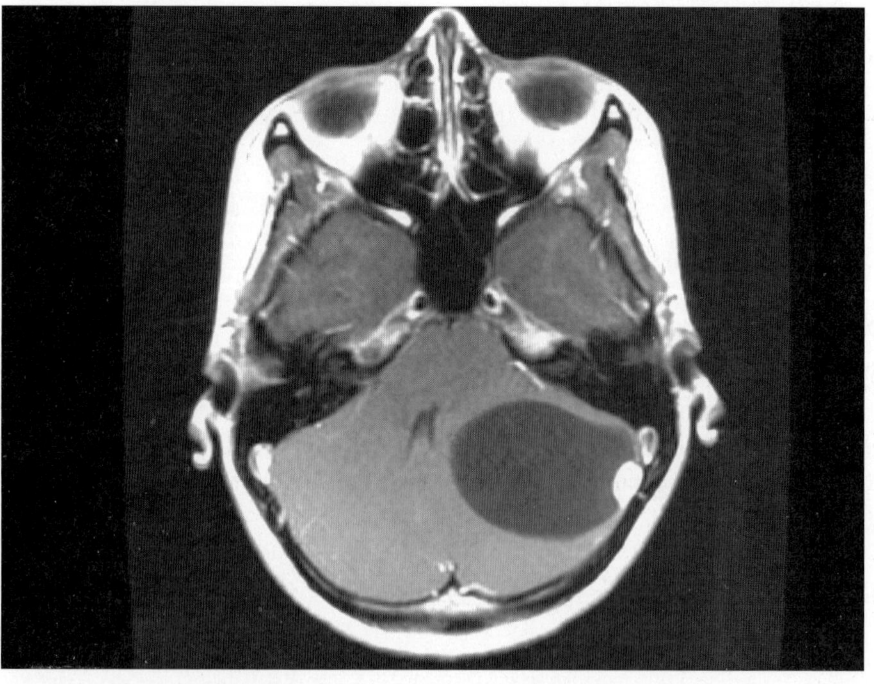

FIGURE 7.10. Hemangioblastoma. Cyst with enhancing mural nodule (sagittal MRI).

Metastatic CNS Tumors

Typically involve the gray-white matter junction. MRI and CT demonstrate ring-enhancing lesion with central necrosis and surrounding edema.

- Most common:
  - Lung
  - Breast
  - Melanoma
  - Renal
  - Colorectal tumors
- Most likely to hemorrhage:
  - Renal
  - Choriocarcinoma
  - Melanoma
  - Thyroid

Metastatic tumors can also involve the CSF pathways and cause leptomeningeal disease (lung and breast most common, but any tumor can spread to the leptomeninges).

KEY FACT

Metastatic lung cancer is the most common brain tumor.

Symptoms/Exam

- Focal neurological dysfunction due to mass effect or edema.
- Headache.
- Seizure.
- Symptoms of leptomeningeal disease:
  - Focal findings due to cranial nerve, spinal nerve root, or cauda equina involvement.
  - Meningeal symptoms (especially nausea and headache).
  - Hydrocephalus due to obstruction of arachnoid granulations.

Diagnosis

- Contrast-enhanced CT or MRI scan.
- CSF for leptomeningeal disease.

Treatment

- Multimodality: Resection, whole brain XRT, radiosurgery.
- Corticosteroids for cerebral edema.
- Leptomeningeal disease → XRT of symptomatic regions and intrathecal chemotherapy (methotrexate, cytarabine).
- Leptomeningeal solid tumors respond poorly to therapy; lymphoma/leukemia responds better and is often curable.

Paraneoplastic Syndromes

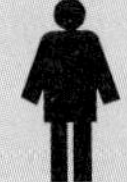

A 64-year-old woman with a history of metastatic breast cancer presents with diplopia. What test do you order next? Contrast-enhanced MRI brain, followed by spinal fluid exam to assess for leptomeningeal involvement (if no significant mass effect on MRI).

- Immune-mediated neurological disorders, typically presenting before cancer is detected.

TABLE 7.5. Paraneoplastic Neurologic Syndromes

Antibody	Most Common Tumors	Syndrome
Anti-Hu	Small cell lung cancer (SCLC)	Limbic encephalitis Encephalomyelitis Sensory neuropathy/ganglionopathy (similar to Sjögren's associated ganglionopathy)
Anti-Yo (PCD-1)	Ovarian, breast, lung	Cerebellar degeneration
PCD-2	Lung, ovarian	Cerebellar degeneration
Anti-Tr	Hodgkin lymphoma	Cerebellar degeneration
Anti-NMDA	Ovarian teratoma	Limbic encephalitis
Anti-amphiphysin or GAD	SCLC and breast	Stiff man syndrome (muscle spasms and rigidity)
Anti-voltage–gated potassium channel (VGKC)	Lung, thymoma	Isaac syndrome (muscle hyperexcitability), limbic encephalitis
Anti-voltage-gated calcium channel (VGCC)	SCLC	Lambert-Eaton syndrome (proximal fatiguing weakness)
Anti-Ma	Lung, testicular	Limbic encephalitis
Anti-Ri	Neuroblastoma	Opsoclonus-myoclonus
Anti-CRMP-5	Lung	Optic neuropathy (blindness)
Anti-acetylcholine-receptor Low density lipoprotein receptor-related protein 4 (LRP4) antibodies Anti-muscle specific tyrosine kinase autoantibodies (anti-MuSK)	Thymoma	Myasthenia gravis
Anti-MAG	IgM monoclonal gammopathies (MGUS, Waldenström macroglobulinemia)	Peripheral neuropathy, usually with distal weakness and ataxia

- Summarized in Table 7.5. Limbic encephalitis and encephalomyelitis can present with focal neurologic deficits, occasional CSF pleocytosis, abnormal T2 signal on MRI, and occasionally seizures (Figure 7.11). Antibodies frequently not detected; diagnosis often relies on recognition of the clinical syndrome.

Treatment

Immunosuppression/immunomodulation, including plasmapheresis, intravenous immune globuin, rituximab, and tumor-directed chemotherapy.

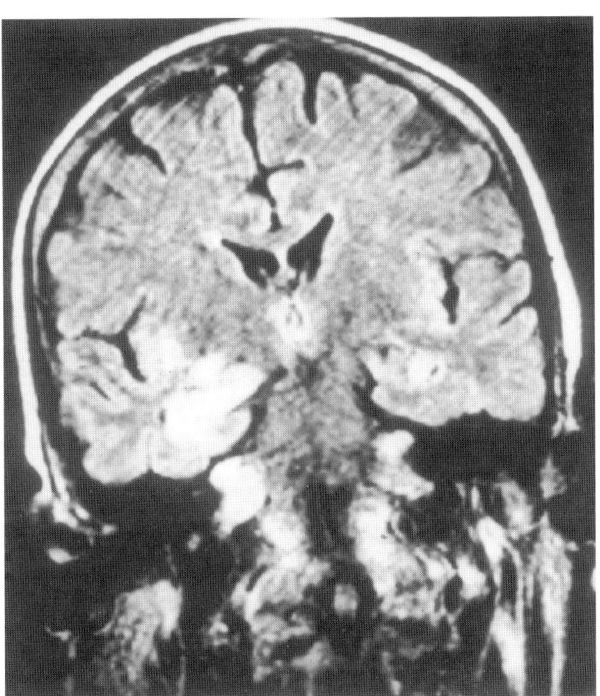

FIGURE 7.11. Paraneoplastic limbic encephalitis. Coronal FLAIR MRI from a woman with associated lung cancer and a mild pleocytosis. Note FLAIR hyperintensity of the medial temporal lobes. (Reproduced, with permission, from Ropper AH, Brown RH. *Adams and Victor's Principles of Neurology*, 8th ed. New York: McGraw-Hill, 2005: 585.)

NOTES

CHAPTER 8

Neuro-ophthalmology and Neuro-otology

Devin D. Mackay, MD
Beau B. Bruce, MD, PhD

Afferent Visual System Disorders

Neuro-ophthalmic disorders can be divided into those affecting the afferent visual system (primarily vision) vs. those affecting the efferent visual system (primarily anisocoria and extraocular motility). As in all of neurology, localization is critical and afferent disorders can occur in the retina, optic nerve, optic chiasm, optic tract, visual radiations, or visual cortex.

RETINA

Light traverses the full thickness of the retina to reach photoreceptors (rods and cones) lying on the retinal pigment epithelium (the outermost and most posterior layer of the retina). The photoreceptors transduce light into electrical signals that are transmitted to ganglion cells (in the inner retina) via the bipolar cells. Horizontal and amacrine cells are modulating interneurons of the retina. The axons of the ganglion cells synapse in the lateral geniculate ganglion (see Figure 8.1).

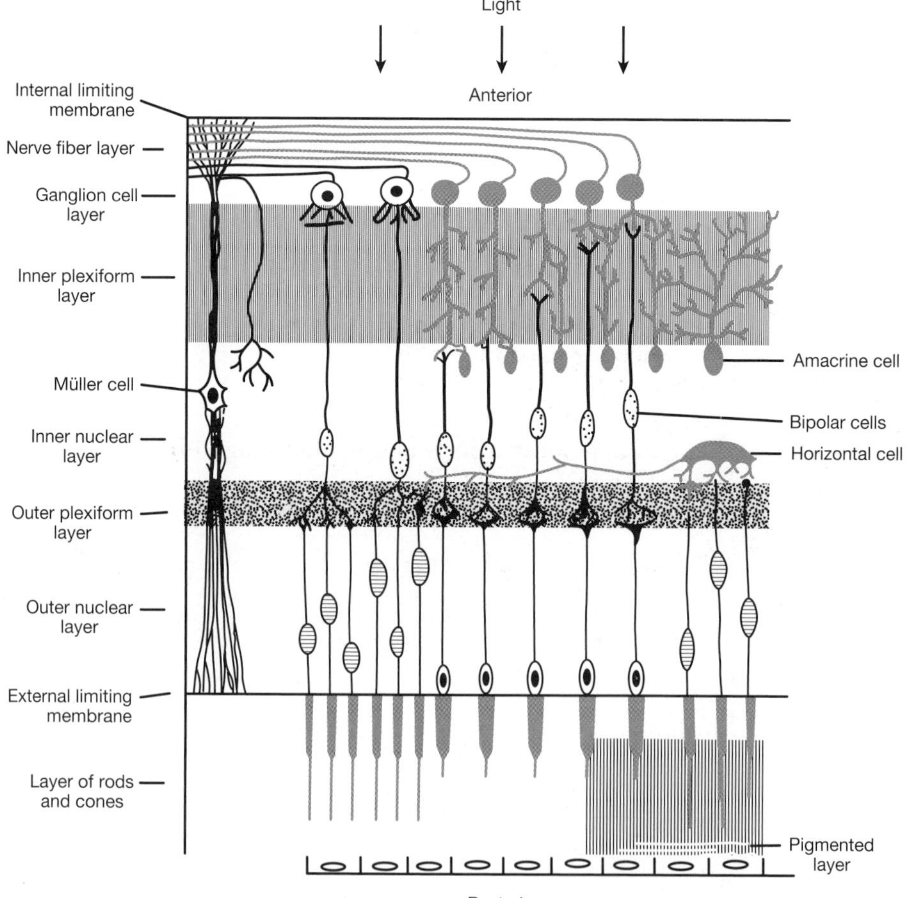

FIGURE 8.1. Diagram of the cellular elements of the retina. Light entering the eye anteriorly passes through the full thickness of the retina to reach the rods and cones (the light sensitive cells and first system of retinal neurons). Impulses arising in these cells are transmitted by the bipolar cells (second system of retinal neurons) to the ganglion cell layer. The third system of visual neurons consists of the ganglion cells and their axons, which run uninterruptedly through the optic nerve, chiasm, and optic tracts, synapsing with cells in the lateral geniculate body. (Reproduced, with permission, from Ropper AH, Brown RH. *Adams and Victor's Principles of Neurology*, 8th ed. New York: McGraw-Hill, 2005: 206.)

Central Retinal Artery Occlusion

Associated with carotid arteriosclerosis, giant cell arteritis, and other vasculitides.

Symptoms and Signs

- Sudden unilateral painless (usually profound) visual loss, often preceded by transient monocular blindness (amaurosis fugax).
- Macular "cherry red spot" and retinal whitening; retinal veins normal, but arteries very attenuated (see Figure 8.2), and may show "boxcarring" with intermittent segmental filling of arteries.

Treatment

Consult ophthalmology emergently regarding appropriate interventions (currently no class I treatment evidence, eg, IV/IA tissue plasminogen activator [tPA] has not been shown to be effective in clinical trials, but research is ongoing). However, patients primarly require immediate stroke evaluation because they are at high risk for subsequent cerebral infarction.

Paraneoplastic Retinopathies

Subacute bilateral visual loss associated with cancer. Retina may appear normal, especially early.

- Cancer-associated retinopathy (CAR):
  - Affects rods and cones; may be associated with antibodies to retinal proteins, such as recoverin.
  - Rods mediate black-and-white and primarily peripheral vision; disease causes photopsias, poor vision at night and in dim conditions, constriction of visual field.
  - Cones mediate color vision and primarily central vision; disease causes decreased visual acuity, decreased color vision, central scotoma.
  - Most frequent malignancy: Small cell lung cancer.
  - Steroids may transiently improve vision.
- Melanoma associated retinopathy (MAR):
  - Affects only rods (preserving visual acuity, color vision, and central visual field but affecting night vision and peripheral field).
  - Associated with melanoma, nearly always after diagnosis, and most frequently after metastatic disease has developed.

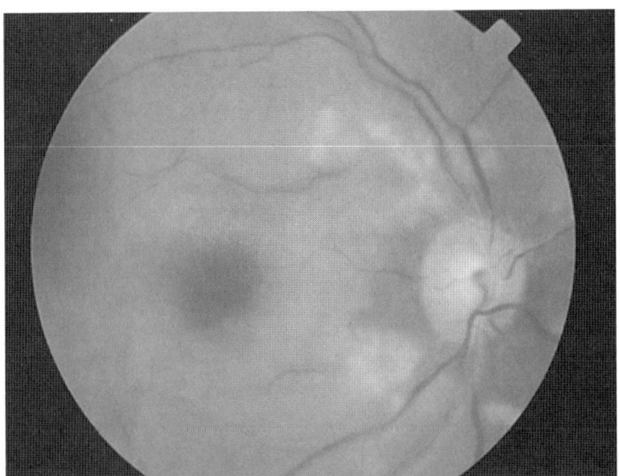

FIGURE 8.2. Central retinal artery occlusion. (Also see Color Plate.) Note the lack of blood column in retinal arteries (veins still have blood inside), cherry red spot, and retinal whitening. (Reproduced, with permission, from Tintinalli JE, Kelen GD, Stapczynski JS. *Tintinalli's Emergency Medicine: A Comprehensive Study Guide,* 6th ed. New York: McGraw-Hill, 2004: Figure 238-17.)

Neuroretinitis

- Acute, usually unilateral, mild to moderate visual loss.
- Disc edema, followed by macular stellate exudates (macular star, Figure 8.3).
- Most frequently associated with Bartonella henselae ("cat scratch disease"), but other causes include syphilis, Lyme disease, sarcoidosis, and toxoplasmosis.
- Not associated with multiple sclerosis.

OPTIC NERVE

Retinal ganglion cell axons converge on the optic nerve head and pass through the lamina cribrosa, after which they become myelinated. The optic nerve and retina consist of central nervous system (CNS) neurons, so they are susceptible to CNS diseases such as multiple sclerosis (MS). They do not regenerate like peripheral nerve.

Anterior Ischemic Optic Neuropathy (AION)

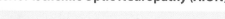

An 80-year-old man presents with sudden, painless vision loss in the right eye associated with swelling of the right optic nerve. What are the next tests? What treatment should you be considering? ESR and CRP, steroids.

Acute painless unilateral visual loss, usually age > 50. Typically, visual loss takes the form of an altitudinal (usually inferior) visual field defect often affecting central acuity. Optic disc edema must be present acutely and may only involve a portion of the optic disc (Figure 8.4).

There are two forms of AION:

- Nonarteritic:
  - Most common, usually in diabetes, hypertension.
  - Sudden, unilateral, painless, profound visual loss in a patient with a small cup-to-disc ratio ("disc at risk").
  - If contralateral cup-to-disc ratio > 0.2, consider giant cell arteritis in patients > 50 and hypercoagulability/other causes in younger patients.

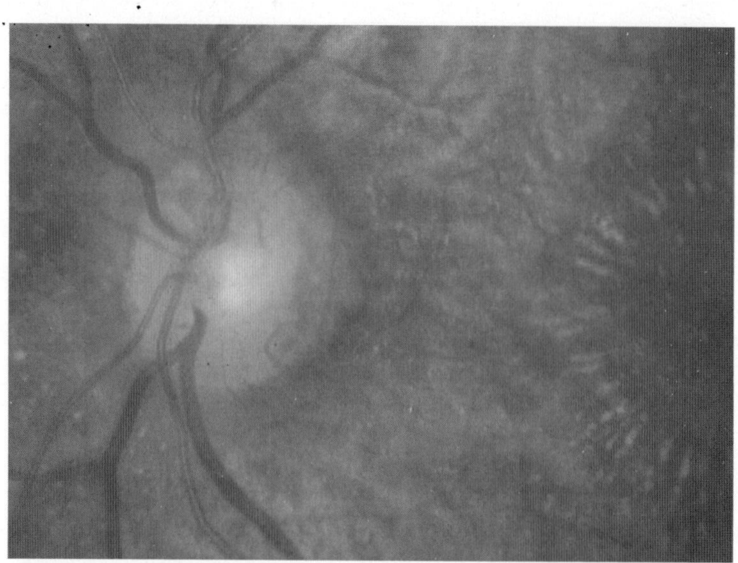

FIGURE 8.3. Neuroretinitis. (Also see Color Plate.) Note the mild optic nerve head edema and the exudates in a starlike pattern in the macula.

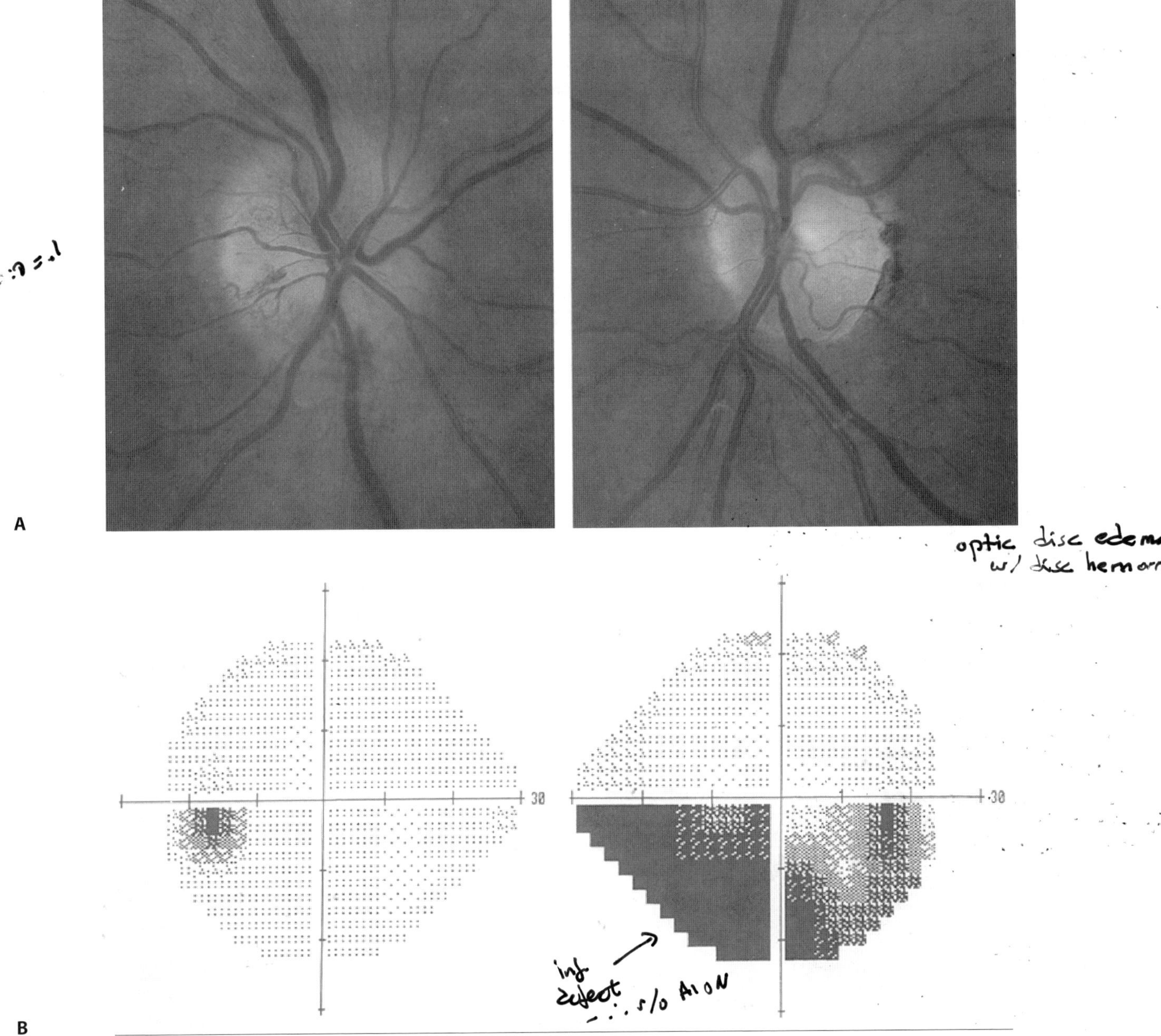

FIGURE 8.4. Anterior ischemic optic neuropathy. (Also see Color Plate.) **A:** Right anterior ischemic optic neuropathy: The right eye (photo on the left above) shows optic disc edema with disc hemorrhages. The left optic nerve has a small cup-to-disc ratio (0.1) seen in most cases of nonarteritic AION. **B:** Right inferior altitudinal defect (remember visual fields are "reversed" from the typical orientation of other medical images) typical of a right anterior ischemic optic neuropathy. (Reproduced, with permission, from Biousse V, Newman NJ. *Neuro-ophthalmology Illustrated.* New York: Thieme, 2009: 197, Figure 8.19B.)

- Arteritic:
  - Caused by giant cell arteritis in patients > 50.
  - Headache, scalp tenderness in 75% of cases.
  - Jaw claudication is the most specific sign.
  - Erythrocyte sedimentation rate (ESR) and C-reactive protein (CRP) rarely normal.
  - Administer steroids immediately while arranging biopsy to confirm diagnosis.
  - Contralateral optic neuropathy will develop in 48 hours in one-third of cases, and within 1 week in another one-third.

KEY FACT

Giant cell arteritis (GCA) is a relatively common cause of AION in patients older than 50. Left untreated, GCA is frequently blinding within days, but when properly considered in the differential of acute visual loss, steroids are a sight-saving treatment.

Optic Neuritis (ON)

A 24-year-old woman presents with subacute visual loss in the left eye associated with pain on eye movements. Her vision is 20/200, and the rest of her exam (including the funduscopic examination) is normal. What is the most important test to obtain? MRI of the brain.

Acute/subacute, central, unilateral visual loss with painful eye movements.

- Acute demyelinating:
  - Most common cause.
  - Typically, painful eye movements (> 90%), nadir over days to 2 weeks, some recovery within 30 days.
  - Two-thirds of ON cases are retrobulbar and therefore produce no disc swelling.
  - If typical ON, magnetic resonance imaging (MRI) to assess the future risk of the development of MS and guide need for disease-modifying therapy.
  - Risk of MS at 15 years with one or more lesions, 56%; 0 lesions, 22%.
- Key treatment guidelines:
  - IV steroids → oral taper as per Optic Neuritis Treatment Trial (ONTT): Quicker recovery of vision, unchanged final visual outcome.
  - ON with two or more MRI lesions, IV steroids delay the onset of MS (although same MS risk by 3 years).
  - Oral steroids alone increase risk of recurrent optic neuritis and should not be prescribed.
  - Risk of MS at 5 years with three or more lesions on MRI, 51%; 1–2 lesions, 37%; 0 lesions, 16%.
  - If there are two or more lesions present on the MRI, treatment with interferon-β_{1a} (Avonex) in addition to IV steroids reduces the 3-year risk of MS by 44%.
- Atypical features (lower MS risk, need to exclude alternatives):
  - Retinal exudates or hemorrhages.
  - Neuroretinitis (discussed above).
  - Marked optic nerve swelling.
  - No light perception vision at onset.
  - Consider antinuclear antibody (ANA), fluorescent treponemal antibody absorption test (FTA-ABS), angiotensin-converting enzyme (ACE), Lyme disease, West Nile virus, ehrlichiosis, Leber optic neuropathy, chest x-ray, and lumbar puncture (LP).

KEY FACT

Oral steroids alone increase the risk of recurrence of ON and should not be prescribed.

Papilledema

- Bilateral optic disc edema due to increased ICP.
- Visual acuity typically normal until late or when very severe. However, peripheral field defects may occur early and patient may be unaware, so formal visual testing should always be obtained.
- Optic nerve edema has features of obscured disc vessels and a relatively preserved optic cup until late.
- Hemorrhages and exudates are also frequently present (Figure 8.5).
- **Symptoms of increased ICP:** Headache, nausea, vomiting, transient visual obscurations (brief transient visual loss usually associated with coughing/Valsalva maneuver, or changes in position), pulsatile tinnitus, diplopia (from cranial nerve [CN] VI palsies).

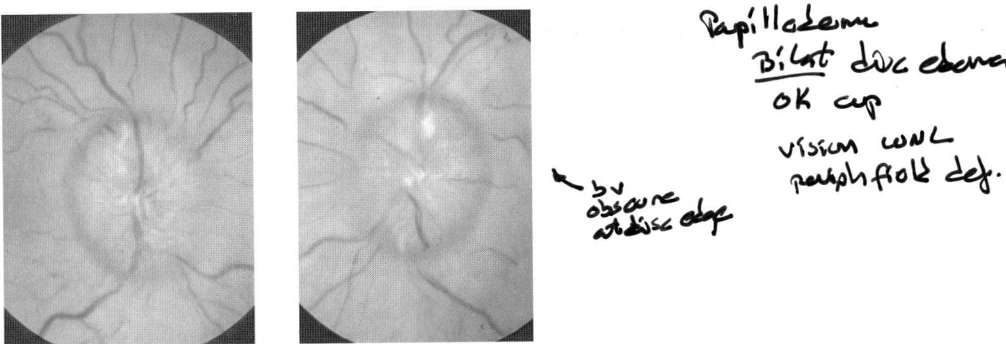

FIGURE 8.5. Papilledema. Note the vessel obscuration at the disc margins with associated hemorrhages and exudates. Note that the optic cup is preserved. (Reproduced, with permission, from Riordan-Eva P, Whitcher JP. *Vaughan & Asbury's General Ophthalmology*, 16th ed. New York: McGraw-Hill, 2003: 275.)

- Idiopathic intracranial hypertension (pseudotumor cerebri):
  - Typically young (20–30), obese women.
  - Sometimes associated with vitamin A (ie, Accutane) and tetracycline antibiotics, among many others.
  - Diagnosis of exclusion requires:
    - Elevated opening pressure (> 25 cm H_2O).
    - Normal MRI of the brain.
    - However, note that radiologic signs of chronically-elevated intracranial pressure may be present, such as posterior flattening of the globes, dilated and tortuous optic nerve sheaths, empty or partially-empty sella, and transverse venous sinus stenosis.
    - Normal CSF.
    - Computed tomography (CT) or MR venogram to exclude venous sinus thrombosis.
    - Treated with acetazolamide and initial diagnostic LP. If progressive visual loss with medical therapy, surgical management with a CSF shunting procedure (ventriculoperitoneal shunt, lumboperitoneal shunt) or optic nerve sheath fenestration should be pursued.

Hereditary Optic Neuropathies

- (Autosomal) dominant optic atrophy:
  - Most common inherited optic neuropathy.
  - Slow bilateral visual loss (approximately one line of vision per decade), frequently first noted at school age but can go undiagnosed for years.
  - Examine family members for optic nerve pallor.
  - Usually central/cecocentral visual field deficits (see Figure 8.6 B, E).
  - Leber hereditiary optic neuropathy:
    - Rare mitochondrial optic neuropathy (maternally transmitted); for unclear reasons typically affects young adult males more than women.
    - Acute visual loss first in one eye and then the second, usually within weeks but always ≤ 1 year.
    - Acute phase: Characteristic hyperemic optic nerve fiber layer with telangectatic and tortuous peripapillary vessels.
    - Cecocentral scotomas typical.

Toxic/Nutritional Optic Neuropathies

Typically, bilateral central/cecocentral visual field defects and color deficiencies.

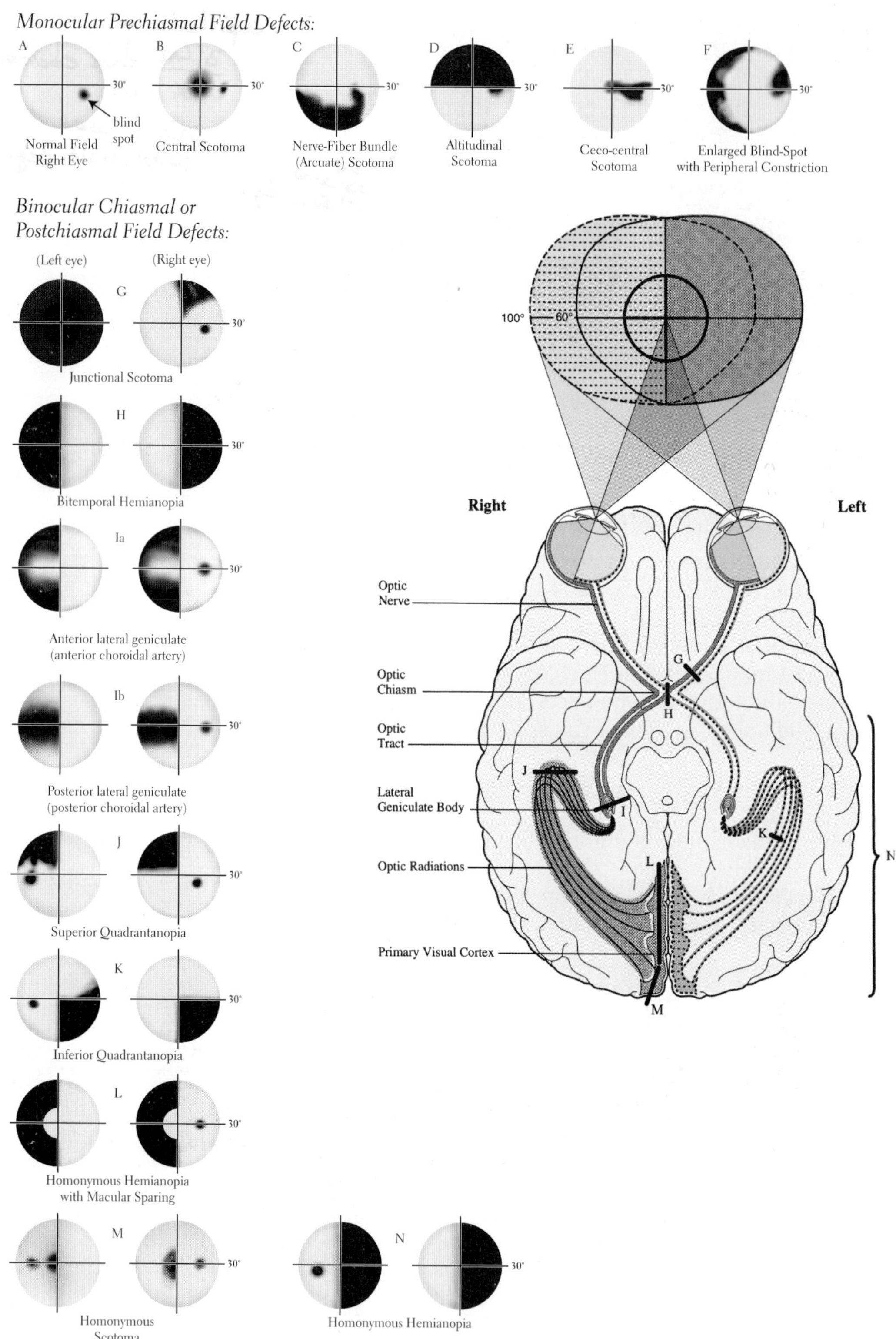

FIGURE 8.6. Localization of visual field deficits. Note that lesions of the posterior occipital lobe can cause a homonymous defect of just central (macular) vision because the occipital lobe is topographically arranged, with central vision located in the posterior half of the occipital lobe and peripheral vision progressively more anteriorly.

- Vitamin B_{12} or copper deficiency.
- Methanol (can be severe, within 24 hours postingestion as MeOH → formaldehyde by alcohol dehydrogenase). Improper distillation of alcohol (moonshine) can produce dangerous concentrations of methanol; sometimes moonshine is distilled in old radiators made of lead which is also neurotoxic.
- Ethambutol (usually after several months of treatment).
- Other medications and exposures: amiodarone, linezolid, cobalt, toluene (glue-sniffing).

Compressive Optic Neuropathies

Can be caused by any type of mass lesion compressing the optic nerve. Key examples include:

- Foster-Kennedy syndrome: Intracranial mass, such as an olfactory groove meningioma plus:
  - Ipsilateral optic pallor (direct compression of optic nerve).
  - Contralateral disc edema (increased ICP).
  - Anosmia from mass effect on the olfactory nerve.
- Optic nerve sheath meningioma:
  - Typically in middle-aged women (like other meningiomas).
  - Slowly progressive optic neuropathy.
  - **MRI of orbits** with contrast and fat saturation (imaging technique that suppresses orbital fat signal, allowing examination of intraorbital contents).
  - **Treatment:** Stereotactic radiation, without biopsy, because surgical procedures nearly always result in visual loss.
- Pituitary adenoma:
  - Can compress an optic nerve or the optic chiasm.
  - Usually slowly progressive visual loss in one eye or a bitemporal visual field defect.
  - However, when the tumor outstrips its blood supply, a hemorrhagic infarction can occur (pituitary apoplexy). Pituitary apoplexy is, in addition to the visual loss, frequently accompanied by headache and ophthalmoplegia. It is a life-threatening condition due to acute hypopituitarism.
- Optic nerve glioma:
  - Appears before the age of 15 in > 85% of cases.
  - Strongly associated with neurofibromatosis I.
  - Usually extremely slow growing with little visual progression.
  - Follow-up rather than more aggressive treatments is generally appropriate unless there is evidence of a malignant course.

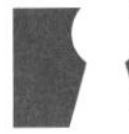

KEY FACT

Routine MRI can miss optic nerve sheath meningiomas; specific orbital imaging is required. Biopsy almost always causes some visual loss and should be avoided in typical cases.

Congenital Optic Neuropathies

Various congenital abnormalities are seen in Table 8.1.

Optic Pathways/Visual Fields

See Figure 8.6.

Pupillary Reflex and Disorders

The pupillary reflex traverses both afferent and efferent visual systems and can be affected by disorders affecting either system. Thus, we will discuss it here before proceeding to other efferent disorders. See Table 8.2 for a summary of pupil abnormalities in coma.

TABLE 8.1. Congenital Optic Disc Anomalies

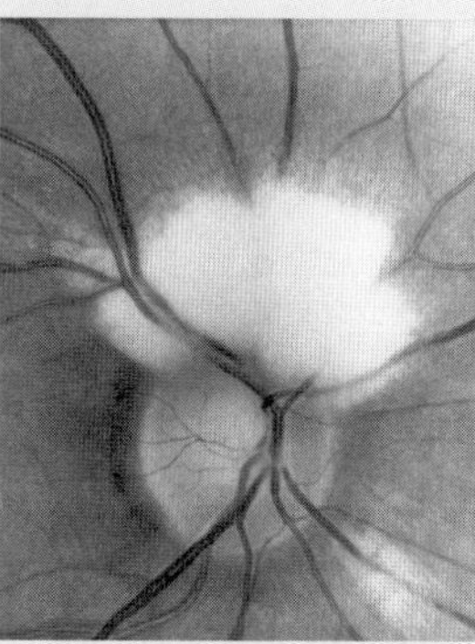 (Reproduced, with permission, from Riordan-Eva P, Whitcher JP. *Vaughan & Asbury's General Ophthalmology,* 16th ed. New York: McGraw-Hill, 2003: 276.)	**Myelinated nerve fibers:** ■ Retinal ganglion cells typically unmyelinated after crossing the lamina cribrosa, but small areas of myelination can persist. ■ White patches with a characteristic "feathered" border. ■ No clinical significance but can be confused with true papilledema.
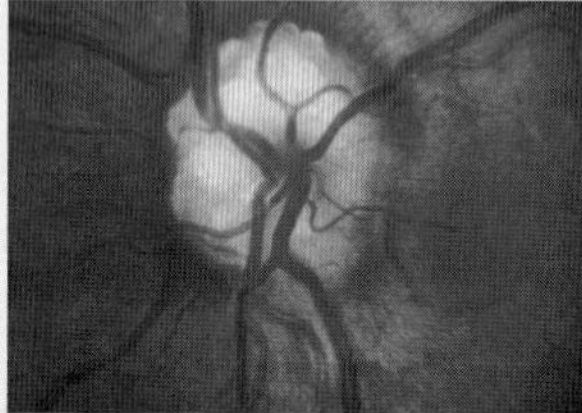 (Reproduced, with permission, from Kasper DL, Braunwald E, Fauci AS, et al. *Harrison's Principles of Internal Medicine,* 16th ed. New York: McGraw-Hill, 2004: Figure 14-25.)	**Drusen:** ■ Round, irregular excrescences on the optic nerve head. ■ Can be "buried" and cause only optic nerve elevation. ■ Can cause vision loss by a variety of mechanisms.
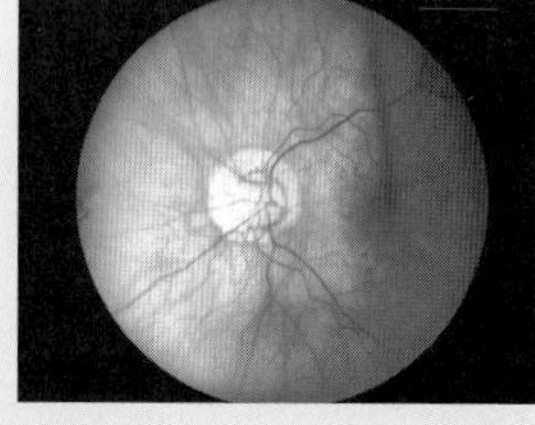 (Reproduced, with permission, from Riordan-Eva P, Whitcher JP. *Vaughan & Asbury's General Ophthalmology,* 16th ed. New York: McGraw-Hill, 2003: Figure 14-21.)	**Optic nerve hypoplasia:** ■ Figure shows "double ring sign": two variable rings of pigment surrounding a small optic nerve. ■ Commonly associated with septo-optic dysplasia, which can cause sudden death in children from corticotropin deficiency due to pituitary abnormalities. ■ MRI and endocrine evaluation required.
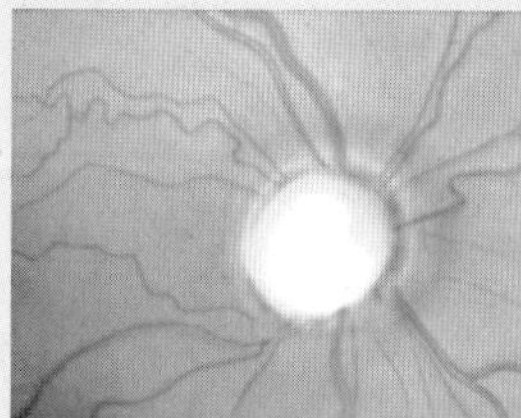 (Reproduced, with permission, from Riordan-Eva P, Whitcher JP. *Vaughan & Asbury's General Ophthalmology,* 16th ed. New York: McGraw-Hill, 2003: Figure 14-23.)	**Optic nerve coloboma:** ■ Dysgenesis of the optic nerve. ■ Associated with other ocular, neurologic, and systemic anomalies such as Walker-Warburg and Aicardi syndromes.

TABLE 8.2. Pupils in Coma

Localization	Pupils	Tips
Encephalic/diencephalic	Small, reactive.	Large pupils require sympathetic activity; ∴ lethargy or encephalopathy → small pupils.
Early uncal herniation (third nerve palsy)	One (unilateral) or both (bilateral or severe unilateral) pupils fixed and dilated.	The uncus pressing the midbrain portion of the third nerve against contralateral tentorium can be falsely localizing.
Midbrain	Midposition, fixed.	Two M's.
Pons	Pinpoint.	Two P's.

NORMAL PUPILLARY LIGHT REFLEX (FIGURE 8.7)

The pupillary light reflex can be divided into an afferent (incoming light signal) arc and an efferent (outgoing pupillary motor control) arc. Lesions in the afferent arc cause relative afferent pupillary defects; lesions in the efferent arc cause anisocoria.

- **Afferent arc:**
  - Light → retina → optic nerve → optic chiasm → optic tract; runs alongside visual fibers, until just before lateral geniculate nucleus, where fibers detour (bypassing the lateral geniculate nucleus) to:
  - Brachium of the superior colliculus → synapses on pretectal nuclei.

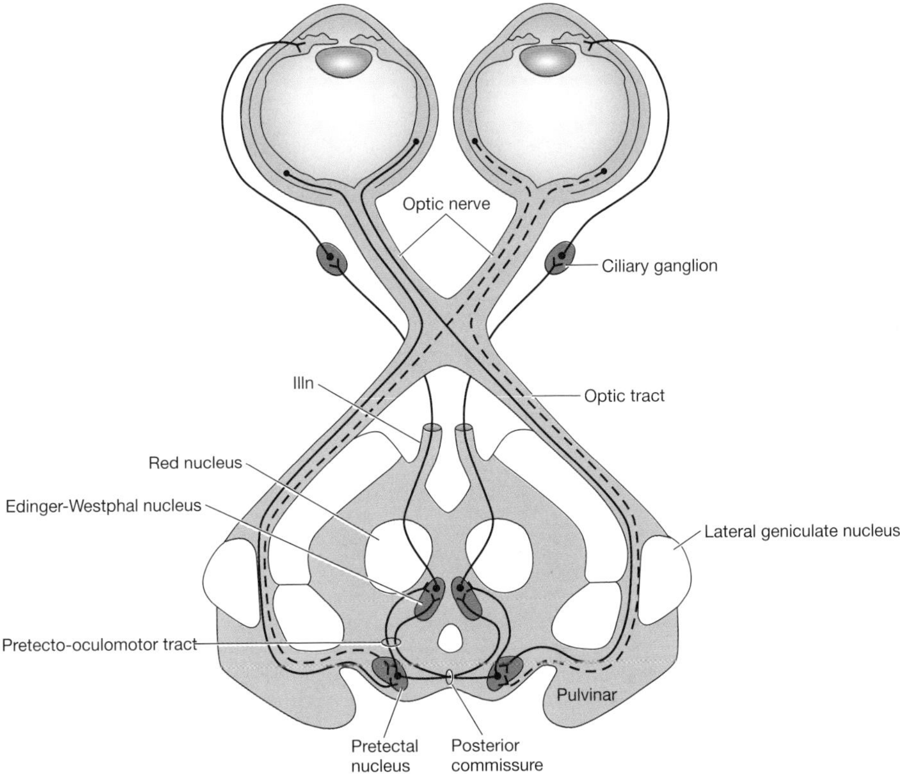

FIGURE 8.7. Pupillary light reflex pathway. (Reproduced, with permission, from Ropper AH, Samuels MA. *Adams & Victor's Principles of Neurology*, 9th ed. NewYork: McGraw-Hill, 2003: 285.)

- Pretectal nuclei → symmetric bilateral inputs to the Edinger-Westphal nuclei (crossing fibers travel via the posterior commissure).
- **Efferent arc:** Edinger-Westphal nuclei (part of CN III nuclei) → CN III → ciliary ganglion → pupillary constrictors.

RELATIVE AFFERENT PUPILLARY DEFECT (RAPD, "MARCUS GUNN PUPIL")

Both pupils constrict incompletely when light is shined into the eye on the abnormal side. Unilateral afferent lesion causes no anisocoria because pretectal nuclei supply symmetric bilateral input to Edinger-Westphal nuclei (Figure 8.8).

- Observed using "swinging flashlight test."
- Abnormal side dilates when the light is shined into it because less light reaches the efferent arc via the damaged afferent arc.
- An RAPD is usually due to a defect anterior to the optic chiasm, but a small RAPD can occur in optic tract lesions. Type of visual field defect distinguishes prechiasmatic RAPD (monocular defect) and postchiasmatic optic tract RAPDs (binocular defect).

LIGHT-NEAR DISSOCIATION

- Poor constriction to light despite relatively preserved constriction to near stimuli ("accommodates, but doesn't react"). Occurs because 90% of the fibers responsible for pupillary constriction are devoted to the near reflex, making it easier to damage the pupillary light reflex than the near reflex.
- **Argyll Robertson pupils:** Small, irregular, poorly light-reactive pupils with light-near dissociation. A classic type of pupil with light-near dissociation

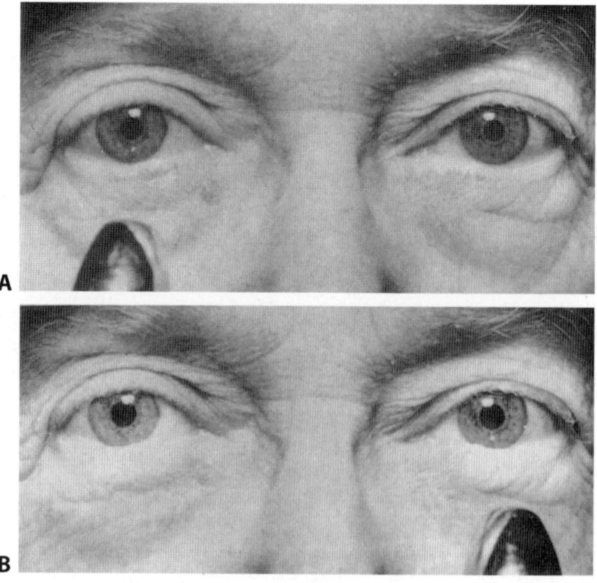

FIGURE 8.8. Left Relative Afferent Pupillary Defect. Note how both pupils are larger in frame B compared with A. This is a left relative afferent pupillary defect because less light is entering through the afferent pathways of the patient's left eye (less light is reaching the brain through this side so the pupils are larger). Remember that this could represent a problem on either side of the brain, but most frequently represents an ipsilateral optic nerve problem. There is no anisocoria because of symmetric input from the afferent arc to both Edinger-Westphal nuclei. (Reproduced, with permission, from Kasper DL, Braunwald E, Fauci AS, et al. *Harrison's Principles of Internal Medicine,* 16th ed. New York: McGraw-Hill, 2004: Figure 25-2.)

due to neurosyphilis, but more common in diabetic neuropathy, chronic Adie pupils, and Perinaud syndrome.

Efferent Visual System Disorders

Efferent system disorders are characterized by anisocoria or extraocular movement disturbances.

ANISOCORIA

Asymmetric pupils are caused by unilateral pathology (or medication) causing either a too-large pupil or a too-small pupil; the first task is to identify which pupil is abnormal. Isolated anisocoria without ptosis or ophthalmoplegia is typically not an emergency. A diagnostic approach to anisocoria is shown in Figure 8.9.

Which pupil is abnormal? If the asymmetry is worse in dim light, the small pupil is abnormal (failure to dilate). If the asymmetry is worse in bright light, the large pupil is abnormal (failure to constrict).

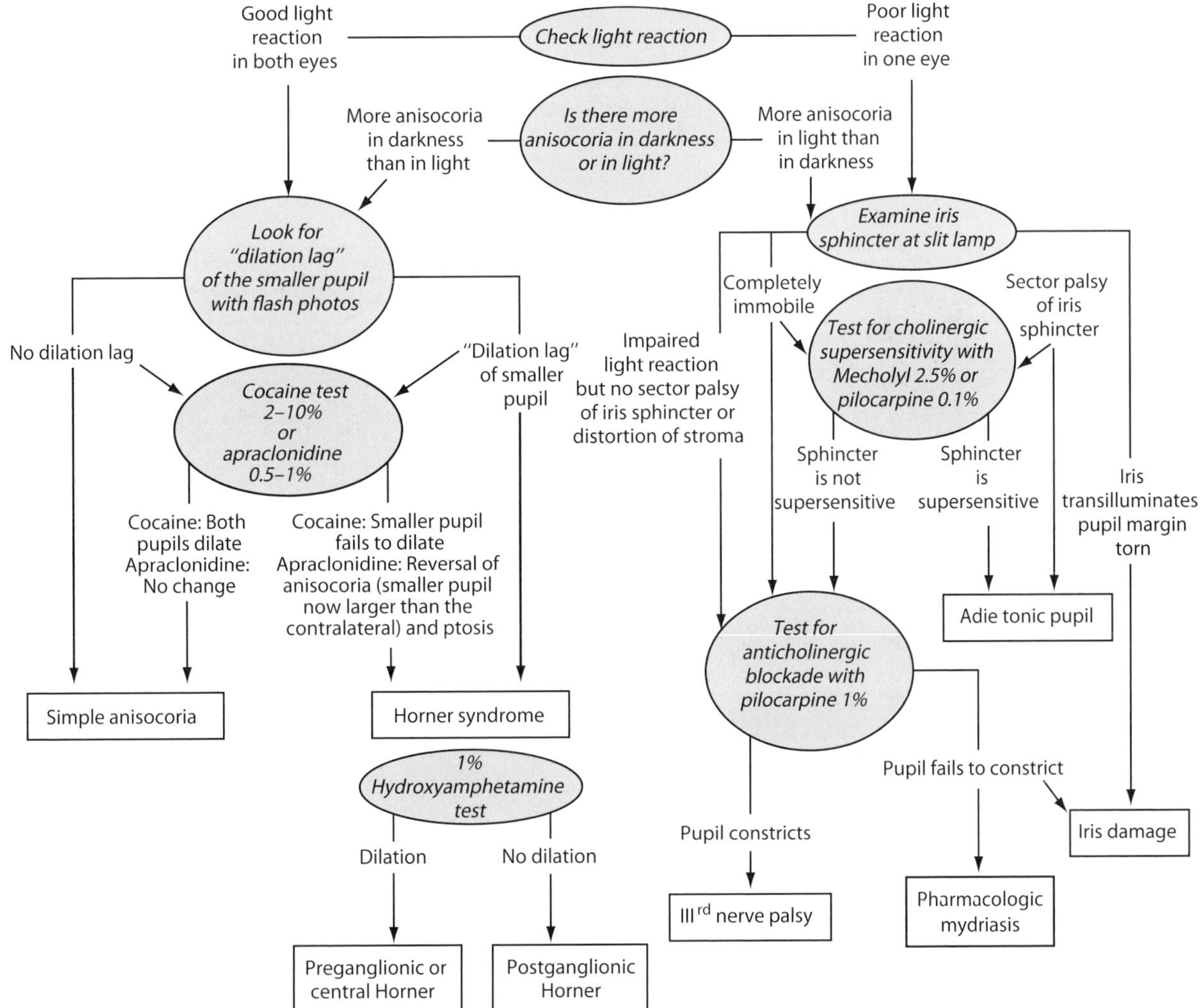

FIGURE 8.9. Diagnostic approach to anisocoria. Ropper AH, Samuels MA. *Adams and Victor's Principles of Neurology,* 9th ed. New York: McGraw-Hill, 2005: 244.)

Abnormally Small Pupil

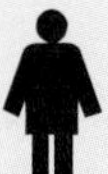

A 45-year-old man presents with a smaller pupil (more noticeable in the dark) and mild ptosis on the left side. He noticed it 2 days ago after he developed severe neck pain. What is the most concerning diagnosis? Carotid dissection.

Horner syndrome, also known as oculosympathetic palsy, is an abnormally small pupil and ptosis, with or without facial anhidrosis, due to a lesion in the sympathetic pathways shown in Figure 8.10.

- A Horner pupil dilates slowly and incompletely after several seconds in dim light ("dilation lag").
- Ptosis of the upper lid is usually mild because sympathetic pathways only contribute to lid elevation via Müller muscle (CN III and levator palpebrae do the rest).
- Sometimes small "upward" ptosis of the lower lid occurs (there is a sympathetically innervated muscle in both upper and lower lids).
- Physiologic ("simple") anisocoria:
  - Approximately 20% of normal people have a small anisocoria (< 0.4 mm), and it often fluctuates.
  - Differentiated from Horner by dilation to cocaine 4%, and by lack of ptosis or anhidrosis.
  - Other causes of an abnormally small pupil include: ocular mechanical causes (eg, previous ocular surgery or adhesions from uveitis) and pharmacologic constriction (eg, pilocarpine drops).

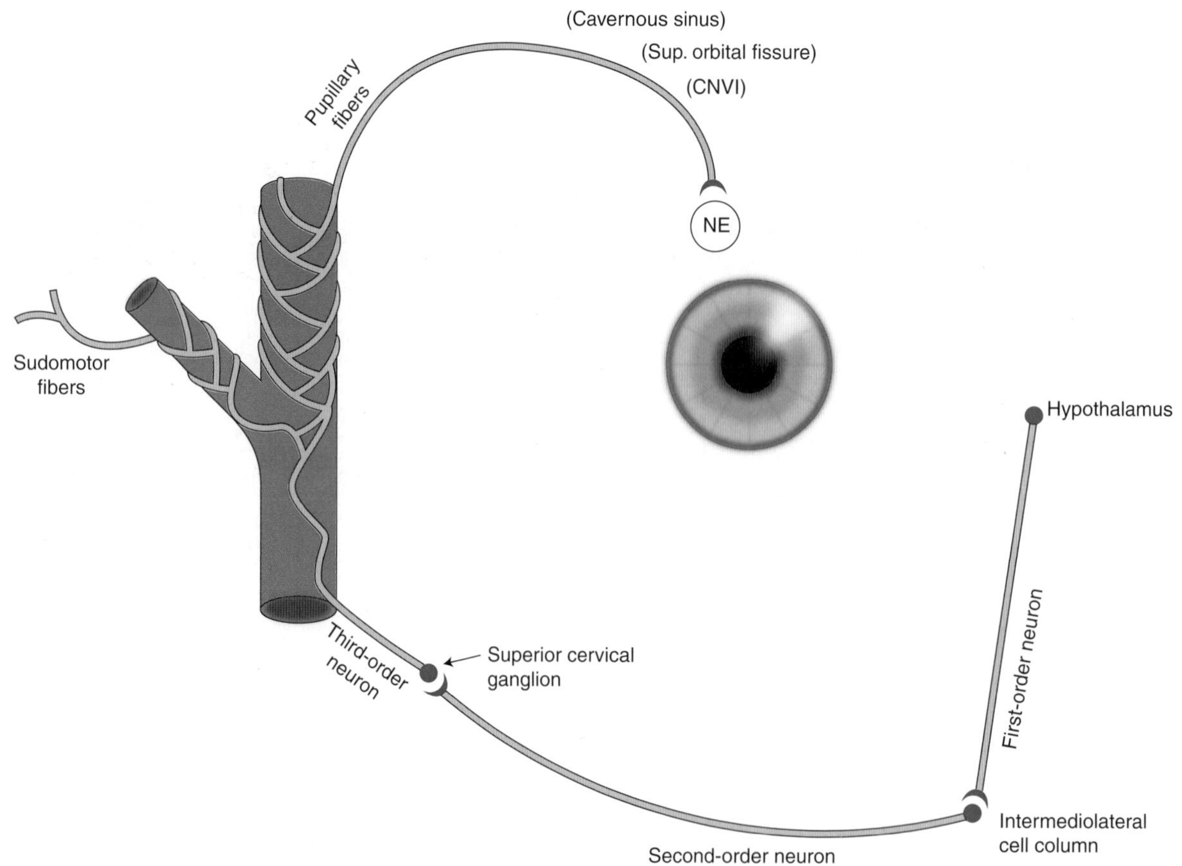

FIGURE 8.10. The oculosympathetic pathway: Critical to the localizing of a Horner syndrome.

Questions to ask when localizing a Horner pupil.

Question 1: Is there oculosympathetic palsy (a Horner pupil)?
Answer: Cocaine 4% (inhibits NE reuptake) dilates a sympathetically innervated pupil, but dilates any Horner pupil poorly or not at all. More recently, apraclonidine 0.5% or 1% has been used in the place of cocaine. In the normal setting, its stronger α_2- than α_1-adrenergic effect causes constriction of the pupil. However, when there is disruption of the sympathetic pathway, α_1 receptors are upregulated (denervation hypersensitivity) on the pupil dilator muscles and then apraclonidine will instead cause dilation of the Horner pupil.

Question 2: Is the lesion preganglionic (1st or 2nd order neurons) or postganglionic (3rd order neurons)?
Answer: Hydroxyamphetamine 1% stimulates NE release from a healthy 3rd order neuron, but in a Horner pupil due to an injury to 3rd order neurons (as in carotid dissection) the pupil will not dilate. First-order neuron lesions are almost always associated with other neurolgic signs (as in the lateral medullary syndrome). A major concern in second-order neuron lesions is an apical lung mass.

Question 3: If the lesion is postganglionic, is it proximal or distal to the internal carotid artery?
Answer: Sudomotor fibers to the face travel via the external carotid artery. Facial anhidrosis suggests a proximal lesion. The most worrisome third-order neuron Horner syndrome is carotid dissection.

Abnormally Large Pupil

A 32-year-old woman presents complaining of a large right pupil she noticed in the mirror this morning. She has no other complaints. On exam there is no ptosis or extraocular movement abnormalities. The pupil does not react to light. What is the next bedside test? Checking to see if the pupil constricts to a near target.

Abnormally large pupils typically have abnormal light reflexes.

- Third nerve palsy:
- Isolated mydriasis without ptosis or extraocular muscle weakness is rarely CN III palsy.
- Complete: Prominent ptosis (levator weakness), eye "down and out" (weakness of superior rectus, inferior oblique, medial rectus). Consider:
  - Aneurysm (posterior communicating artery is classic).
  - Pituitary apoplexy.
  - Giant cell arteritis.
  - Meningeal syndromes (eg, tuberculosis, sarcoid, carcinomatous, and lymphomatous).
- Pupil-sparing: Ptosis and CN III weakness,
  - Classically due to diabetic infarction.
  - Spares the pupillary fibers located on the outside portion of the nerve (see also below, under Disordered Motility of Extraocular Muscles).
- **Adie tonic pupil:**
  - Isolated, large, sluggish ("tonic") pupil.
  - Light-near dissociation.
  - Probably viral/postviral autoimmune damage to ciliary ganglion (parasympathetic) neurons.
  - Damage to ciliary ganglion often incomplete, causing sectoral papillary paralysis and papillary irregularity.
  - Constricts to dilute (0.1%) pilocarpine—which doesn't constrict normal pupils—because of postsynaptic receptor hypersensitivity.
  - A longstanding Adie pupil can become small and irregular ("Argyll Robertson appearance").
- **Adie syndrome:** Adie pupil plus absent/reduced deep tendon reflexes.

KEY FACT

Isolated mydriasis without ptosis or EOM weakness is rarely due to CN III palsy.

- **Pharmacologic pupil (atropinic mydriasis):** Large, sluggish pupil due to scopolamine, albuterol, ipratropium, plants such as belladonna, jimson weed, and the like. Does not constrict to undiluted pilocarpine (1%) due to pharmacologic blockade.
- **Traumatic pupil:** Blunt eye trauma can disrupt the pupillary musculature or the parasympathetic fibers leading to a dilated pupil. This can also be seen following similar injuries from intraocular surgery.

PTOSIS AND OTHER LID DISORDERS

- Distinguishing ptosis of Horner syndrome from third nerve palsy:
  - CN III: Weakness of levator → severe ptosis, upper lid only. CN III never causes isolated ptosis.
  - Horner: Weakness of Müller muscle → mild upper and sometimes small "upward" lower lid ptosis with a small pupil.
- **Mechanical ptosis:** Due to dehiscence of levator aponeurosis. Associated with age, long-standing contact lens wear. Asymmetric lid creases are seen.
- **Lagophthalmos:** Incomplete eye closure during gentle eyelid closure, as when sleeping. Can occur in Bell's palsy. Requires treatment with corneal lubrication.
- **Blepharospasm:** Brief bilateral involuntary eye closure. Can be triggered/worsened by bright light. Seen in some dystonias and other movement disorders. Can be helped with botulinum toxin.
- **Eyelid apraxia:** Most associated with blepharospasm, seen in other conditions (Parkinson, progressive supranuclear palsy). Difficulty opening the eyelids, which appear only gently closed. Patients elevate eyebrows and forehead in an attempt to open the eyes.
- **Lid lag:** While pursuing a visual target moving slowly from superior to inferior, the lid will lag slightly behind its normal position (in normal patients the lid is always at the limbus ready to protect the cornea). Associated with thyroid eye disease (see below).
- **Lid twitch:** "Cogan lid twitch" can be seen in myasthenia gravis. After looking downward, when gaze returns to midposition the lid "jumps" higher before settling into position. (Resting the levator allows brief return of normal function in a myasthenic.)

DISORDERED MOTILITY OF EXTRAOCULAR MUSCLES (EOMs)

Ophthalmoparesis and ophthalmoplegia can be caused peripherally by mechanical interference with movement or disease of muscle, neuromuscular junction, or motor nerves.

- Restrictive/muscle:
  - Thyroid eye disease: Proptosis, lid retraction, lid lag (Figure 8.11). Inferior rectus, medial rectus most commonly involved. Can have normal thyroid function; can develop after treatment of Graves disease. Enlarged EOMs on orbital imaging studies.
  - Other muscle-related causes: congenital (congenital fibrosis of extraocular muscles, Duane syndrome), mitochondrial myopathies (eg, Kearns-Sayre syndrome, progressive external ophthalmoplegia).
- **Neuromuscular junction:** Ocular findings (eg, fluctuating ptosis, weakness of eye closure, Cogan lid twitch, diplopia) are the initial manifestation in ~75% of patients with myasthenia gravis. Of these, 20% of cases remain purely ocular.
- **Nerve:**
  - Third nerve palsy (Figure 8.12): See also above, under Pupillary Reflex and Disorders. "Pupil-sparing" CN III palsy (ptosis and EOM weakness

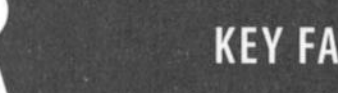

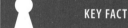

KEY FACT

"Pupil-sparing CN III palsy" suggests nerve infarction and a benign prognosis. But only consider this when the CN III palsy is otherwise complete, since even aneurysms can cause partial CN III palsies that "spare the pupil."

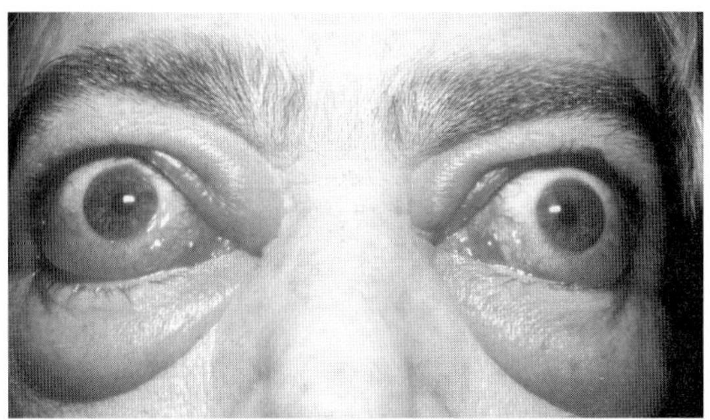

FIGURE 8.11. Thyroid eye disease. (Reproduced, with permission, from Riordan-Eva P, Whitcher JP. *Vaughan & Asbury's General Ophthalmology*, 17th ed. New York: McGraw-Hill, 2008: Figure 15-23A.)

is complete, but pupil normal) is due to microvascular nerve infarction. Greater risk in age > 50, diabetes, and hypertension. Typically intensely painful, with severe ptosis and weakness of CN III–innervated EOMs, but pupil is unaffected. Improvement is typically dramatic within 4–6 weeks (full recovery by 3 months).

- Sixth nerve palsy (Figure 8.13): Horizontal diplopia worsened by gaze directed toward the ipsilateral side, resulting in an esotropia. Note that not all normal patients "bury the sclera" on lateral gaze. A Horner syndrome + sixth nerve palsy = possible cavernous sinus lesion. If isolated, usually microvascular in older patients, and in young patients, often not suggestive of an emergent condition. Other causes include trauma, increased ICP, compression, meningeal or cavernous sinus process. Cavernous carotid aneurysms/fistula.
- Fourth nerve palsy: Subtle vertical or oblique diplopia, worsened by Gazing in the Opposite direction or Tilting the head in the Same direction (mnemonic: "it GOTS worse") (see Figure 8.14).
  - Superior oblique muscle primarily intorts the eye, but also contributes to depression and abduction. When the eye is adducted, the superior

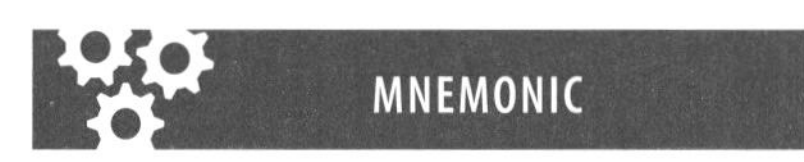

MNEMONIC

Gazing in the **O**pposite direction or **T**ilting the head in the **S**ame direction make diplopia due to a fourth nerve palsy worse ("it **GOTS** worse").

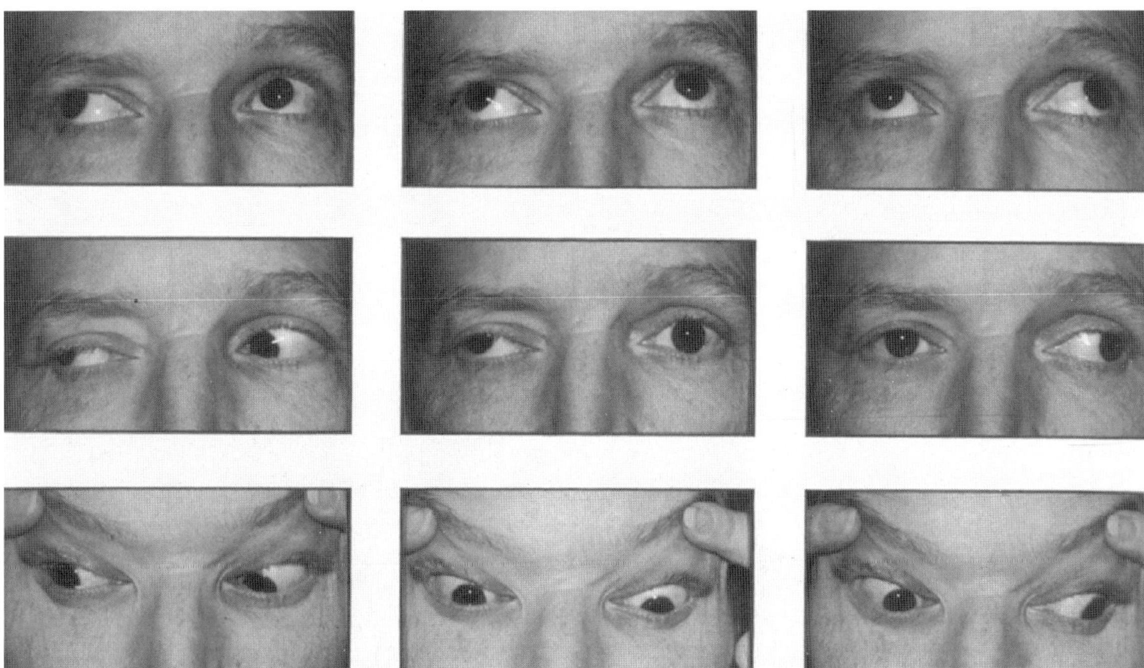

FIGURE 8.12. Right third nerve palsy. (Also see Color Plate.) Note the ptosis and limitation in the movement of the right eye upward, downward, and inward. (Reproduced, with permission, from Biousse V, Newman NJ. *Neuro-ophthalmology Illustrated*. New York: Thieme Medical Publishers, 2009: 392.)

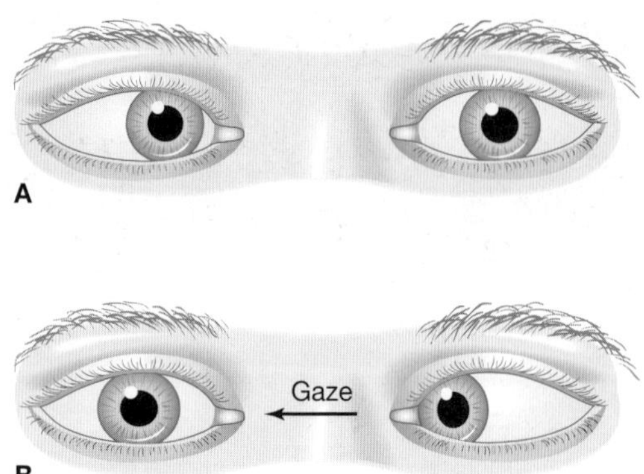

FIGURE 8.13. Right sixth nerve palsy. A: In primary gaze the patient has an esotropia (eyes turned inward). **B:** When the patient looks to the right the right eye is unable to abduct. (Reproduced, with permission, from Aminoff MJ, Greenberg DA, Simon RP. *Clinical Neurology,* 6th ed. New York: McGraw-Hill, 2005: Figure 4-16.)

oblique depresses it. It also contributes to some abduction, but this is primarily done by CN VI via the lateral rectus.

- Most commonly idiopathic.
- Can be congenital—patients tend to compensate into adulthood; head tilt on old photographs.
- Frequently traumatic—CN IV most common cause of diplopia after closed head trauma (even minor).
- Other: Nerve infarction, mass lesions, and meningeal processes. Isolated CN IV rarely due to emergent processes like aneurysms.
- Remember that the superior oblique significantly depresses the eye only when it is adducted (by CN III via the medial rectus). So testing CN IV involves adducting and depressing the eye, even though the superior oblique depresses and abducts the eye. In a third nerve palsy the

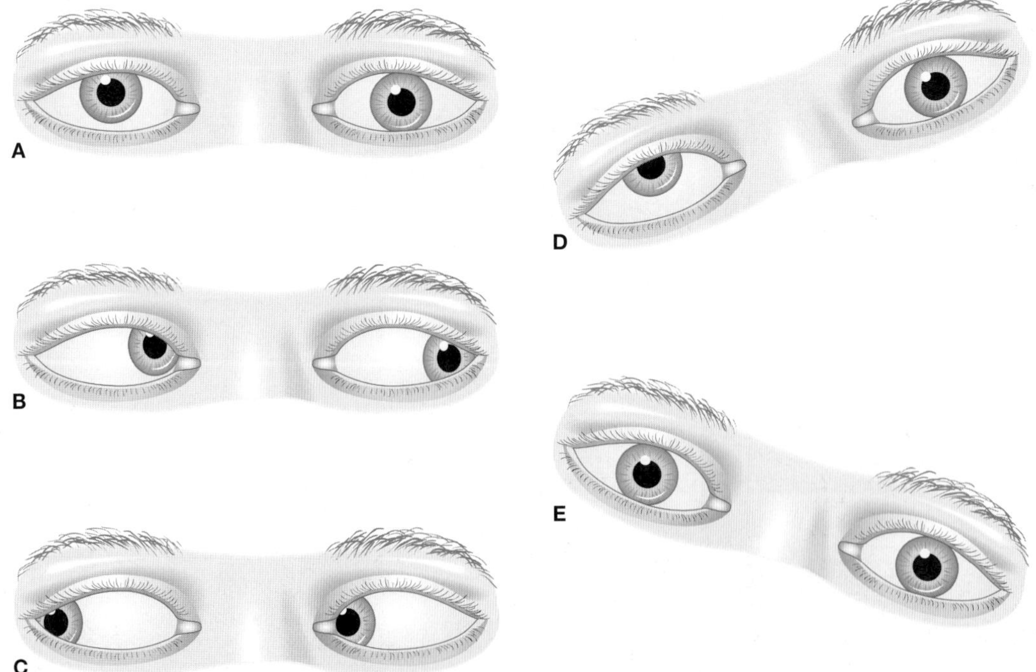

FIGURE 8.14. Right fourth nerve palsy. A: Primary gaze: affected (right) eye elevated and abducted. **B:** Contralateral gaze: affected eye is elevated and incompletely adducted. **C:** Ipsilateral gaze. **D:** Ipsilateral tilt: worsens diplopia. **E:** Contralateral tilt: improves diplopia. (Reproduced, with permission, from Aminoff MJ, Greenberg DA, Simon RP. *Clinical Neurology,* 6th ed. New York: McGraw-Hill, 2005: Figure 4-15.)

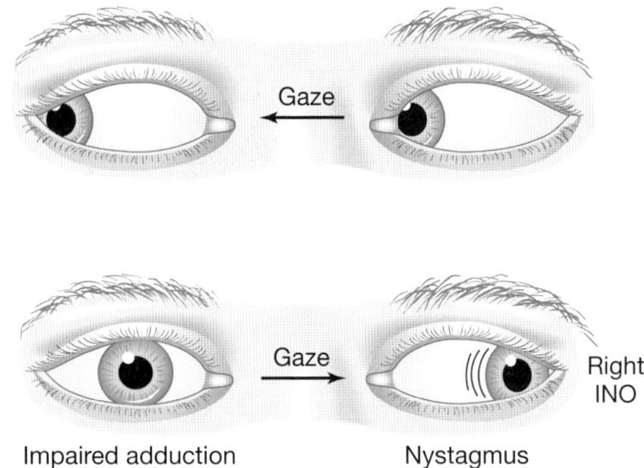

FIGURE 8.15. Right internuclear ophthalmoplegia. The patient is able to look to the right without difficulty but on left gaze has impaired adduction of the right eye and abducting nystagmus of the left eye. (Reproduced, with permission, from Aminoff MJ, Greenberg DA, Simon RP. *Clinical Neurology*, 6th ed. New York: McGraw-Hill, 2005: Figure 4-17.)

eye cannot be adducted. Thus, CN IV function is tested by abducting the eye (with the normal CN VI function) and looking for intortion when the patient looks down.

INFRANUCLEAR VERSUS SUPRANUCLEAR OPHTHALMOPLEGIA

With supranuclear ophthalmoplegia, the patient is unable to move the eye(s) in a given direction voluntarily, but during passive head movement during visual fixation, the eyes can move.

- Nuclear third nerve palsy: Dorsal midbrain process causing ipsilateral CN III palsy plus contralateral ptosis and upgaze limitation.
  - CN III subnuclei for superior recti are located contralaterally. These fibers decussate immediately so nuclear lesion → bilateral upgaze impairment.
  - Insult to the single caudal central nucleus serving both levator muscles → bilateral ptosis.
- Internuclear ophthalmoplegia (INO): Damage to the ipsilateral medial longitudinal fasciculus. See Figures 8.15 and 8.16.
- Horizontal gaze palsy: Ipsilateral nuclear CN VI palsy. See Figure 8.16.
- One-and-a-half syndrome: Damage to ipsilateral CN VI and medial longitudinal fasciculus (MLF). See Figure 8.16.
- Upgaze paralysis occurs with lesions of the posterior commissure or pretectal area and is part of Parinaud dorsal midbrain syndrome (upgaze palsy, lid retraction, light-near dissociation, and convergence-retraction nystagmus).
- Downgaze paralysis occurs with bilateral lesions in the rostral interstitial nucleus of the MLF.
  - Vascular supply: Posterior thalamosubthalamic paramedian branch of the PCA.
  - Can occur in association with thalamic infarcts.
  - Up- and downgaze palsies seen in Whipple disease, progressive supranuclear palsy, diffuse upper brain stem disorders.
- Skew deviation: Vertical deviation of the eyes not caused by infranuclear lesions (eg, CN III or IV palsy). Caused by lesions in the cerebellum, brain stem, and vestibulo-ocular pathways. Most common in lateral medullary syndromes in which vestibular pathways are affected. Skew deviations may improve when the patient is lying flat because unopposed utricular input from the normal side is removed.

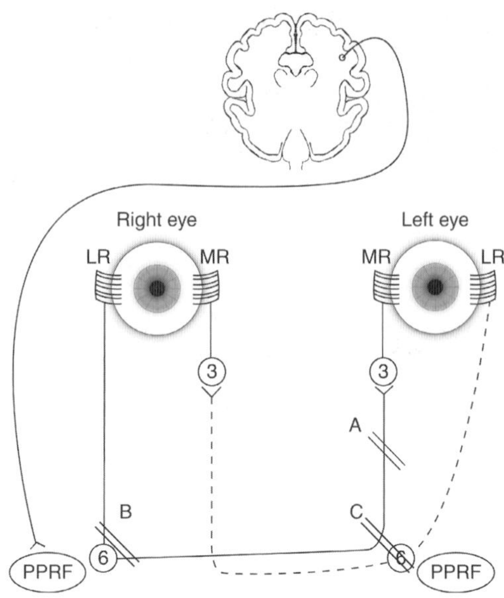

FIGURE 8.16. INO, horizontal gaze palsy, and one-and-a-half syndrome. A: Left INO: Damage to the left MLF causes inability of the left eye to adduct when gazing to the right, but the left eye can adduct when converging. Right-beating nystagmus in the right eye results because the right eye tends to drift back in an attempt to stay aligned with the weak left eye. **B:** Right horizontal gaze palsy: Damage to the right sixth nerve nucleus causes inability of either eye to gaze rightward due to the right sixth nerve nucleus' direct control of the ipsilateral lateral rectus and its indirect control of contralateral medial rectus by connections to the third nerve nucleus via the MLF. **C:** Damage to the left 6th nerve nucleus and the adjacent passing fibers of the left MLF causes a left "one-and-a-half" (left horizontal gaze palsy and INO): Both eyes unable to look left and left eye unable to look right.

- Ocular tilt reaction (OTR): Normally when tilting the head, both eyes counter-roll in the opposite direction (contralateral eye falls, ipsilateral eye rises). The OTR (abnormal) is a triad of spontaneous (1) skew deviation, (2) cyclotorsion of both eyes, and (3) paradoxical head tilt toward the lower eye. Caused by damage anywhere along the vestibular pathways/connections.

Hearing Loss and Tinnitus

SENSORINEURAL VERSUS CONDUCTIVE HEARING LOSS

- **Sensorineural:**
  - Disease from cochlea to CN VIII.
  - Air conduction (AC) > bone conduction (BC)—normal pattern.
  - Weber test: Louder in the normal ear.
- **Conductive:**
  - Disease of tympanic membrane or ossicles → failure to conduct vibration to cochlea.
  - BC > AC.
  - Weber test: Louder in the abnormal ear (no distracting environmental noise).

TINNITUS

- Occurs in up to a third of adult population.
- Suggests lesion (eg, tumor) along auditory pathway when louder than environmental sounds.
- Vestibulo-ocular reflex (VOR): Steady ocular fixation while head is rotated.
- Cancellation of VOR: Normal = no nystagmus if patient fixates on their thumb while being turned in a rotating chair. Nystagmus suggests lesion of cerebellar pathways.

PERIPHERAL CAUSES OF DIZZINESS AND NYSTAGMUS

Peripheral versus Central Vertigo

- Central:
  - Milder (unless due to a vascular event).
  - Nystagmus: Direction changing (fast phase → gaze).
  - Can be positional, but no latency; may last > 1 minute; does not fatigue.
- Peripheral:
  - Typically more severe, associated with vomiting.
  - Nystagmus: Direction fixed.
  - Can be positional, has onset latency; fatigues.

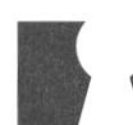

KEY FACT

Peripheral vertigo ≠ "benign" vertigo! It can be caused by mass lesions (eg, cerebellopontine angle tumors) and cranial neuropathies.

Benign Paroxysmal Positional Vertigo (BPPV)

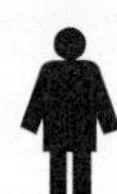

A 60-year-old woman presents with brief, intermittent dizziness triggered only by lying down or sitting up in bed. What is an effective treatment to consider that is directed at the underlying pathophysiology? Epley maneuver.

- Transient (usually < 60 seconds) vertigo provoked by position change.
- Short (usually < 10 seconds) latency onset after provocative maneuver (eg, Dix-Hallpike).
- Fatigable: Effect reduced with repetition.
- Caused by **canalolithiasis**—stimulation of the semicircular canal by debris floating in the endolymph.
- Canaliths in posterior canal (most common) diagnosed with the Dix-Hallpike maneuver (Figure 8.17) and treated with the Epley maneuver (Figure 8.18).

Vestibular Neuronitis/Labyrinthitis

- Subacute onset of severe vertigo, often vomiting. Presumed viral/postviral cause.
- Usually improves in < 1 week; may recur.
- Vertigo only: Neuronitis.
- Vertigo and hearing loss: Labyrinthithis.

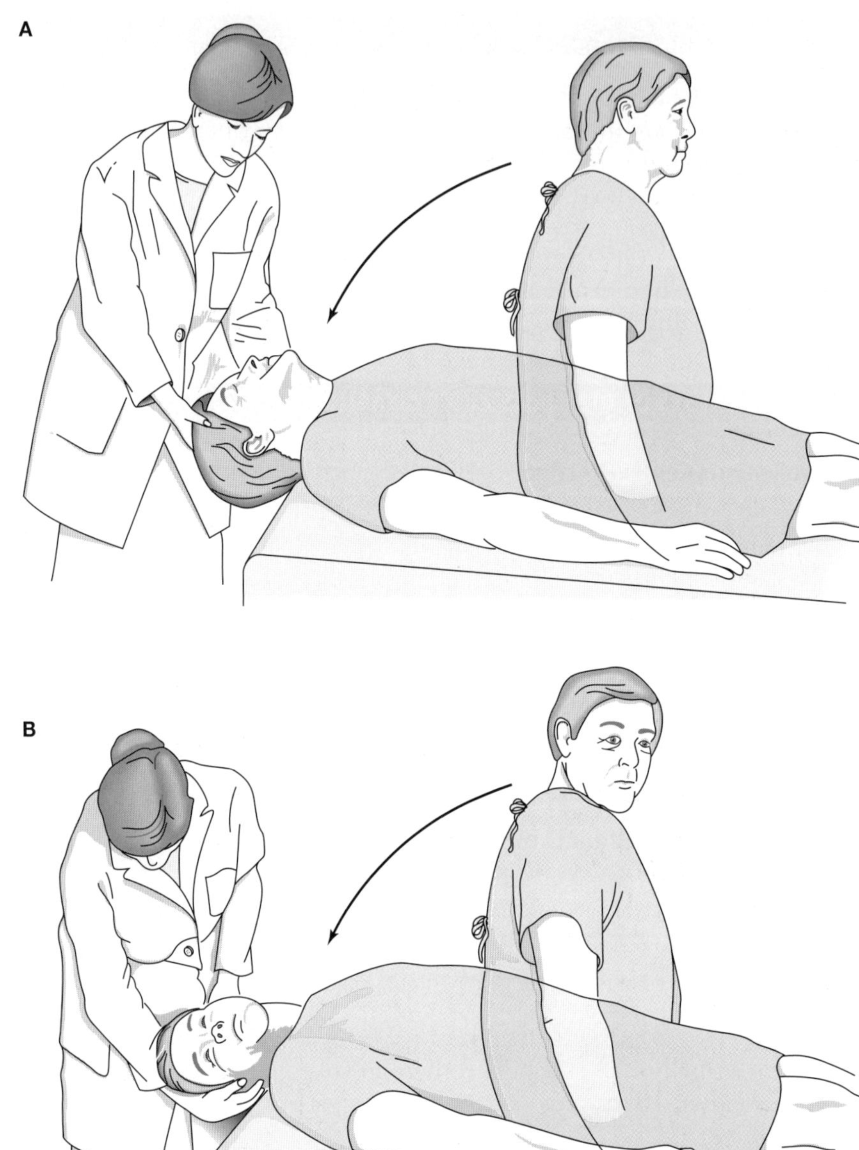

FIGURE 8.17. Dix-Hallpike maneuver, a test for positional vertigo and nystagmus. The patient is seated on a table with the head and eyes directed 45 degrees to the left (A), and is then quickly lowered to a supine position with the head hanging over the table edge, 45 degrees below horizontal. The patient's eyes are then observed for nystagmus, and the patient is asked to report any vertigo. The test is repeated with the patient's head and eyes turned 45 degrees to the right (B). (Adapted, with permission, from Aminoff MJ, Greenberg DA, Simon RP. *Clinical Neurology*, 6th ed. New York: McGraw-Hill, 2005: 104.)

Ménière Disease

- Recurrent attacks of vertigo, tinnitus, and progressive low-frequency hearing loss.
- Tinnitus or deafness may be absent during the initial attacks.
- No established effective treatment; can try low-salt diet, diuretics, steroids, then various surgical treatments if these fail.

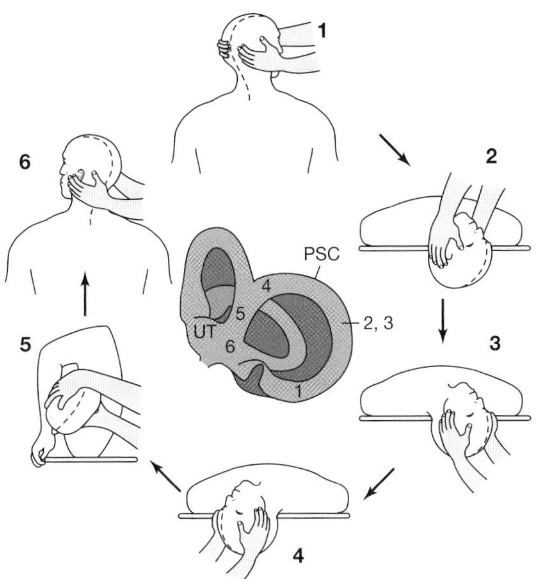

FIGURE 8.18. Epley maneuver—repositioning treatment for benign positional vertigo resulting from canalolithiasis. In the example shown, repositioning maneuvers are used to move endolymphatic debris out of the posterior semicircular canal (PSC) of the right ear and into the utricle (UT, where they belong!). The numbers (1–6) refer to both the position of the patient and the corresponding location of debris within the labyrinth. The patient is seated and the head is turned 45 degrees to the right (1). The head is lowered rapidly to below the horizontal (2); the examiner shifts position (3); and the head is rotated rapidly 90 degrees in the opposite direction, so it now points 45 degrees to the left, where it remains for 30 seconds (4). The patient then rolls onto the left side without turning the head in relation to the body and maintains this position for another 30 seconds (5) before sitting up (6). This maneuver may need to be repeated until nystagmus is abolished. The patient must then avoid the supine position for at least 1–2 days. (Adapted, with permission, from Aminoff MJ, Greenberg DA, Simon RP. *Clinical Neurology*, 6th ed. New York: McGraw-Hill, 2005: 109.)

Vestibulotoxicity

- Progressive unsteadiness caused by drugs or toxins; aminoglycosides most common.
- Little nystagmus or vertigo due to bilateral pathology.

Localizing Nystagmus

Jerk nystagmus is characterized by direction of the fast phase, but caused by a disorder of slow gaze. Table 8.3 describes various forms of nystagmus and their localizing value.

Here's one way to conceptualize the significance of jerk nystagmus: the eyes are slowly "dragged" in an abnormal direction or because of vestibular imbalance. They then have to "jerk back" in order to maintain the desired gaze direction.

TABLE 8.3. Types of Nystagmus and Localizing Value

Type of Nystagmus	Description	Localization
Downbeat	Fast phase downward. Usually most noticeable on down or lateral gaze.	Cervicomedullary junction.
Upbeat	Fast phase upward.	Posterior fossa.
Rebound	Horizontal, gaze-evoked; few beats of nystagmus in the opposite direction upon return to primary position.	Cerebellum.
Brun	Large amplitude, low frequency with ipsilateral gaze. Small amplitude, high frequency with contralateral gaze.	Cerebellopontine angle.
Periodic alternating	Horizontal—first in one direction, then stops, changes direction, usually cycles over 3 minutes.	Nodulus of cerebellum.
Convergence-retraction	Rapid convergence and retraction movements on upgaze.	Dorsal midbrain (part of Parinaud syndrome).
See-saw	One eye intorts and falls as the other extorts and rises, then alternates sides like a see-saw.	Optic chiasm.
Sensory	Pendular, in children with vision problems.	Visual loss.
Congenital motor	Horizontal pendular and jerk nystagmus. Less with convergence. Often latent worsening (see below). Sometimes compensatory head turn and head shaking.	Associated with many visual pathway disorders but not caused by visual loss. Isolated in some children.
Spasmus nutans	Dissociated, asymmetric (occasionally monocular), high-frequency, low-amplitude pendular nystagmus. Age 6–12 months and lasting about 2 years. Often associated with torticollis and titubation.	Benign, but rule out visual pathway lesion.
Latent	Occurs only when the other eye is occluded.	Congenital, usually related to impaired development of binocular vision pathways (thus frequently associated with a history of amblyopia or strabismus).
Induced	Induced by a variety of stimuli, eg, sound ("Tullio phenomenon") or Valsalva.	Usually associated with vestibular disorders.

OCULAR OSCILLATIONS

Various disorders of fast eye movements (saccades) are of localizing value. These are described in Table 8.4.

TABLE 8.4. Ocular Oscillations and Their Localizing Value

Name	Description	Localization/Significance
Square wave jerks	Paired saccades with a brief intersaccade latency.	Cerebellar disease, progressive supranuclear palsy, and multiple system atrophies.
Opsoclonus	Continuous random directional saccades.	Posterior fossa, seen as a paraneoplastic syndrome associated with neuroblastoma; other toxic, metabolic paraneoplastic syndromes of cerebellum and pons.
Ocular flutter	Back-to-back horizontal saccades.	Posterior fossa (cerebellum or paramedian pontine reticular formation).
Ocular bobbing	Fast downward with slow upward return.	Pons.
Oculopalatal tremor (myoclonus)	Pendular oscillation of the eyes and palate (patients report a "clicking noise").	Inferior olive hypertrophy after insult within Mollaret triangle (inferior olive, red nucleus, dentate nucleus).
Oculomasticatory myorhythmia	Dissociated pendular vergence with simultaneous jaw contractions.	Whipple disease.

NOTES

CHAPTER 9

Stroke and Neurocritical Care

Matthew A. Koenig, MD, FNCS

Ischemic Stroke

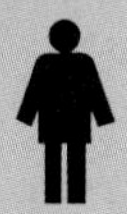

A 69-year-old man presents with acute onset of left-sided weakness. When he woke up at 6 AM, he was unable to get out of bed. He called for his wife, who found him confused and unable to move his left side. He was in his usual state of health prior to going to bed at 11 PM the previous night.

On exam, his head and gaze are deviated to the right. Cranial nerves II through XII demonstrate left-sided lower facial droop with diminished gag. Motor examination shows 0/5 strength in the left arm and leg with ↑ tone. Right-sided strength is 5/5 throughout. Reflexes are 3+ in the left arm and leg, 2+ in the right arm and leg, and a Babinski reflex is present in the left foot. The patient seems to neglect his left hand. His speech is monotone, but there does not appear to be any aphasia. What is the differential diagnosis? What tests should be done?

This is a dense, left hemiplegia with left neglect, confusion, and lack of normal prosody and speech. It is a classic presentation for a right proximal middle cerebral artery infarction. This artery supplies the right posterior frontal lobe, the right parietal lobe, and the right anterior temporal lobe. A CT should be done immediately to exclude an intracerebral hemorrhage. He is not a tissue plasminogen activator (tPA) candidate because the time of symptom onset is unknown. The workup should include a search for an embolic source, such as paroxysmal atrial fibrillation or cervical carotid atherosclerosi. His treatment should include an antiplatelet medication.

Ischemic stroke → sudden onset of a focal neurological deficit referable to the central nervous syndrome. Ischemic stroke can be divided into thrombotic and embolic etiologies.

GENERAL PRINCIPLES AND ETIOLOGIES

- Embolic strokes are maximal at onset, more likely to be multiple, and more likely to be associated with headache. Middle cerebral artery (MCA) strokes are the most common embolic strokes. Atrial fibrillation, dilated cardiomyopathy, thrombophilic states, patent foramen ovale, and recent cardiac procedures or angiography are all red flags for embolic disease.
- Thrombotic strokes are more likely to have a progressive or stuttering course and may be sensitive to fluctuations in blood pressure.
- Lacunar strokes may be embolic or thrombotic and are more likely to have a stuttering course.
- Posterior circulation strokes, particularly involving the basilar artery territory, are more likely to have a slowly evolving course over several hours, with progressive loss of brain stem nuclei related to thrombus propagation.
- Watershed strokes, especially from large vessel insufficiency (ie, carotid near-occlusion), typically have a progressive or stepwise course with deficits accumulating over hours to days.
- Headache associated with embolic stroke tends to be temporal in MCA strokes and retro-ocular in posterior circulation strokes.

ANTERIOR CIRCULATION STROKE SYNDROMES

- **MCA stroke syndromes:**
  - **M1 occlusion:** Face/arm/leg hemiplegia (due to infarction of the internal capsule), hemianesthesia, and homonymous hemianopsia (due to infarction of the lateral geniculate body), eye deviation toward the lesion, aphasia or anosognosia/neglect. Usually embolic.
  - **Superior division:** Anterior/superior MCA territory → face = arm > leg weakness and sensory loss, motor aphasia, eye deviation toward the lesion. Usually embolic.
  - **Inferior division:** Posterior temporal, parietal, angular regions → superior quadrantanopia or homonymous hemianopia, sensory aphasia or neglect; lesions to nondominant parietal lobe may cause an isolated agitated delirium with sensory deficits that are obscured by delirium.
  - **Bilateral perisylvian strokes (anterior opercular):** Facio-glosso-pharyngo-masticatory diplegia (anarthria without aphasia).
- **Anterior cerebral artery (ACA) stroke syndromes:**
  - Supplies anteromedial frontal lobe, anterior four-fifths of corpus callosum; deep branches supply anterior limb of internal capsule, inferior head of caudate, anterior globus pallidus (including artery of Huebner).
  - Both ACAs may arise from a single ACA origin, occlusion of which → paraplegia, incontinence, abulia, motor aphasia, and personality changes (abulic, psychomotor slowing, depression).
  - Anterior choroidal artery: Direct branch of the internal carotid artery (ICA) supplies the internal segment of the globus pallidus and posterior limb of the internal capsule and optic tract. Occlusion → hemiplegia, hemisensory loss, and homonymous hemianopia, sparing cognition and language.
  - **Gerstmann syndrome:** Dominant inferior parietal lobule/angular gyrus stroke → finger agnosia, left/right confusion, acalculia, agraphia.
  - **Ideomotor apraxia:** Dominant parietal lobe stroke → bilateral inability to perform complex, learned movements with preserved understanding of the intended movement.
  - **Ideational apraxia:** Dominant parietal lobe stroke → bilateral inability to perform complex, learned movements with impaired understanding of the intended movement.
  - **Limb-kinetic apraxia:** Dominant premotor or parietal stroke → bilateral clumsiness of skilled acts with preserved understanding of the intended movement.
  - **Dressing apraxia:** Nondominant parietal lobe stroke → loss of topographical and spatial orientation resulting in inability to dress in an organized, goal-directed manner.
  - **Constructional apraxia:** Nondominant parietal lobe stroke → loss of topographical and spatial orientation, resulting in inability to dress in an organized, goal-directed manner.

POSTERIOR CIRCULATION STROKE SYNDROMES

A 60-year-old Chinese man presents with sudden onset of nausea, vomiting, vertigo, and ataxia. Approximately 4 hours ago, he was working in his garden when he had acute-onset dizziness and nausea and began vomiting. He was unable to walk back to his house from his yard because of tremendous unsteadiness, and his wife called 911. Paramedics came to the scene and noted that he looked quite ill, but when they brought him to the emergency room they noted that his vital signs were stable. The patient's vertigo and vomiting were somewhat improved by lying down. There was no evidence of photophobia, and he did not have a history of migraine headaches.

On neurological review of systems, he also complained of numbness of the left side of his face and he also noted a hoarse quality to his voice. He denied any similar symptoms in the past. He denied any head injuries or recent illnesses.

The most likely diagnosis is posterior circulation stroke. The acute nausea, vomiting, vertigo, and mild ataxia could be symptoms of acute labyrinthitis. However, he does have risk factors for stroke, including age, ethnicity, heavy smoking history, and hypertension. In this case, we are concerned about a posterior circulation stroke. The patient is demonstrating signs and symptoms referrable to the lateral pons and cerebellum.

- **Anton syndrome:** Bilateral cortical blindness with normal-appearing optic disks and preserved pupillary light reflexes, with denial of blindness and visual hallucinations.
- **Balint syndrome:** Bilateral occipitoparietal border zone strokes → simultagnosia (inability to synthesize disparate images within the visual field into a coherent whole), optic ataxia (inability to reach targets under visual guidance), gaze apraxia (inability to direct gaze at a target or scan a visual field).
- **Peduncular hallucinosis:** Stroke of the midbrain in the vicinity of the cerebral peduncles related to posterior cerebral artery (PCA) occlusion → purely visual hallucinations that are well formed, complex, appear cartoonish and nonthreatening, and are perceived as unreal by the patient.
- **Prosopagnosia:** Bilateral ventromesial occipitotemporal strokes → inability to recognize and identify familiar faces, interpret facial expressions, or judge age or gender based on facial features.
- **Homonymous hemianopia with macular sparing:** Occipital lesion sparing the region of the occipital pole supplied by collateral circulation from the inferior division of the MCA.
- **Alexia without agraphia:** Dominant occipital lobe and splenium of the corpus callosum due to dominant PCA stroke → disconnection of preserved input from left visual field from language centers but preservation of connection between language centers and motor centers.
- **Weber syndrome:** Midbrain stroke due to PCA thrombus → ipsilateral cranial nerve (CN) III lesion and contralateral hemiparesis.
- **Claude syndrome:** Midbrain stroke due to PCA thrombus → ipsilateral CN III lesion and contralateral ataxia/tremor.
- **Benedikt syndrome:** Midbrain stroke due to PCA thrombus → ipsilateral CN III lesion and contralateral hemiparesis and ataxia/tremor.
- **Wallenberg syndrome:** Lateral medullary stroke due to vertebral or posterior inferior cerebellar artery (PICA) thrombus → ipsilateral CN V, IX, X, XI palsy; Horner syndrome; cerebellar ataxia; contralateral pain and temperature loss of the body; vertigo; nausea; hiccups.
- **Palatal tremor (myoclonus):** Stroke in the dentato-rubro-olivary triangle of Guillain-Mollaret (usually pontine tegmentum) → palatal tremor that persists during sleep and is audible to patient.
- Thalamoperforate arteries (branches of PCA) → inferior, medial, and anterior thalamus; may cause hemiballismus if subthalamic nucleus is infarcted.
- Thalamogeniculate arteries (branches of PCA) → lateral geniculate body and central/posterior thalamus.

- **Thalamic syndrome of Dejerine and Roussy:** Thalamic ventral posterolateral nucleus (VPL)/ventral posteromedial nucleus (VPM) stroke → hemisensory loss followed by painful paresthesias after weeks to months.

LACUNAR SYNDROMES

- **Pure motor hemiplegia:** Internal capsule or ventral pontine stroke.
- **Pure sensory stroke:** Lateral thalamic stroke.
- **Clumsy hand–dysarthria:** Paramedian midpontine stroke.
- **Ipsilateral hemiparesis–ataxia:** Pons, midbrain, or internal capsule stroke.

BRAIN STEM LESIONS

- As a rule of thumb, the following tips on brain stem localization should be used:
  - Crossed face and body signs (motor or sensory) suggest a brain stem lesion.
  - CN III–IV are in the midbrain, V–VIII in the pons, and IX–XII in the medulla. Exceptions are that CN V actually runs from the midbrain to approximately C4 in the spinal cord with vibration sense in the mesencephalic nucleus, light touch in the chief sensory nucleus (pons), and pain/temperature sense in the medulla/cervical cord (spinal nucleus).
  - All CN nuclei are ipsilateral to the nerve except CN IV and the superior rectus subnucleus of CN III, which cross contralaterally.
  - The root of CN VII encircles the nucleus of CN VI, so nuclear CN VI lesions may cause a peripheral-appearing facial palsy.
  - The nucleus of CN III is divided into subnuclei for each function (eg, extraocular muscles and levator palpebrae, and pupilloconstrictors) with

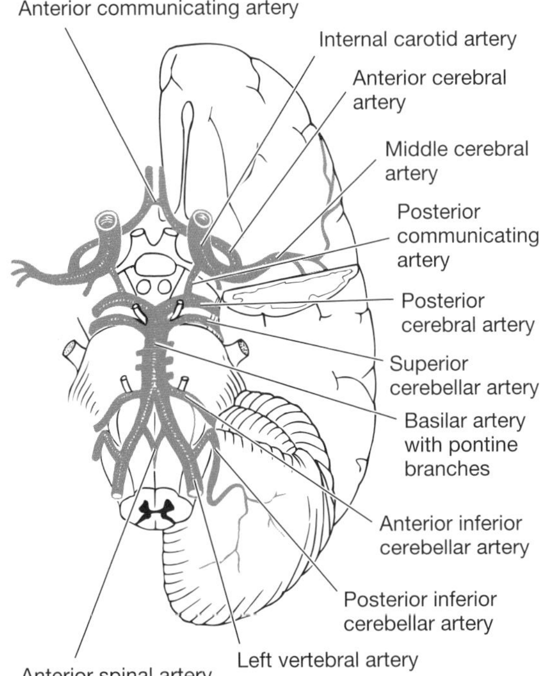

FIGURE 9.1. Anatomy of the circle of Willis in relation to the brain stem and cranial nerves. (Reproduced, with permission, from Ropper AH, Brown RH. *Adams and Victor's Principles of Neurology*, 8th ed. New York: McGraw-Hill, 2003: Figure 12-2.)

contralateral innervation of the superior rectus muscle and bilateral innervation of the levator palpebrae. A true nuclear CN III lesion will therefore cause ipsilateral ophthalmoplegia (sparing the lateral rectus and superior oblique), contralateral upgaze palsy, and bilateral ptosis.

- Sensory nuclei and subnuclei are located laterally within the brain stem, and motor nuclei are located medially, so lateral pontine and medullary syndromes result in ipsilateral sensory deficits depending on the structures involved, sparing motor function.
- Rough brain stem localization, as required on the board examination, can be easily undertaken with the number of nuclei involved and whether they are primarily sensory or motor nuclei.

Pathophysiology

- Normal cerebral blood flow: 55 mL/100 g/min. Critical threshold for functional impairment 23 mL/100 g/min, < 12 mL/100 g/min → infarction.
- Mean arterial pressure (MAP) between 50 and 150 mm Hg is within the autoregulatory curve (Figure 9.2), pial vessels dilate and constrict to maintain constant brain perfusion. MAP < 50 mm Hg → ischemia. MAP > 150 → cerebral edema. Autoregulatory curve is shifted to the right with chronic hypertension.

DIAGNOSTIC TESTS

- Head CT will show subtle signs of stroke such as cortical effacement or loss of grey-white distinction after ~6 hours from stroke onset, but significant hypodensity is often not present for 24 hours; other subtle signs include spontaneous hyperdensity along an occluded proximal MCA (hyperdense MCA sign) or MCA branches within the Sylvian fissure (MCA dot sign).
- MRI is the gold standard for imaging stroke (Figure 9.3A, B); hyperintensity on diffusion-weighted imaging and hypointensity on apparent diffusion coefficient maps may be present within 30 minutes of stroke onset and remain so for ~1 week.
- Magnetic resonance angiography (MRA)/computed tomographic angiography (CTA)/cerebral angiography: Indicated when clinical suspicion of large vessel dissection, intracranial atherosclerosis, vasculitis, moyamoya, or fibromuscular displasia.

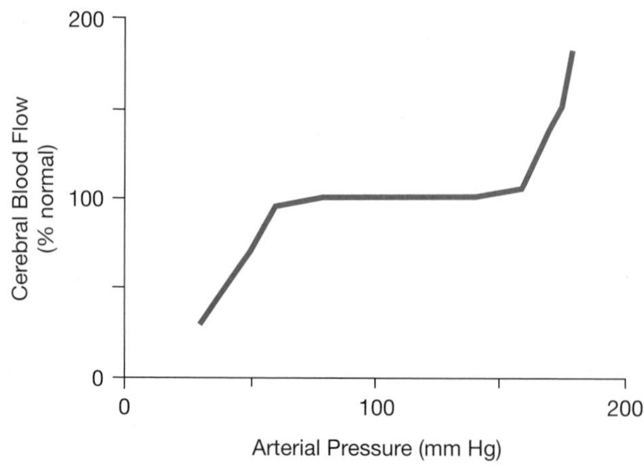

FIGURE 9.2. Hypothetical autoregulatory curve demonstrating stable cerebral blood flow at MAP between 50 and 150 mm Hg. (Reproduced, with permission, from Hall JB, Schmidt GA, Wood LDH. *Principles of Critical Care*, 3rd ed. New York: McGraw-Hill, 2005: Figure 65-5.)

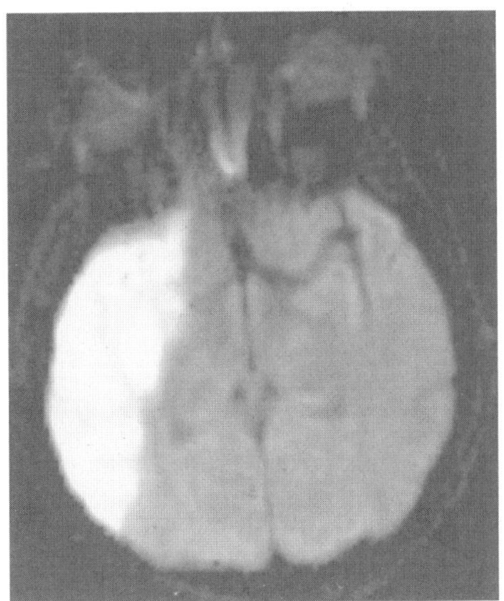

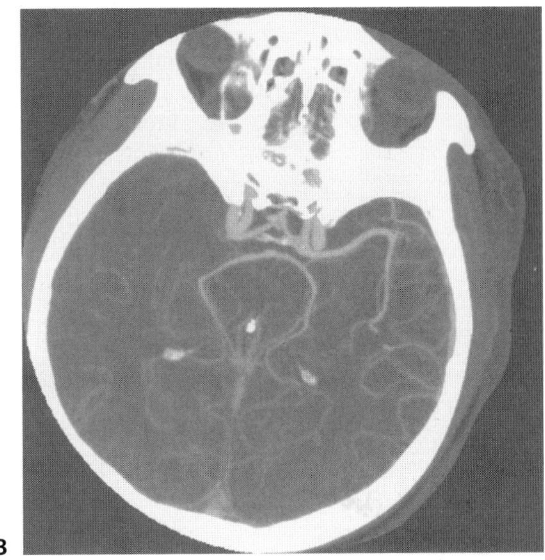

FIGURE 9.3. Diffusion-weighted MRI (A) showing acute ischemic stroke related to right MCA occlusion (B). (Reproduced, with permission, from Ropper AH, Brown RH. *Adams and Victor's Principles of Neurology*, 8th ed. New York: McGraw-Hill, 2005:666.)

- Echocardiography: Transthoracic or transesophageal, indicated for evaluation of dilated cardiomyopathy, apical thrombus, valvular thrombus or endocarditis, patent foramen ovale, aortic arch atherosclerosis.
- Cardiac telemetry: Indicated for evaluation of paroxysmal atrial fibrillation.
- Carotid Doppler ultrasonography/CTA/MRA/angiography: Indicated to exclude cervical carotid stenosis.
- Thrombophilia evaluation: Indicated for unexplained stroke in young/healthy patients, family history of thrombophilia, or clinical suspicion of hypercoagulable state.

CAUSES OF STROKE

Atrial Fibrillation

- Turbulent/static blood clots within dilated left atrium or atrial appendage → embolic stroke (MCA territory most common).
- Treated with warfarin, a direct thrombin inhibitor, or a direct factor Xa inhibitor unless contraindicated.
- Multiple clinical trials demonstrate superiority of warfarin over aspirin for primary and secondary prevention of stroke in patients with atrial fibrillation (SPAF II).
- Recent clinical trials have demonstrated non-inferiority and lower hemorrhagic complication rates for direct thrombin inhibitors and direct factor Xa inhibitors compared to warfarin for primary prevention of stroke in patients with non-valvular atrial fibrillation.
- Rate control and anticoagulation now recommended over rhythm control.
- Anticoagulation recommended for paroxysmal and chronic atrial fibrillation.

Vertebral or Carotid Dissection

- Intimal tear of the vertebral or carotid artery at the skull base resulting in stenosis or occlusion of the parent or feeder vessels and potential distal embolization, typically associated with neck pain with a "tearing" quality.

- **Diagnosis:** T1 fat-saturated axial noncontrast MRI showing bilateral internal carotid arteries (Figure 9.4); also may be demonstrated by CTA, MRA, or angiography (Figure 9.5).
- **Treatment:** Best practice has not been determined by clinical trials. Treatments include IV heparin followed by warfarin for up to 6 months (not based on strong evidence), anti-platelet medications, and endovascular coil sacrifice.
- May result from minor neck hyperextension or trauma; classic examples are roller-coaster ride, whiplash injury, painting the ceiling, rock climbing, and chiropractic manipulation.
- **Risk factors:** Fibromuscular dysplasia, collagen diseases, Marfan disease.

Patent Foramen Ovale

- Congenital anomaly resulting in paradoxical embolization of venous thrombi via a right → left shunt due to failure of closure of the fetal foramen ovale.
- May be diagnosed by bubble transcranial Doppler (TCD) or echocardiography showing right-to-left movement of bubbles (not absorbed by the lungs) with Valsalva maneuver or spontaneously.
- Present in 15% of the normal population and 50% of patients with cryptogenic stroke.
- Highest risk for stroke with large defect, spontaneous right-to-left shunt, and concurrent atrial septal aneurysm.
- Statistically associated with migraine.
- Surgical closure is currently considered experimental therapy and clinical trial results have been inconclusive to date.
- Unclear whether anticoagulation is superior to antithrombotic therapy.

Carotid Stenosis

- Atherosclerosis of the cervical internal carotid artery just distal to the carotid bifurcation, caused by turbulent blood flow and resulting in distal emboli, typically in the MCA territory.
- Prior neck radiation is a risk factor.
- Carotid bruit is 60–80% specific for carotid stenosis > 50% among patients with stroke or transient ischemic attack (TIA, symptomatic bruit).

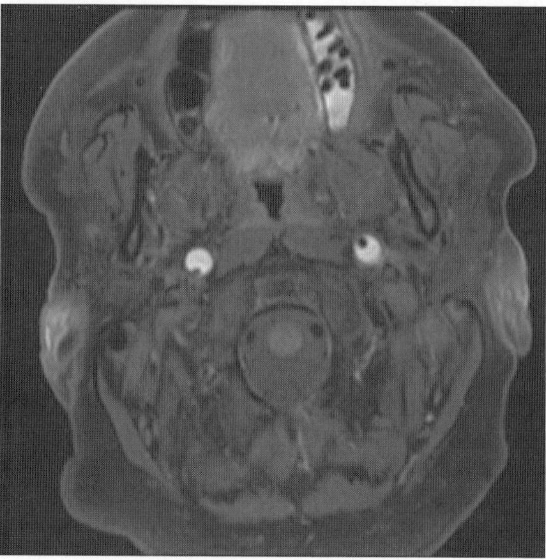

FIGURE 9.4. Axial T1-weighted MRI with fat saturation showing dissected bilateral internal carotid arteries. T1 hyperintensity that is shown is due to thrombus within the false lumen of the vessel. (Reproduced, with permission, from Ropper AH, Samuels MA, Klein JP. *Adams and Victor's Principles of Neurology*, 10th ed. New York: McGraw-Hill Education, 2014: 828.)

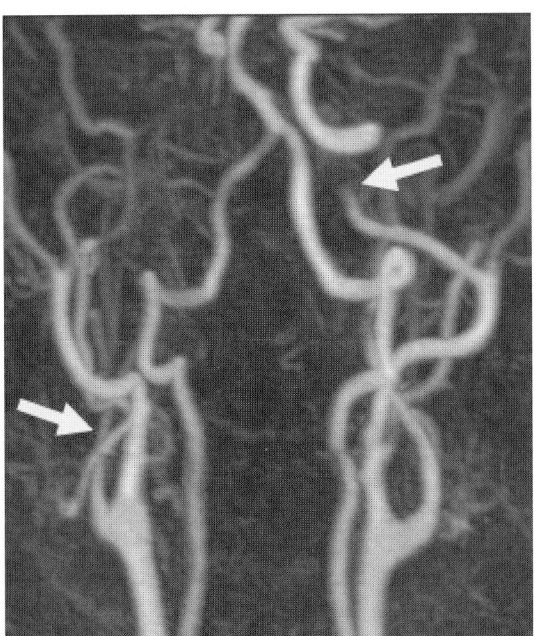

FIGURE 9.5. Angiogram showing dissection of bilateral internal carotid arteries distal to the bifurcation. (Reproduced, with permission, from Ropper AH, Samuels MA, Klein JP. *Adams and Victor's Principles of Neurology,* 10th ed. New York: McGraw-Hill Education, 2014: 828.)

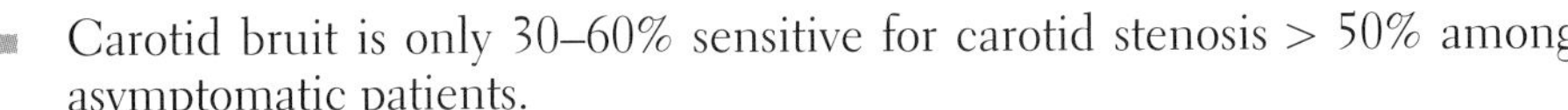

- Carotid bruit is only 30–60% sensitive for carotid stenosis > 50% among asymptomatic patients.
- **North American Symptomatic Carotid Endarterectomy Trial (NASCET):** > 70% symptomatic carotid stenosis (stroke or TIA) in same arterial distribution, recommend elective carotid endarterectomy for low-risk patients at centers with high surgical volume (< 6% complication rate).
- **Asymptomatic Carotid Atherosclerosis Study (ACAS):** > 60% asymptomatic carotid stenosis.
- Carotid stenting remains an experimental therapy but may be considered in patients with prior neck surgery, cancer, or radiation or those with unfavorable anatomy for endarterectomy such as a high carotid bifurcation.
- **Complications of carotid endarterectomy:** Hyperperfusion syndrome → ispsilateral headache, focal seizure activity, and focal neurological deficits caused by cerebral edema or hemorrhage from acute reperfusion, usually associated with postoperative hypertension.

Intracranial Atherosclerosis

- Focal atherosclerosis of the large intracranial vessels of the circle of Willis → recurrent strokes or TIAs in the same vascular territory or blood pressure–dependent focal neurological deficits.
- More common in African-Americans and Asians, whereas extracranial atherosclerosis is more common in Caucasians.
- Until recently, recommended treatment with anticoagulation but Warfarin Aspirin Symptomatic Intracranial Disease (WASID) Trial showed no difference between aspirin and warfarin in stroke rates.
- Diagnosed by MRA, CTA, or angiography.

Dilated Cardiomyopathy

- Turbulent blood flow within dilated ventricle → embolic stroke, typically in the MCA distribution.
- Highest risk for embolic stroke with ejection fraction (EF) < 20%.

- Warfarin previously recommended with EF < 20%, but recent clinical trials failed to show superiority of warfarin over aspirin for primary stroke prevention in patients with dilated cardiomyopathy.

Watershed Infarcts

- Ischemic stroke involving the watershed region between two vascular territories due to focal or generalized reduction in perfusion pressure.
- Most commonly occurs between the MCA and ACA territories → bilateral infarcts along the medial cortical and subcortical regions → bilateral proximal arm/leg and trunk weakness (man-in-barrel syndrome).
- Also occurs between deep and superficial branches of MCA with ICA (Figure 9.6A) or proximal MCA occlusion → internal border zone stroke.
- Occurs with systemic hypotension or focal arterial stenosis/occlusion (Figure 9.6B).

Primary Central Nervous System (CNS) Vasculitis

- Autoimmune, inflammatory disease of medium- and small-caliber cerebral arteries in the absence of other systemic vasculitic manifestations → subacute presentation of headache and progressive/stepwise neurological deficits.
- Equal gender distribution, onset usually in 40s and 50s.
- May have nonspecific markers of inflammation such as elevated ESR.
- MRI shows nonspecific white matter disease and is rarely normal.
- Angiography may show "beading" of blood vessels similar to vasospasm (Figure 9.7).
- Brain and meningeal biopsy is gold standard but still only ~75% sensitive.
- Cerebrospinal fluid (CSF) may have aseptic meningitis pattern, but may be normal.
- Must be distinguished from reversible cerebral vasoconstriction syndrome (Call-Fleming syndrome), which tends to occur in young women with an acute presentation of headache, focal neurological deficits, ischemic strokes, and/or spontaneous convexity subarachnoid hemorrhage. Call-Fleming syndrome may be associated with pregnancy, analgesic overuse, sympathomimetic decongestant medications, or oral contraceptives.

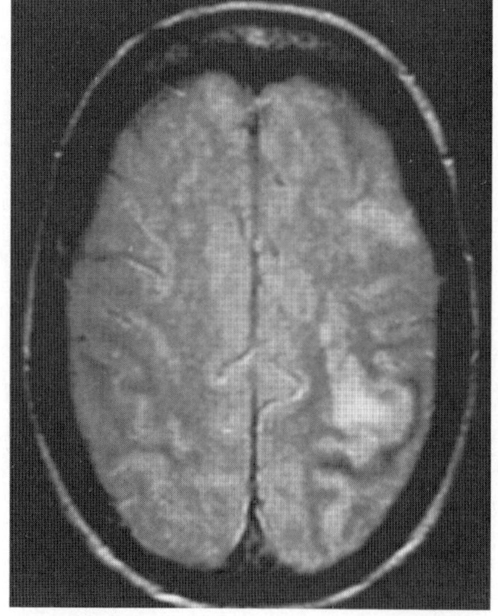

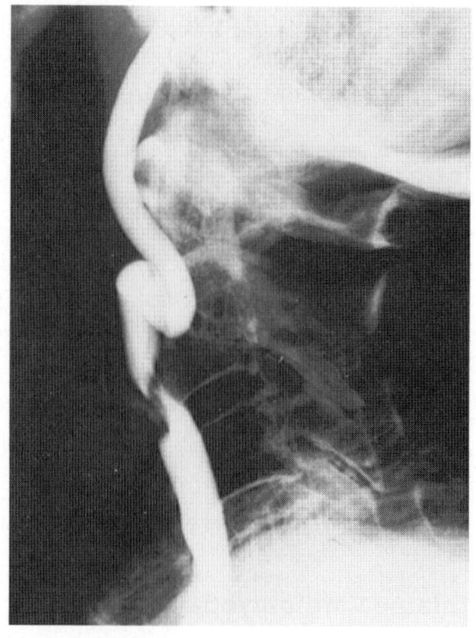

FIGURE 9.6. Axial fluid attenuation inversion recovery (FLAIR) MRI (A), showing left watershed stroke related to tight stenosis of the left internal carotid artery (B). (Reproduced, with permission, from Ropper AH, Brown RH. *Adams and Victor's Principles of Neurology,* 8th ed. New York: McGraw-Hill, 2005: 689.)

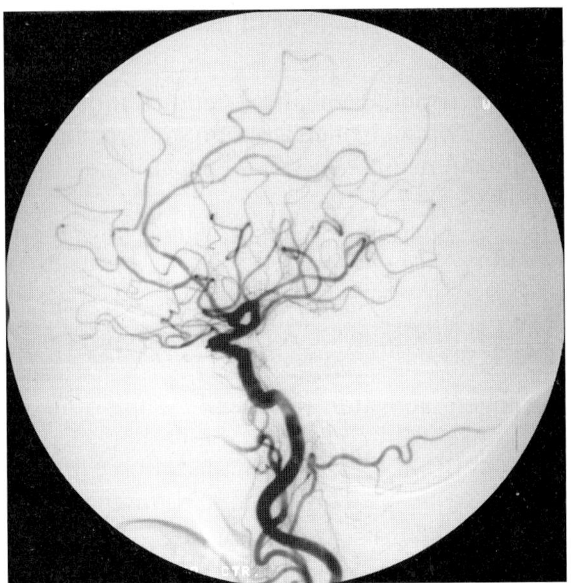

FIGURE 9.7. Angiogram showing focal regions of stenosis in the anterior circulation, as occurs in primary CNS vasculitis and vasospasm after subarachnoid hemorrhage. (Reproduced, with permission, from Ropper AH, Brown RH. *Adams and Victor's Principles of Neurology*, 8th ed. New York: McGraw-Hill, 2005: 731.)

Thrombophilic States

- Antithrombin III deficiency.
- Prothrombin G21201A mutation.
- Methylenetetrahydrofolate reductase (MTHFR) deficiency.
- Factor C or S deficiency.
- Lupus anticoagulant syndrome/anticardiolipin antibodies.
- Fabry disease.
- Hyperhomocysteinemia.
- Factor V Leiden.
- Oral contraceptives.

Mitochondrial Myopathy, Encephalopathy, Lactic Acidosis, and Strokes (MELAS)

- Genetically heterogeneous syndrome caused by mitochondrial mutation, most commonly involving the *MTTL* gene.
- Syndrome of episodic migraine-like headache and cyclic vomiting with focal neurological deficits and seizure.
- May have sensorineural hearing loss, pigmentary retinopathy, and myopathy (hallmarks of mitochondrial disease).
- Symptom onset between ages 10 and 25 in most cases, rarely in older adults.
- Elevated peripheral and CSF lactate.

Cerebral Autosomal Dominant Arteriopathy with Subcortical Infarcts and Leukoencephelopathy (CADASIL)

- Onset in middle age.
- Autosomal-dominant inheritance pattern.
- Stepwise progression of recurrent focal neurological deficits related to subcortical infarcts → dementia and pseudobulbar palsy, often associated with seizures, migraine headache, and psychiatric features.
- Caused by mutation of the *NOTCH3* gene.
- MRI shows bilateral, confluent white matter hyperintensities (nonspecific).
- Diagnosis requires skin biopsy with monoclonal antibody testing for *NOTCH3*.

Fibromuscular Dysplasia

- Onset in middle age.
- Renovascular hypertension, renal artery stenosis, and internal carotid stenosis often associated with spontaneous aneurysm formation and dissection.
- Caused by noninflammatory fibrosis and hyperplasia, usually involving the arterial intimal layer.
- Angiogram shows chain-of-lakes pattern, which may be difficult to distinguish from vasculitis.

ACUTE TREATMENT

- **Tissue plasminogen activator (tPA):** FDA approved for treatment of acute ischemic stroke within 3 hours of onset. Recent guidelines also support off-label use of tPA within the extended time window of 3–4.5 hours. Should be offered to all patients without contraindications to tPA. Activates plasminogen, which cleaves fibrin.
  - tPA group is 32% more likely to have no or minimal deficit at 90 days than controls; no difference at 24 hours.
  - There is a 6% rate of intracranial hemorrhage (ICH); 3% rate of fatal ICH.
  - Indications: Ischemic stroke within 3 hours of symptom onset, a significant clinical deficit based on the National Institutes of Health Stroke Scale (NIHSS), no hemorrhage on head CT, clear time of onset.
  - Contraindications: Rapidly resolving deficits, seizure at onset, prior stroke or head trauma < 3 months, major surgery > 14 days, prior ICH, sustained systolic blood pressure > 185 and/or diastolic blood pressure > 110 despite treatment, gastrointestinal or urinary tract hemorrhage < 21 days, noncompressible arterial puncture < 7 days, elevated prothrombin time (PT)/partial thromboplastin time (PTT), platelets < 100,000, glucose < 50 or > 400.
  - Relative contraindications: NIHSS > 22, CT evidence of established infarct that involves more than one-third of MCA territory.
  - Additional contraindications in the extended time window (3–4.5 hours): age > 80, combination of prior stroke and diabetes, and NIHSS score > 25.
  - Menstruation is not a contraindication to tPA.
  - Do not give tPA to patients who awoke with symptoms unless last seen normal within the appropriate time window for treatment.
  - There is a 5% risk of angioedema, which tends to be facial and orolingual; higher risk in patients taking angiotensin-converting enzyme (ACE) inhibitors, likely due to excess bradykinin release.
- **Aspirin:** Antithrombotic action due to inhibition of platelet function by acetylation of the platelet cyclooxygenase (COX), which prevents binding of arachidonic acid and results in an irreversible inhibition of platelet-dependent thromboxane formation.
  - Appropriate dose unclear; trials range from 81 to 1600 mg/day.
  - Chinese Acute Stroke Trial (CAST): 160 mg/day, starting within 48 hours of stroke onset → recurrent stroke 1.6% in aspirin group versus 2.3% in controls, death 5.0% in aspirin group versus 5.4% in controls; no ↑ in ICH.
  - International Stroke Trial (IST): 300 mg/day, starting within 48 hours of stroke onset → recurrent stroke 2.8% in aspirin group versus 3.9% in controls; no ↑ in ICH.
  - Unclear if aspirin should be given within 24 hours when tPA is given.
- **Heparin:** Binds to antithrombin III to ↑ inactivation of thrombin and factor Xa.
  - No clear indication for intravenous heparin, subcutaneous heparin,

low-molecular-weight heparins, or heparinoids in the treatment of acute stroke.

- May safely be withheld for a week in patients with large stroke and atrial fibrillation.
- No reduction in early stroke recurrence in all patients with acute ischemic stroke.
- IV heparin still used for carotid/vertebral dissection, stroke-in-evolution, posterior circulation occlusion, "crescendo" TIA, but not strictly evidence-based.

- **Other treatments:**
  - Peptic ulcer prophylaxis with H_2 blocker or $5HT_3$ blocker.
  - DVT prophylaxis with subcutaneous heparin or low-molecular-weight heparin.

PRIMARY AND SECONDARY PREVENTION OF STROKE

- Antiplatelet agents: Aspirin, clopidogrel, ticlopidine, adenosine/aspirin.
- Statins/HMG CoA (3-hydroxy-3-methylglutaryl-coenzyme A) reductase inhibitors.
- Smoking cessation.
- Treatment of hypertension (ACE inhibitor and thiazide diuretic preferred).
- Tight glycemic control.

Intracerebral Hemorrhage

A 70-year-old man presents with a complaint of sudden onset of right-sided weakness today. There was no loss of consciousness or head trauma. He also complains of headache, mostly left-sided. He is brought to the emergency department by his wife, who also noted confusion and slurring of his speech. Past medical history is notable for hypertension, as well as a history of melanoma. He takes metoprolol and a baby aspirin.

His initial blood pressure is 187/105. On exam, cranial nerves are intact. There is ↑ tone in the left upper extremity. A pronator drift is noted on the left side. Weakness is noted in the left upper extremity. Reflexes are brisk on the left side, and a Babinski sign is present on the left. He is alert and oriented × 3. Speech, naming, and recall are intact. A head CT demonstrates a 6 mL hyperdense lesion in the right putamen. What is the differential diagnosis? The most likely diagnosis is spontaneous intracerebral hemorrhage (ICH). Hemorrhagic melanoma metastasis is another possibility but the location and blood pressure values are more typical of a hypertensive ICH.

GENERAL PRINCIPLES

- Occurs most commonly in putamen (50%) followed by cortex, thalamus, cerebellum, and pons, respectively.
- Blood pressure is the number one modifiable risk factor.
- ICH volume expands within the first 4 hours in one-third of cases.
- Hematocrit effect on CT/MRI in anticoagulated patients → layering of clotted blood posteriorly while supine.
- Predictable evolution of blood products seen on T1 and T2 MRI (Table 9.1).

MNEMONIC

It Be	
Isointense on T1,	
Bright on T2	0–7
I-Ddy	
Isointense on T1,	
Dark on T2	7–3
Bi-Ddy	
Bright on T1,	
Dark on T2	3–7
Ba-By	
Bright on T1,	
Bright on T2	7–3
Doo-Doo	
Dark on T1,	
Dark on T2	3+

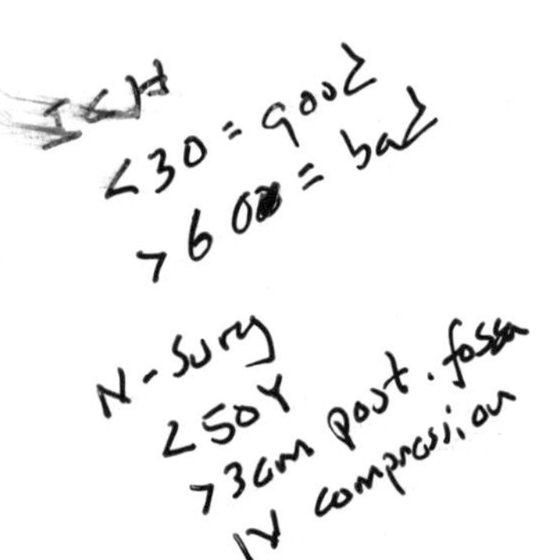

TABLE 9.1. Evolution of MRI Signal Intensity of Hemorrhage

T1 MRI	T2 MRI	Time	Hemoglobin (Hgb)
Isointense	Bright	0–7 hours	OxyHgb
Isointense	Dark	7 hours–3 days	DeoxyHgb
Bright	Dark	3–7 days	Extracellular metHgb
Bright	Bright	7 days–3 weeks	Intracellular metHgb
Dark	Dark	> 3 weeks	Hemosiderin

- Prognosis from ICH is influenced by hematoma volume, initial pulse pressure, age, initial Glasgow Coma Scale (GCS) score, and presence of intraventricular blood.
- Hematoma volume < 30 cc is associated with potential for good neurological outcome (depending on location); > 60 cc portends poor prognosis.
- Indications for neurosurgical consultation: Posterior fossa hemorrhage > 3 cm in maximal diameter or significant mass effect on the fourth ventricle or rapidly expanding superficial supratentorial ICH in a young patient (age < 50) with a declining neurological exam.
- **Complications:** Cerebral herniation, hydrocephalus (due to mass effect on third or fourth ventricle or intraventricular extension [Figure 9.8]), seizures (up to 25% of ICH, more common with cortical ICH; prophylactic anticonvulsant use is controversial).

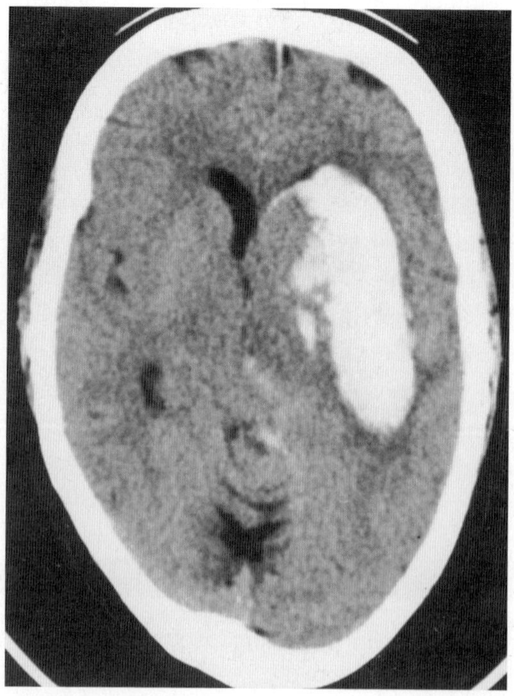

FIGURE 9.8. Noncontrast head CT showing ICH in the left putamen with intraventricular extension. (Reproduced, with permission, from Ropper AH, Brown RH. *Adams and Victor's Principles of Neurology*, 8th ed. New York: McGraw-Hill, 2005: 711.)

LESS COMMON CAUSES OF ICH

- **Cerebral amyloid angiopathy:** Deposition of beta-amyloid in the media and adventitia of small and medium-sized arteries of the cerebral cortex and meninges:
  - Risk factors: Advanced age (typically 80s), Alzheimer dementia, Down syndrome (earlier onset).
  - Typical presentation: New ICH in demented patient; cortical ICH in the absence of significant hypertension, silent microbleeds seen best on gradient echo or susceptibility-weighted MRI sequences (Figure 9.9).
- **Arteriovenous malformation (AVM):** Tangle of abnormal, tortuous arteriovenous fistulas that lack an intervening capillary bed and are separated by a nidus of brain tissue; most commonly supratentorial (extending from subcortical region to the ventricle in a wedge shape) but can occur anywhere; present with headache, seizures, or hemorrhage; 2% annual hemorrhage rate, 10–20% recurrence rate in first year after hemorrhage; best seen on MRI (Figure 9.10), angiogram (Figure 9.11) 60% sensitive.
- **Cavernous hemangioma:** Cluster of thin-walled veins without significant arterial feeders or intervening brain tissue; infratentorial in 50%, multiple in 10%, and familial (autosomal dominant) in 5%; hemorrhage rate 1–2%/year; best seen on MRI (Figure 9.12), angiographically silent.
- **Underlying tumor:** Most common tumors that bleed are breast, lung, thyroid, renal cell, melanoma, and choriocarcinoma.

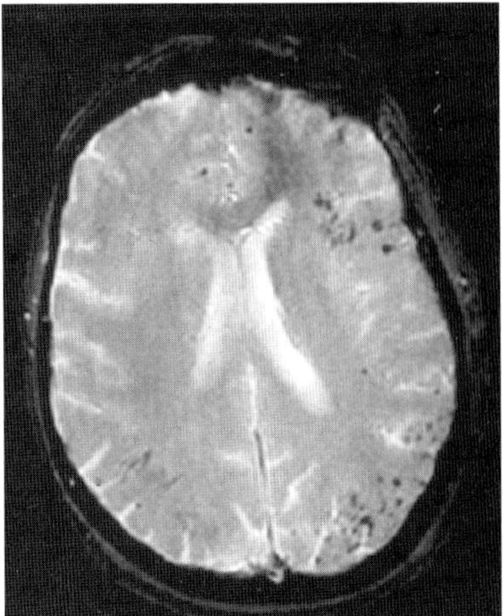

FIGURE 9.9. Axial gradient echo MRI showing numerous punctuate hemorrhages in amyloid angiopathy.

(Reproduced, with permission, from Walker DA, Broderick DF, Kotsenas AL, Rubino FA. Routine use of gradient-echo MRI to screen for cerebral amyloid angiopathy in elderly patients. *American Journal of Roentgenology* 182:1549, 2004.)

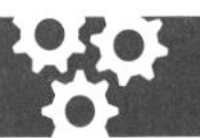

MNEMONIC

Most common tumors that bleed—Breast, Lung, Thyroid, Kidney, and Melanoma

BLT with
Ketchup and
Mayo

Cerebral Venous Thrombosis

Thrombosis of dural venous sinuses → elevated intracranial pressure, cerebral edema, ischemia, and hemorrhage. Symptoms and findings are caused by

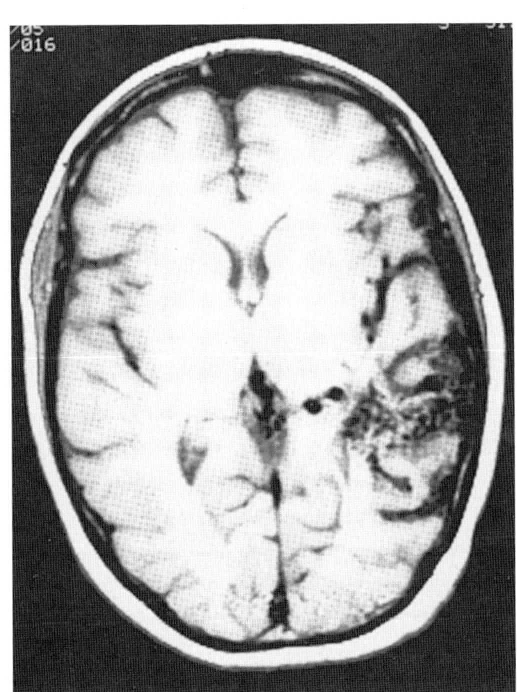

FIGURE 9.10. Axial T1-weighted MRI showing flow voids from a left temporal AVM.

(Reproduced, with permission, from Ropper AH, Brown RH. *Adams and Victor's Principles of Neurology*, 8th ed. New York: McGraw-Hill, 2005: 724.)

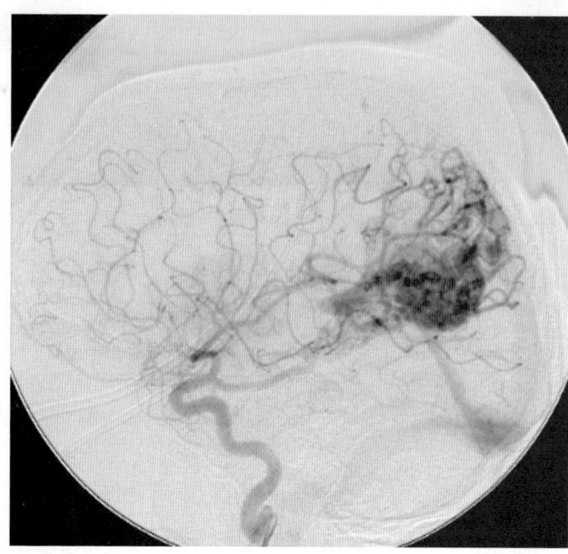

FIGURE 9.11. Angiogram showing feeding arteries from a left temporal AVM. (Reproduced, with permission, from Ropper AH, Brown RH. *Adams and Victor's Principles of Neurology*, 8th ed. New York: McGraw-Hill, 2005: 724.)

impedance of venous drainage of blood and CSF. Most commonly involves the superior sagittal sinus, but may involve any venous sinus. Should be suspected in young patients (30s and 40s) with focal neurological deficits and signs of elevated intracranial pressure (ICP).

Symptoms

- Headache: Worse while dependent or with straining.
- Nausea/vomiting.
- Meningismus with or without fever.
- Focal neurological deficits.
- Visual blurring or blindness.

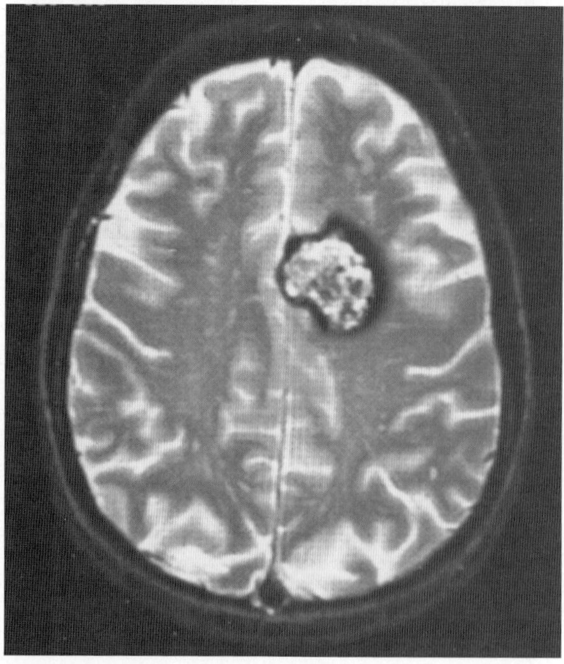

FIGURE 9.12. Axial T2-weighted MRI showing a hemosiderin ring surrounding hemorrhage of various ages (popcorn sion) from a cavernous hemangioma. (Reproduced, with permission, from Ropper AH, Brown RH. *Adams and Victor's Principles of Neurology*, 8th ed. New York: McGraw-Hill, 2005: 726.)

EXAM

- Papilledema.
- Nuchal rigidity (if associated with infectious causes).
- Rheumatological findings (arthritis, rash) if associated with lupus or inflammatory bowel disease.
- Mastoid tenderness (if associated with mastoiditis).
- Tympanic erythema (if associated with otitis media).
- Bruises (if associated with skull fracture).
- ↑ skin turgor (if associated with dehydration).
- Coma (especially with thrombosis of deep sinuses or severe intracranial hypertension).

DIAGNOSIS

- Brain CT: Presence of diffuse cerebral edema and slitlike ventricles or focal edema in the region of the thrombosed sinus. Superior sagittal sinus thrombosis → bilateral vasogenic and cytotoxic edema of the posterior frontal lobes with or without hemorrhage. Straight sinus thrombosis → bilateral edema with or without hemorrhage of the thalami, resulting in coma. On noncontrast CT, spontaneous hyperdensity may be present in the thrombosed sinus. On contrast-enhanced CT, an empty delta sign may be present where contrast does not fill the sinus.
- Brain MRI: Magnetic resonance venogram (MRV) reveals absent flow in thrombosed sinus. Midsagittal T1 without gadolinium (Figure 9.13A) shows spontaneous hyperintensity in the region of the sinus, when this structure is thrombosed. Gadolinium-enhanced coronal or sagittal MRI shows an empty delta sign in the thrombosed sinus.
- Search for underlying cause: Dehydration, mastoiditis or otitis media, meningitis, skull fracture, lupus, congenital or acquired thrombophilia, inflammatory bowel disease (ulcerative colitis or Crohn disease), sickle cell disease, compression by local mass (meningioma), remote malignancy, pregnancy, or oral contraceptives.

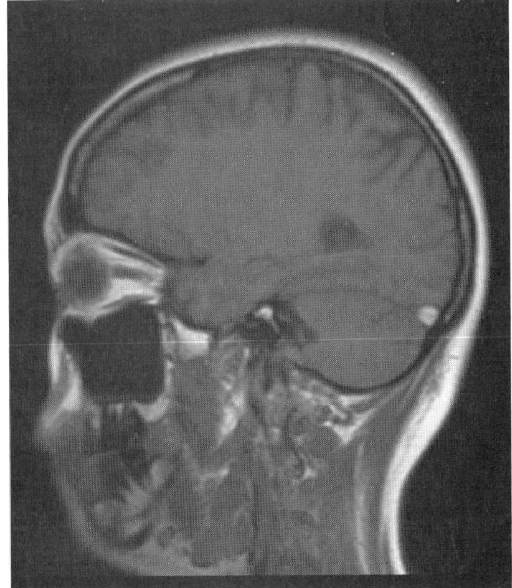
A

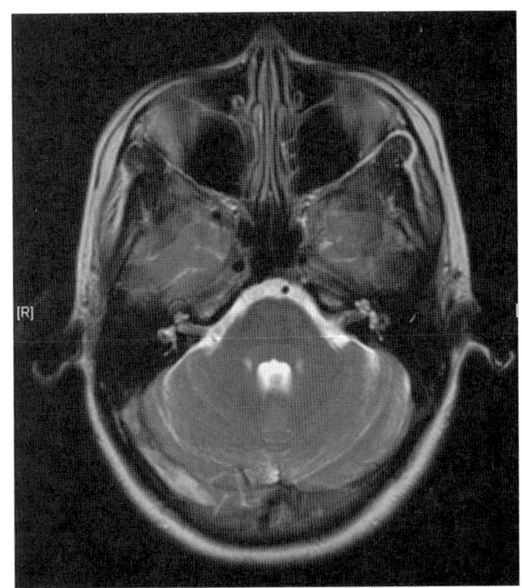

B

FIGURE 9.13. Sagittal T1 weighted (A) and axial T2-weighted (B) noncontrast MRI showing spontaneous hyperintensity in the right transverse sinus from venous thrombosis.

TREATMENT

- Hydration and treatment of the underlying process.
- Anticoagulation with intravenous heparin is the gold standard therapy even in the presence of venous hemorrhage and safety has been demonstrated in clinical trials.
- CSF diversion may be required for intracranial hypertension.

COMPLICATIONS

- Blindness due to elevated intracranial pressure.
- Thrombus propagation → hemorrhage.
- Coma due to cerebral edema, ICP elevation, or mass effect.

Subarachnoid Hemorrhage

Presence of blood in the CSF-filled space underlying the arachnoid layer of the meninges, related to trauma or rupture of a vascular structure. The most common cause of subarachnoid hemorrhage (SAH) is head trauma. In the absence of trauma, rupture of a cerebral aneurysm or arteriovenous malformation should be suspected. The most common locations for aneurysms include posterior communicating artery, anterior communicating artery, middle cerebral artery, and basilar artery (in order).

SYMPTOMS

- Sudden-onset headache ("worst headache of my life").
- Meningismus.
- Fever.
- Nausea/vomiting.
- Seizures.
- Coma.
- Patients complain of new-onset headache within the preceding 1–7 days in about 30% of cases, likely due to sentinel leak prior to major aneurysm rupture.

EXAM

- Nuchal rigidity.
- Papilledema (if hydrocephalus present).
- Focal neurological deficits (if intraparenchymal hemorrhage present).

DIAGNOSIS

- Noncontrast head CT (Figure 9.14) is 90–95% sensitive for SAH within 24 hours of symptom onset, but sensitivity declines by about 10% per day thereafter. Hyperdense blood is evident in the basal cisterns outlining the circle of Willis in aneurysmal SAH. Reflux of blood into the ventricles also occurs frequently.
- Presence of blood in the Sylvian fissure suggests MCA aneurysms.
- For anterior communicating artery aneurysms, a "flame-shaped" intraparenchymal jet of blood may be present in the gyrus rectus.
- Primary intraventricular hemorrhage without significant subarachnoid blood is suggestive of an underlying AVM or venous hemorrhage rather than an aneurysm.
- Isolated subarachnoid blood in the perimesencephalic basal cistern is suggestive of venous hemorrhage and does not require exclusion of an aneurysm unless the index of suspicion is high.

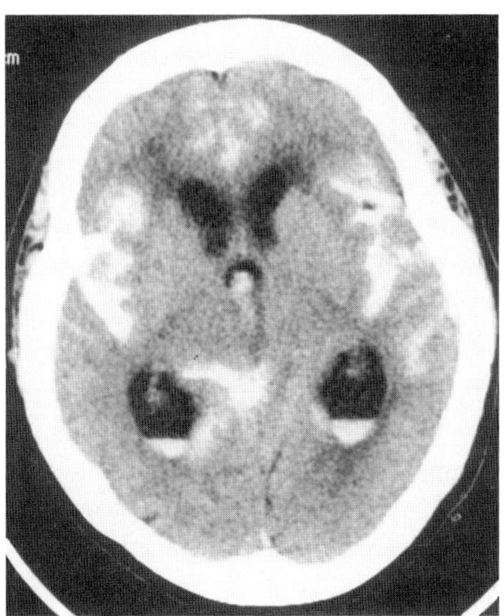
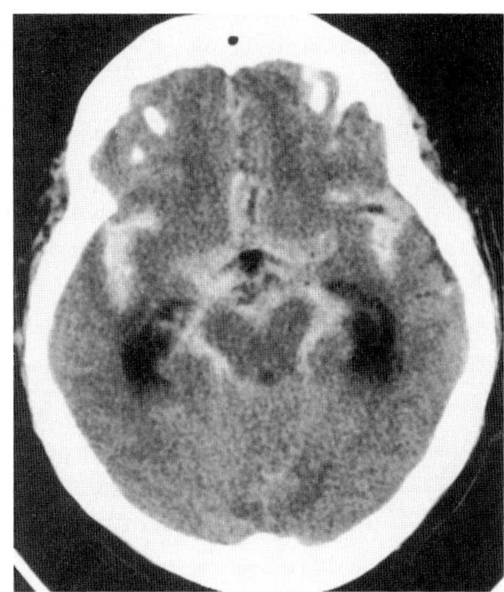

FIGURE 9.14. Noncontrast head CT showing subarachnoid hemorrhage and intraventricular extension with early hydrocephalus. (Reproduced, with permission, from Ropper AH, Brown RH. *Adams and Victor's Principles of Neurology*, 8th ed. New York: McGraw-Hill, 2005: 719.)

- Isolated subarachnoid blood around the convexity is suggestive of traumatic hemorrhage or rupture of a mycotic aneurysm. Spontaneous convexity SAH is also commonly reported in reversible cerebral vasoconstriction syndrome (Call-Fleming syndrome).
- If the head CT is unrevealing or equivocal and the index of suspicion for SAH remains high, an LP should be performed. CSF should be centrifuged and examined against a white backdrop or with a spectrophotometer for xanthochromia. If the CSF appears blood tinged, a cell count should be performed on the first and last tubes to determine if the number of erythrocytes ↓ with CSF drainage (suggestive of traumatic LP). CSF protein may be high and glucose low, especially with more remote symptom onset. Bloody CSF is unlikely to clot in the collection tubes with true SAH, unlike traumatic LP.
- Brain MRI fluid attenuation inversion recovery (FLAIR) sequences demonstrate hyperintensity (failure to suppress the CSF signal) within the sulci with SAH. This finding has similar sensitivity to head CT within 24 hours of symptom onset.
- Cerebral angiography remains the gold standard test for locating cerebral aneurysms.

Treatment

- Securing the aneurysm with clipping or coiling should be performed as early as possible. In clinical trials, immediate aneurysm occlusion resulted in better outcomes compared to delayed therapy.
- Prior to securing the aneurysm, the risk of rerupture should be minimized by aggressive blood pressure control, anticonvulsant medications, stool softeners, and avoidance of unnecessary procedures or stressors.
- Nimodipine 60 mg every 4 hours for 21 days improved mortality and functional outcome but did not ↓ the incidence of angiographic vasospasm.
- Avoidance of dehydration, but not prophylactic hypervolemia, may ↓ the incidence of vasospasm.
- Current recommendation for unruptured aneurysms is coiling or clipping for anterior circulation aneurysms > 7 mm, posterior circulation aneurysms > 3 mm, any remote aneurysm in a patient with prior aneurysm rupture, or

a rapidly enlarging aneurysm. Otherwise, observation with serial angiography is an option.

Complications

- Cardiomyopathy: Contraction band necrosis results in stress cardiomyopathy (apical ballooning and global hypokinesis on echocardiography) possibly related to cathecholamine toxicity.
- Neurogenic pulmonary edema.
- Hydrocephalus (communicating or obstructive): May require CSF diversion.
- Cerebral vasospasm: Days 1–21 (peak 4–10), monitor for new onset of focal neurological deficits and with serial transcranial Doppler ultrasonography; treat with hemodynamic augmentation and/or balloon angioplasty.
- Seizures.
- Aneurysm rerupture: Mortality > 50% in most series.

Intracranial Pressure

- Normal physiologic parameters:
  - Intracranial volume: 1400–1700 mL.
    - Brain parenchyma 80%.
    - CSF 10% (150 mL).
    - Blood 10%.
  - CSF produced by the choroid plexus at 20 mL/hr (450–500 mL/day).
  - Normal intracranial pressure < 15 mm Hg.
- **Monroe-Kellie doctrine:** Overall volume of the cranial vault cannot change, hence an ↑ in the volume of one component, or the presence of pathologic components, necessitates the displacement of other structures, an ↑ in ICP, or both.
  - The compliance relationship between changes in volume of intracranial contents and ICP is nonlinear, and compliance ↓ as the combined volume of the intracranial contents.
  - Early compensatory mechanisms include (1) displacement of CSF out of the cranial vault and (2) ↓ in the volume of the cerebral venous blood via venoconstriction and extracranial drainage.
  - When these compensatory mechanisms have been exhausted, significant ↑ in pressure develops, with small ↑ in volume → abnormally elevated ICP.

INTRACRANIAL HYPERTENSION (> 20 mm Hg)

- Common causes: Space-occupying lesions (tumors, hemorrhage), diffuse brain edema (meningitis, brain trauma, anoxia), hydrocephalus.
- Relationship between cerebral perfusion and intracranial pressure: Pathological outcomes secondary to high ICP are caused by lowering of cerebral perfusion pressure (CPP) and cerebral blood flow (CBF).
  - CPP = MAP – ICP (where MAP is mean arterial pressure).
  - CBF = (CAP – JVP) ÷ CVR (where CAP is carotid arterial pressure, JVP is jugular venous pressure, and CVR is cerebrovascular resistance).
  - CBF is constant secondary to autoregulation at CPP range of 50–100, but this may not be true in pathological states such as following brain trauma.
  - Low CPP may → ischemia but elevated CPP (> 120) may → hypertensive encephalopathy and hydrostatic cerebral edema, shifting of au-

toregulatory curve to the right allows for higher tolerance for elevated CPP/MAP in chronically hypertensive patients.

- Clinical manifestations:
  - Headache (worse with dependency/cough/Valsalva, better when upright).
  - Papilledema.
  - Depressed level of consciousness.
  - Signs and symptoms secondary to herniation (pupillary dilatation, extensor posturing).
  - Cushing triad (hypertension, bradycardia, respiratory depression).

CEREBRAL HERNIATION SYNDROMES (FIGURE 9.15)

- **Subfalcine herniation:** Lateral displacement of the medial frontoparietal cortex below the dural reflection of the falx cerebri.
  - Due to cortical space-occupying lesion → lateral displacement of cortex.
  - Compression of the ACA traveling over the tentorial incisure → ipsilateral medial frontoparietal infarct and contralateral leg weakness.
  - Rapid onset of midline shift > 1 cm results in loss of consciousness.
- **Transtentorial (uncal) herniation:** Lateral and caudal displacement of the medial temporal lobe through the tentorial incisure, resulting in compression of the midbrain.
  - Due to supratentorial space-occupying lesions → downward and lateral displacement of the temporal lobe.
  - Compression of CN III → ipsilateral fixed/dilated pupil.
  - Midbrain shift results in compression of the contralateral cerebral peduncle against the rigid tentorial incisure → ipsilateral hemiparesis (Kernohan notch phenomenon, false localizing sign).
  - Compression of the PCA traveling over the tentorial incisure → ipsilateral occipital infarct and contralateral homonymous hemianopia.

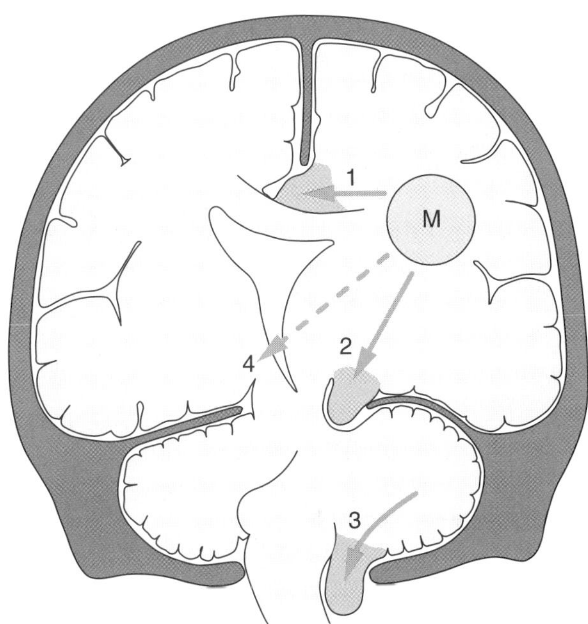

FIGURE 9.15. Schematic of cerebral herniation syndromes, including subfalcine (1), transtentorial (2), and cerebellar (3). Compression of the contralateral cerebral peduncle at Kernohan notch (4) is also shown. (Reproduced, with permission, from Ropper AH, Brown RH. *Adams and Victor's Principles of Neurology*, 8th ed. New York: McGraw-Hill, 2005: 310.)

TABLE 9.2. Stages of Coma

Location	Respiration (Figure 9.16)	Pupils	Doll Eyes	Posturing
Bilateral cortex	Cheyne-Stokes	Normal/reactive	Present	Localize/flexor
Midbrain—upper pons	Central hyperventilation	Dilated/fixed	Present	Flexor
Lower pons	Apneustic	Small/fixed	Absent	Extensor
Medulla	Ataxic	Midsized/fixed	Absent	None

- **Central herniation:** Bilateral transtentorial herniation resulting in loss of consciousness, bilateral weakness/posturing, and bilateral fixed/dilated pupils.
- **Cerebellar herniation:** Caudal displacement of the cerebellar tonsils into the foramen magnum.
  - Due to infratentorial space-occupying lesions → caudal displacement of the cerebellum.
  - Compression of the medulla → loss of consciousness, quadriplegia, respiratory failure.
  - Does not result in fixed/dilated pupil.
  - Compression of fourth ventricle → obstructive hydrocephalus.

ICP MONITORING

- Indications:
  - GCS 3–8 and abnormal CT scan or
  - Comatose patients with normal CT if 2/3 conditions:
    - Age > 40 years.
    - Unilateral or bilateral motor posturing.
    - Systolic blood pressure (SBP) < 90 mm Hg.
- Modalities:
  - Intraventricular: Provides access for CSF drainage but ↑ risk of infection (meningitis, ventriculitis) up to 20%, more common if left in for > 5 days.
  - Intraparenchymal: Fiberoptic tranducers have less infection risk (< 1%) but does not provide access for CSF drainage, tendency to lose accuracy after a few days (drift), cannot be recalibrated.

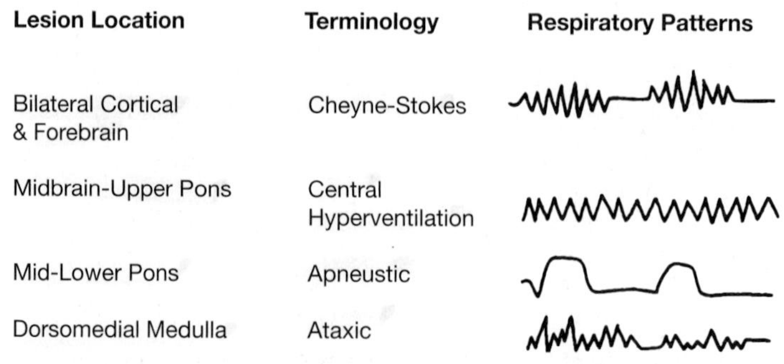

FIGURE 9.16. Schematic of respiratory patterns at different levels of brain stem injury in coma. (Reproduced, with permission, from Hall JB, Schmidt GA, Wood LDH. *Principles of Critical Care*, 3rd ed. New York: McGraw-Hill, 2005: Figure 67-1.)

    - Subarachnoid: Fluid calibrated, low risk if hemorrhage/infection but tend to become obstructed.
    - Noninvasive: TCD for pulsatility index.
- Waveforms (Figure 9.17):
    - P1: Percussion wave due to cardiac systole transmitted to the choroid plexus → CSF secretion.
    - P2: Compliance or tidal wave due to restriction of ventricular expansion by rigid skull, normally lower amplitude than P1 but may be higher amplitude than P1 in patients with poor ventricular compliance.
    - P3: Dicrotic wave due to closure of the aortic valve (corresponds to arterial dicrotic notch).
    - Lundborg A waves (plateau waves): Dangerous, sudden, sustained elevation of ICP to > 50 mm Hg for 5–20 minutes; demonstrates poor compliance.
    - Lundborg B waves: – Rhythmic oscillations in ICP every 1–2 minutes.
    - Lundborg C waves: Rhythmic oscillations in ICP every 4–8 minutes.

TREATMENT

- Emergent airway, breathing, and circulation (ABCs): Secure airway, assess need for mechanical ventilation.
- Treat the cause: Surgical removal of space-occupying lesion.
- Hyperosmolar therapy: Mannitol bolus 0.5–1g/kg IV, target serum osmolarity 300–310 mOsm/L (risk of acute tubular necrosis with serum osmolarity > 320); may → paradoxical worsening of midline shift secondary to greater efficacy on the side of brain with intact blood-brain barrier in patients with large strokes.
- Steroids (only for vasogenic edema, contraindicated in brain trauma and stroke).
- Hyperventilation: Target PCO_2 to 28–32 mm Hg, rapidly reduces ICP through vasoconstriction → decreasing volume of intracranial blood, short-lived effect on ICP, slow normalization of respiratory rate on ventilator to avoid rebound effect.
- Ventricular CSF drainage with a goal ICP < 20. Lumbar drainage contraindicated in the setting of mass lesions or midline shift, but may be effective in cryptococcal meningitis, idiopathic intracranial hypertension (pseudotumor cerebri), and communicating hydrocephalus.

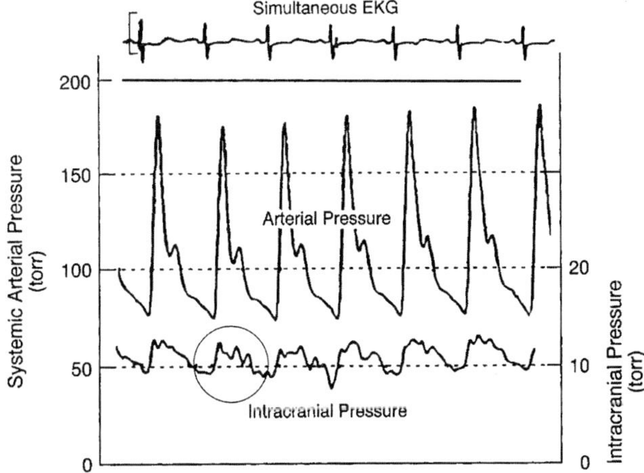

FIGURE 9.17. ICP waveform tracing showing P1, P2, and P3 waves in relation to the cardiac cycle and arterial pressure tracing. Elevation of P2 above P1 suggests poor intracranial compliance. (Reproduced, with permission, from Hall JB, Schmidt GA, Wood LDH. *Principles of Critical Care,* 3rd ed. New York: McGraw-Hill, 2005: Figure 65-1.)

- Pharmacological coma: Using barbiturates or propofol titrated to specific ICP goals, acts by reducing brain metabolism and demand ($CMRO_2$). Side effects include ↑ risk of infection, myocardial suppression, propofol infusion syndrome (lactic acidosis, rhabdomyolysis, and heart failure).
- Therapeutic hypothermia: Evidence for improved neurological recovery following cardiac arrest, not reproduced in other settings (brain trauma, stroke); slow rewarming to prevent rebound ICP elevation.
- Decompressive hemicraniectomy: Option in patients < 60 years old with likelihood of good outcomes based on clinical and radiological criteria.
- Supportive measures: Elevate head of bed to 30 degrees, treat fever (metabolic demand), glycemic control (worsen cerebral edema), sedation, control or prevent seizures.

HYDROCEPHALUS

Dilatation of the ventricles secondary to obstruction of CSF pathways, impaired venous absorption, or ↑ CSF production.

- Noncommunicating hydrocephalus: Obstruction of ventricular system (colloid cyst, mass effect from ICH) (see Figure 9.18).
- Communicating hydrocephalus: Occlusion of arachnoid granulations → decreased CSF absorption (meningitis, SAH).
- **Symptoms:** Headache, vomiting, lethargy.
- **Signs:** Limited upgaze, bilateral CN VI palsy, papilledema.
- **Management:**
  - Emergent ABCs, especially if hydrocephalus evolves acutely.
  - Intraventricular catheter for drainage/ICP monitoring.
  - Lumbar drain or serial LP only in communicating hydrocephalus (risk of herniation in noncommunicating hydrocephalus).
  - Definitive procedure: CSF diversion/implanted shunt.

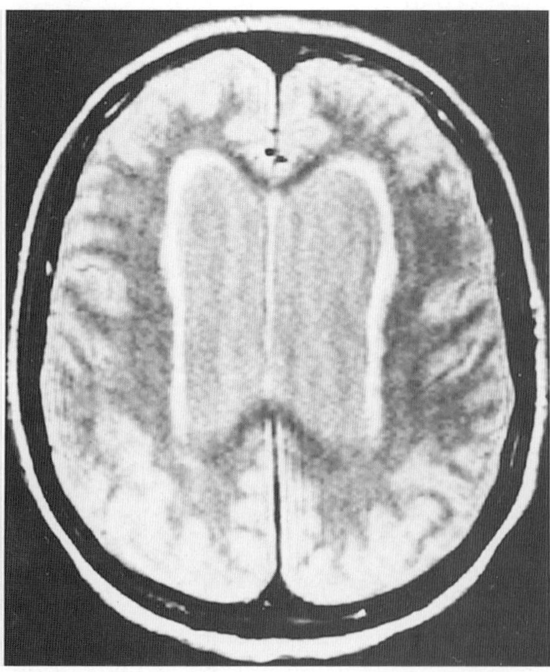

FIGURE 9.18. Axial proton density MRI showing ventriculomegaly, sulcal compression, and transependymal flow due to obstructive hydrocephalus. (Reproduced, with permission, from Ropper AH, Brown RH. *Adams and Victor's Principles of Neurology*, 8th ed. New York: McGraw-Hill, 2005: 534.)

- **Special conditions:** Normal pressure hydrocephalus—ventriculomegaly with normal opening pressure on LP.
  - **Symptoms:** Triad of wet (incontinence), wacky (dementia), and wobbly (gait disturbance).
    - Magnetic (apraxic) gait: Feet being "stuck" to floor, ↓ stride length and height, postural instability, wide-based (parkinsonian gait is narrow-based).
    - Urinary symptoms: Urgency early in disease process, incontinence later.
    - Dementia: Subcortical dementia with psychomotor slowing, ↓ attention and apathy.
  - **Etiology:** ↓ reabsorption of CSF, may be primary (unknown etiology) or secondary to history of subarachnoid hemorrhage, chronic meningitis, etc.
  - **Differential diagnosis:** Dementia with Lewy bodies, vascular dementia, Alzheimer disease, parkinsonism.
  - **Diagnosis:**
    - CT/MRI shows ventriculomegaly disproportionate to cortical atrophy.
    - High-volume LP (35–50 cc) with gait and cognitive testing before and 30–60 minutes after LP.
  - **Treatment:** CSF shunting → 60% improvement in gait; negative predictors are advanced dementia, idiopathic NPH, and symptoms > 6 months.

SPONTANEOUS INTRACRANIAL HYPOTENSION

Low ICP due to spontaneous or traumatic chronic CSF leakage.

- **Symptoms and signs:** Headache (migrainous quality, worse when upright, improved by dependency), vomiting, cranial neuropathy (CN VI most common).
- **Etiology:** Postoperative (ie, transsphenoidal hypophysectomy), post-LP, skull base fracture, idiopathic (usually due to spontaneous spinal dural tear).
- **Diagnosis:** Contrast-enhanced sagittal or coronal T1 MRI showing uniform pachymeningeal thickening and enhancement, sagging of cerebellar tonsils into foramen magnum, and sagging of diencephalon below optic nerves (Figure 9.19).
- **Treatment:** Directed toward locating and repairing site of CSF leak, blood patch for post-LP leak.

HYPERTENSIVE ENCEPHALOPATHY

Hydrostatic cerebral edema, typically involving the occipital lobes, due to extravasation of water through leaky vascular endothelium in hypertensive emergency.

- **Symptoms and signs:** Headache (similar character to hydrocephalus), vomiting, cortical blindness (visual blurring or loss with preserved papillary light reflex and no papilledema), lethargy, or coma.
- **Etiology:** Extreme hypertension results in leakage of water across the vascular endothelium into brain parenchyma; posterior circulation territories are particularly susceptible because of looser endothelial junctions.
- **Differential diagnosis:** Eclampsia (may occur without extreme hypertension or seizures), reversible posterior leukoencephalopathy syndrome (RPLS) due to idiosyncratic reaction to immunosuppressive transplant drugs (ie, cyclosporine, tacrolimus).

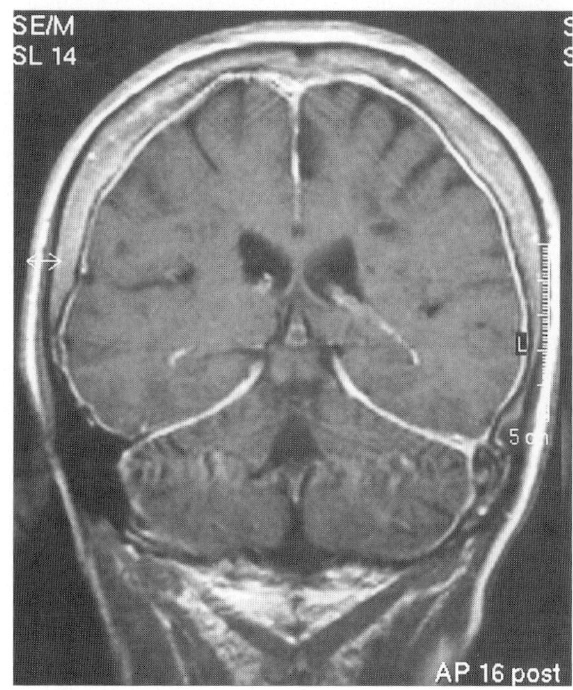

FIGURE 9.19. Coronal contrast-enhanced T1-weighted MRI showing diffuse thickening and enhancement of the pachymeninges in intracranial hypotension due to CSF leak. (Reproduced, with permission, from Ropper AH, Brown RH. *Adams and Victor's Principles of Neurology,* 8th ed. New York: McGraw-Hill, 2005: 542.)

- **Diagnosis:** CT or MRI shows symmetric vasogenic edema in the occipital lobes with or without hemorrhage in a patient with extreme hypertension (Figure 9.20).
- **Treatment:** Gradual ↓ of blood pressure (25% within first 24 hours) to avoid precipitating cerebral or cardiac ischemia in chronic hypertensives, delivery (eclampsia), discontinuation of causative drug (RPLS).

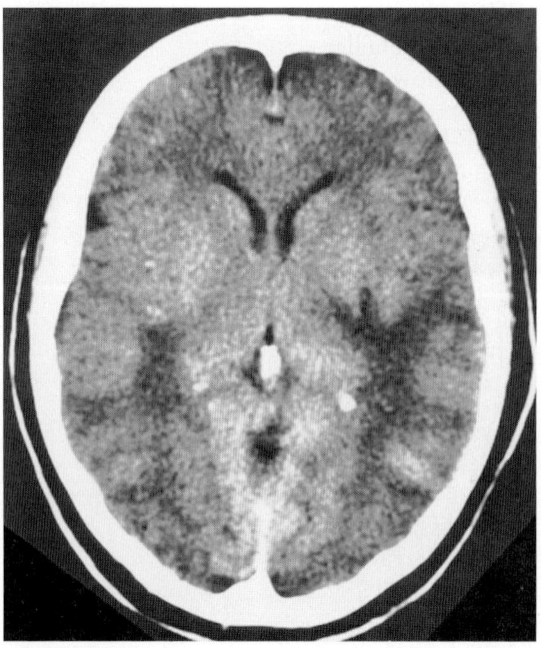

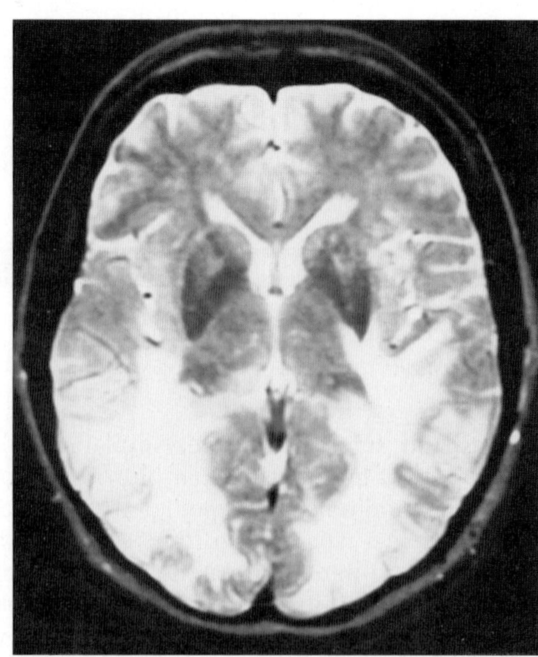

FIGURE 9.20. Axial CT (left) and T2-weighted MRI showing symmetric vasogenic edema in the occipital regions in hypertensive encephalopathy or reversible posterior leukoencephalopathy syndrome (RPLS). (Reproduced, with permission, from Ropper AH, Brown RH. *Adams and Victor's Principles of Neurology,* 8th ed. New York: McGraw-Hill, 2005: 729.)

Traumatic Brain Injury (TBI)

Etiology

- < 75 years of age: Most commonly associated with motor vehicle collision.
- > 75 years of age: most commonly secondary to falls.
- Alcohol related: 50%.
- Violence related: 20%.

Clinical Subtypes

- **Mild TBI:** No loss of consciousness (LOC) or LOC for a few seconds, symptoms of headache, blurry vision, tinnitus, confusion, loss of appetite, insomnia, mood fluctuations, and memory problems. Initial GCS 13–15.
- **Moderate TBI:** Loss of consciousness at onset, lethargy, persistent headache, nausea and vomiting, disorientation, agitation and other personality changes, incoordination, seizures, and neurological deficits. Initial GCS 9–12.
- **Severe TBI:** Stuporous or comatose, clinical signs of herniation, severe focal neurological deficits, worsening neurological exams, recurrent seizures. Initial GCS 3–8.
- **Concussion:** Mild TBI resulting in headache, brief LOC, and amnesia or other transient neurological symptoms such as dizziness without radiographic findings.
  - Grade I: No LOC, transient confusion or other symptoms < 15 minutes.
  - Grade II: no LOC, transient confusion or other symptoms > 15 minutes.
  - Grade III: LOC for any duration.
- **Epidural hematoma:** Hemorrhage between the dura and skull periosteum, typically due to tearing of the middle meningeal artery associated with temporal bone fracture.
  - Emergency neurosurgical evaluation, often necessitating urgent evacuation.
  - Head CT: Convex (lens shaped) hyperdensity that does not cross skull suture lines (Figure 9.21).
  - Classical lucid interval (initial loss of consciousness due to force on the brain stem arousal centers followed by improvement in alertness followed by loss of consciousness due to mass effect from the expanding hematoma).
- **Subdural hematoma:** Tearing of bridging veins (venous sinuses) due to shearing forces with trauma associated with rotational acceleration/deceleration (falls and assaults).
  - May occur without a blow to the head (ie, whiplash injury) in older patients due to movement of an atrophic brain with respect to the dura.
  - Management may be expectant in minimally symptomatic patients with small or chronic lesions, surgical evacuation in symptomatic patients.
  - Head CT: Concave hyperdensity that crosses skull suture lines, subacute lesions are isodense and hypodense lesions are chronic (Figure 9.22).
  - Chronic subdural hematomas are susceptible to repeat bleeding due to friable vessels within chronic, fibrous membranes that develop.
- **Cerebral contusions:** Parynchymal bruising of brain due to blunt head trauma.
  - Coup/contre-coup injuries: Blows to the back of the head result in contusion of the orbital frontal and anterior temporal lobes as brain strikes the rigid orbital plate and sphenoid wing, respectively.
  - Tend to "blossom" (hematoma enlargement due to coalescence of microhemorrhages in injured brain tissue) within first 24 hours.

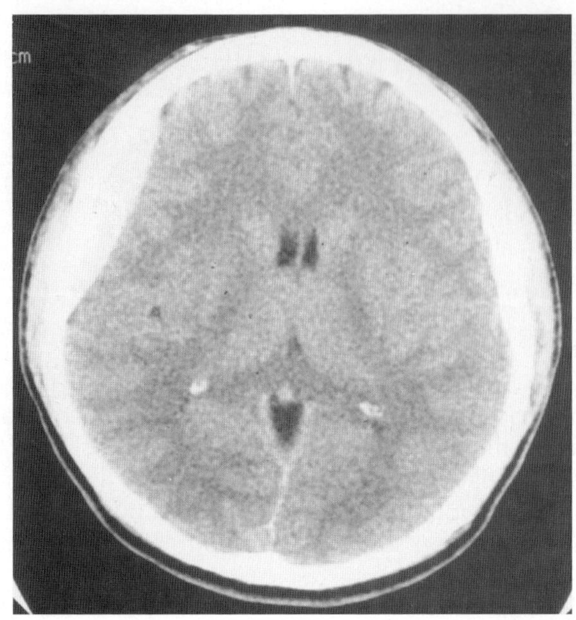

FIGURE 9.21. Noncontrast head CT showing a right-sided epidural hematoma. (Reproduced, with permission, from Ropper AH, Brown RH. Adams and Victor's Principles of Neurology, 8th ed. New York: McGraw-Hill, 2005: 758.)

- **Diffuse axonal injury (DAI):** Acceleration/deceleration injury → shearing/tearing of axons, typically seen with rotational/angular as opposed to linear forces.
  - Most commonly occurs at gray-white junction and large white matter tracts such as the corpus callosum and middle cerebral peduncles.
  - Head CT: Multiple, punctate white matter hyperdensities measuring 1–15 mm at gray-white junction and white matter tracts (Figure 9.23A); classical finding is normal or near-normal CT in comatose patient.

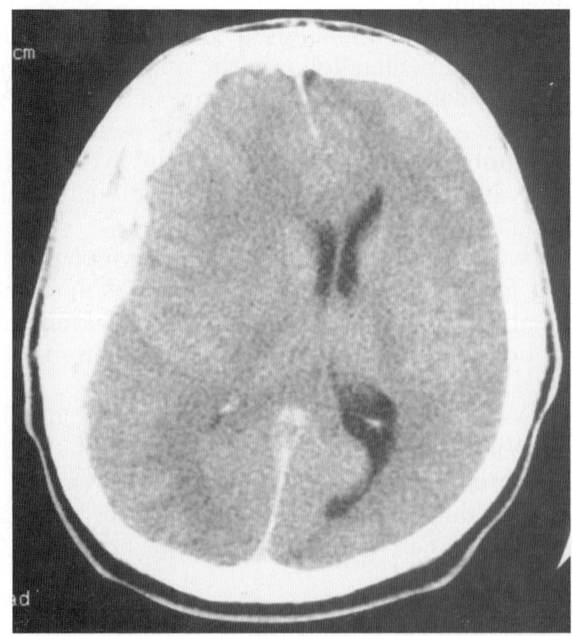

FIGURE 9.22. Noncontrast head CT showing an acute right-sided subdural hematoma resulting in shift of midline structures and early hydrocephalus. (Reproduced, with permission, from Ropper AH, Brown RH. *Adams and Victor's Principles of Neurology,* 8th ed. New York: McGraw-Hill, 2005: 246.)

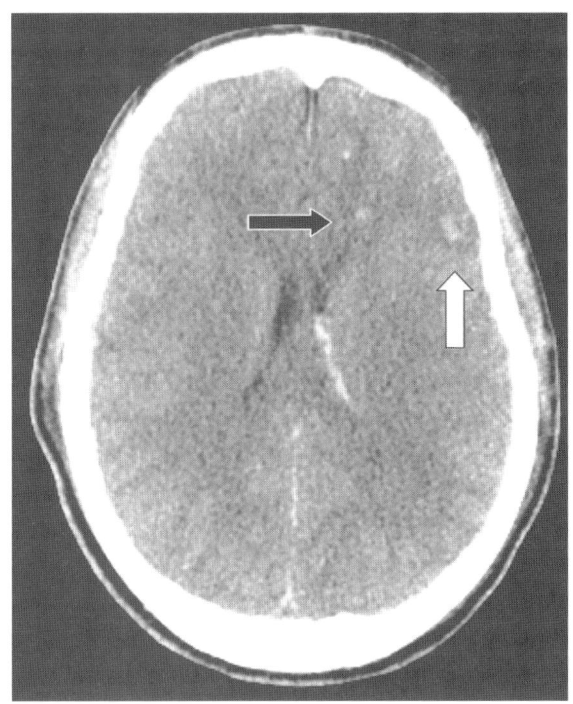
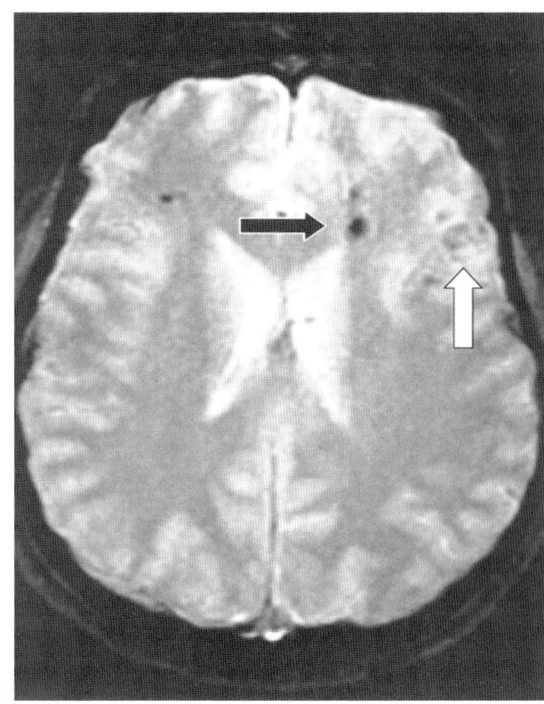

FIGURE 9.23. Noncontrast head CT (A) and axial gradient echo MRI (B) showing hemorrhage in white matter tracts in diffuse axonal injury (DAI). (Reproduced, with permission, from Ropper AH, Brown RH. *Adams and Victor's Principles of Neurology*, 8th ed. New York: McGraw-Hill, 2005: 753.)

- Head MRI: Gradient echo and susceptibility-weighted sequences reveals multiple punctuate hemorrhages (hypointensities) in white matter tracts and subcortical gray matter (Figure 9.23B). DAI lesions may also restrict diffusion.
- Outcomes poor in over 90% (severe disability, persistent vegetative state [PVS], death).
- Grade 1: Diffuse injury without focal component.
- Grade 2: Diffuse injury with focal damage (corpus callosum, etc).
- Grade 3: Diffuse damage and focal brain stem lesions.

Treatment

- Emergent ABCs: Assess need for airway control, look for signs of hemodynamic instability, evaluate for possible sources of bleeding, which may be overt or subtle (bruising in blunt injury).
- Stabilize C-spine at all times including securing airway (if indicated).
- Indications for intubation: GCS ≤ 8, major extracranial injuries, respiratory failure, circulatory shock, imminent need for operative management, combativeness.
- Avoid prophylactic hyperventilation secondary to risk of reducing CBF.
- C-spine clearance: 5–10% of TBI patients have occult C-spine injuries.
- In awake, nonintoxicated patient with no distracting injuries: three-view C-spine x-ray and clinical clearance are adequate.
- In a comatose patient not expected to awaken for > 72 hours, C-spine CT to exclude fracture and MRI to exclude ligamentous injury missed in 25% of patients with CT or x-ray alone.
- Cerebral perfusion pressure (CPP) goal > 60 (changed from prior goal of CPP > 70 based on similar neurological outcomes but higher incidence of acute respiratory distress syndrome [ARDS] in CPP > 70 group) and ICP goal < 20.

- Seizure prophylaxis recommended for 1 week in setting of moderate to severe TBI, reduces risk of seizures in first week but not later development of epilepsy.
- Steroids not associated with any clinical benefit in human trials with trend toward ↑ mortality and worse outcomes.
- Hyperglycemia associated with worse neurological outcomes but target glucose range is undefined.
- Fever is independently associated with poor outcome, but therapeutic hypothermia did not improve outcome in clinical trials.
- Nutrition: Severe TBI patients require 140% of expected caloric needs due to ↑ metabolic demands.

Outcomes

- Prognosis correlates with initial GCS and clinical severity of TBI.
- Severe TBI associated with high incidence of severe disability, epilepsy, and hydrocephalus.
- **Postconcussion syndrome:** Headache, dizziness, memory problems, difficulty concentrating, sleep dysfunction, restlessness, irritability, apathy, depression, and anxiety (any three).
- **Dementia pugilistica:** Cognitive decline and parkinsonism associated with repetitive head trauma.
- **Second impact syndrome:** Head trauma days or weeks after a concussion, before initial symptoms have resolved, may be fatal due to refractory generalized cerebral edema from vascular leakiness.
- **Sports-related concussion:** Symptoms of concussion include: headache, phonophobia, photophobia; changes in reaction time, balance, and coordination; changes in memory, judgment, speech, and sleep; brief LOC (present in only 10% of concussions). Immediate assessment for concussion should use standard assessment tools. Players with suspected concussion should be immediately removed from play until evaluated by a licensed healthcare professional with expertise in concussion management. The period of maximal risk for second concussion is 10 days.

Spinal Cord Trauma

- Compressive myelopathy after trauma to the spine presents acutely as spinal shock: Areflexia, flaccid paralysis, loss of sphincter tone, urinary retention, autonomic instability, hypotension due to peripheral vasodilation, and numbness to all sensory modalities below the level of injury (sensory level).
- Spinal cord contusion may present as central cord syndrome due to venous congestion of the central spinal cord: Disproportionate weakness of the upper extremities (especially hands) > lower extremities, sensory level with sparing of sacral sensation, urinary retention, and other signs of myelopathy.
- Use of high-dose solumedrol in spinal cord trauma is controversial and recent guidelines do not recommend routine use of steroids in spinal cord trauma.
- Autonomic instability often requires frequent monitoring of blood pressure and electrocardiogram, especially during patient manipulation, bowel movements, etc.
- Recent guidelines recommend avoidance of hypotension in spinal cord trauma with an option of hemodynamic augmentation to maintain MAP > 85 mm Hg for 7 days in order to maximize spinal cord perfusion.
- In chronic spinal cord injury, upper motor signs are present, and urinary retention is usually succeeded by spastic urinary incontinence.

Intensive Care Management of Neurological Diseases

GUILLAIN-BARRÉ SYNDROME

- Commonly associated with ventilatory failure and autonomic dysfunction.
- **Criteria for intubation:**
  - Vital capacity < 15 mL/kg (< 1 L in average adult).
  - Negative inspiratory force (NIF) < 25 mL/kg.
  - 30% decrement in forced vital capacity (FVC) or NIF over 24 hours.
  - Evidence of severe uncompensated respiratory acidosis on blood gas.
  - Severe bulbar involvement with inability to control secretions → airway compromise.
- **Predictors of respiratory failure:**
  - Time of onset to admission < 7 days.
  - Inability to cough.
  - Inability to stand.
  - Inability to lift the elbows.
  - Inability to lift the head off the pillow.
  - Elevated liver enzymes.
  - In those with four predictors, mechanical ventilation is required in > 85%.
- **Autonomic dysfunction:** Severe autonomic dysfunction present in 20%, mostly in patients who develop severe weakness and respiratory failure.
  - Tachy- or bradycardia, urinary retention, hyper- or hypotension, cardiac arrhythmia, ileus, and hyper- or hypothermia.
  - Need close cardiac and hemodynamic monitoring, especially during plasmapheresis; avoid hypovolemia; watch for postural hypotension.

MYASTHENIC CRISIS

- Severe decompensation of disease, → respiratory failure and need for mechanical ventilation, often associated with bulbar dysfunction.
- Criteria for intubation and mechanical ventilation same as Guillain-Barré syndrome and other neuromuscular causes of respiratory failure.
- Treated with plasmapheresis, intravenous immune globulin (IVIG), or steroids.
- Rapid initiation of high-dose steroids → transient clinical worsening of weakness and respiratory failure in 50% of patients.
- Precipitating factors:
  - Infection (urinary tract infection, pneumonia).
  - Noncompliance with medications.
  - Rapid tapering of myasthenia drugs.
  - Anesthetic agents and neuromuscular blockers for surgery.
  - Concomitant use of medications that ↓ neuromuscular transmission (aminoglycosides, fluorquinolones, beta blockers, calcium channel blockers, anticonvulsants, etc).

NEUROLEPTIC MALIGNANT SYNDROME (NMS)

- Tetrad of fever, rigidity, mental status changes, and autonomic instability.
  - Fever > 38° C is essential for diagnosis, > 40° C seen in almost half of patients.
  - Lead pipe muscle rigidity seen in majority of patients.

- Mental status change is typically first sign, usually agitated delirium.
- Autonomic instability: Tachycardia, extreme variability of blood pressure.

- **Lab abnormalities:** Rhabdomyolysis → elevated creatine kinase and creatinine, leukocytosis, hyperkalemia, myoglobinuria, and low serum iron.
- Occurs in 1–3% of patients taking neuroleptics; seen more commonly with high-potency neuroleptics such as haloperidol.
  - Idiosyncratic; can occur with first dose or after several years of use.
  - Higher risk with higher doses, rapid dose escalation, parenteral administration.
- **Host risk factors:** Underlying psychosis, catatonia, concomitant use of lithium. NMS is occasionally secondary to antiemetic use or rapid discontinuation of chronic dopamine agonist medications for parkinsonism (levodopa).
- **Management:** Discontinuation of causative agent, hydration, temperature reduction, dantrolene or bromocriptine.

SEROTONIN SYNDROME

- Syndrome triggered by selective serotonin reuptake inhibitors (SSRIs); triad of mental status changes, autonomic hyperactivity, and neuromuscular abnormalities.
- **Symptoms and signs:** Similar to NMS.
- Additional signs include ataxia, hyperreflexia, myoclonus, and shivering.
- Symptom onset typically < 24 hours of starting or changing drug (unlike NMS).
- **Management:** Discontinuation of causative agent, benzodiazepines, cyproheptadine (specific antidote).

SURVIVORS OF CARDIAC ARREST

- Negative predictors of outcome in comatose survivors:
  - Burst suppression, generalized suppression, or unreactive alpha coma on electroencephalogram (EEG) > 24 hours after resuscitation.
  - Bilaterally absent cortical N20 potentials on median nerve somatosensory evoked potential (SSEP) > 24 hours after resuscitation (100% specific for PVS or death).
  - Fixed and dilated pupils, absent corneal reflexes, and/or no motor activity other than extensor posturing > 72 hours after resuscitation.
  - Myoclonic status epilepticus.
  - Elevated serum neuron-specific enolase.
  - Absence of these findings is not specific for good neurological outcome (majority of patients have poor outcome regardless of EEG and SSEP results).
- **Myoclonic status epilepticus:** Generalized, symmetric, nonrhythmic myoclonic jerks occurring within the first 48 hours after resuscitation in comatose patients.
  - Believed to reflect severe cortical injury, not seizure activity.
  - Often time-locked to bursts in burst-suppression EEG (Figure 9.24).
  - Usually stimulus-sensitive—by suctioning, position change, etc.
  - Typically resolve spontaneously within 3–5 days.
  - Highly refractory to anticonvulsant drugs, often requiring anesthetic agents, if control is required (ie, interferes with mechanical ventilation).

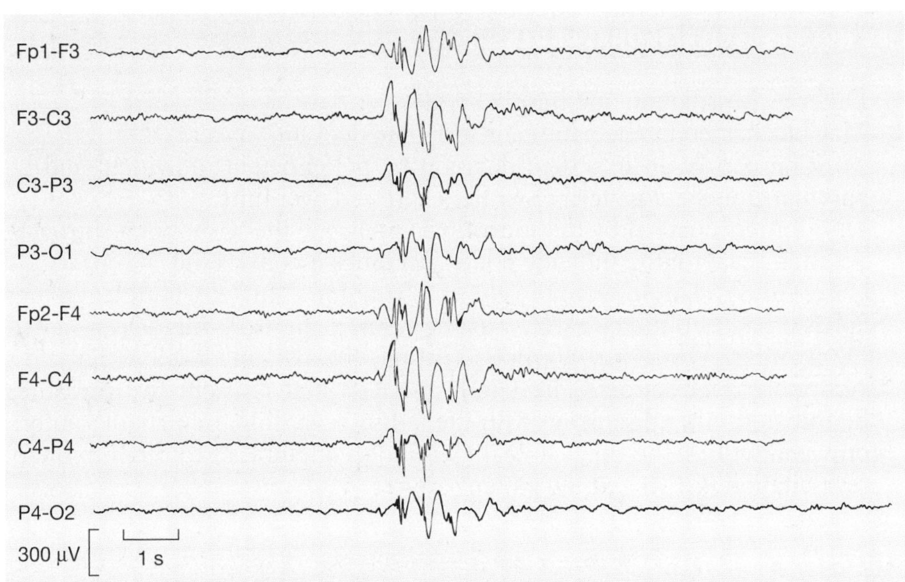

FIGURE 9.24. Burst-suppression EEG after cardiac arrest. (Reproduced, with permission, from Aminoff MJ, Greenberg DA, Simon RP. *Clinical Neurology*, 6th ed. New York: McGraw-Hill, 2005: Figure 8-4.)

- **Postanoxic myoclonus (Lance-Adams syndrome):** Action myoclonus occurring in chronic survivors of cardiac arrest.
  - Asymmetric myoclonic jerks brought out by volitional movement.
  - Distinct syndrome from myoclonic status epilepticus; does not necessarily portend poor prognosis for recovery.
  - Begins weeks to months after cardiac arrest and persists.
  - Difficult to control but may respond to benzodiazepines, valproic acid, levetiracetam, barbiturates, etc.

Ethical Issues and End-of-Life Care

BRAIN DEATH

- Brain death declaration procedures differ according to state laws and hospital policies.
- Absence of sedative/paralytic drugs, chemical intoxication, severe metabolic derangements, and hypothermia.
- Absence of all brain stem reflexes and cortical activity.
- No respiratory effort despite elevation of $PaCO_2$ to > 60 mm Hg and a 20 mm Hg rise from baseline in apnea testing.
- Legally accepted determination of death; no further need for consent to withdraw supportive measures such as mechanical ventilation (except where specifically mandated by state laws).
- Case: An 80-year-old woman presents with massive ICH and fulfills criteria for brain death. After formal declaration of death, the family requests that the patient remain on mechanical ventilation in hopes that she will improve. After discussion with the family and the hospital ethics committee, the decision is made to remove the patient from the ventilator after the family is given a reasonable opportunity to spend time with the patient.

DO NOT RESUSCITATE (DNR) ORDERS

- Differ by jurisdiction and hospital policy.
- May be enacted by the patient or surrogate decision maker.
- Must be part of an informed decision by a competent individual and be part of a consistent pattern of wishes expressed over time.
- DNR orders enacted by the individual supersede the wishes of a surrogate decision maker if the individual later becomes incompetent.
- Case: An 85-year-old woman is hospitalized for a stroke, which leaves her aphasic and hemiparetic. Her nursing home paperwork includes a signed DNR order. While her family is visiting, the patient develops pulseless ventricular tachycardia. The family requests that resusctitative measures be initiated. After discussion with the family regarding the patient's autonomy and wishes, the medical team withholds attempts at cardiopulmonary resuscitation (CPR) and the patient expires.

TRANSFER OF PATIENTS

- Emergency Medical Transportation and Active Labor Act (EMTALA) dictates that tertiary hospitals have an obligation to transfer patients who require a higher level of care regardless of the patient's ability to pay when:
  - The referring hospital is incapable of delivering required care.
  - The accepting hospital is capable of providing this care.
  - The accepting hospital has the resources and capacity to accept the patient.
  - The patient is medically stable for transfer.
- Case: A community hospital does not have a neurologist on staff and the emergency department physician has not been trained to evaluate patients for thrombolytic therapy. The physician calls to refer a patient with signs of acute ischemic stroke of 30 minutes' duration to your tertiary hospital. The patient does not have medical insurance. The accepting hospital has experience providing tPA, a neurologist on call to the emergency department, and the capacity to accept the patient. The patient is medically stable for transfer, which is arranged on an emergency basis.

MEDICAL FUTILITY

- Determination by the medical team that no therapy will result in improvement of a patient's medical condition and death is imminent, usually invoked when no surrogate decision maker is available.
- No uniform legal definition.
- Rarely invoked against patient/family request for treatment.
- Complicated ethical situations should provoke consultation with available family and the hospital ethics committee.
- Case: An 80-year-old man with advanced glioblastoma multiforme develops bacterial meningitis after a surgical procedure. He develops septic shock despite adequate antibiotic coverage, which is refractory to medical therapies. The medical team believes that further medical therapy would be unlikely to result in meaningful recovery and contemplates withdrawal of supportive measures. In this situation, the prognosis should be discussed with the patient's family and surrogate decision makers and advance directives consulted if applicable. If the family wishes to continue medical care that is believed to be futile, the hospital ethics committee should be consulted.

CHAPTER 10

Neurological Infections

Michael S. Rafii, MD, PhD

Meningitis

A 27-year-old right-handed male presents with a fever and altered mental status. He has a 4-day history of a flulike illness, fever, myalgias, and a severe headache, which progressed to nausea and vomiting. He initially thought that he might have a stomach flu, so he stayed home from work and tried to drink lots of fluids. However, the fever persisted and the headache worsened. On the day of presentation, his girlfriend noticed that he was quite lethargic and difficult to arouse and called the paramedics.

A CBC is 19,500 white cells, electrolytes are within normal limits, blood glucose is 100. A head computed tomography (CT) scan without contrast is normal. The next best test to get is a lumbar puncture (LP) with opening pressure of 270 mm of water observed, protein of 150, glucose of 15, cell count of 2400, 95% polymorphonuclear cells. Gram stain and culture are sent and pending. (The head CT was done first to rule out cerebral edema, which may prohibit LP.)

The patient should be immediately started on IV antibiotics for presumed bacterial meningitis.

Inflammation or infection of the meninges, usually caused by bacteria, viruses, or fungi, but occasionally caused by other infectious agents or noninfectious conditions.

Symptoms

Depend on the etiology of the meningitis, but typically include fever, headache, and irritability.

Exam

Clinical signs include evidence of meningeal irritation, including nuchal rigidity, Kernig sign, and Brudzinski sign.

- **Kernig sign:** Passive flexion of the patient's hip and extension of the knee causes the patient to flex his or her neck.
- **Brudzinski sign:** Passive flexion of the neck causes the patient to flex his or her legs.
- Both of these signs occur because when the meninges are irritated, placing a stretch on them produces pain, causing the patient to take an action to relieve that stretch.

Diagnosis

- By definition, inflammation must be present, so spinal fluid examination will reveal a pleocytosis (see Table 10.1).
- Patients with meningitis may have elevated intracranial pressure (ICP); perform head CT prior to LP to assess the safety of the procedure.

Differential Diagnosis

- Systemic infection or sepsis; trauma or closed head injury or child abuse; multiple metabolic abnormalities (hypoglycemia, ketoacidosis, electrolyte imbalance, uremia, toxic exposure); seizure, brain tumor, subarachnoid hemorrhage, intracranial hemorrhage, epidural abscess.
- Recurrent meningitis: Cerebrospinal fluid (CSF) leak, HIV, Mollaret (herpes simplex virus, type 2 [HSV-2]), inflammatory (noninfectious).

- Chronic meningitis and cranial nerve palsy: Lyme disease, syphilis, tuberculosis, sarcoidosis.

BACTERIAL MENINGITIS

Symptoms

- Typically include fever, headache, photophobia, nausea, vomiting, irritability, and lethargy, proceeding to further clouding of consciousness and, ultimately, death.
- The course is frequently fulminant, with rapid neurologic deterioration; therefore, initiation of appropriate antibiotic treatment must not be delayed.

Exam

- Evidence of meningeal irritation, though this can be lacking in children, the elderly, and the deeply comatose.
- Fever may be ≥ 103°F or higher.
- Focal neurological signs may also appear.

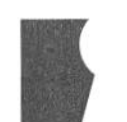

KEY FACT

Antibiotics may be started up to several hours before CSF is obtained without affecting culture results.

Differential Diagnosis

See Table 10.2 for the most common etiologies of bacterial meningitis in various demographic groups.

Diagnosis

- CSF exam showing a predominantly neutrophilic pleocytosis is strongly suggestive; should prompt broad-coverage antibiotic treatment; however, in the proper clinical setting, do not delay treatment in order to obtain CSF.
- Because many types of bacteria can cause enough brain edema to make an LP hazardous, consider brain imaging prior to CSF exam.
- No currently available tests to confirm the identity of the causative organism are fast enough to base initial treatment on their findings. The main value of these tests is to confirm the clinical diagnosis.
- CSF Gram stain and culture are about 70% sensitive; antibiotics do not

TABLE 10.1. CSF Examination in Meningitis

	Normal Values	Bacterial	Viral	Fungal
Opening pressure (mm Hg)	50–80	Elevated (100–300)	Normal or slightly elevated (80–100)	Elevated
Pleocytosis (WBCs/mm³)	0–5	Usually > 1000	Usually > 100	Usually > 100
% Neutrophils	0	> 50%	< 20%	Variable
Protein (mg/dL)	20–45	Usually > 100	Usually > 45	Variable
Glucose (mg/dL)	Two-thirds of serum glucose	↓	Normal	Often very ↓
Other tests		Gram stain and culture	Viral polymerase chain reaction (PCR)	India ink, culture, cryptococcal antigen

TABLE 10.2. Common Causes of Bacterial Meningitis

Age	Bacteria
Neonates (< 1 year old), due to exposure in the birth canal	Group B streptococci and gram-negative enteric bacilli, particularly *Escherichia coli.*
Children ≥ 1 year old and adults	*Streptococcus pneumoniae* and *Neisseria meningitidis.*
Elderly (> 50 years old)	*S pneumoniae* and gram-negative bacilli, including *Haemophilus influenzae, E coli, Enterobacter,* and *Pseudomonas.*
Recurrent meningitis, CSF leak, head trauma, due to skin and nasopharyngeal colonization	*S pneumoniae* and nontypeable *H influenzae.*
Pneumonia (adults 18–50 years old)	*S pneumoniae.*
Chronic lung disease	*Pseudomonas.*
Chronic urinary tract infection	*E coli* or *Enterobacter.*
Sinusitis, otitis media	Nontypeable *H influenzae, S pneumoniae.*
Immunosuppressed and/or elderly	*Listeria monocytogenes.*
Neurosurgical patients	*S pneumoniae,* nontypeable *H influenzae,* and *S aureus.*

change the sensitivity if the culture is obtained within 4 hours of antibiotic initiation.

Meningococcal Meningitis

- Caused by a gram-negative diplococcus, *Neisseria meningitidis.*
- Typically associated with a rash, which can vary from petechial to purpuric (see Figure 10.1). Such a rash, together with fever and hypotension/shock, is strong evidence for this infection.

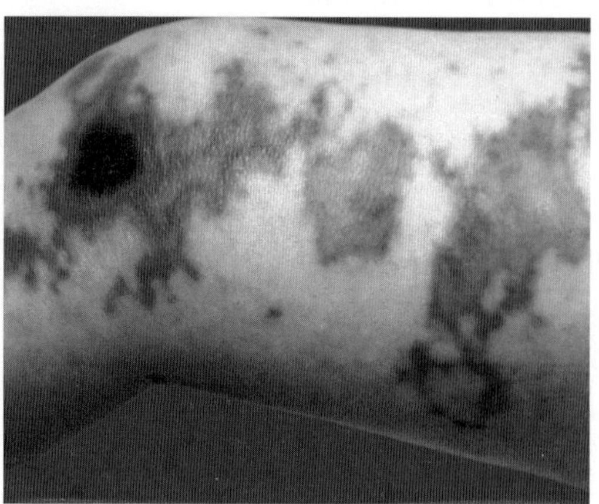

FIGURE 10.1. Acute meningococcal rash. (Also see Color Plate.) (Reproduced, with permission, from Wolff K, Johnson RA, Saavedra AP. *Fitzpatrick's Color Atlas & Synopsis of Clinical Dermatology,* 7th ed. New York: McGraw-Hill Education, 2013. Figure 25-57.)

- Highly effective vaccines protect against serotypes that cause approximately 75% of cases.
- Bacterial antigen can be detected from CSF, but detection from serum or urine is unreliable. Blood and CSF cultures are usually positive, but false negatives can occur for all these tests, so the clinician should not be dissuaded from the diagnosis by negative tests if the clinical presentation is suggestive.
- Waterhouse-Friderichsen syndrome (WFS) or hemorrhagic adrenalitis is a disease of the adrenal glands most commonly caused by the bacterium *Neisseria meningitidis.*
- The infection leads to massive hemorrhage into 1 or (usually) both adrenal glands.
- Characterized by overwhelming bacterial infection meningococcemia, low blood pressure and shock, disseminated intravascular coagulation (DIC) with widespread purpura, and rapidly developing adrenocortical insufficiency.

Pneumococcal Meningitis

- Caused by *Streptococcus pneumoniae*, gram-positive cocci that tend to grow in chains.
- Leading cause of bacterial meningitis worldwide; accounts for significant morbidity and mortality in all age groups.
- Often, a history of productive cough, dyspnea, and constitutional symptoms in the days prior to onset of meningitis-like symptoms. Concomitant pneumonia is common. Pneumonia is often associated with bacteremia and, therefore, with meningitis.
- *S pneumoniae* is also a common cause of otitis media and acute sinusitis, which can provide a source of meningitis, by either hematogenous spread or direct extension.
- It is an encapsulated organism and patients with various underlying conditions, including asplenic states, cancer, alcoholism, malnutrition, and diabetes mellitus are at ↑ risk of infection.
- Highly effective vaccines protect against serotypes that cause approximately 80% of cases of pneumococcal meningitis.
- Both blood and CSF cultures will usually be positive. Bacterial antigen, particularly capsular polysaccharides can also be detected from serum, CSF, and urine.

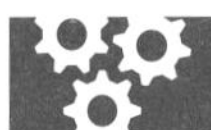
MNEMONIC

Strep = **strip: Strep**tococci usually grow in chains or **strip**s.

Haemophilus Meningitis

- Caused by gram-negative coccobacilli that will frequently be seen on Gram stain of the CSF.
- Prior to development of a vaccine for *H influenzae* type b (Hib), Hib was the leading cause of bacterial meningitis in children < 5 years old in the United States.
- Both nasopharyngeal colonization and meningitis due to this organism have now been nearly eradicated in infants and children who are routinely vaccinated, but still must be strongly considered in any patient from developing countries where Hib vaccine may not be readily available.
- Frequent history of an upper respiratory tract infection preceding onset of meningitis, with hematogenous spread.
- Hib is an encapsulated organism, so patients with splenectomy (functional or surgical) are at ↑ risk.
- The vaccine works only against type b *H influenzae.* Non–type b *H influenzae* can also cause meningitis, is also encapsulated, manifests similarly to Hib meningitis, and is ↑ in the United States.

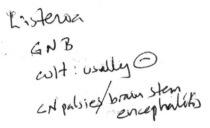

MNEMONIC

The **Grapes** of **Staph** (like the "Grapes of Wrath"): **Staph**ylococci are frequently seen in **grape**-like clusters.

- Unencapsulated, nontypeable strains also cause meningitis, but usually by direct extension from a focus of infection, such as sinusitis or otitis media. Other risk factors include head trauma, neurosurgical procedure, or other cause of CSF leak, and nontypeable *H influenzae* is therefore a common cause of recurrent bacterial meningitis.
- Both blood and CSF cultures will usually be positive. The capsular polysaccharide of Hib can be detected from serum, CSF, and urine by multiple methods, which are usually more rapid than culture and may be useful in patients with sterile cultures.
- *H influenzae* meningitis was once the leading cause of acquired mental retardation in the United States, but this has now been almost completely eliminated due to the vaccine.

Staphylococcal Meningitis

- Caused by gram-positive cocci that tend to grow in clusters, like grapes (see Figure 10.2).
- Leading cause of bacterial meningitis in patients with CSF shunts or following neurosurgical procedures or neurological trauma.

Listeria Meningitis

- Caused by gram-positive rods, but CSF Gram stain and culture are frequently negative.
- *Listeria* meningitis is often associated with a brain stem encephalitis, so patients will frequently have cranial nerve palsies.
- Unlike other bacterial meningitides, the CSF pleocytosis is usually lymphocytic in nature, and CSF glucose is often normal.
- Associated with improper handling of food and consumption of unpasteurized milk and raw vegetables.

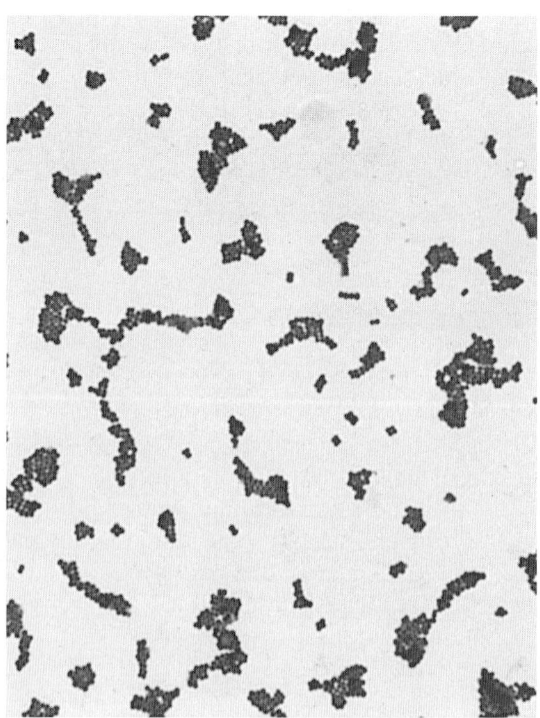

FIGURE 10.2. Gram stain of *Staphylococcus aureus* showing gram-positive cocci in clusters. (Reproduced, with permission, from Brooks GF, Carroll KC, Butel, JS, Morse SA. *Jawetz, Melnick, & Adelberg's Medical Microbiology*, 24th ed. New York: McGraw-Hill, 2007: Figure 14-1.)

Tuberculous Meningitis

- Caused by the acid-fast bacillus (AFB) *Mycobacterium tuberculosis* (see Figure 10.3).
- Especially in developing countries, this is a very common cause of meningitis and other neurological complications, including cerebral tuberculomas, spinal arachnoiditis, radiculomyelopathy, and transverse myelitis.
- Basilar meningitis with cranial neuropathies.
- TB is often seen in association with HIV, and manifestations may be worse in patients with HIV, but TB is common even in patients without HIV. TB is also often associated with malnourishment, alcoholism, and crowded living conditions such as jails and homeless shelters.
- Often proceded by weeks of general malaise and other nonspecific constitutional symptoms. Chest x-ray may show evidence of pulmonary TB, and diagnosis may be made by sputum AFB smear.
- CSF pleocytosis is often lymphocytic, protein is elevated, and glucose is extremely low.
- CSF AFB smear and culture are frequently negative, or may take weeks to grow.
- Caseating granulomas on pathology.
- Optimal treatment regimen is undefined and empirical but usually includes some combination of isoniazid, rifampin, pyrazinamide, ethambutol, and streptomycin.
- Prognosis depends on the stage at which treatment is initiated: Good if started early, poor if started late.

TB
acid fast bacillus
CSF: lympho
↓↓ gluc

TREATMENT

- When bacterial meningitis is suspected, antibiotic treatment must be initiated emergently, even without identification of the causative organism.
- Treatment is usually directed primarily against S *pneumoniae* and N *meningitidis*, the most common causes of community-acquired meningitis.

Meningitis Empiric Tx
→ s. pneum
n. meningitides

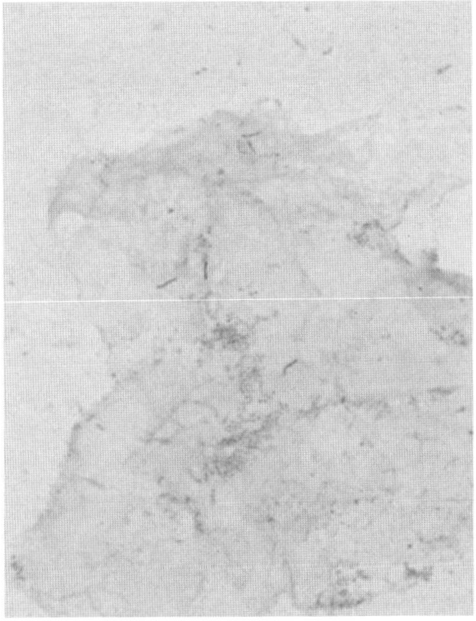

FIGURE 10.3. Acid-fast bacillus smear showing *M tuberculosis*. (Also see Color Plate.) (Courtesy of the CDC, Atlanta. Reproduced, with permission, from Kasper DL, Braunwald E, Fauci AS, et al. *Harrison's Principles of Internal Medicine,* 16th ed. New York: McGraw-Hill, 2005: 954.)

- Doses (higher than for other indications):
  - Vancomycin 15 mg/kg IV q6h (up to 2 g/day), plus
  - *Either* cefotaxime 50 mg/kg IV q4–6h (maximum 2 g IV q4h) *or*
  - Ceftriaxone 50–100 mg/kg IV q12h (maximum 2 g IV q12h).
- Dexamethasone 0.15 mg/kg q6h given 15–20 minutes prior to antibiotics for the first 4 days of therapy may also be beneficial for initial treatment of community-acquired bacterial meningitis, though this recommendation is still controversial.
- For coverage of *Listeria:* Ampicillin 2 g IV q4h is often added in patients over 50 or in the immunosuppressed.
- Narrow antibiotic coverage when speciation and sensitivities are available.
- Total duration of therapy is 10–14 days.
- Current intensive care techniques offer great benefit for patients with bacterial meningitis.

Complications

- Early diagnosis and initiation of appropriate antibiotic therapy dramatically reduces mortality and morbidity.
- Acute complications include: Subdural effusion, empyema, ischemic or hemorrhagic stroke, cerebritis, ventriculitis, abscess, hydrocephalus, seizures.
- Permanent neurological sequelae include: behavioral and developmental difficulties, mental retardation, hearing loss, seizures, motor deficits, ataxia.

Prognosis

Overall, 20–25% fatality rate, but depends greatly on how quickly antibiotics are started.

ASEPTIC MENINGITIS

In this condition, the patient has typical signs and symptoms of meningitis and CSF exam reveals a pleocytosis, but no organism can be cultured from the CSF.

Causes

- Viral infection most common, but can occur with other neuroinflammatory conditions (central nervous system [CNS] or metastatic malignancy, sarcoidosis, Sjögren, Behçet, various vasculitides).
- Drug-reactions also common (nonsteroidal anti-inflammatory drugs [NSAIDs], intravenous immune globulin [IVIG], antibiotics, carbamezepine).
- Nonviral infections, including partially treated bacterial meningitis, brucellosis, *Listeria*, *Mycoplasma*, syphilis, borreliosis (Lyme), leptospirosis, *Rickettsia*, parasites, fungi, and TB.

Diagnosis

- In the majority of cases, no specific organism is ever identified.
- Common etiologic organisms include enteroviruses, coxsackieviruses, echoviruses, and arboviruses. Enteroviruses and herpesviruses can be tested for by polymerase chain reaction (PCR) techniques.
- Most noninfectious neuroinflammatory conditions that can cause meningitis will be associated with other systemic or neurological manifestations, which will serve as a clue to the need for assessing these conditions.
- The nonviral infectious causes can usually be cultured if proper condi-

tions and enough time are allowed. History will usually provide clues to risk factors for these relatively rare infections.

TREATMENT

- Viral meningitis is usually a self-limited infection and requires only supportive care and symptomatic treatment of pain.
- Unlike HSV-1 encephalitis, HSV-2 meningitis is a benign condition, but treatment with acyclovir or valacyclovir may ↓ risk of recurrence.
- If a noninfectious neuroinflammatory condition is diagnosed, it should be treated with appropriate immunosuppression, while nonviral infectious conditions can often be treated with appropriate antimicrobials.

PROGNOSIS

Long-term complications are rare with most viral meningitides. With nonviral and/or noninfectious etiologies, the overall prognosis is dependent on the underlying condition.

FUNGAL MENINGITIS

- Can present with an acute, fulminant course or with a chronic course.
- Most patients will be immunocompromised, usually by HIV infection, malignancy, posttransplant immunosuppression, diabetes, or steroid use.

DIFFERENTIAL DIAGNOSIS

- *Cryptococcus:* See section on neurological complications of HIV.
- *Coccidioides:* Found in southwestern United States, Mexico, Central and South America; exposure to soil dust (construction, farmers); CSF pleocytosis will often include an eosinophilia.
- *Histoplasma:* Found in Mississippi and Ohio river valleys; exposure to bat and bird droppings (exploring caves, cleaning chicken coops).
- *Blastomyces:* Found in same areas as *Histoplasma* but also in upper Midwest and Great Lakes regions.
- *Candida:* Seen in premature neonates possibly related to vaginal yeast infection of mother.

DIAGNOSIS

Depends on the particular fungus.

- Most will grow on the media typically used in clinical microbiology laboratories, although sometimes large volumes and/or multiple specimens are required.
- Many can also be observed with India ink staining of the CSF.
- Antigen and/or antibody testing can be used for some. Histoplasma antigen is usually present in the urine.

TREATMENT

- Depends on the sensitivities of the particular infecting organism: Amphotericin B, fluconazole, itraconazole, voriconazole, caspofungin.
- Empiric antifungal therapy (usually with amphotericin B) is sometimes reasonable in high-risk patients who are severely ill with meningitis, but without an identified bacterial organism.

PROGNOSIS

- Prior to the development of amphotericin B, most fungal infections of the nervous system were fatal, although sometimes after a chronic course.

- With proper treatment, mortality can be reduced to ≤ 30% for most of these organisms.

Cerebral Abscess

Symptoms

- The classic triad of brain abscess is fever, headache, and focal neurological symptoms, but only a minority of patients actually has all 3 of these.
- Brain abscess usually presents as an acute to subacute mass lesion.
- Symptoms of elevated ICP include headache, nausea, and vomiting, which may worsen with Valsalva maneuver or when the patient lies down.
- Seizures occur and are often generalized; they should have a focal onset, but this may not be easily apparent by history or observation.
- Historical risk factors for cerebral abscess will usually provide a clue to the diagnosis for the astute clinician.

Exam

- Fever is helpful but is often not present or is attributed to other causes.
- Focal neurological signs are also often absent or may be extremely subtle.
- Papilledema is frequently absent because the abscess evolves too rapidly for this sign to appear.

Differential Diagnosis

- *Staphylococcus aureus:* Usually associated with a penetrating head wound or neurosurgical procedure; may also be seen in association with bacterial endocarditis.
- *Streptococcus:* Often arises from sinusitis or dental infections.
- Anaerobes: Include *Bacteroides, Actinomyces, Clostridium.*
- Gram-negative rods: Include *Haemophilus, Pseudomonas, Escherichia coli, Enterobacter*; often seen in neonates and the immunocompromised and with an associated meningitis.
- Other:
  - *Aspergillus, Mucor:* Usually due to direct extension from the sinuses in a patient with immunocompromise or diabetes and is fulminant and fatal.
  - *Nocardia:* A gram-positive, weakly AFB-positive, branching rod often seen in the immunocompromised but can be in the immunocompetent.
  - About 20–30% of cerebral abscesses are due to multiple organisms, in which case the abscess is usually associated with sinusitis or otitis.

Diagnosis

- Brain magnetic resonance imaging (MRI) with contrast is the test of choice: Demonstrates ring-enhancing lesion (see Figure 10.4); head CT with contrast can be used if MRI is not available, but is not as sensitive.
- CSF exam is usually unhelpful, and LP may cause brain herniation and death; CSF exam is usually normal or may show a nonspecific mild pleocytosis, and CSF cultures are rarely positive.
- Peripheral WBC may be normal or elevated.
- Blood cultures are rarely positive.

Treatment

- Broad antibiotic coverage should be initiated, usually with a third-generation cephalosporin and metronidazole. In the setting of a neurosurgical

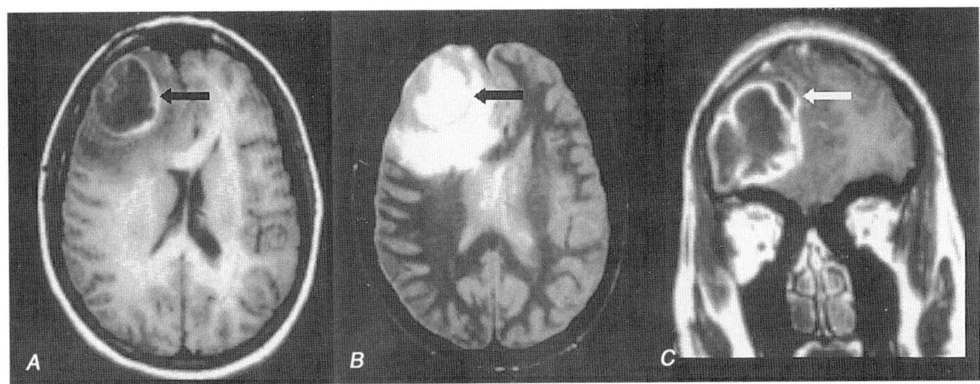

FIGURE 10.4. Cerebral abscess. Note the surrounding edema on T1 (A) and T2 (B) imaging and the prominent enhancement after gadolinium administration (C). (Courtesy of Joseph Lurito, MD. Reproduced, with permission, from Kasper DL, Braunwald E, Fauci AS, et al. *Harrison's Principles of Internal Medicine,* 16th ed. New York: McGraw-Hill, 2005: 2486.)

procedure or head trauma, vancomycin should be used to cover *Staphylococcus.* Coverage can be narrowed when speciation and sensitivities are available. Total duration of therapy is 4–8 weeks, depending on clinical course and follow-up imaging.

- Surgical aspiration or excision is often required.
- Supportive care, including control of surrounding edema and elevated ICP and seizures, is essential.

Complications

- Early diagnosis and initiation of appropriate antibiotic therapy dramatically reduces mortality and morbidity.
- Acute complications include intraventricular rupture, which substantially worsens prognosis, hydrocephalus, seizures.

Prognosis

Overall, 5–10% fatality rate, but long-term complications frequently include behavioral and learning problems, seizures, hydrocephalus, and residual focal neurological deficits.

Spinal Epidural Abscess

Usually seen in patients with diabetes, back trauma (even minor trauma), IV drug abuse, immunocompromise (including pregnancy), and following back surgery.

Symptoms

- Spinal epidural abscesses usually present acutely or subacutely and represent a neurological emergency.
- The initial symptom is usually a localized, severe pain on the back over the site of the abscess. This may be followed by radicular pain and then by myelopathic symptoms as the abscess compresses the spinal cord.
- Myelopathic symptoms include incoordination due to loss of position sense, gait ataxia, stiffness, and spasms in the legs due to impairment of the cortical spinal tract, numbness below a spinal level, and loss of bowel and bladder control.

Exam

- Fever is helpful but is often not present or is attributed to other causes.
- The patient will usually have focal pain to percussion over the spine.
- Myelopathic signs include loss of position and vibration sense, upper motor neuron signs, and a spinal sensory level.

Differential Diagnosis

- *Staphylococcus aureus:* The most common etiological agent.
- *Staphylococcus epidermidis:* Associated with neurosurgical procedures.
- *Streptococcus.*
- Anaerobes: Especially *Bacteroides.*
- Gram-negative rods: Especially *Pseudomonas* and *E coli.*
- Tuberculosis: Can cause chronic epidural abscess and is associated with HIV infection and injection drug use.
- Rare causes: *Aspergillus, Nocardia, Echinococcus, Brucella.*
- About 10% are due to multiple organisms.
- Intracranial epidural abscesses are rare and usually associated with sinusitis.

Diagnosis

- Spine MRI with contrast is the test of choice; CT myelography can be used if MRI is not available, but is not as sensitive and risks introducing the organism into the subarachnoid space and causing meningitis.
- CSF exam is usually unhelpful; it is usually normal or may show a nonspecific mild pleocytosis, and CSF cultures are rarely positive.
- Peripheral WBC may be normal or elevated.
- Blood cultures are positive about half the time.

Treatment

- Early diagnosis and treatment significantly reduces mortality and morbidity.
- Almost always requires urgent open surgery for debridement; sometimes CT-guided aspiration can be used.
- Broad antibiotic coverage should be initiated, usually with a third-generation cephalosporin and vancomycin.
  - If gram-negative organisms are suspected, use gentamicin; the epidural space lies outside the blood-brain barrier.
  - Metronidazole if anaerobes are suspected.
- Coverage can be narrowed when speciation and sensitivities are available.
- Total duration of therapy is 4–8 weeks, depending on clinical course and follow-up imaging.

Prognosis

Overall, 5–15% fatality rate; residual deficits depend on degree and duration of acute neurological deficit, degree of cord compression, and length of abscess.

Subdural Empyema

Symptoms

- Subdural empyemas usually present acutely, with progressive neurological decline over hours to days.

- Initial symptoms usually include focal or generalized head pain, which may worsen with Valsalva maneuver or lying down.
- As the empyema progresses, there may be generalized change in mental status, followed by focal neurological deficits often attributable to an entire cerebral hemisphere or posterior fossa.
- Many patients will have seizures.

EXAM

- Fever is present in the majority of cases. Focal neurological signs include hemiplegia and aphasia.
- Papilledema is frequently absent because the empyema evolves too rapidly for this sign to appear.

DIFFERENTIAL DIAGNOSIS

The organisms associated with a subdural empyema are similar to those associated with a cerebral abscess.

DIAGNOSIS

- Brain MRI with contrast is the test of choice: Demonstrates subdural fluid collection, often with associated mass effect and midline shift.
- Head CT with contrast can be used if MRI is not available; it is better at detecting injury to adjacent bone, but not as sensitive for detecting the empyema.
- Films should be carefully evaluated for presence of associated cerebral abscess, osteomyelitis, sinusitis, and/or otitis.
- CSF exam is usually unhelpful and lumbar puncture may cause brain herniation and death; CSF exam is usually normal or may show a nonspecific mild pleocytosis, and CSF cultures are rarely positive.

COMPLICATIONS

- Early diagnosis and initiation of appropriate antibiotic therapy dramatically reduces mortality and morbidity.
- Acute complications include meningitis, brain abscess, and septic intracranial venous thrombosis.

TREATMENT

- Immediate surgical drainage is almost always indicated.
- Antibiotic treatment and supportive care is the same as for cerebral abscess.

PROGNOSIS

Overall, 10–25% fatality rate, with up to 30% of survivors having severe residual neurological deficits.

Neurological Sequelae of Infectious Endocarditis

- Infection of the heart valves is frequently caused by *Staphylococcus* or *Streptococcus* species, with *S aureus* often being the cause in those who have neurological complications.
- Injection drug users and individuals with prosthetic heart valves are at ↑ risk.

SYMPTOMS/EXAM

- Fevers, chills.
- May have signs and symptoms of bacteremia or sepsis.
- A heart murmur can usually be detected. The organism embolizes from the heart valve to the periphery and also into the brain.
- In the hands and feet: Osler nodes, Janeway lesions (Figure 10.5), and splinter hemorrhages can be observed.
- In the eye: Roth spots (Figure 10.6) can be seen.
- In the brain: Mycotic aneurysms form, → strokes and cerebral abscesses; neurological presentation is usually with a sudden-onset focal neurological deficit consistent with a septic infarction or stroke.
- Ruptured mycotic aneurysms present with severe headache and declining level of consciousness, as with a subarachnoid hemorrhage; such rupture is rare, but it is usually fatal.
- Patients may also present with signs and symptoms of meningitis due to hematogenous seeding of the meninges in these bacteremic patients.

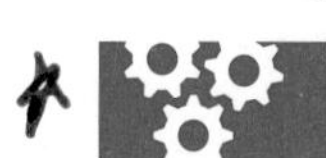

MNEMONIC

High-Tech Lab Re ults Point At Endocarditis

Hematuria
Thrombocytopen
Leukocytosis or le copenia
Red blood cell ca
Proteinuria
Anemia
Elevated ESR

DIAGNOSIS

- Blood cultures are positive in 85–95% of cases. If endocarditis is suspected, take 3 sets of blood cultures 1 hour apart, before antibiotics.
- Echocardiography, especially transesophageal echocardiogram (TEE), has high sensitivity and specificity for detecting the vegetation on the valve.
- Brain imaging and CSF analysis can be used to help determine the nature of neurological involvement.
- Conventional angiography can be used to define the presence of mycotic aneurysms.

TREATMENT

- Proper choice of antibiotics depends on the isolated organism.
- Rapid treatment minimizes the risk of neurological sequalae.
- Broad-spectrum treatment is often started, followed by appropriate narrowing of coverage; total duration of antibiotic treatment is usually 4–6 weeks.
- Surgical treatment of the infected valve is sometimes required, especially if the patient develops congestive heart failure.
- Anticoagulation must **not** be used in patients with septic cardiac emboli, because of high risk of hemorrhage in the brain.
- Coiling, clipping, or stenting is sometimes used for treatment of mycotic aneurysms.

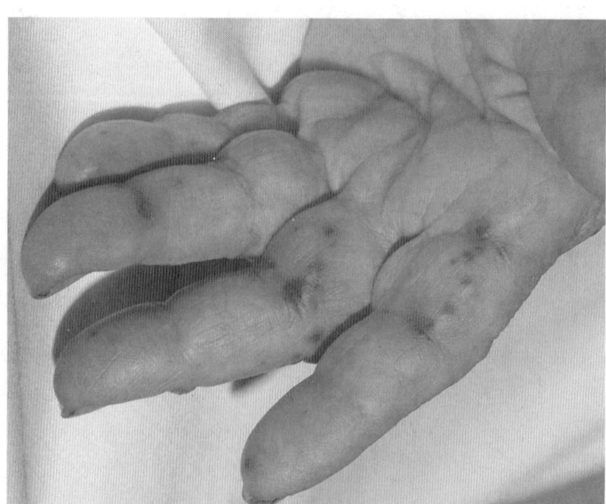

FIGURE 10.5. Janeway lesions. (Also see Color Plate.) (Reproduced, with permission, from Wolff K, Johnson RA. *Fitzpatrick's Color Atlas and Synopsis of Clinical Dermatology*, 5th ed. New York: McGraw-Hill, 2005: 636.)

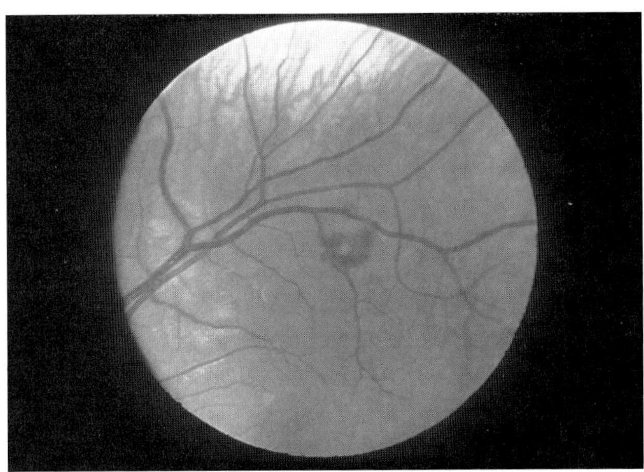

FIGURE 10.6. Roth spot. (Also see Color Plate.) (Reproduced, with permission, from Knoop KJ, Stack LB, Storrow AB. *Atlas of Emergency Medicine*, 2nd ed. New York: McGraw-Hill, 2002: 80. Photographer: William E. Cappaert, MD.)

Prognosis

Now that infected heart valves can be repaired or replaced, neurological sequelae are a leading cause of mortality in patients with infectious endocarditis.

HIV-Associated Conditions

A 38-year-old, HIV-positive man is evaluated because of increasing difficulty with ambulation over the past 3 months. He reports slowly worsening stiffness in his lower extremities. He also has noticed episodes of urinary frequency and urgency over the past 2 months. On examination, the patient displays a mild paraparesis of his lower extremities with spasticity and brisk reflexes in the left patella and ankle, as well as bilateral upgoing toes. Sensory examination shows moderate loss of proprioception in the legs, but no sensory level. A CSF analysis demonstrates a protein of 63 mg/dL, white cells 10/mm^3, 100% lymphocytes, and a glucose of 65. CSF viral and bacterial studies are negative. Vitamin B_{12} level is normal, as is an MRI of the cervical, thoracic, and lumbar spine with and without gadolinium contrast.

The most likely diagnosis is AIDS-associated vacuolar myelopathy. The patient described in this vignette has insidiously progressive lumbar myelopathy because of the spastic paraparesis, bladder dysfunction, and corticospinal as well as posterior column dysfunction without sensory level and a normal MRI. The differential diagnosis includes CMV myelopathy, which presents as an acute radiculomyelitis with pain and flaccid paraplegia with urinary incontinence. The patient in this case does not have signs of radicular pain and is actually slow in the progression of the disease. HIV myelitis can appear acute or subacute. It is a complication of HIV infection but it typically presents with a transverse myelitis–type picture, which results in a sensory level. AIDS associated vacuolar myelopathy is a slowly progressive disease. It occurs in about 30% of all patients with AIDS; however, only a minority present symptoms. These patients present late in the course of the illness; they may report bladder dysfunction or mild paraparesis, and the examination typically demonstrates a spastic asymmetric paraparesis, increased reflexes in the lower extremities, at times with clonus, and no sensory level. The CSF shows a mild pleocytosis with elevated protein.

HIV

ASEPTIC MENINGITIS

- Frequently occurs at initial infection/seroconversion.
- Lymphocytic pleocytosis with 20–300 cells.
- HIV test will usually still be negative.
- May be associated with cranial neuropathies.

ACUTE/CHRONIC INFLAMMATORY DEMYELINATING POLYNEUROPATHY (CIDP)

- A syndrome that is clinically indistinguishable from idiopathic Guillain-Barré syndrome (GBS), and sometimes evolving into CIDP, can occur, usually at initial infection/seroconversion.
- Any patient with GBS should be tested for HIV at presentation and, if negative, tested again 3 months later; treatment with IVIG or plamapheresis is effective.

DISTAL PAINFUL SENSORIMOTOR POLYNEUROPATHY

A length-dependent, small-fiber neuropathy caused by HIV itself is clinically indistinguishable from a toxic neuropathy caused by the D-drug (ddI, ddC, d4T, and 3TC). D-drugs believed to cause neuropathy due to mitochondrial toxicity.

Symptoms

Predominantly marked by distal symmetric burning pain of feet and hands; numbness and paresthesias in the same pattern.

Exam

- Stocking-glove sensory loss.
- Achilles reflex usually ↓.

Differential Diagnosis

Diabetic small-fiber peripheral neuropathy.

Diagnosis

- Clinical in patient with known HIV.
- Electromyogram (EMG)/nerve conduction velocity (NCV) may show axonal neuropathy, but is often normal because evaluates only large nerve fibers.
- Skin biopsy to assess small nerve fibers will confirm diagnosis.

Treatment

- Cessation of D-drugs will usually ameliorate symptoms.
- Symptomatic therapies include antiepileptic drugs, tricyclic antidepressants, and serotonin and norepinephrine reuptake inhibitors (SNRIs).

MULTIPLE MONONEUROPATHIES

Symptoms/Exam

- The most common mononeuropathy is facial nerve palsy.
- Other cranial neuropathies occur.
- Mononeuritis multiplex occurs as simultaneous or sequential involvement

of multiple peripheral nerves; → symptoms in variable dermatomal distributions.

DIFFERENTIAL DIAGNOSIS

Herpes zoster, neurosyphilis, hepatitis C vasculitis, cryoglobulinemia, lymphoma, cytomegalovirus infection, polyarteritis nodosa, invasion of the nerves by lymphoma or Kaposi sarcoma.

DIAGNOSIS

Sural nerve biopsy often necessary to evaluate for vasculitis, cytomegalovirus (CMV), or lymphoma.

MYOPATHIES

- Myositis at HIV seroconversion or later in the disease course; clinically similar to polymyositis in HIV-negative patients.
- A form of nemaline rod myopathy, with slowly progressive weakness and muscle wasting.
- Toxic myopathy caused by zidovudine (AZT), resolves when AZT is discontinued.
- **Diagnosis:** Muscle biopsy.

VACUOLAR MYELOPATHY

- CD4 counts < 200.
- **Symptoms:**
  - Progressive spastic paraparesis, weakness.
  - May have dorsal column dysfunction or other sensory loss, usually more prominent in the legs than arms.
  - Bowel and bladder involvement.

ENCEPHALOPATHY AND AIDS DEMENTIA COMPLEX

- Most common neurological syndrome in HIV infection: Prevalence 15–30%; annual incidence approximately 5%.
- Highly active antiretroviral therapy (HAART) has significantly ↓ incidence of severe forms; mild forms persist, and prevalence has risen as more patients live longer with HIV.
- This is the most common form of dementia worldwide in people under age 40, striking in prime adult working years, having a large socioeconomic impact.
- Neuroprotective strategies beyond HAART are badly needed, but all clinical trials of such agents so far have failed.

KEY FACT

Mild forms of HIV neurocognitive impairment can have large impact on a patient's quality of life, but may not be easily recognized unless the physician looks carefully.

SYMPTOMS/EXAM

- HIV dementia is termed *subcortical*, marked by a classic triad of cognitive, motor, and behavioral manifestations.
- Psychomotor slowing is hallmark of the cognitive deficits, although patients also have memory deficits.
- Motor manifestations include parkinsonism and other extrapyramidal signs and symptoms.
- Behavioral symptoms include apathy and social withdrawal.
- Degree of dementia can vary from asymptomatic with subtle signs on formal neurocognitive testing to severe dementia with inability to sustain a

complex conversation, marked slowing, and inability to walk unassisted, and eventually mutism, paraplegia, incontinence, and death.

Differential Diagnosis

- Early stages of HIV dementia often misdiagnosed as depression, anxiety, effects of substance abuse, B_{12} deficiency.
- In later stages, differential includes CNS opportunistic infections, such as toxoplasmosis, neurosyphilis, cryptococcal, or tuberculous meningitis; cytomegalovirus encephalitis; CNS lymphoma; and progressive multifocal leukoencephalopathy (PML).

Diagnosis

- CSF examination: May show mild lymphocytic pleocytosis.
- Brain MRI will typically show patchy periventricular T2 bright changes (see Figure 10.7), which pathologically represents disruption of blood-brain barrier.
- Neuropsychological testing can demonstrate a specific pattern of neurocognitive deficit typical of HIV dementia as opposed to other dementias and can also help quantify the severity.

Treatment

HAART should be initiated. If already in place, consideration should be given to changing regimen to one with greater CNS penetration.

Prognosis

Without treatment, dementia is rapidly progressive and death usually occurs in 6 months. With treatment, mild chronic dementia persists.

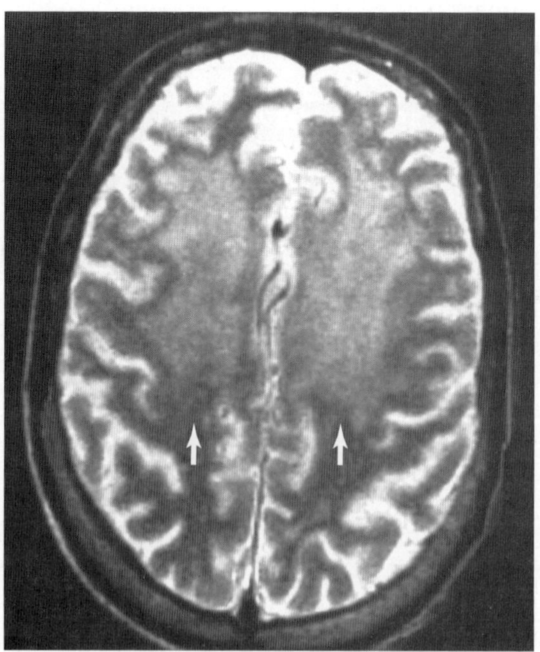

FIGURE 10.7. Brain MRI of a patient with HIV dementia showing bilateral T2 bright white matter changes. (Reproduced, with permission, from Aminoff MJ, Greenberg DA, Simon RP. *Clinical Neurology*, 6th ed. New York: McGraw-Hill, 2005: 58.)

HIV-Associated Opportunistic Infections

A 31-year-old right-handed man with a history of HIV infection developed headaches and right-sided weakness progressing over the course of 3 weeks. Physical examination demonstrates some mild right hemiparesis with increased reflexes, a right Babinski, and a fever of 102°F. The MRI of the brain with contrast shows a single ring-enhancing lesion in the left basal ganglia with some surrounding vasogenic edema. A positron emission tomography (PET) scan is also performed, which demonstrates hypoactivity corresponding to the same area. His CD4 lymphocyte count is 15/μL, and serum testing for *Toxoplasmoa gondii* serology is positive. What is the appropriate treatment for this patient?

Start antitoxoplasmosis therapy with no steroids. In this vignette, the differential diagnosis of a bone/brain lesion in an HIV-positive patient with low CD4 count with positive toxoplasmosis serology includes toxoplasmosis encephalitis and primary central nervous system lymphoma. Although the patient's head MRI does not present classic multiple space-occupying, enhancing lesions of toxoplasmosis, the combination of positive serology, a CD4 count < 200/μL, and diminished activity on PET scanning is more suggestive of toxoplasmosis encephalitis than lymphoma. The appropriate treatment is instituting an empiric antibiotic therapy for toxoplasmosis and follow-up imaging. If the patient shows clinical and radiological response to the antibiotic therapy, he can be presumed to have CNS toxoplasmosis. The patient should be maintained on suppressive antibiotics for the remainder of his life after finishing the initial treatment. If the patient does not show improvement on antibiotics after 2 weeks, he should have a stereotactic biopsy. The empiric use of corticosteroids is not recommended for toxoplasmosis. The addition of corticosteroids has not been shown to improve neurological outcome in these patients and may in fact diminish the diagnostic validity of biopsy in the case of CNS lymphoma.

CNS CRYPTOCOCCOSIS

- Caused by the fungus *Cryptococcus neoformans*, an encapsulated yeast.
- In AIDS patients, usually occurs with CD4 counts < 100. Can also be seen in patients with cancer, especially leukemia and lymphoma, and with immunosuppression from other causes.

KEY FACT

Immunocompromised patients with meningitis may lack the typical meningitic signs and symptoms seen in immunocompetent patients with meningitis.

Symptoms/Exam

- Usually manifests as meningitis, with headache, mental status changes, and cranial nerve palsies, but usually also involves brain parenchyma, so there may be other focal neurological signs and symptoms.
- Obvious meningeal signs may be lacking because of a lack of inflammatory response in the immunosuppressed.

Differential Diagnosis

TB meningitis, bacterial meningitis, viral encephalitis, meningitis caused by other fungi, other CNS opportunisitic infections.

KEY FACT

CSF cryptococcal antigen titers are useful for monitoring treatment response, and should ↓ with successful treatment. Serum titers are **not** useful.

KEY FACT

Serial LPs can be lifesaving in patients with cryptococcal meningitis.

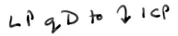

Diagnosis

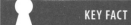

- Cryptococcal antigen in the CSF is sensitive and specific for detecting the organism's polysaccharide capsule.
- India ink staining of CSF may show budding yeast with a thick capsule (see Figure 10.8), but < 50% sensitive.
- CSF often shows a lymphocytic pleocytosis, high protein, low glucose, and elevated opening pressure, but changes may be mild or absent due to the patient's immunosuppression.
- Brain imaging may show hydrocephalus and parenchymal nodules (cryptococcomas).

Treatment

- Two weeks of amphotericin B plus flucytosine, followed by 8 weeks of fluconazole 400 mg/day, followed by fluconzole 200 mg/day until immune reconstitution.
- In patients with an opening pressure > 25 cm water, daily LPs are recommended to relieve the pressure, as long as brain imaging does not raise concern for impending herniation.
- A temporary lumbar drain may be used instead of daily spinal taps.
- Intraventricular shunting is sometimes used in cases of obstructive hydrocephalus.

Complications

↑ ICP can be severe and fatal.

CNS LYMPHOMA

- Caused by Epstein-Barr virus (EBV) infection of B lymphocytes.
- Occurs with CD4 counts < 100.

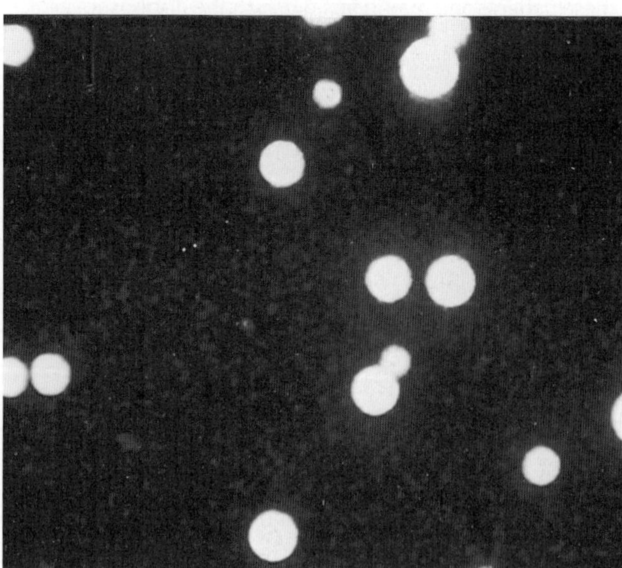

FIGURE 10.8. India ink preparation from a patient with cryptococcal meningitis demonstrating the budding yeast form with prominent capsule. (Also see Color Plate.) (Courtesy of Morse et al. *Atlas of Sexually Transmitted Diseases*. London: Mosby-Wolfe; 1990. Reproduced, with permission, from Knoop KJ, Stack LB, Storrow AB. *Atlas of Emergency Medicine*, 2nd ed. New York: McGraw-Hill, 2002: 688.)

SYMPTOMS/EXAM

- Focal neurological deficits.
- Mental status changes.

DIFFERENTIAL DIAGNOSIS

- The biggest consideration is CNS toxoplasmosis.
- Frequently, patients with a compatible presentation are treated for toxoplasmosis, and if there is no improvement within 2 weeks, strong consideration is given to a lymphoma diagnosis.

DIAGNOSIS

- Brain MRI will typically demonstrate a unifocal ring-enhancing lesion, although it can be multifocal (see Figure 10.9).
- CSF EBV PCR has high sensitivity and specificity for the diagnosis of CNS lymphoma in HIV patients, but not in HIV-negative patients.
- Malignant cells may also be present in CSF.

TREATMENT

Cranial radiotherapy and methotrexate.

PROGNOSIS

Median survival < 6 months.

CNS TOXOPLASMOSIS

- Infection caused by *Toxoplasma gondii*, a small intracellular parasite.
- Occurs with CD4 counts < 100. Congenital forms also occur, usually causing periventricular calcification.

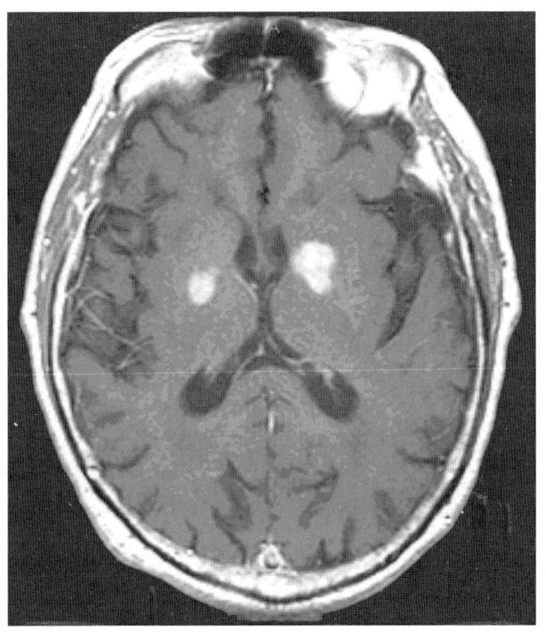

FIGURE 10.9. Brain MRI of a patient with CNS lymphoma demonstrating multifocal gadolinium enhancing lesions. (Reproduced, with permission, from Kantarjian HM, Wolff RA, Koller CA. *MD Anderson Manual of Medical Oncology*. New York: McGraw-Hill, Figure 30-8.)

SYMPTOMS/EXAM

Focal neurological deficits and mental status changes.

DIFFERENTIAL DIAGNOSIS

- The biggest consideration is CNS lymphoma.
- Frequently, patients with a compatible presentation are treated for toxoplasmosis, and if there is no improvement within 2 weeks, strong consideration is given to a lymphoma diagnosis.

DIAGNOSIS

- Brain MRI typically demonstrates multifocal ring-enhancing lesions, although can be unifocal (see Figure 10.10).
- Single photon emission computed tomography (SPECT) and PET imaging and *Toxoplasma* serologies may help differentiate CNS toxoplasmosis from CNS lymphoma.

TREATMENT

Pyrimethamine, sulfadiazine, and folinic acid.

PROGNOSIS

Rapid response to proper treatment.

CYTOMEGALOVIRUS ENCEPHALITIS

- Occurs with CD4 counts < 50.
- **Symptoms:**
  - Rapidly progressive mental status changes.
  - CMV can also cause a myeloradiculitis and a retinopathy.
- **Differential diagnosis:** HIV dementia tends to evolve much more slowly.
- **Diagnosis:** CMV PCR in the CSF is very sensitive and specific.
- **Treatment:** Ganciclovir and/or foscarnet.
- **Prognosis:** Poor.

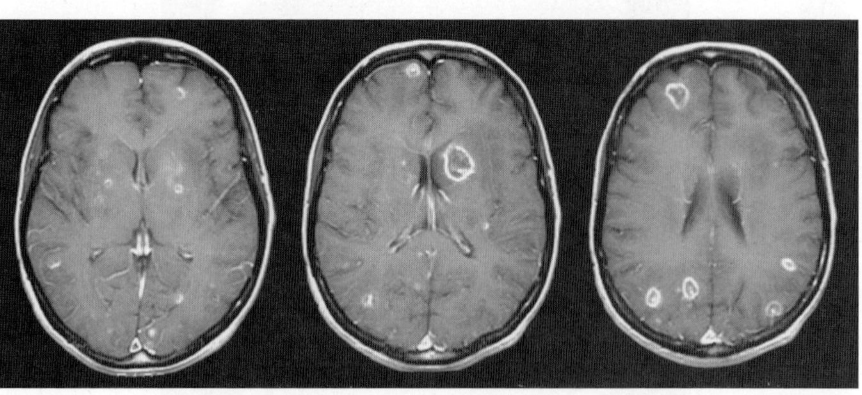

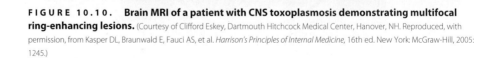

FIGURE 10.10. Brain MRI of a patient with CNS toxoplasmosis demonstrating multifocal ring-enhancing lesions. (Courtesy of Clifford Eskey, Dartmouth Hitchcock Medical Center, Hanover, NH. Reproduced, with permission, from Kasper DL, Braunwald E, Fauci AS, et al. *Harrison's Principles of Internal Medicine,* 16th ed. New York: McGraw-Hill, 2005: 1245.)

PROGRESSIVE MULTIFOCAL LEUKOENCEPHALOPATHY (PML)

- Caused by reactivation of latent JC virus.
- CD4 counts < 200. Can also occur in cancer patients (especially leukemia and lymphoma), and in patients who have been immunosuppressed for organ transplants. Recently associated with immunomodulatory monoclonal antibodies, such as natalizumab and rituximab.

Symptoms

- Highly variable depending on the parts of the brain that are affected.
- Personality change, cognitive decline, hemiparesis or hemisensory deficits, visual field cuts or cortical blindness, aphasias, brain stem, and cerebellar symptoms.

Diagnosis

Brain MRI reveals multifocal, nonenhancing white matter lesions.

Treatment

Reversal of immunosuppression; in AIDS patients this is accomplished by introducing HAART.

Prognosis

Usually fatal and those who survive are left with permanent, severe neurological injury.

IMMUNE RECONSTITUTION INFLAMMATORY SYNDROME (IRIS)

- Occurs when effective HAART is initiated and restored immune system reacts vigorously to the presence of an opportunistic infection, causing inflammatory injury.
- Paradoxical clinical deterioration in the setting of ↑ CD4 count and ↓ HIV viral load.
- Can occur in patients with cryptococcal meningitis or PML, or even in patients without overt opportunistic infection, presumably in response to subclinical opportunistic infection or to HIV itself.
- **Treatment:** Supportive; steroids sometimes used in life-threatening IRIS.
- **Prognosis:** Poor in short term but good if the patient survives acute illness.

Human T-Lymphotropic Virus-1 (HTLV-1)

- Also known as "tropical spastic paraparesis" or HAM/TSP.
- **Symptoms:** Progressive myelopathic signs and symptoms.
- **Incidence:** Endemic to Caribbean and Japan, transmitted by blood or sexually.
- **Diagnosis:** Serology useful in patients from nonendemic areas, but not in patients from endemic areas because they are likely to have asymptomatic HTLV and an alternative explanation for the myelopathy.
- **Treatment:** Only symptomatic and supportive therapies available.
- **Complications:** HTLV-1 infection can also cause T-cell leukemia.

Herpes Simplex Encephalitis

A 48-year-old female presents with an episode of sudden staring, turning her head to the right, smacking her lips, and then a generalized tonic-clonic type of movement where her body goes stiff and then there is a back-and-forth movement of her arms. This episode lasted about 3 minutes. She does not recall anything that happened prior to or during the event and remained confused 20 minutes later. Her friend says that she had not been recently ill, she'd had no recent injuries, but she had been "stressed out." They say that she had been having "zoning out" spells for a few days prior to this event. Past history is remarkable for hypothyroidism. She is currently taking synthroid and has no known drug allergies.

CT scan shows a poorly circumscribed, hypointense, left temporal lobe lesion with small foci of hemorrhage and minimal surrounding edema.

The most likely diagnosis is HSV encephalitis. The subacute onset with a poorly circumscribed, unilateral temporal lobe lesion with some edema is concerning for HSV encephalitis.

Caused by herpes simplex virus type 1, except in neonates where it is associated with maternal genital HSV type 2.

Symptoms

- Presents, as with any encephalopathy or encephalitis, with mental status and behavioral changes.
- Often a prodromal viral-like illness including fever, general malaise, headache, neck stiffness.
- Because organism has predisposition to temporal lobes, patients often have profound memory loss and seizures.
- There may be olfactory and gustatory hallucinations.

Exam

Focal neurological signs including motor signs and cranial neuropathies.

Diagnosis

- CSF examination: Since this infection causes hemorrhagic encephalitis, the presence of nonclearing (atraumatic) red blood cells strongly suggests the diagnosis in the proper clinical setting; predominantly lymphocytic pleocytosis is nonspecific.
- HSV PCR of CSF has high sensitivity and specificity and is thus the diagnostic test of choice.
- Brain MRI will typically show T2 bright changes and edema in temporal, cingulate, and orbitofrontal lobes (see Figure 10.11).
- Electroencephalogram (EEG) may show temporal spikes or periodic lateralized epileptiform discharges (PLEDs).

Treatment

Intravenous acyclovir 10 mg/kg q8h should be started immediately in any patient with a compatible clinical presentation, and continued for 14–21 days if diagnosis confirmed.

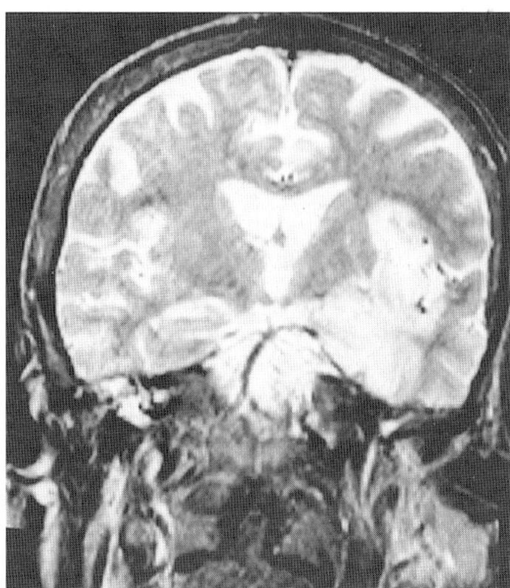
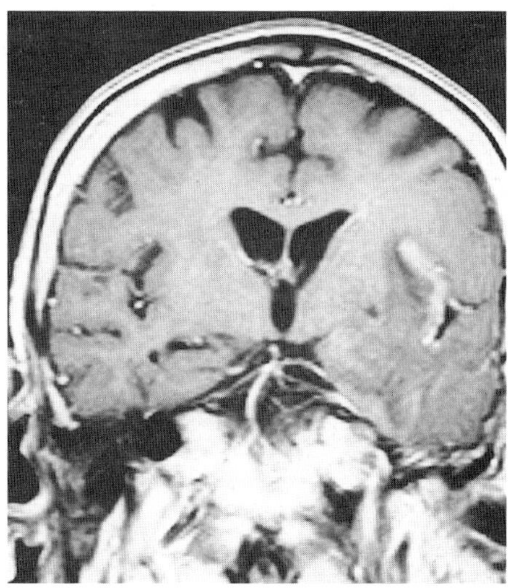

FIGURE 10.11. Brain MRI of a patient with herpes simplex encephalitis demonstrating extensive involvement of the left temporal lobe and insular cortex. (Reproduced, with permission, from Ropper AH, Brown RH. *Adams and Victor's Principles of Neurology*, 8th ed. New York: McGraw-Hill, 2005: 639.)

KEY FACT

Acyclovir must be started in any patient with possible viral encephalitis, and continued until herpes encephalitis is excluded.

Complications

Survivors frequently have severe problems with forming new memories, persistent neurocognitive deficits, and seizures.

Prognosis

Fifty percent severe morbidity or mortality, especially if treatment is delayed.

West Nile Encephalitis

Symptoms/Exam

- Presents, as with any encephalopathy or encephalitis, with mental status and behavioral changes.
- Often a prodromal viral-like illness including fever, general malaise, headache, neck stiffness.
- West Nile can also cause a flaccid paralysis, similar to poliomyelitis.
- West Nile paralysis and West Nile encephalitis may or may not occur together in the same patient.

Diagnosis

- Positive West Nile serology and a compatible clinical presentation.
- CSF examination: Nonspecific lymphocytic pleocytosis.

Treatment

Supportive.

Prognosis

Mortality low, but persistent deficits common.

Subacute Sclerosing Panencephalitis

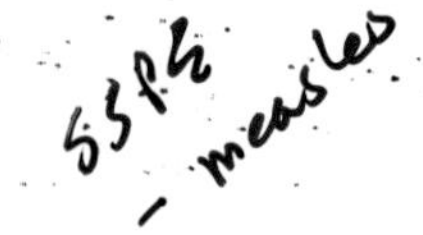

- Rare complication of measles, usually in young children, now even more rare because of measles vaccination.
- Presentation: Gradually worsening cognitive decline, often first manifesting as poor school performance, progressing to behavioral problems, seizures, motor manifestations, coma, death usually 1–3 years after onset.

Other Viral Encephalitides

- No specific organism is isolated for most encephalitides of presumed viral etiology.
- St. Louis encephalitis is relatively common.
- Eastern and Western Equine encephalitis rarely affects humans.
- Powasan encephalitis is very rare.
- The above are all transmitted by mosquitoes, except Powasan, which is transmitted by the tick.
- **Treatment:** Supportive only.

Poliomyelitis

- Infection of lower motor neurons by an enterovirus, transmitted by fecal-oral route.
- Extremely rare in United States because of widespread use of polio vaccine, but historically was common cause of paralysis of 1 or more extremities, and still occurs in underdeveloped countries.
- **Symptoms:**
  - Mild flulike illness; myalgias; aseptic meningitis, which usually resolves with no further problems.
  - Paralytic poliomyelitis: Rapid limb and bulbar weakness, most patients recover completely, but some have residual weakness and atrophy of 1 or more extremities.
- **Diagnosis:** Serological testing, viral isolation from stool; virus is rarely if ever isolated from CSF.
- **Treatment:** Supportive/symptomatic only.
- **Prognosis:** Mortality rate 5–10%.

Rabies

Caused by rhabdovirus.

SYMPTOMS/EXAM

- Transmitted by bite of rabid animal, most commonly a bat, but found in any mammal, including dogs, raccoons, and skunks. The patient may not even realize he or she was bitten, especially if it was by a bat.
- There is prolonged incubation period, usually 20–60 days, from time of bite to onset of rabies symptoms. During this time, virus spreads along peripheral nerves from site of inoculation into central nervous system.

- Prodromal symptoms last a few days and include fever, chills, malaise, fatigue, insomnia, anorexia, headache, anxiety, irritability.
- About one-half develop pain, paresthesias, or pruritus at or close to bite site, which may reflect infection of the dorsal root ganglia.
- Encephalitic (furious) rabies affects about 80%. This is the classic/stereotypical form, in which patients have episodes of hyperexcitability alternating with periods of relative lucidity. They may have aggressive behavior, confusion, hallucinations, and seizures.
- Autonomic dysfunction is common and includes hypersalivation, sweating, and piloerection. Fever may occur.
- About one-half develop hydrophobia; not truly fear of water, but avoidance of swallowing, because they have painful spasms and difficulty swallowing. On attempts to swallow, they experience contractions of the diaphragm and other inspiratory muscles, which last for 5–15 seconds. Subsequently, the sight, sound, or even mention of water (or of any liquids) may trigger the spasms.
- A draft of air on the skin may have the same effect (aerophobia).
- The disease progresses through paralysis, coma, multisystem organ failure, death.
- Paralytic (flaccid) rabies affects about 20%. Flaccid muscle weakness develops early in course of disease, usually beginning in the bitten extremity and spreading to other extremities and facial muscles. Sphincter involvement, pain, and sensory disturbances also occur. Hydrophobia is uncommon, although bulbar and respiratory muscles eventually involved. Patients with paralytic rabies usually survive longer than those with the encephalitic form.

Differential Diagnosis

- Often misdiagnosed as psychiatric or laryngopharyngeal disorder.
- Pseudorabies or rabies hysteria has been reported, usually due to fear of rabies after an animal bite.
- Other viral encephalitides may have similar signs and symptoms, but generally without hydrophobic spasms.
- Rabies has been misdiagnosed as Creutzfeldt-Jakob disease (CJD).
- Tetanus can cause laryngospasm along with spasm and rigidity of diffuse muscles, but usually not associated with encephalopathy.
- Paralytic rabies has been misdiagnosed as Guillain-Barré; bladder dysfunction and fever are more common in rabies.

Diagnosis

- Rabies virus RNA can be detected by PCR from brain, saliva, and CSF.
- Antirabies antibodies are usually not present until 10 days after symptom onset, by which time death may occur.
- Rabies virus can occasionally be cultured from saliva or CSF.
- Rabies antigen may be detected in skin biopsies from site of exposure or from nape of the neck.

Treatment

- After clinical symptoms emerge, supportive only.
- Postexposure prophylaxis (PEP) can prevent onset of clinical rabies and subsequent death. PEP includes both active and passive immunization. Five doses of rabies vaccine are given in the deltoid or anterolateral thigh, with first dose as soon as possible after exposure, and subsequent doses on days 3, 7, 14, and 28 after the first dose.
- Passive immunization with human rabies immunoglobulin is given to provide protection before active immunity develops. It should be given at

same time as first dose of active vaccine, but can be given within 7 days of that dose.
- After local wound care, the wound should be infiltrated with the immunoglobulin and the remainder of the dose given in the gluteal muscle.

KEY FACT

Because rabies is fatal if not treated until after clinical symptoms start, postexposure prophylaxis should be initiated in any patient with an animal bite and continued until rabies is definitively excluded.

Prognosis

Uniformally fatal after symptom onset.

Varicella-Zoster

- Also known as "shingles."
- **Symptoms:**
  - Vesicular rash in a dermatomal pattern, usually on one side of body along the course of 1 or more cutaneous nerves (Figure 10.12).
  - Frequently painful or pruritic, rash may follow onset of pain by a few days.
  - Spontaneous reactivation of latent varicella-zoster virus (VZV), which, after an initial infection usually as a child (chickenpox), lies dormant in dorsal root ganglia of spinal nerves or fifth cranial nerve.
- **Incidence:** ↑ with age and immunosuppression.
- **Diagnosis:** Usually clinical, but can do Tzanck prep from a vesicle, which will show multinucleated giant cells and can be cultured or stained for virus.
- **Complications:** Ophthalmic zoster can result in blindness.
- **Treatment:**
  - Acyclovir, valacyclovir, or famciclovir, started as soon as possible and no later than 3 days after onset of rash, shortens duration of illness and ↓ incidence of postherpetic neuralgia. Steroids sometimes used, but their benefit is unclear.
  - Rarely, VZV can involve the CNS, usually as encephalitis or myelitis. Diagnosis can be made by PCR of CSF.

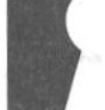

KEY FACT

Severe dermatomal pain, without rash, often heralds onset of shingles.

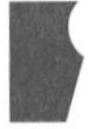

KEY FACT

Lesions on the tip of the nose indicate involvement of the ophthalmic division of the trigeminal nerve, and such patients should have an urgent ophthalmologic consult.

RAMSAY HUNT SYNDROME

VZV rash in auditory canal with ipsilateral lower facial nerve palsy, usually with loss of taste on anterior two-thirds of ipsilateral tongue, often with tinnitus and vertigo. Deafness may occur.

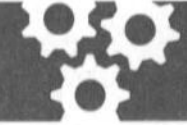

MNEMONIC

Ramsay **H**unt: Etiology, **R**eactivated **H**erpes zoster; complication, **R**educed **H**earing.

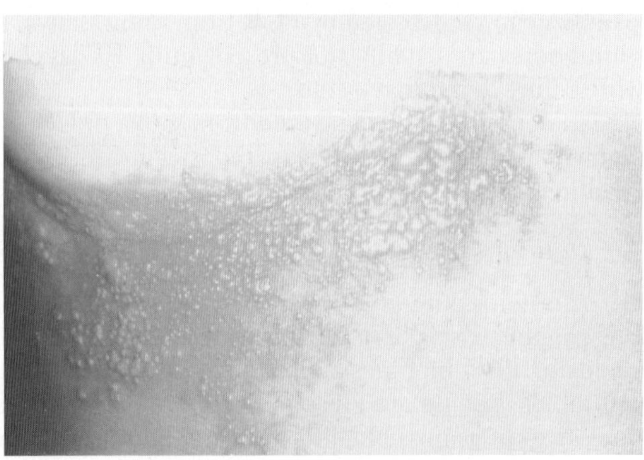

FIGURE 10.12. Dermatomal herpes zoster rash. (Reproduced with permission from Twersky JI, Schmader K. Chapter 129. Herpes Zoster. In: Halter JB, Ouslander JG, Tinetti ME, Studenski S, High KP, Asthana S. eds. *Hazzard's Geriatric Medicine and Gerontology*, 6e. New York, NY: McGraw-Hill; 2009. Figure 129-2.)

Complications of Ramsay Hunt syndrome may include:

- Permanent hearing loss and facial weakness: For most patients, the hearing loss and facial paralysis associated with Ramsay Hunt syndrome is temporary. However, it can become permanent for some people.
- Eye damage: The facial weakness caused by Ramsay Hunt syndrome may make it difficult for eyelid closure. Incomplete eyelid closure can lead to corneal injury.

POSTHERPETIC NEURALGIA

- Persistent neuropathic pain in a dermatome previously affected by shingles.
- Symptomatic treatments with antiepileptic drugs, tricyclic antidepressants, or SNRIs may be useful, but condition is often severely painful and treatment resistant.

Leprosy

- Infection of peripheral nerves by *Mycobacterium leprae.*
- Transmitted person-to-person, usually by prolonged direct contact.
- **Symptoms:** Paroxysmal neuralgic pain initially; numbness later.
- **Diagnosis:**
  - Skin or nerve biopsy usually reveals presence of AFB; serological and PCR-based tests are available.
  - EMG/NCV reveals mixed axonal-demyelinating neuropathy.
- **Treatment:** Triple therapy with dapsone, rifampin, and clofazimine for up to 2 years.

MNEMONIC

LEP*rosy*

Loss of sensation of affected skin/**L**oss of function (paralysis)
Enlargement of affected superficial nerves (tender too)
Positive identification of *M leprae* under microscope

Neuro-Lyme Disease

- *Borrelia burgdorferi* transmitted by bite of *Ixodes* tick, also known as deer tick. Ticks are tiny, ranging in size from the period at the end of this sentence to a sesame seed, depending on phase of life cycle.
- Dog ticks are much larger, do not transmit Lyme disease, but are often reported by patients who are concerned they have Lyme disease; the astute doctor should not take this as evidence of Lyme disease.
- Lyme disease is markedly overdiagnosed in this country, especially in nonendemic areas. *Ixodes* ticks and *Borrelia burgdorferi* are found in the Northeast, mid-Atlantic, and upper Midwest, and not in the Southwest.
- Other *Borrelia* species can cause Lyme disease in Europe and Asia.
- Transmission usually occurs in late spring or summer.

Symptoms/Exam

- Lyme disease causes wide variety of symptoms. Erythema migrans rash occurs at time of initial infection, looks like a bull's eye, with a pale center, surrounded by a red ring (see Figure 10.13). Rash expands in diameter over several days before resolving. After organism has disseminated, patients sometimes develop numerous small bull's-eye rashes.
- Migratory myalgias, arthralgias, fatigue, and general malaise common.
- Most common neurological involvement is facial palsy, sometimes bilaterally. Other cranial nerve palsies may also be seen.
- Headache and aseptic meningitis are also common.

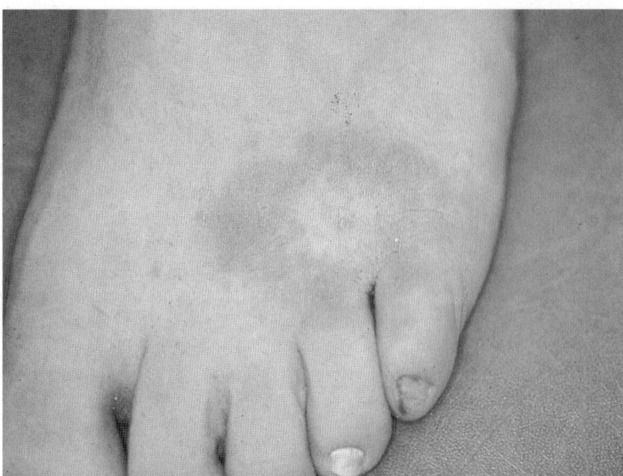

FIGURE 10.13. Erythema migrans. (Also see Color Plate.) This pathognomonic enlarging rash of Lyme disease forms at the site of the tick bite and consists of an outer ring where spirochetes can be found, an inner ring of clearing, and sometimes an area of central erythema as well. (Courtesy of Timothy Hinman, MD. Reproduced, with permission, from Knoop KJ, Stack LB, Storrow AB. *Atlas of Emergency Medicine,* 2nd ed. New York: McGraw-Hill, 2002: 399.)

KEY FACT

The erythema migrans rash is often missed and resolves in 3–4 weeks even without treatment.

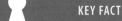

- Although neuro-Lyme disease can mimic multiple sclerosis, this is rare, and most patients who are diagnosed with MS-like Lyme disease actually have MS.

Diagnosis

- As with any condition, history trumps all else, and description of appropriate rash, together with exposure to a tick environment, should prompt treatment. However, many patients are concerned about Lyme disease, and will describe a rash that may *not* be typical of erythema migrans. Patients also may not see the rash.
- If pretest probability is intermediate, serum enzyme-linked immunosorbent assay (ELISA) is used for screening (high sensitivity, low specificity), and diagnosis is confirmed with Western blot (lower sensitivity, but high specificity).
- Western blot must be performed and interpreted by standardized and validated CDC protocols and criteria; a number of laboratories around the country use nonvalidated standards that result in a high false-positive rate and results from these laboratories should not be relied upon.
- IgM Western blot should only be used to make a diagnosis in the acute setting; if patient is believed to have contracted Lyme disease > 1 month before testing, then only the IgG Western blot result is valid.
- If serum is negative, then patient cannot have neuroborreliosis and CSF antibodies need not be tested.
- If serum is positive and there is clinical concern for neurological involvement, then CSF Western blot should be tested.
- A CSF lymphocytic pleocytosis, elevated protein, normal glucose should also be present in a patient with active neuro-Lyme disease.
- If pretest probability is low (nonspecific complaints with no objective findings), serologic testing is not indicated and patients should not be treated because positive test results will likely be false positives.
- PCR testing in plasma is sensitive, but no guidelines exist for its use, and PCR testing of the CSF is **not** useful.

KEY FACT

CNS Lyme disease should be diagnosed and treated only in patients with appropriate CSF test results, performed in a reliable laboratory.

TREATMENT

- Oral doxycycline is effective for non-neurological Lyme disease and probably for Lyme meningitis and facial nerve palsies; IV ceftriaxone is needed for more severe CNS involvement.
- The most common cause of apparent antibiotic failure in Lyme disease is misdiagnosis.
- Prevention includes use of insect repellant with DEET and careful examination and washing of body after exposure to tick environment, because transmission requires > 24 hours of tick attachment.

COMPLICATIONS

Following confirmed and appropriately treated Lyme disease, some patients develop a poorly defined syndrome of subjective complaints, including depression, memory and concentration problems, myalgias, and fatigue. These patients do not benefit from repeated or prolonged antibiotics.

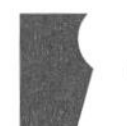

KEY FACT

It is clear that additional or prolonged courses of antibiotics provide no compelling sustained benefit for Lyme disease and carry significant risk.

Neurosyphilis

Treponema pallidum is sexually transmitted and causes a wide variety of symptoms.

SYMPTOMS/EXAM

- Neurological involvement occurs during tertiary syphilis, usually months to years after initial infection; often asymptomatic.
- Chronic meningitis is most common neurological manifestation, in up to 25% of cases.
- Focal symptoms and signs may occur due to granuloma, or "gumma," formation.
- Stroke may occur secondary to vasculitic involvement.
- *Tabes dorsalis* refers to involvement of dorsal columns with loss of proprioception and vibration sensation, which can → severe gait disturbance and/or incoordination. Argyll Robertson pupil may be seen (irregular, small pupil that accommodates but does not respond to light).

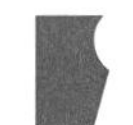

KEY FACT

Argyll Robertson pupil is like a prostitute: it will accommodate, but not react. Common sign in syphilis, often carried by prostitutes.

DIAGNOSIS

- CSF exam demonstrates lymphocytic pleocytosis (usually mild), elevated protein, and positive Venereal Disease Research Laboratory (VDRL) test.
- Serum VDRL and rapid plasma reagin (RPR) are nontreponemal tests that are nonspecific, but useful for screening. Fluorescent treponemal antibody absorption test (FTA-ABS) is specific treponemal antibody test used to confirm positive VDRL or RPR.
- CSF VDRL is specific but not sensitive for neurosyphilis.
- Positive serum FTA-ABS and positive CSF VDRL is sufficient to diagnose neurosyphilis. A patient with positive serology and neurological signs and symptoms should be treated for presumed neurosyphilis, especially if there is a CSF pleocytosis, even if CSF VDRL is negative.

TREATMENT

- Penicillin G 4 million units IV q4h for 10–14 days.
- Monitor CSF at 6 weeks, 3, 6, 12, and 24 months. VDRL titer should ↓ at least fourfold within 9 months of treatment. If clinical signs or symptoms persist or recur, or titer does not ↓ fourfold, patient should be treated again for presumed treatment failure or reinfection.

Amoebiasis

- Infection usually caused by *Naegleria fowlerii.*
- Amoeba reach the CNS through cribriform plate while patient swims in freshwater lake, often jumping or diving such that water is forced up the nose.
- **Symptoms:** Rapidly progressive encephalitis.
- **Diagnosis:** Hemorrhagic pleocytosis with organisms usually seen in CSF.
- **Treatment:** Amphotericin B and rifampin.
- **Prognosis:** Usually fatal.

Rocky Mountain Spotted Fever

- *Rickettsia rickettsii* transmitted by bite of *Dermacentor* tick. Type of dog tick, much larger, and more likely for patient to discover, than the tick that transmits Lyme disease.
- Despite name of disease, *Dermacentor* ticks and *Rickettsia rickettsii* are broadly distributed, with most common areas being mid-Atlantic and South Central states.
- Transmission usually occurs in late spring or summer.
- **Symptoms:** Usually diagnosed by internist based on presence of fever and maculopapular rash starting on wrists and ankles (see Figure 10.14), spreading centripetally, and evolving into petechial or purpuric rash. Neurologist may become involved because of severe headaches, significant mental status changes, → coma and ultimately death if the diagnosis not made.
- **Diagnosis:** Treatment should be started based on clinical presentation. Confirmation of diagnosis can be obtained by serological testing and/or biopsy of skin lesions.

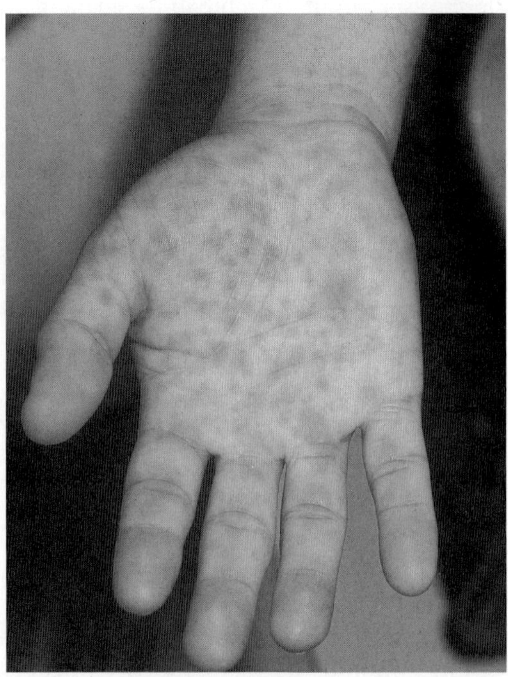

FIGURE 10.14. The rash of Rocky Mountain spotted fever starts in the distal extremities and spread centripetally. (Also see Color Plate.) (Reproduced, with permission, from Knoop KJ, Stack LB, Storrow AB, Thurman RJ. *The Atlas of Emergency Medicine,* 3rd ed. New York, McGraw-Hill Education, 2010. Photographer: Daniel Noltkamper, MD.)

- **Differential:** Meningococcemia and viruses can also cause rash and meningitis.
- **Treatment:** Doxycycline or chloramphenicol.
- **Prognosis:** Usually fatal within 8–15 days of symptom onset if left untreated; full recovery if properly treated.

KEY FACT

Think of Rocky Mountain spotted fever and start treatment early in any patient with a recent tick bite who presents with fever, headache, and/or myalgias.

Prion-Related Diseases

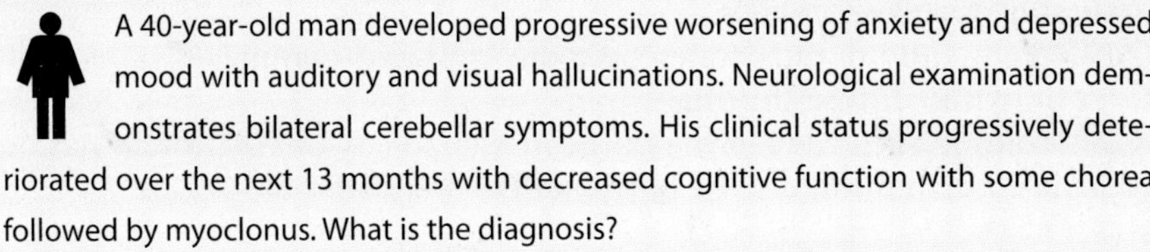

A 40-year-old man developed progressive worsening of anxiety and depressed mood with auditory and visual hallucinations. Neurological examination demonstrates bilateral cerebellar symptoms. His clinical status progressively deteriorated over the next 13 months with decreased cognitive function with some chorea followed by myoclonus. What is the diagnosis?

Creutzfeldt-Jakob disease (CJD). The classic or sporadic CJD is a rapidly progressive multifocal dementia, usually with myoclonus. The onset usually occurs between the ages of 45 and 75, with the peak onset between 60 and 65. Around 70% of patients die within 6 months of onset. Prodromal symptoms include fatigue, insomnia, depression, weight loss, and headaches, but mental deterioration and myoclonus frequently present with some extrapyramidal signs, cerebellar ataxia, and cortical blindness. The most remarkable neuropathological feature of CJD is the PrP protein abnormality and the CSF finding of 14-3-3 protein in the CSF, as well as at times diffusion-weighted imaging demonstrating diffusion restriction either in the cortical ribbon or in bilateral thalamic areas.

CREUTZFELDT-JAKOB DISEASE (CJD)

- Caused by an infectious protein with no nucleic acid component.
- CJD occurs worldwide at a rate of about 1 case per million population per year.
- Mean age for sporadic or classic CJD is 65. Duration of illness until death is about 6 months.
- CJD occurs sporadically, but has been transmitted iatrogenically via corneal transplants, human growth hormone, and neurosurgical instruments; such instruments can only be decontaminated with autoclaving or bleach.
- Also transmitted among Fore tribes of New Guinea via ritualistic cannibalism, in which case disease is termed kuru.
- There are other rare genetic forms, such as Gerstmann-Straussler disease and fatal familial insomnia.

Symptoms/Exam

- The hallmark of most prion disese is rapidly progressive dementia.
- Other symptoms include personality changes, anxiety, depression, paranoia, obsessive-compulsive symptoms, hallucinations, and psychosis.
- Patients will also often develop motor manifestions, including both pyramidal and extrapyramidal signs and symptoms.
- Startle myoclonus is common, but often does not appear until late in disease course.

Differential Diagnosis

- Reversible causes of encephalopathy should be excluded.
- CJD can sometimes be confused for other types of dementia, such as frontotemporal dementias and dementia with Lewy bodies disease.

Diagnosis

- **Pathology:**
  - Demonstrates spongiform encephalopathy with extensive vacuolization, especially of cortex and deep gray matter.
  - Special cautions must be taken to prevent transmission when brain biopsy is done on any patient with suspected prion disease.
- Brain MRI will typically show ↑ T2 signal in caudate, putamen, cortex, and thalamus (see Figure 10.15). Diffusion weighted imaging (DWI) is the most sensitive. In about 25% of cases, DWI shows only cortical hyperintensity; in about 70%, cortical and subcortical abnormalities; and in 5%, only subcortical anomalies.
- EEG frequently demonstrates periodic triphasic complexes, and evolves over time into diffuse slowing.
- CSF examination: May have nonspecific changes; 14-3-3 protein has been associated with prion disease but is neither sensitive nor specific.

Treatment

Supportive only.

Prognosis

Uniformally fatal, with death usually within 12 months.

VARIANT CJD AND BOVINE SPONGIFORM ENCEPHALOPATHY

- Form of prion disease transmitted to humans via consumption of infected beef (mad cow disease).
- Age of onset usually younger than in sporadic CJD. Psychiatric manifestations typically precede neurologic manifestations, and patients are usually initially thought to have primary psychiatric disorder.
- Neurologic symptoms develop about 6 months after psychiatric onset, and include dementia, akinetic mutism, painful sensory symptoms, ataxia, involuntary movements.
- EEGs show nonspecific slowing and do not show typical triphasic complexes of sporadic CJD.
- Brain MRI usually demostrates T2 bright signal in bilateral pulvinar.

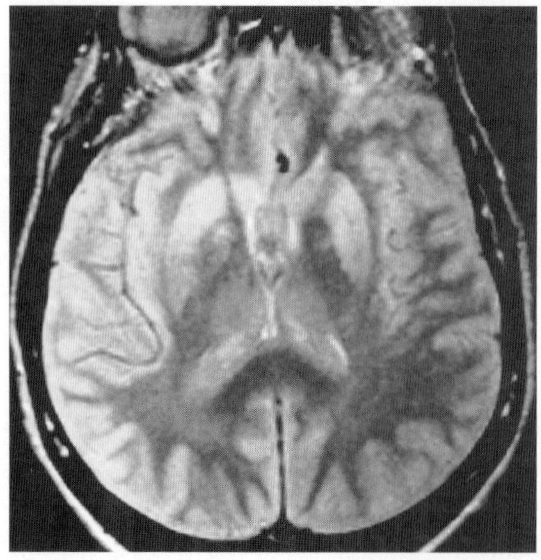

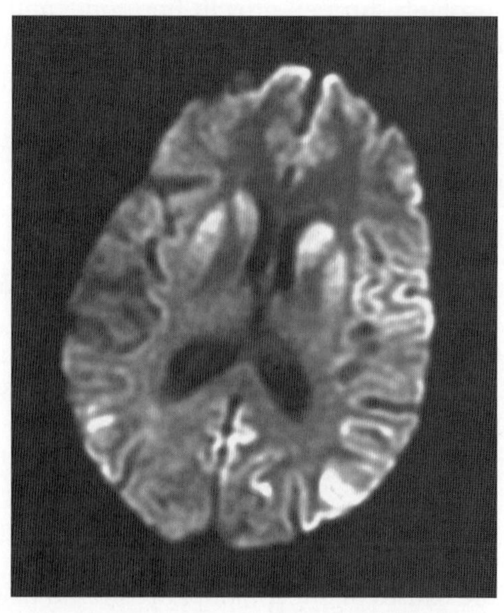

FIGURE 10.15. Typical brain MRI findings of a patient with Creutzfeldt-Jakob disease demonstrating T2 and DWI signal changes in the basal ganglia and cortical ribbon. (Reproduced, with permission, from Ropper AH, Brown RH. *Adams and Victor's Principles of Neurology*, 8th ed. New York: McGraw-Hill, 2005: 655.)

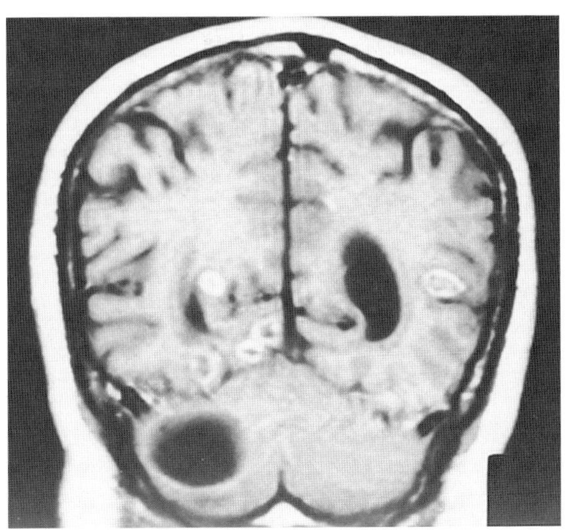

FIGURE 10.16. Contrast-enhanced head CT of a patient with neurocysticercosis demonstrating numerous enhancing and calcified cysts. (Courtesy of A. Gean. Reproduced, with permission, from Aminoff MJ, Greenberg DA, Simon RP. *Clinical Neurology*, 6th ed. New York: McGraw-Hill, 2005: Figure 32-8.)

Neurocysticercosis

- Infection usually caused by parasite, *Taenia solium*, acquired by fecal-oral route.
- Endemic to Central and South America and being seen with ↑ frequency in the United States among immigrants from that part of the world.
- **Symptoms:** Extremely common cause of seizures worldwide.
- **Diagnosis:** Brain imaging reveals multiple calcified cysts (Figure 10.16).
- **Treatment:** Albendazole or praziquantel, sometimes with steroids; anticonvulsants as needed.

NOTES

CHAPTER 11

Neuromuscular Disease

Thomas I. Cochrane, MD, PhD

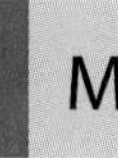

Molecular Anatomy and Physiology

PERIPHERAL NERVE

Peripheral nerves are classified by diameter and myelination (Tables 11.1 and 11.2).

- Larger fibers are faster.
- Myelinated fibers faster (saltatory conduction between nodes of Ranvier).
- Motor fibers are larger, more heavily myelinated.
- Nociceptive and autonomic fibers are smaller, thinly myelinated.
- Different sensory receptors have different functions:
  - Pacinian corpuscles: Deep pressure, touch, high-frequency vibration.
  - Meissner corpuscles: Light touch.
  - Merkel discs: Low-frequency vibration, light touch.
  - Ruffini endings: Skin stretch and movement along skin.
  - Free nerve endings: Temperature, pressure, pain.
- Location of selected myelin-associated proteins (CNS vs PNS):
  - Myelin protein zero (MPZ, P0): PNS.
  - Myelin associated glycoprotein: CNS and PNS.
  - Peripheral myelin protein 22 (PMP22): PNS.
  - Myelin-oligodendrocyte glycoprotein (MOG): CNS.
  - Oligodendrocyte-myelin glycoprotein (OMgp): CNS.

NEUROMUSCULAR JUNCTION (NMJ)

Key features of the NMJ are illustrated in Figure 11.1.

- Motor axon depolarization opens P/Q-type voltage-gated calcium channel (VGCCs) → influx of Ca^{2+}.
- Ca^{2+} mediates synaptic vesicle binding, release of acetylcholine (ACh).
- ACh binds to ACh receptors (not voltage-dependent) at the muscle fiber end plate → muscle membrane depolarization.
- Acetylcholinesterase (AchE) degrades ACh into acetyl-CoA and choline.

MUSCLE

- Muscle consists of:
  - **Myofibers:** Syncytial cells spanning the length of the muscle, containing **myofilaments** of actin and myosin. Connective tissue around myofibers is **endomysium.**
  - Myofibers bundled in **fascicles,** surrounded by **perimysium.**
  - Hundreds of fascicles make up a muscle, surrounded by **epimysium.**

TABLE 11.1. Classification and Myelination of Motor Nerves

To skeletal muscle (extrafusal)	Aα, Aβ	Larger	More myelin
To skeletal muscle (intrafusal)	Aβ, Aγ	↓	↓
Preganglionic autonomic fibers	B		
Postganglionic autonomic	C	Smaller	Less myelin

TABLE 11.2. Classification and Myelination of Sensory Nerves

Muscle spindle afferents	Aα, Aβ	Ia, II	Larger	More myelin
Golgi tendon organs	Aα	Ib	↓	↓
Touch	Aα, Aβ	Ib, II		
Pressure	Aα, Aβ	Ib, II		
Vibration	Aβ, Aγ	II		
Pain and temperature	Aδ, B, C	III, IV	Smaller	Less myelin

Note: The Roman numeral classification applies to sensory nerves only.

- Myofibers are extrafusal or intrafusal:
  - **Extrafusal fibers:** Contraction across joints. **Type I:** Slow-twitch, fatigue resistant, naturally darker, low in glycogen, high in oxidative enzymes. High in acid-stable ATPase (stains dark at pH 4.2). **Type II:** Fast-twitch, more glycogen and myophosphorylase. High in alkaline-stable ATPase (stains dark at pH 9.4).
  - **Intrafusal fibers:** Myofibers within **muscle spindle** or **Golgi tendon organ.** Coupled with sensory stretch/tension receptors. Involved in stretch reflexes and maintenance of tone (Figure 11.2).

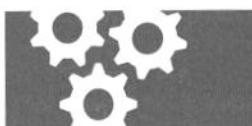

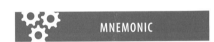

MNEMONIC

One Slow Red Ox: Type I (**one**) fibers are **Slow** twitch, and stain **red** because of **ox**idative enzymes.

Disorders of Roots, Plexus, and Nerve

A 73-year-old man presents with several years of gradual, symmetric numbness and tingling that started in his toes. The numbness now reaches about halfway up his foreleg. What feature of the exam would most convincingly show that his problem is peripheral, not central?

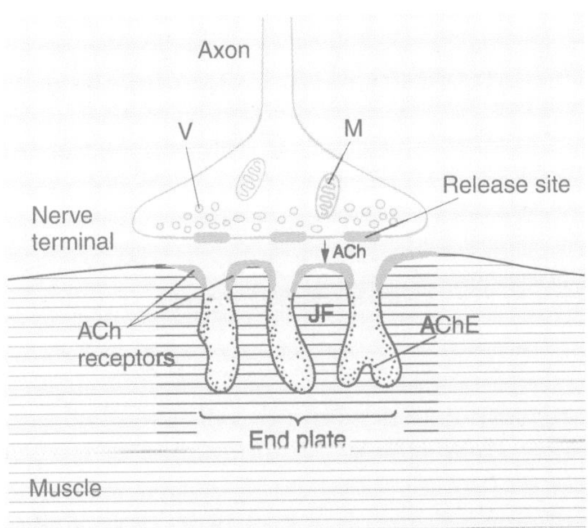

FIGURE 11.1. Overview of the neuromuscular junction. ACh, acetylcholine. JF, junctional folds. V, vesicle. M, mitochondrion. (Reproduced, with permission, from Morgan GE, Mikhail MS, Murray MJ. *Clinical Anesthesiology*, 4th ed. New York: McGraw-Hill, 2006: Figure 9-1.)

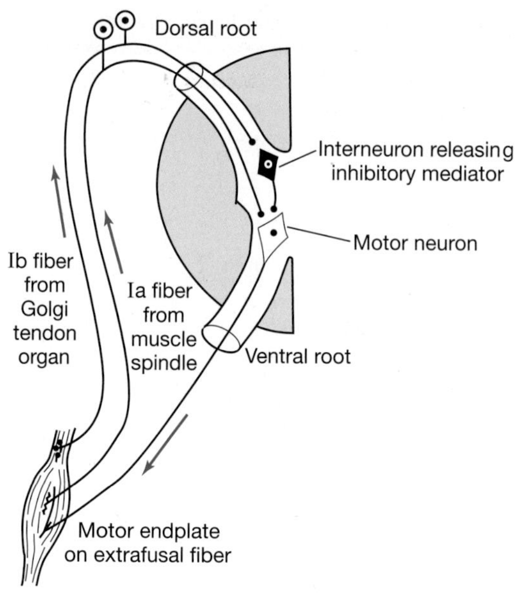

FIGURE 11.2. Tendon reflex arc. (Reproduced, with permission, from Ganong WF. *Review of Medical Physiology,* 22nd ed. New York: McGraw-Hill, 2005.)

Diminished or absent ankle reflexes. Though this presentation is most likely a distal symmetric polyneuropathy, this patient's symptoms could conceivably be related to a central problem (eg, dorsal column dysfunction due to B_{12} deficiency).

APPROACH TO NEUROPATHIES

A suggested scheme for categorizing neuropathies is shown in Table 11.3.

DISTAL SYMMETRIC SENSORY > MOTOR POLYNEUROPATHIES

- Slow, symmetric, distal onset of paresthesias, hypesthesias.
- Length-dependent symptoms, begin in feet. (Early hand involvement suggests non-length-dependent or central nervous system [CNS] problem).
- Most common category of polyneuropathy.

DIFFERENTIAL DIAGNOSIS

- Diabetes ~30%.
- Alcohol ~30%.
- Idiopathic ~30%.
- Amyloidosis.
- B_1, B_{12} deficiency.
- Confluent vasculitis (onset usually multifocal).

DIAGNOSIS

- Extent of investigation depends on index of suspicion.
- Electromyography (EMG)/nerve conduction studies (NCS) usually just confirmatory.
- "Straightforward" (onset age > 50, starts in feet, symmetric, slowly progressive, mild distal weakness):
    - Fasting blood sugar or HbA_{1c}.

TABLE 11.3. Differential Diagnosis of Neuropathies

Distal Symmetric Sensory and Motor	Multifocal Motor and Sensory	Sensory Neuronopathy/Ganglionopathy
Diabetes	**Immune-mediated**	Sjögren syndrome
Alcohol/drugs/toxins	Vasculitis	Vitamin E, B_6 deficiency/excess
Idiopathic	Brachial neuritis (neuralgic amyotrophy)	Paraneoplastic (anti-Hu, rarely anti-CV2)
Paraprotein-related	Sarcoidosis	Toxic (cisplatin, etoposide, nucleoside analogues)
Amyloidosis	CIDP/MMN	**Frequent/prominent autonomic involvement**
Vitamin B_{12}, vitamin E, thiamine	**Infectious**	Diabetic neuropathies
Confluent vasculitis	Lyme disease	AIDP/CIDP
Diffuse motor > sensory[a]	HIV-associated CMV	Amyloidosis
AIDP, CIDP	Leprosy	HSAN
Osteosclerotic myeloma	Herpes zoster	Porphyria
Drugs (amiodarone, gold, perhexilene)	**Infiltrative**	HIV-related autonomic neuropathy
Inherited (SMA, CMT, KD, FALS)	Diabetic amyotrophy (may be vasculitic)	Idiopathic pandysautonomia
Acute intermittent porphyria	Amyloidosis	
Acute arsenic	Lymphomatous infiltration	
Diphtheria	**Hereditary**	
	CMTX/HNPP	

[a]Consider NMJ, muscle disorder.

AIDP, acute inflammatory demyelinating polyneuropathy; CIDP, chronic inflammatory demyelinating polyneuropathy; CMT, Charcot-Marie-Tooth disease; CMTX, Charcot-Marie-Tooth disease, X-linked; CMV, cytomegalovirus; FALS, familial amyotrophic lateral sclerosis; HIV, human immunodeficiency virus; HNPP, hereditary neuropathy with liability to pressure; HSAN, hereditary sensory and autonomic neuropathy; KD, Kennedy disease; MMN, multifocal motor neuropathy; SMA, spinal muscular atrophy.

  - Vitamin B_{12} levels. If low normal, consider homocysteine, methylmalonic acid levels.
  - Thyroid function tests.
  - Serum protein electrophoresis (SPEP) and immunofixation.
- Not straightforward (age < 50, somewhat asymmetric onset, diffuse or proximal involvement, prominent weakness):
  - All the above, plus: Creatinine; erythrocyte sedimentation rate (ESR), antinuclear antibody (ANA), rheumatoid factor (RF); HIV testing; liver function tests (LFTs): If abnormal, hepatitis B and C serologies; consider anti-ssA (Ro), anti-ssB (La) antibodies.

DIFFUSE MOTOR > SENSORY NEUROPATHIES

Symptoms and Signs

- Weakness and hyporeflexia with little or no sensory disturbance.
- Weakness roughly symmetric.
- Consider category whenever onset is rapid or weakness prominent/proximal.

Differential Diagnosis

- Acute/chronic inflammatory demyelinating polyneuropathy (AIDP/CIDP).
- Osteosclerotic myeloma.
- Drugs (amiodarone, gold, perhexilene).
- Inherited (Charcot-Marie-Tooth disease [CMT], spinal muscular atrophy [SMA], Kennedy disease [KD], familial amyotrophic lateral sclerosis [ALS]).

- Acute intermittent porphyria.
- Acute arsenic.
- Diphtheria.

INVESTIGATIONS

As in distal symmetric sensory neuropathies, plus:

- Consider cerebrospinal fluid (CSF) cells and protein.
- EMG/NCS helpful in documenting demyelination.

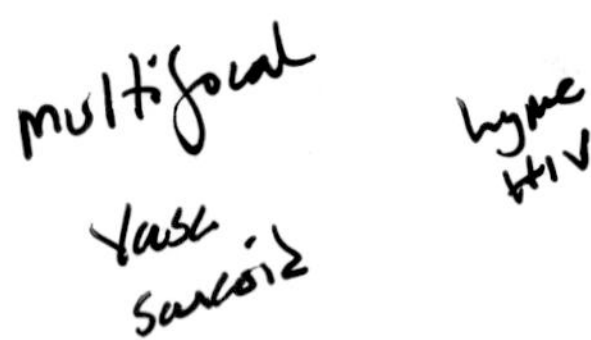

MULTIFOCAL MOTOR AND SENSORY NEUROPATHIES

SYMPTOMS AND SIGNS

- Asymmetric weakness and sensory loss in named nerves/portions of plexus.
- Consider this category in patients with a new mononeuropathy.

DIFFERENTIAL DIAGNOSIS

- **Immune-mediated:**
  - Vasculitis.
  - Brachial neuritis (also called neuralgic amyotrophy).
  - Sarcoidosis.
  - Multifocal CIDP, multifocal motor neuropathy.
- **Infectious:**
  - Lyme disease.
  - HIV-associated cytomegalovirus (CMV).
  - Leprosy.
  - Herpes zoster.
- **Infiltrative:**
  - Diabetic amyotrophy.
  - Amyloidosis (also causes length-dependent small-fiber neuropathy).
  - Lymphomatous infiltration.
- **Hereditary:**
  - CMT X (mutation in Connexin-32).
  - Hereditary neuropathy with liability to pressure palsies (HNPP).

INVESTIGATIONS

All of the above, plus:

- Lyme antibodies.
- ANCA, cryoglobulins.
- If HIV positive, check for CMV antigenemia.
- Chest x-ray (sarcoidosis).
- CSF cells and protein.
- EMG/NCS can confirm a multifocal/asymmetric process.
- Nerve biopsy helpful when vasculitis or amyloidosis suspected.

SENSORY NEURONOPATHIES

- Profound loss of proprioception → pseudoathetosis, sensory drift.
- Disease of the sensory cell body: **Neuronopathy** or **ganglionopathy.**
- Consider when sensory disturbance is non-length-dependent, with prominent ataxia and no weakness.
- Relatively rare.

Differential Diagnosis

- Sjögren syndrome.
- Vitamin E deficiency.
- Vitamin B_6 deficiency/excess.
- Paraneoplastic (anti-Hu, rarely anti-CV2).
- Toxic (cisplatin, etoposide, nucleoside analogues).

Investigations

As for multifocal neuropathies, plus:

- Vitamin E levels.
- Vitamin B_6 levels.
- Anti-ssA (Ro) and anti-ssB (La) antibodies.
- Consider anti-Hu antibodies and a search for malignancy.

NEUROPATHIES THAT COMMONLY HAVE AUTONOMIC INVOLVEMENT

Ask about:

- Cardiovascular (resting tachycardia, orthostasis, exercise intolerance).
- Gastrointestinal (gastroparesis, constipation, diarrhea).
- Genitourinary (recurrent urinary tract infection, erectile dysfunction, incontinence/nocturia/urgency/hesitancy).
- Skin (mottling/discoloration, sudomotor dysfunction).
- Visual (blurring, impaired night vision).
- Other (impaired thermoregulation).

Differential Diagnosis

- Diabetes (very common, usually mild).
- AIDP/CIDP (common in AIDP, can be severe/life threatening).
- Amyloidosis (very common, can be severe).
- Hereditary sensory and autonomic neuropathy (rare).
- Porphyria.
- HIV-related autonomic neuropathy.
- Idiopathic pandysautonomia.

COMPRESSIVE/TRAUMATIC RADICULOPATHIES, PLEXOPATHIES, AND FOCAL NEUROPATHIES

Anatomy of roots, plexus, and nerves is covered extensively on the boards. Memorization of a diagram like Figure 11.3, including root supply of commonly tested muscles, is very high yield.

Cervical Radiculopathies

Symptoms (see Table 11-4)

- Pain in neck, shoulder, arm—often vague localization.
- Sensory disturbance: Hypesthesia, paresthesias in dermatomal distribution.
- Weakness: Myotomal.
- Reflexes reduced: Biceps, brachioradialis (C5 or C6), triceps (C7).

Diagnosis

- Spurling sign: Neck extension and rotation toward symptomatic side reproduces radicular symptoms.

MNEMONIC

I'M THAT DIM!

Infectious: HIV, Lyme disease, hepatitis B and C
Metabolic: Diabetes, hypothyroidism
Traumatic: Entrapment, shear injury
Hereditary: CMT, familial amyloid, porphyria
Autoimmune: Connective tissue (Sjögren, SLE, RA), sarcoidosis, vasculitis, GBS
Toxins: Heavy metals (lead, thallium, arsenic), chemotherapy
Diet (Nutrition:) B_{12}, thiamine, alcohol
Immunoglobulins: Monoclonal proteins, cryoglobulinemia, primary and secondary amyloidosis
Malignancy: Compression, meningeal carcinomatosis, paraneoplastic

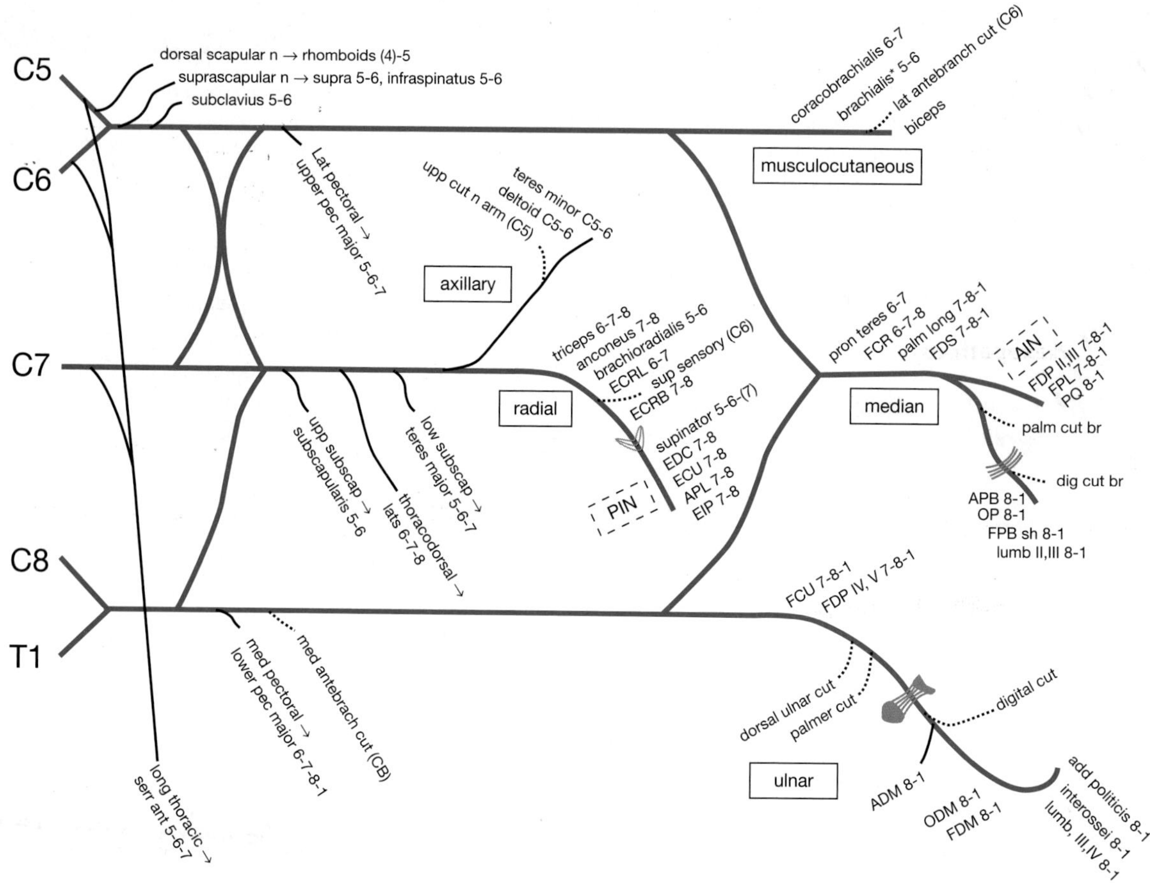

FIGURE 11.3. Brachial plexus. PIN, posterior interosseous nerve. AIN, anterior interosseous nerve. The arcade of Frohse is pictured on the radial nerve; the carpal tunnel is pictured on the median nerve; and Guyon canal is pictured on the ulnar nerve.

- NCS/EMG: NCS can help differentiate radiculopathy from plexopathy (sensory nerve action potentials [SNAPs] are preserved in radiculopathy).
- MRI or CT myelography.
- Most common cause is compression by disk protrusion, ligament hypertrophy, spondylolisthesis.

TABLE 11.4. Cervical Radiculopathies

Root	Weakness	Sensory Disturbance	Notes
C3/C4	Rarely hemidiaphragm.	Posterolateral scalp, behind the ear.	Rare.
C5	Rhomboids, shoulder abduction, shoulder external rotation, elbow flexion.	Shoulder, upper lateral arm.	
C6	Shoulder abduction, shoulder external rotation, elbow flexion, forearm pronation, wrist extension, radial wrist flexion.	Lateral forearm, digits 1 and 2.	
C7	Forearm pronation, wrist flexion, finger extension.	Digit 3; patient reports of pain/sensory abnormality in "the whole hand" common.	Most common.
C8/T1	Finger abduction, thumb opposition, thumb abduction.	Digits 4 and 5, medial forearm and arm.	

Treatment

- Mild radiculopathies do not require specific treatment.
- Approximately 80% recover within a month; 90% within 3 months.
- Physical therapy (PT) and exercise.
- Epidural steroid injections (ESIs).
- Indications for surgical decompression:
  - Moderate-severe weakness.
  - Worsening weakness/sensory loss.
  - Severe pain unresponsive to conservative measures.

Upper Brachial Plexopathies

Symptoms/Exam

- Weakness: C5–6-innervated muscles (deltoid, supra/infraspinatus, biceps, brachialis; very proximal injury; serratus anterior and/or rhomboids).
- Sensory disturbance: Shoulder and lateral arm.

Causes

- Birth injury ("**Erb-Duchenne palsy**") due to traction of the head and neck away from the shoulder.
- Any injuries involving downward displacement of the shoulder/arm and/or lateral displacement of the head and neck.

Treatment

- Physical therapy, prevention of contractures.
- Nerve grafting can be considered when severe and focal.

Lower Brachial Plexopathies

Symptoms/Exam

- Weakness of C8–T1-innervated muscles (the intrinsic hand muscles).
- Sensory disturbance of the medial arm, forearm, fourth and fifth digits.
- Horner syndrome if T1 root is affected.
- Clue to lower trunk lesion: Atrophy of thenar eminence with sensory loss in medial hand/fingers.

Causes

- **Klumpke palsy:** Birth injury due to forced abduction of the arm.
- Any trauma involving forced abduction of the arm.
- Open thoracotomy (lung surgery, cardiac surgery).
- Neurogenic **thoracic outlet syndrome (nTOS):** Compression by cervical rib or fibrous band between lateral process of C7 and first rib.
- Pancoast tumor (apical lung cancer).

Treatment

- Decompression of nTOS.
- Physical therapy, prevention of contractures.
- Nerve grafting can be considered when severe and focal.

Upper-Limb Focal Neuropathies

- **Long thoracic nerve:**
  - Traumatic or as part of brachial neuritis.
  - Weakness of serratus anterior → scapular winging.
  - Treatment conservative; if winging is painful, can consider surgical scapula fixation.

- **Axillary nerve:**
  - Usually traumatic or as part of brachial neuritis.
  - Weakness: Shoulder abduction/external rotation.
  - Sensory disturbance: Lateral upper arm.
- **Radial nerve:**
  - Usually traumatic/compressive.
  - Weakness of elbow extension, wrist extension, supination, finger extension, and radial sensory loss, depending on location:
    - Axilla (eg, crutches): Weakness of all radial muscles, sensory loss in posterior arm/forearm/hand.
    - Spiral groove of humerus (eg, fracture, compression/"**Saturday night palsy**"): Spares elbow extension; sensory loss in posterior hand.
    - **Arcade of Frohse:** Posterior interosseous nerve entrapment (see Figure 11.3). Wrist drop, finger drop, no sensory loss.
- **Median nerve:**
  - Compression syndromes: Ligament of Struthers (fibrous band between distal humerus and medial epicondyle); antecubital fossa, under lacertus fibrosus; within pronator teres; within carpal tunnel (carpal tunnel syndrome).
  - Anterior interosseous neuropathy: Anterior interosseous nerve (AIN) supplies pronator teres (PT), flexor pollicis longus (FPL), and flexor digitorum profundus (FDP) to digits 2 and 3, no sensory. Weakness of pronation especially when arm is extended. Weakness of flexion in distal joint of digits 1, 2, and 3. Can be traumatic or part of brachial neuritis. Clinical signs:
    - **Tinel sign:** Positive if percussion of a nerve reproduces symptoms.
    - **Phalen sign** (in carpal tunnel syndrome): Wrists held in flexed posture for 60 seconds. Positive if symptoms reproduced/worsen.
- **Ulnar nerve:**
  - Cubital tunnel at the elbow.
  - Guyon canal at the wrist.
  - Clinical signs associated with ulnar neuropathy:
    - **Benediction sign** (ulnar claw hand): When extending fingers, fourth and fifth digits hyperextend at metacarpophalangeal (MCP) joint due to weakness of fourth and fifth lumbricals → inability to extend distal interphalangeal (DIP)/proximal interphalangeal (PIP) joints fully.
    - **Wartenberg sign:** At rest, the fifth digit is slightly abducted due to weakness of third palmar intraosseous (IO).
    - **Froment sign:** Curled thumb when trying to pinch. (Thumb adduction and index abduction weakness → weak pinch. To compensate, median-innervated FPL causes thumb flexion).

Lumbosacral Radiculopathies (Table 11-5)

A 45-year-old woman presents several days after the acute onset of low back and leg pain. She has electrical, lancinating paresthesias over her lateral foreleg and dorsal foot, and feels like she's "dragging" her foot. What localizations should be considered, and what features will help distinguish the possibilities?

Peroneal neuropathy is consistent with this patient's foot drop and sensory disturbance. Although the history of back pain argues against this possibility, always check ankle inversion in patients with foot drop. A peroneal neuropathy should not cause inversion weakness. A partial sciatic neuropathy could cause this patient's symptoms,

TABLE 11.5. Clinical Manifestations of Lumbosacral Radiculopathies

Root	Weakness	Sensory Disturbance	Notes
L2/L3/L4	Hip flexion, adduction, knee extension.	Hip, thigh, medial leg.	Rare. Differential: Femoral, obturator neuropathies and diabetic amyotrophy.
L5	Ankle and toe extension, ankle inversion.	Paresthesias/numbness lateral leg and dorsomedial foot.	Most common. Usually caused by L4 disk protrusion, although L3 and L5 disks possible.
S1	Toe extension/flexion, foot plantar flexion, hip extension.	Posterolateral calf and foot (usually plantar aspect).	Usually caused by L5 disk.
S2/S3/S4	Bowel, bladder, and sexual dysfunction, loss of bulbocavernosus reflex and rectal tone.	Perineal and anal sphincter region.	

although the acute onset and associated back pain make it less likely. An L5 radiculopathy would explain the symptoms, and seems to fit the presentation neatly. Nerve conduction studies and EMG can help distinguish sciatic neuropathy and L5 radiculopathy in tough cases.

Symptoms

- Dermatomal pain/paresthesias. Severe sensory loss is unusual.
- Myotomal weakness. Paralysis rare—muscles supplied by ≥ 2 roots.
- Reflexes reduced: L3 or L4—knee jerk. S1—ankle jerk.

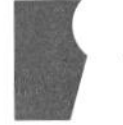

KEY FACT

Tibialis anterior (supplied by L4/L5, sciatic nerve, common peroneal, deep peroneal nerve) is the only muscle below the knee with a contribution from the L4 root.

Causes

- Common: Disk herniation, facet or ligament hypertrophy, spondylolisthesis, osteophytes, synovial cysts.
- Less common: Tumor, infectious masses.

Treatment

- Physical therapy, exercises to promote flexibility and core strength.
- Epidural steroids.
- Decompressive surgery: When weakness severe or worsening, sometimes when pain is intractable and persistent.

Lumbosacral Plexopathies

- **Symptoms:** Weakness and sensory loss ≥ 1 root or nerve territory; can be difficult to distinguish from multiple LS radiculopathies.
- **Causes:**
  - Neuralgic amyotrophy (diabetic or idiopathic; pathophysiology may be microvasculitis).
  - Vasculitic.
  - Infectious (zoster, Lyme disease).
  - Traumatic/compressive: Abdominal/pelvic surgery, obstetric, retroperitoneal tumor or hematoma, aortic/iliac aneurysm.

Lower-Limb Focal Neuropathies

- **Lateral femoral cutaneous nerve (meralgia paresthetica):**
  - **Symptoms:** Numbness of lateral thigh (medial thigh involvement suggests more proximal lesion (femoral, LS plexus, L3 root).
  - **Causes:** Entrapment/pressure along inguinal ligament, tight belts/waistbands, rapid weight gain, excessive/prolonged flexion of the hip (eg, giving birth).
- **Femoral neuropathy:**
  - **Symptoms:** Weakness of hip flexion, knee extension, sensory disturbance over anterior/medial thigh, medial leg, and ankle.
  - **Causes:** Trauma/compression (eg, femur fracture, hip dislocation, tumor, obstetric trauma), retroperitoneal/iliopsoas hematoma (femoral nerve traverses the muscle), vascular/vasculitic (eg, neuralgic amyotrophy).
- **Obturator neuropathy:**
  - Weakness of hip adduction, internal rotation.
  - Sensory disturbance over medial thigh.
  - Same causes as femoral neuropathies.
- **Sciatic neuropathy:**
  - **Symptoms:** Weakness of hip extension, knee flexion, ankle and toe extension/flexion, inversion and eversion. Sensory disturbance possible in tibial and peroneal territories (entire lower leg and foot).
  - **Causes:** Most common: compression at sciatic notch or proximal thigh (eg, surgical, pelvic/hip/femur fracture, hematoma, tumor, etc). Peroneal (lateral) division of sciatic nerve is more susceptible to injury.
- **Tibial neuropathy:**
  - **Symptoms:** Weakness of ankle and toe plantar flexion, ankle inversion. Sensory disturbance over lateral ankle (sural territory), sole of foot.
  - **Causes:** Compression/tumor in popliteal fossa/posterior calf. Medial ankle at flexor retinaculum ("tarsal tunnel syndrome")—loss in plantar, calcaneal, but not sural distribution.
- **Peroneal neuropathy:**
  - **Symptoms:** Weakness of ankle dorsiflexion and eversion, toe extension. Ankle inversion is not weak—test with ankle at 90 degrees. Sensory disturbance over lateral leg (distal two-thirds) and dorsal/lateral foot.
  - **Causes:** Compression, stretch, or trauma to common peroneal nerve at the fibular head; prolonged/repeated leg-crossing; prolonged crouch (eg, catcher in baseball); ganglion cyst/tumors of popliteal fossa.

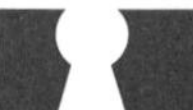

KEY FACT

In foot drop, weakness of ankle inversion distinguishes peroneal neuropathy from L5 radiculopathy or sciatic neuropathy. Tibialis posterior (L5–S1, sciatic nerve, tibial nerve) is not weak in peroneal neuropathy.

IMMUNE-MEDIATED NEUROPATHIES

Acute Inflammatory Demyelinating Polyradiculoneuropathy (AIDP) or Guillain-Barré Syndrome (GBS)

Epidemiology

- Most common neurological cause of acute generalized weakness.
- Annual incidence ~2 in 100,000.
- Slight male predominance.
- Any age except infancy; incidence highest in adulthood.

Symptoms and Signs

- Rapidly developing generalized (proximal and distal) weakness. Facial and eyelid weakness is common.
- Tingling/numbness in hands, feet, and later face, usually mild.
- Early hand, trunk, or face involvement is important clue to a non-length-dependent process such as AIDP.

- Respiratory insufficiency or failure in approximately one-third.
- Autonomic instability (eg, tachycardia, bradycardia, orthostasis, sweating abnormalities, pupil changes, urinary retention) sometimes severe.
- LFT abnormalities common (exclude viral hepatitis).
- Low back pain and proximal thigh/buttock pain common.
- If symptoms progress > 4 weeks, consider CIDP.
- See Table 11.6 for AIDP variants.

Pathophysiology

- T-cell mediated autoimmunity → multifocal demyelinating polyradiculoneuropathy.
- Approximately two-thirds parainfectious.
- Antecedent illness, trauma, or vaccination in prior month are common.
- Sometimes antibodies against *Campylobacter jejuni* (32%), CMV (13%), Epstein-Barr virus (EBV) (10%), *Mycoplasma* (5%).
- HIV and influenza occasionally implicated.
- **Histopathology:** Perivascular mononuclear infiltrates and segmental/multifocal demyelination; variable axonal loss. Predilection for ventral nerve roots.
- **Laboratory evaluation:**
  - NCS: Demyelinating findings—motor slowing, temporal dispersion, conduction block; abnormal F-wave responses; often normal early.
  - CSF albuminocytologic dissociation (high protein, normal WBCs). CSF often normal, especially in first 2 weeks.
  - If CSF WBC > 10–15, consider infectious/malignant polyradiculopathy.
  - MRI can show enhancement of nerve roots.
- **Treatment:**
  - Respiratory monitoring and support: FVC < 15 mL/kg, inability to count to 20 in 1 breath—consider ICU monitoring, intubation.
  - Treat autonomic instability (especially large swings in blood pressure, heart rate).
  - Intravenous immune globulin (IVIG) or plasmapheresis.
  - Corticosteroids are not effective.

KEY FACT

Early hand, trunk, or face involvement is important clue to a non-length-dependent neuropathy such as AIDP, and CNS pathology should be considered.

TABLE 11.6. AIDP Variants

Variant	Features	Notes
Miller-Fisher variant	Ophthalmoplegia, gait ataxia, areflexia +/− mild limb weakness.	Associated with *C jejuni,* IgG against GQ1b gangliosides.
Pharyngeal-cervical-brachial +/− ophthalmoparesis	Ptosis, neck and respiratory weakness, +/− ophthalmoparesis.	Reflexes decreased in the arms, can be preserved in legs. Consider botulism.
Acute pandysautonomia	Primarily autonomic dysfunction.	Consider thallium toxicity.
Acute motor-sensory axonal neuropathy (AMSAN)		
Acute motor axonal neuropathy (AMAN)		Most common in rural China, summer months—association with diarrheal infections.
Polyneuritis cranialis	Multiple cranial neuropathies.	Consider skull-base processes (sarcoid, TB, lymphoma).

- Mild cases may not need treatment.
- Sensory involvement typically resolves quickly; prognosis is good for mild to moderate cases.

Chronic Inflammatory Demyelinating Polyneuropathy (CIDP)

- Diffuse, roughly symmetric weakness and hyporeflexia developing over ≥ 8 weeks.
- Sensory symptoms usually mild.
- Can be monophasic, relapsing-remitting, or chronically progressive.
- Association with lymphoma/leukemia, infections (eg, HIV), autoimmune disorders.
- Asymmetric/multifocal variant: **Multifocal CIDP (mCIDP),** or **multifocal acquired demyelinating sensory and motor (MADSAM) neuropathy.**
- Prognosis good—95% improve with immunotherapy.
- Relapse rate almost 50% over 4 years.
- **Treatment:**
  - Corticosteroids (eg, oral prednisone).
  - Plasma exchange, IVIG, azathioprine, cyclosporine.
  - Cyclophosphamide only in the most severe and refractory.

Multifocal Motor Neuropathy (MMN)

- Cramps and fasciculations, followed by slowly progressive focal weakness.
- Typically affects 1 or more individual named nerves, arms more common than legs. Wrist drop, intrinsic hand weakness, foot drop common.
- Slowly progressive.
- No sensory loss.
- Patients typically > 40 years, male-to-female ratio 3:1.
- **Investigations/pathophysiology/treatment:**
  - Asymmetric immune-mediated demyelinating motor neuropathy.
  - Some association with anti-GM1 antibodies.
  - Conduction block/focal demyelination on NCS distinguishes MMN from ALS (MMN much rarer).
  - Responds to IVIG, but not to corticosteroids.

Autoimmune Sensory Neuronopathy (Ganglionopathy)

- Acute-subacute, severe generalized (non-length-dependent) sensory loss (especially vibration, proprioception).
- Profound ataxia and pseudoathetosis.
- Associated with anti-ganglioside antibodies, especially GD1b.
- **Differential diagnosis:**
  - Sjögren syndrome.
  - Paraneoplastic (especially anti-Hu antibodies).
  - Idiopathic.
  - Vitamin E, B_6 deficiency/excess, some chemotherapy (discussed in their sections).

VASCULITIC NEUROPATHIES

- **Symptoms and signs:**
  - Classic: multiple mononeuropathies ("mononeuritis multiplex").
  - Acute/subacute multifocal weakness/sensory loss in nerve territories.
  - Almost always associated with painful (burning) paresthesias.

- **Pathology:**
  - Vasculitis can be classified as primary (see Table 11.7) or secondary.
  - Transmural inflammation.
  - Necrosis of epineurial or perineurial blood vessels.
  - Deposition of immunoglobulin and membrane attack complex (MAC).
  - Normal nerve fascicles next to ischemic fascicles.

Secondary Vasculitis

- Vasculitis caused by connective tissue diseases: Sjögren, rheumatoid arthritis (RA), systemic lupus erythematosus (SLE), scleroderma/CREST syndrome (calcinosis, Raynaud phenomenon, esophageal dysfunction, sclerodactyly, telanciectasia), mixed connective tissue disease.
- Infection-related vasculitis: Varicella-zoster virus VZV, HIV, CMV, hepatitis B virus (HBV), hepatitis C virus (HCV).
- Malignancy-associated vasculitis: Most common are small cell lung cancer and lymphoma. Associated neuropathies are not necessarily vasculitic (can be autoantibodies directed against PNS epitopes).
- Drug-induced hypersensitivity vasculitis: Complement-mediated leukocytoclastic vasculitis.
- Cryoglobulinemia-associated vasculitis.

Brachial Neuritis (Neuralgic Amyotrophy, Parsonage-Turner Syndrome)

- **Symptoms:**
  - Acute onset of severe neuropathic pain (sharp, stinging, electrical, etc) in shoulder/shoulder girdle, sometimes arm and hand.

TABLE 11.7. Primary Vasculitis and Neuropathies

Type	Neuropathy?	Other Features
Large-vessel		
Giant-cell/temporal arteritis	Yes	ESR elevated in 97%.
Takayasu arteritis	No	
Medium-vessel		
Polyarteritis nodosa	Yes	Most common necrotizing vasculitis; 50–70% have neuropathy. Renal, hepatic, skin, GI involvement common. Orchitis and constitutional symptoms are classic.
Kawasaki disease	No	May precede development of systemic vasculitis.
Isolated PNS angiitis	Yes	
Pauci-immune small-vessel		
Wegener granulomatosis	Yes	cANCA, glomerulonephritis, granulomatous upper and lower respiratory involvement.
Churg-Strauss syndrome	Yes	pANCA, usually respiratory involvement (rhinitis, sinusitis, asthma), peripheral eosinophilia.
Microscopic polyangiitis	Yes	Similar to PAN, but lung involvement.
Immune-complex small-vessel		
Henoch-Schönlein purpura	No	
Cryoglobulinemic vasculitis	Yes	

cANCA, circulating anti-neutrophil cytoplasmic antibody; ESR, erythrocyte sedimentation rate; GI, gastrointestinal; PAN, polyarteritis nodosa; pANCA, perinuclear anti-neutrophil cytoplasmic antibody; PNS, peripheral nervous system.

- Intense pain lasts days to weeks, replaced by weakness (usually proximal), with little sensory disturbance.
- Good prognosis; nearly 90% with functional recovery at 3 years.

- **Pathophysiology:**
  - Unclear; probably microangiopathic/autoimmune.
  - Male predominance, unilateral in two-thirds of patients.
  - Antecedent/concurrent illness in ~50%.
  - Rarely hereditary (see hereditary neuropathies).

Diabetic Lumbosacral Radiculoplexopathy (Bruns-Garland Syndrome, Diabetic Amyotrophy)

- **Symptoms:**
  - Severe, acute unilateral hip, thigh, low back pain, with mild tingling/numbness, worsening over days, then resolving.
  - Weakness/atrophy develops over days to weeks, lasts weeks to months, occasionally permanent.
  - Association with diabetes; sometimes preceded by rapid weight loss.
- **Pathophysiology:** May be microangiopathic due to endothelial damage.
- **Laboratory:** CSF protein normal to mildly elevated, CSF WBCs normal. ESR can be elevated.
- **Treatment:** Prednisone can help pain; use caution in diabetes.

Peripheral Neurosarcoidosis

- **Symptoms:**
  - Relapsing and remitting multiple mononeuropathies (especially cranial nerves) with or without simultaneous myositis.
  - Approximately 5% of patients with systemic sarcoidosis (lungs, hilar adenopathy, uveitis, liver, spleen, parotids) develop CNS or PNS disease.
- **Diagnosis:**
  - Chest x-ray: Hilar adenopathy.
  - Angiotensin-converting enzyme (ACE) levels unhelpful.
  - Histopathology: Noncaseating granulomas within and around peripheral nerves and associated blood vessels.

Isaac Syndrome

Symptoms

- Progressive and widespread muscle stiffness.
- Muscle twitching (myokymia) and cramps/carpopedal spasm.
- Persists during sleep.
- Fluctuating in severity over weeks to months.
- Sometimes hyperhidrosis.
- Sometimes encephalopathy, insomnia.

Laboratory

- Antibodies against voltage-gated potassium channels (VGKC).
- Cramps, fasciculations, neuromyotonia on EMG.

Pathophysiology

- Spontaneous or paraneoplastic (small cell cancer, thymoma, lymphoma).
- Association with other autoimmune diseases.

Treatment

- Some respond to immunomodulation (eg, IVIG, plasma exchange, corticosteroids).
- Na^+ channel blockade (eg, carbamazepine, phenytoin) helps symptoms.

Stiff-Person Syndrome

Symptoms

- Progressive rigidity and spasms of the trunk and limbs, with or without encephalomyelitis.
- Spasms worsened by stimulation, startle, emotions.
- Thirty percent develop diabetes.

Laboratory

- Antiglutamic acid decarboxylase (GAD) antibodies in 60%.
- Some have anti-amphiphysin antibodies.
- Creatine kinase (CK) levels can be elevated.

Pathophysiology

- GAD synthesizes gamma-aminobutyric acid (GABA) from glutamic acid; reduced inhibition of upper motor neurons → hyperactivity.
- GAD present in pancreatic islet cells → diabetes.
- Spontaneous or paraneoplastic (especially lymphoma, small cell lung cancer, colon, breast).
- Associated with other autoimmune disorders (myasthenia gravis, thyroiditis, SLE, RA).

Treatment

- GABA-ergic medications (eg, diazepam, gabapentin).
- Baclofen (PO or intrathecal).
- Immunomodulation (eg, IVIG, plasma exchange, corticosteroids) can occasionally help.

INFECTIOUS NEUROPATHIES

Leprosy

Symptoms

- Three disease types (lepromatous, tuberculoid, and borderline) based on clinical and histopathologic features (see Table 11.8).
- Diagnosis typically made via skin or nerve biopsy.

TABLE 11.8. Classification of Leprosy

	Lepromatous	Borderline	Tuberculoid
Skin findings	Many small macules/papules. Predominates in cooler areas of the skin (eg, face, limbs).	Intermediate	Several large plaques, erythematous with central pallor and anesthesia. Raised edges.
Neuropathy	Diffuse dissemination → distal symmetric polyneuropathy more common than focal neuropathies.	Intermediate	Focal involvement and robust immune response → focal neuropathies, especially ulnar at the elbow, median in the forearm, peroneal at the fibular head, superficial radial nerve, and greater auricular nerve.
Cell-mediated immunity	Impaired; Th2 response predominant (IL-4, IL-5, IL-10).	Intermediate	Intact; TH1 response and macrophage activity predominant (IL-2, gamma-interferon).
Histopathology	Fite-Faraco stain for organisms shows abundant mycobacteria, and few inflammatory cells are identified.	Intermediate	Fite-Faraco stain typically negative. Robust inflammatory response with granulomas and multinucleated giant cells.

Epidemiology

- Most common cause of neuropathy in the world.
- Common in third-world settings (eg, Southeast Asia, South America, Africa).
- Some regions of the United States (eg, Texas, Hawaii, Florida).
- Armadillos = natural reservoir.
- Transmitted by contact and via nasal droplets.
- Most who are infected develop immunity without disease.

Lyme Neuropathies

> A 42-year-old man presents with several days of bilateral facial weakness, causing labial dysarthria, drooling, and incomplete eye closure. The remainder of his neurological exam is normal. Two weeks ago, he completed a weeklong hike along the Appalachian Trail. What is the likely diagnosis, and what testing should be done to exclude alternatives?
>
> Lyme disease, Stage 2, is most likely, especially given the history of potential exposure to infected ticks. Lyme serology can confirm the diagnosis; TB, sarcoidosis, and other meningeal processes (eg, lymphoma, carcinoma) should be considered.

Symptoms

- **Stage 1:**
  - Early infection/erythema migrans.
  - Expanding erythematous rash with central pallor (bull's eye).
- **Stage 2:**
  - Disseminated Lyme.
  - Hematogenous spread → cranial neuropathies (especially CN VII) and radiculopathies.
  - Less commonly focal neuropathy/plexopathy.
  - CNS and cardiac complications occur in stages 2 and 3.
- **Stage 3:**
  - Chronic Lyme.
  - Late-stage/chronic untreated Lyme can result in distal symmetric polyneuropathy.

Epidemiology

- In the United States, caused by spirochete *Borrelia burgdorferi.*
- Transmitted by tick bite after 24–48 hours of tick attachment.
- Endemic in Northeast and western Great Lakes (especially Wisconsin, Minnesota).
- Symptoms most common from May to September.
- Long incubation period: Consider Lyme year-round.

HIV Neuropathies

Various presentations:

- Chronic and progressive distal symmetric sensory > motor polyneuropathy, usually in patients who meet criteria for AIDS.
- AIDP or CIDP—even at seroconversion (check HIV in suspected AIDP/CIDP, especially if CSF pleocytosis).
- Polyradiculopathy, most commonly lumbosacral, probably due to neuronal CMV infection and inflammation.

- Multiple mononeuropathies: HIV, HIV-associated CMV, and hepatitis B or C → vasculitic process/mononeuritis multiplex.
- Sensory neuronopathy: Severe ataxia, prominent sensory disturbance and paresthesias.

Human T-Lymphotropic Virus-1 (HTLV-1)

Typically causes tropical spastic paraparesis (due to a myelopathic process), but occasionally causes a sensory > motor polyneuropathy and/or a myopathy.

CMV

In immunocompromised patients, CMV typically causes acute polyradiculopathy (especially lumbosacral) or multiple mononeuropathies.

EBV

Most strongly associated with AIDP but can cause cranial neuropathies, polyradiculopathies, multiple mononeuropathies.

Herpes/VZV

Symptoms

- **Shingles/zoster:** Painful sensory radiculopathy (thoracic > lumbosacral and cranial roots; cervical roots rare) associated with a vesicular rash.
- Postherpetic neuralgia: Pain/sensory loss > 1 month.
- **Ramsay Hunt syndrome:**
  - Viral reactivation in geniculate ganglion of the facial nerve.
  - Acute/subacute severe facial weakness.
  - Vesicular rash in external auditory canal.
  - Pain is severe around the ear, head, or neck.
  - Taste can be abnormal (dysgeusia).
  - Hyperacusis due to dysfunction of fibers to stapedius.
  - If CN VIII is affected → dizziness and hearing loss.

Cause

- Reactivation of latent infection of dorsal root ganglia neurons.
- VZV can cause cranial neuropathies, myelopathy, encephalitis.

Hepatitis B and C

- Hepatitis-associated vasculitis → mononeuritis multiplex.
- HCV and type III cryoglobulinemia → distal sensory polyneuropathy.

Diphtheria

Symptoms

- Myalgias and fever ~1 week after exposure.
- Approximately 50% develop neuropathy:
- Bulbar weakness (dysarthria, dysphagia, respiratory weakness).
- Autonomic dysfunction can be severe.
- Blurred near vision due to failure of accommodation.
- Generalized polyneuropathy can develop months after acute infection, with distal sensory disturbance/weakness and hyporeflexia.

Pathophysiology

Binding of diphtheria toxin to Schwann cells in nerve roots and dorsal root ganglia → neuropathy.

ENDOCRINOPATHIES

Diabetic Neuropathies

- **Distal symmetric sensory > motor polyneuropathy:**
  - Most common by far.
  - Mix of axonal and demyelinating findings.
  - Possible mechanisms: Impaired metabolism (eg, altered glycosylation of proteins), microangiopathy due to hyperglycemia-induced endothelial damage, autoimmunity.
- **Autonomic neuropathy:**
  - Common, usually mild.
  - Constipation, postprandial bloating, orthostasis, abnormal sweating, dry eyes/mouth, sexual dysfunction.
- **Focal cranial neuropathies** (especially III, VI): Typically acute-subacute orbital pain/headache, followed by ophthalmoparesis (and ptosis with CN III).
- **Thoracoabdominal radiculopathy:**
  - Similar to shingles, but no rash.
  - Focal weakness of abdominal muscles can mimic abdominal hernia.
  - Weakness distinguishes from shingles (typically affects only sensory roots).
- **Diabetic proximal neuropathies:**
  - Brachial neuritis.
  - Lumbosacral radiculoplexopathy.
- **Mononeuropathies:** Compressive—carpal tunnel, ulnar at the elbow, peroneal at fibular head.

Hypothyroidism

- Carpal tunnel syndrome common, may be due to soft-tissue edema.
- Distal symmetric sensory > motor polyneuropathy can occur, but pathophysiology unclear.

SYSTEMIC DISEASES

Uremic Neuropathy

- Distal symmetric sensory > motor polyneuropathy seen in most dialysis patients.
- Urea/other waste products (eg, β_2 microglobulin) are likely cause.

Malabsorption and Gastrointestinal Surgery

- Typically distal symmetric sensory > motor polyneuropathy.
- Most likely cause: Vitamin deficiency, especially B_{12}, E, copper (see Nutritional Neuropathies).
- Autoimmune neuropathies such as AIDP can occur in association with autoimmune GI disorders (eg, Crohn disease, ulcerative colitis).

Critical Illness

- Neuropathy can occur in any critically ill patient.
- Critical-illness myopathy may be more common.
- Either can cause severe weakness, failure to wean from ventilator.
- Risk factors: Multiple organ failure, prolonged use of neuromuscular blocking agents, high-dose corticosteroids.

MALIGNANCIES

- One to 5% of patients with malignancy have clinically evident neuropathy.
- Any carcinoma, most common in lung cancers.
- Lymphoproliferative malignancies.
- Potential causes:
  - Direct invasion (rare).
  - Triggered autoimmunity/paraneoplastic.
  - Paraprotein related.
  - Toxic (chemotherapy, radiation).

Hematologic Malignancies and Paraproteinemias (Table 11.9)

- **Paraproteins:** Excess immunoglobulins, either polyclonal or monoclonal.
- **Monoclonal gammopathies:**
  - Caused by clonal expansion of a plasma cell line (can be non-malignant or malignant).
  - Four times more common in idiopathic peripheral neuropathies than other neuropathies.
- **Pathogenesis of paraproteinemic neuropathy:**
  - Unclear, presumably autoimmune.
  - Nerve infiltration generally only in amyloidosis.
  - Immunomodulation/immunosuppression usually does not affect the course; treatment of a hematologic malignancy can sometimes be helpful.

TABLE 11.9. Paraproteinemic Neuropathies

Disease	Protein	Notes
Multiple myeloma	IgG/IgA (κ > λ)	Distal axonal sensory/motor—fatigue, bone pain, hypercalcemia, anemia.
MGUS	IgG/IgA	Distal axonal sensorimotor (can be demyelinating).
	IgM 50% with anti-MAG antibodies	With ataxia and distal demyelination (distal acquired demyelinating symmetric [DADS] neuropathy).
	IgM 50% without anti-MAG antibodies	
Osteosclerotic myeloma	IgG/IgA (almost always λ)	POEMS/Castleman disease.
Waldenstrom macroglobulinemia	IgM	Anemia, fatigue, lymphoplasmacytoid cells.
Amyloidosis	AL λ:κ ratio 3:1	Early painful sensory and autonomic, commonly with compressive neuropathies (carpal tunnel, ulnar neuropathies).
	AA	Protein A accumulation in RA, connective tissue disease—neuropathy is uncommon.
	FAP	Familial transthyretin, apolipoprotein A-1, or gelsolin mutation.

AA, amyloid composed of protein A; AL, amyloid composed of light chains; FAP, familial amyloid polyneuropathy; MGUS, monoclonal gammopathy of uncertain significance; POEMS, polyneuropathy, organomegaly, endocrinopathy, M-spike, and skin changes.

Multiple Myeloma (MM)

- Monoclonal expansion of plasma cells → monoclonal gammopathy.
- Fatigue, bone pain, hypercalcemia, anemia.
- About two-thirds of neuropathies associated with MM are due to amyloid (AL) accumulation.

Osteosclerotic Myeloma and POEMS

- Approximately 3% myelomas associated with osteosclerotic lesions.
- Approximately 50% have polyneuropathy, with or without features of **POEMS:**
  - **P**olyneuropathy (symmetric).
  - **O**rganomegaly (hepatosplenomegaly, ascites, papilledema).
  - **E**ndocrinopathy (hypothyroidism, gynecomastia, testicular atrophy, amenorrhea).
  - **M**onoclonal gammopathy.
  - **S**kin changes (hyperpigmentation, hypertrichosis, edema, clubbing).
- Associated with elevated vascular endothelial growth factor (VEGF), reduced erythropoetin.
- Other malignancies associated with POEMS: Angiofollicular lymphadenopathy (Castleman disease,) extramedullary plasmacytoma.

Amyloidosis-Related Neuropathy

- Neuropathy: Length-dependent small fiber.
  - Burning, painful distal paresthesias.
  - Autonomic symptoms (orthostasis, edema, GI, sexual dysfunction).
  - Compressive neuropathies (eg, carpal tunnel) due to nerve enlargement.
- Treatment directed at reducing production of monoclonal proteins.

TOXIC NEUROPATHIES

Chemotherapy and Other Medications

- **Taxanes:** Paclitaxel, docetaxel—promote microtubule assembly and interfere with axonal transport, resulting in a length-dependent sensory > motor polyneuropathy.
- **Vinca alkaloids:** Vincristine, vinblastine, vindesine, vinorelbine—interfere with microtubule assembly and axonal transport, resulting in length-dependent sensory > motor polyneuropathy.
- **Platinum agents:** Cisplatin—interferes with DNA repair. Neuropathy predominantly of sensory neurons (cell bodies of the dorsal root ganglia); results in sensory neuropathy with prominent sensory ataxia.
- **Cytosine arabinoside (Ara-C):** Interferes with DNA polymerization. Can cause a pure sensory neuropathy (like platinum). Autoimmune neuropathies (GBS, brachial neuritis) have been described.

Heavy Metals and Industrial Toxins

- **Arsenic:**
  - Acute abdominal pain, nausea, vomiting, diarrhea, then burning distal paresthesias, distal weakness.
  - Axonal sensorimotor neuropathy begins 5–20 days after exposure, progresses over weeks.
  - Proximal and cranial/bulbar weakness when severe.
  - **Mees lines** in the fingernails and toenails develop after weeks.
  - Pancytopenia and basophilic stippling of RBCs.
  - Supportive treatment.

- **Lead:**
  - Slow onset of upper- > lower-limb weakness; classic is wrist and finger drop.
  - Motor axonal neuropathy, usually no sensory complaints.
  - Basophilic stippling of RBCs, microcytosis, and hypochromia.
  - Twenty-four-hour urine lead excretion elevated.
  - Treated with chelation.
- **Mercury:**
  - Primarily motor axonal neuropathy.
  - CNS effects: Encephalopathy, ataxia, psychosis.
- **Thallium:**
  - Severe axonal sensorimotor neuropathy.
  - Burning pain and paresthesias in the feet.
  - Nausea/vomiting and (after weeks) alopecia.
  - When severe, proximal and cranial/bulbar weakness.
  - Anemia, uremia, hepatic dysfunction.
- **Gold:**
  - Rarely used to treat rheumatoid arthritis.
  - Mixed axonal/demyelinating neuropathy, primarily motor.
  - Some distal hypesthesia.
- **Alcohol:**
  - High levels of intake (> 100 g/day for years) → length-dependent axonal sensorimotor polyneuropathy.
  - Due to a direct toxic effect, nutritional deficiency (especially B vitamins, folate), or both.

NUTRITIONAL NEUROPATHIES

B_1 (Thiamine) Deficiency

- Severe malnutrition, historically common in alcoholics.
- Give thiamine to hospitalized patients with altered mental status.
- → beriberi:
  - Neuropathy, primarily axonal, → profound weakness.
  - "Wet": Congestive heart failure (CHF)/extremity edema.
  - "Dry": No CHF, weakness severe.

B_6 (Pyridoxine) Deficiency

- B_6 deficiency seen in alcoholics, severely malnourished patients.
  - Can be induced by isoniazid (treatment of TB), hydralazine.
  - Distal symmetric sensory > motor polyneuropathy.
- B_6 toxicity due to excess supplementation: Acute/subacute sensory neuronopathy (non-length-dependent sensory loss, paresthesias, ataxia).

B_{12} (Cobalamin) Deficiency

Symptoms

- Encephalopathy.
- Combined systems degeneration:
  - Posterior columns: Decreased vibratory and position sense.
  - Corticospinal tracts: Weakness, hyperreflexia, Babinski sign.
- Classically. Macrocytic anemia (masked by folate supplementation).

Pathophysiology

- Cobalamin is a cofactor in DNA synthesis.
- DNA synthesis required for myelin metabolism (see Figure 11.4).

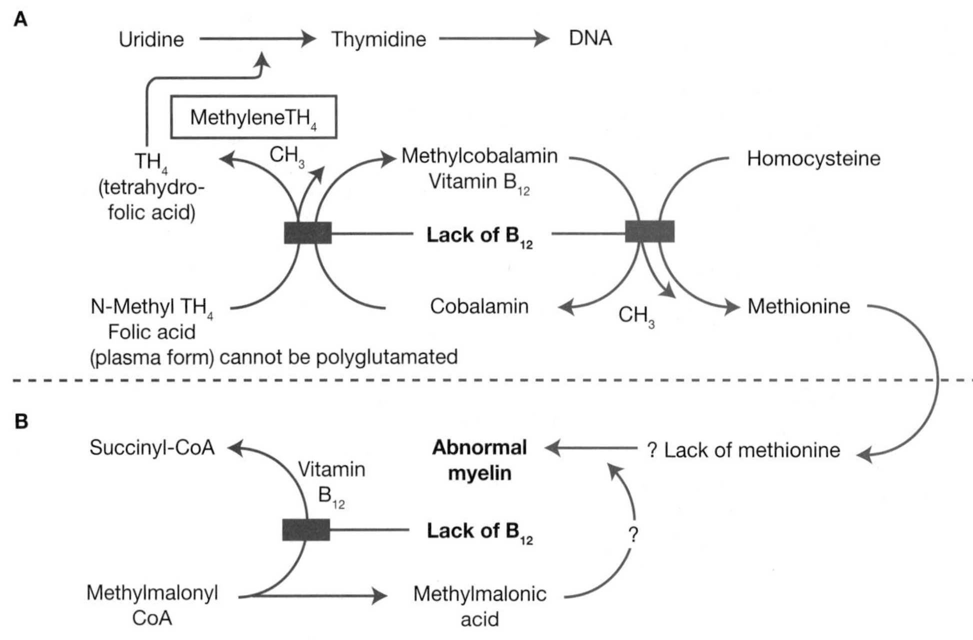

FIGURE 11.4. Role of B_{12} and folate in myelin metabolism. Folate is responsible for demethylation of tetrahydrofolate. "Lack of B_{12} or folate retards DNA synthesis (A), and lack of B_{12} leads to loss of folate, which cannot be held intracellularly unless polyglutamated. B_{12} deficiency also leads to abnormal myelin synthesis, probably via deficiency in methionine production (B)." (Reproduced, with permission, from McPhee SJ, Papadakis MA, Tierney LM Jr. *Current Medical Diagnosis & Treatment 2008,* 47th ed. New York: McGraw-Hill, 2007: Figure 13-1.)

- Dietary deficiency (naturally found in animal flesh only).
- Lack of intrinsic factor (gastrectomy, antibodies against parietal cells → pernicious anemia).
- Disease/resection of terminal ileum.
- Exposure to nitrous oxide (inactivates methylcobalamin).
- Low-"normal" B_{12} levels can cause symptoms and may be associated with elevated levels of methylmalonic acid and homocysteine.

KEY FACT

Nitrous oxide (NO) inactivates methylcobalamin. In patients with subclinical B_{12} deficiency, exposure to NO can cause acute combined systems degeneration. Exposure to NO usually occurs during anesthesia or as an inhaled recreational drug (ie, "whippets").

Treatment

IM B_{12} replacement.

Folic Acid Deficiency

- Symptoms, causes, pathophysiology similar to B_{12} deficiency.
- Macrocytic anemia is strongly associated.
- Pure folate deficiency is very rare.

Vitamin E Deficiency

Symptoms

- Non-length-dependent sensory loss and hyporeflexia.
- Prominent sensory ataxia, gait instability and Romberg sign, pseudoathetosis, "sensory drift."

Pathophysiology

- The fat-soluble vitamins, A, D, E, and K, are absorbed in small intestines.
- Deficiency primarily damages dorsal root ganglia neurons, but also affects other large myelinated nerves.

- Deficiency caused by:
  - Fat malabsorption.
  - Familial abnormalities of lipid metabolism (eg, abetaliproteinemia, Bassen-Kornzweig syndrome).
  - Rare inherited abnormalities of vitamin E metabolism.

IDIOPATHIC AND HEREDITARY NEUROPATHIES, INCLUDING MOTOR NEURON DISEASES

Amyotrophic Lateral Sclerosis (ALS)

Epidemiology

- Annual incidence of 0.5–3 in 100,000.
- Approximately 90% sporadic, 10% familial.
- Two to 3% due to mutation in copper/zinc superoxide dismutase (SOD1).

Pathophysiology

- Unclear combination of genetic and environmental factors.
- Hypotheses as to final pathways:
  - Oxidative stress.
  - Glutamate excitotoxicity.
  - Mitochondrial dysfunction.

Symptoms and Signs

- Slowly progressive weakness.
- Typically asymmetric onset, regional spread, eventually → bulbar and respiratory weakness.
- Many patients have either upper or lower motor neuron (UMN/LMN) dysfunction early in their course, but most go on to develop both.
- Extraocular movements and bowel/bladder sphincter functions typically spared.
- Signs of LMN dysfunction:
  - Atrophy
  - Fasciculations
  - Cramps
- Signs of UMN dysfunction:
  - Slowness.
  - Spasticity.
  - Hyperreflexia (consider reflexes increased when easily elicitable in an atrophied limb).
  - Clonus, spreading, Hoffman/Babinski signs.
  - Pseudobulbar affect (inappropriate laughing/crying).
  - "Frontal release signs" (rooting, snout, glabellar signs).
- Four clinical syndromes:
  - Primary muscular atrophy (~10%): LMN dysfunction without UMN involvement—atrophy and fasciculations without spasticity, slowness, or hyperreflexia.
  - Progressive bulbar palsy (1–2%): Exclusively bulbar LMN dysfunction without UMN or limb involvement—dysarthria and dysphagia without slow, "spastic" quality or hyperreflexia.
  - Primary lateral sclerosis (1–3%): UMN dysfunction alone—weakness, slowness, spasticity, and hyperreflexia without atrophy or fasciculations.
  - "True" ALS: UMN and LMN dysfunction affecting limbs, bulbar, and respiratory muscles—slowness, spasticity, weakness, atrophy, fasciculations, hyperreflexia.

LABORATORY

- EMG/NCS show evidence of motor denervation/reinnervation, without demyelinating findings to suggest multifocal motor neuropathy (MMN).
- CK can be mildly to moderately elevated.

TREATMENT

- Riluzole 50 mg PO bid may add 2–3 months of tracheostomy-free survival, but does not increase overall life expectancy, strength, or quality of life. Possible GI side effects, hepatotoxicity.
- Consider gastrostomy for tube feedings.
- Consider noninvasive ventilation (eg, bilevel positive airway pressure [BiPAP]) and/or tracheostomy.
- Supportive care and treatment of spasticity, constipation, salivation, depression, dysphagia.

Kennedy Disease (X-Linked Bulbospinal Muscular Atrophy)

- Adult-onset (usually third to fifth decade) LMN dysfunction.
- Most severe in bulbar and proximal limb muscles (dysarthria, dysphagia, limb atrophy, and fasciculations).
- Gynecomastia and testicular atrophy.
- Mutation in the androgen receptor gene on chromosome Xq11–12.
- Sensory neuronopathy with low-amplitude SNAPs on NCS (patients only rarely complain of sensory disturbances).

Spinal Muscular Atrophy (SMA)

- Weakness and muscular atrophy, typically with fasciculations.
- Can present at any age.
- Classified by age of onset and severity (Table 11.10).

PATHOPHYSIOLOGY

- Autosomal recessive mutation in the spinal motor neuron (SMN) gene on chromosome 5q.
- Muscle biopsy: Extreme fiber type grouping, grouped atrophy.

Hereditary Neuralgic Amyotrophy

- Recurrent neuralgic amyotrophy ("brachial neuritis").
- Associated with hypotelorism, syndactyly, short stature.
- Rare AD disorder associated with SEPT9 mutation on chromosome 17.

TABLE 11.10. Classification of Spinal Muscular Atrophy

DISEASE	AGE OF ONSET	NOTES
SMA type I (Werdnig-Hoffman)	Birth–6 months	"Floppy baby": Severe weakness, poor feeding, frog-leg posture. Survival measured in years.
SMA type II (intermediate type)	6–18 months	Generalized weakness, sometimes sit unsupported initially. Survival to second or third decade, occasionally longer.
SMA type III (Kugelberg-Welander)	After 18 months, including adulthood	Typically presents in first few decades, prognosis variable. In adulthood, axial and respiratory weakness are common presenting symptoms.

Charcot-Marie-Tooth Disease (CMT; Hereditary Motor and Sensory Neuropathy)

Historically classified by conduction velocity on NCS (demyelinating vs axonal), age of onset, and mode of inheritance.

- **CMT1:**
  - Demyelinating motor and sensory neuropathy.
  - Most common CMT.
  - **Symptoms:** Age of onset varies; usually childhood to early adulthood. Weakness, primarily distal, pes cavus (high arched feet), hammertoes, distal atrophy, foot drop → "steppage" gait, sensory loss all modalities; patients rarely complain, reflexes reduced, tremor in approximately one-third **(Roussy-Levy syndrome).**
  - **Laboratory and special features:** Most autosomal dominant except CMT 1X (X-linked dominant). Motor nerve conduction velocities uniformly < 38 m/s. SNAPs usually low amplitude/unobtainable. No conduction block, temporal dispersion (if present, think CIDP). CSF protein can be elevated. Nerve biopsy: Reduced myelin, Schwann cell proliferation → "onion bulbs."
  - **Various mutations:**
    - CMT 1A: Peripheral myelin protein (PMP-22) duplication 17p11.2–12.
    - CMT 1B: Myelin protein zero (MPZ) on 1q22–23.
    - CMT 1C: Lipopolysaccharaide-induced TNF-α factor (LITAF).
    - CMT 1D: Early growth response 2 (ERG2) on 10q21.1–22.1.
    - CMT 1E: Point mutations in PMP-22.
    - CMT 1F: Neurofilament light chain (NF-L) on 8p13–21.
    - CMT 1X: Connexin-32.
    - HNPP: PMP-22 deletion or MPZ mutation: Also called tomaculous neuropathy; presents in second to third decade; painless numbness/weakness in single nerve territory; most common at compression sites (peroneal nerve at fibular head, ulnar nerve at elbow, median nerve at wrist); reduced reflexes, sometimes pes cavus, hammertoes.
- **CMT2** (axonal motor and sensory neuropathy):
  - **Symptoms:** Similar to CMT1 (distal > proximal weakness, asymptomatic sensory loss). Relatively more atrophy than CMT1. Reflexes often diminished only distally.
  - **Laboratory and special features:** Most are autosomal dominant except CMT 2B1 (AR).
    - CMT 2A1: Microtubule motor kinesin-like protein.
    - CMT 2A2: Mitofusin-2 (MFN2). Most common CMT2. Sometimes optic atrophy, hearing loss, subcortical white matter abnormalities on MRI.
    - CMT 2B1: Lamin A/C. Allelic with LGMD 1B. Nerve biopsy: Axonal atrophy, few/no onion bulbs.
- **Dominant intermediate CMT (DI-CMT):**
  - Intermediate conduction velocities (mild slowing > 38 m/s).
  - Demyelinating and axonal features on biopsy.
  - AD inheritance.
  - Clinical features similar to CMT1/2.
- **CMT3:**
  - Autosomal dominant, severe demyelination, early childhood.
  - Also called Dejérine-Sottas disease.
  - Presents infancy–early childhood with generalized weakness, hyporeflexia, arthrogryposis, respiratory distress.
  - Most due to spontaneous PMP-22, MPZ, or ERG2 point mutations.

- Biopsy: Hypomyelination, prominent onion bulbs.
- Severe cases: Complete lack of myelination, severe generalized weakness, death in infancy.

- **CMT4:** Autosomal recessive, presents in childhood to adulthood.
  - Severe, childhood onset.
  - Delayed motor milestones, pes cavus, scoliosis.
  - Autosomal recessive.
  - Demyelinating or axonal features.

Hereditary Sensory and Autonomic Neuropathy (HSAN)

- **HSAN 1:**
  - Slowly progressive sensory loss in teens to 30s.
  - Primarily small-fiber loss (pain, temperature).
  - Distal skin ulcers, Charcot joints.
  - Mild autonomic dysfunction (bladder dysfunction, reduced distal sweating).
  - AD inheritance.
  - Mutation in serine palmitoyltransferase long chain base 1 (SPTLC1) on 9q22.
- **HSAN 2:**
  - Severe sensory loss and areflexia at birth/early childhood.
  - Distal skin ulcers, Charcot joints.
  - Impaired sweating, bladder dysfunction.
  - AR inheritance.
  - Mutation in PRKWNK1 on 12p13.33.
- **HSAN 3:**
  - Also called Riley-Day syndrome, familial dysautonomia.
  - Presents in infancy.
  - Body temperature fluctuation, blood pressure, repeated vomiting, GI dysmotility, sweating, tonic pupils, orthostatic hypotension.
  - Most common in Ashkenazi Jews.
  - AR inheritance.
  - IKB kinase complex-associated protein (IKAP) on 9q31.
- **HSAN 4:**
  - Presents in infancy/childhood.
  - Insensitivity to pain, self-mutilation, anhidrosis.
  - Mental retardation, risk of hyperthermia.
  - AR inheritance.
  - Tyrosine kinase A nerve growth factor (trkA/NGF) on 3q.
- **HSAN 5:**
  - Congenital indifference (not insensitivity) to pain.
  - Normal sensation otherwise, normal reflexes.

Distal Hereditary Motor Neuropathy (DHMN)

Also called distal spinal muscular atrophy (SMA).

Hereditary Neuropathies Associated with Disorders of Lipid Metabolism

- Metachromatic leukodystrophy
- Krabbe disease
- Fabry disease
- Adrenoleukodystrophy
- Adrenomyeloneuropathy
- Refsum disease
- Tangier disease
- Cerebrotendinous xanthomatosis

Hereditary Neuropathies Associated with Ataxia

- Friedreich ataxia
- Vitamin E deficiency
- Spinocerebellar ataxia
- Abetalipoproteinemia (Bassen-Kornzweig disease)

Other Hereditary Neuropathies

- Ataxia-telangectasia
- Cockayne syndrome
- Giant axonal neuropathy
- Acute intermittent porphyria

Disorders of the Neuromuscular Junction

AUTOIMMUNE DISORDERS

Myasthenia Gravis (MG)

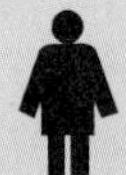

A 21-year-old woman presents with fluctuating ptosis and mild ophthalmoparesis causing blurred and sometimes double vision. She has antibodies against acetylcholine receptors. What further diagnostic testing should be performed?

The diagnosis of ocular myasthenia gravis is established by the classic presentation and AChR antibodies. CT of the chest should be performed to exclude thymoma (which would require surgery).

Epidemiology

- Most common NMJ disorder. Annual incidence of 0.25–2 per 100,000. No seasonal or geographic gradients.
- Early-onset MG (< 40) is about 3 times more common in women.
- Late-onset MG (> 40) is slightly more common in men, and represents more than 60% of new cases.
- Childhood MG is rare but is more common in Asian populations.
- Increased incidence of other autoimmune disorders; ~5% of MG patients have hyperthyroidism.

Symptoms and Signs

- Muscular weakness and fatigability worsening with repeated activities.
- Ptosis, diplopia, dysphagia, dysarthria, dyspnea, weakness of neck extensors (head drop), limb weakness—typically roughly symmetric.
- Occasionally very focal; can remain localized for many years.
- Can be classified as:
  - **Ocular MG** (ptosis and ophthalmoparesis only; see Table 11.11).
  - **Generalized MG** (bulbar, diaphragmatic, limb weakness, +/– ocular weakness).
- **Cogan twitch:** When rapidly looking up, ptotic eyelid briefly opens fully and then returns to the "droop" position.
- **Icepack test:** Cooling eyelid with ice can sometimes improve ptosis.

Pathophysiology

- IgG antibodies against nicotinic acetylcholine receptor (AChR) α_1 subunit.

TABLE 11.11. Neuromuscular Causes of Ptosis and Ophthalmoparesis

LOCALIZATION	DISEASE CATEGORY AND DISEASE	
Peripheral nerve		AIDP (Fisher variant)
Neuromuscular junction	Postsynaptic	Myasthenia gravis
	Presynaptic	Botulism
	Pre- or postsynaptic	LEMS
		Congenital myasthenias
Muscle	Dystrophies	Myotonic dystrophy (ptosis), OPMD
	Mitochondrial myopathies	PEO/KSS
	Congenital myopathies	Centronuclear myopathy
	Hyperthyroidism	Nemaline myopathy (ptosis)

AIDP, acute inflammatory demyelinating polyradiculoneuropathy; KSS, Kearns-Sayre syndrome; PEO, progressive external ophthalmoplegia; LEMS, Lambert-Eaton myasthenic syndrome; OPMD, oculopharyngeal muscular dystrophy.

- Interfere directly with function of the AChR.
- Reduce the number of AchRs.
- "Simplifies" postsynaptic folds, reducing size of muscle end plate.

Laboratory

- Anti-AchR antibodies detectable in ~85–90% of generalized MG, 50–70% of ocular MG, 100% of thymoma-associated MG.
- More than 50% of seronegative patients have antibodies against muscle-specific tyrosine kinase (MuSK).
- More than 10% decrement of CMAP amplitude with 2–3-Hz repetitive nerve stimulation (RNS). Single-fiber EMG (sfEMG): "jitter" and blocking of neuromuscular transmission.
- Edrophonium (Tensilon) test:
  - Short-acting (~5 minutes) cholinesterase inhibitor.
  - Test requires an objective sign (eg, ptosis, ophthalmoparesis) to observe.
  - 2 mg IV test dose, monitor for bradycardia, hypotension, GI side effects (cramping, diarrhea).
  - If test dose tolerated, administer another 8 mg (10 mg total).
  - If significant side effects: 1 mg atropine IV (prepared prior to starting the test).
- Chest CT scan, rule out thymoma.

Treatment

- Anticholinesterase medications: Increase availability of ACh at the NMJ.
  - Pyridostigmine (Mestinon): Onset 30 minutes, peak 2 hours, effect 4–6 hours; up to 120 mg PO q3h; more than 450 mg/day increases likelihood of cholinergic crisis (miosis, salivation, diarrhea, cramps, fasciculations); long-acting preparation at bedtime can improve AM weakness.
- Immunosuppression/immunomodulation:
  - Prednisone: Rapid benefit. High doses can transiently exacerbate symptoms at initiation (2–5% of patients).
  - Azathioprine (Imuran): Benefit can take months. Hepatotoxicity, bone marrow suppression (monitor CBC, LFTs), pancreatitis. Idiosyncratic reaction (fever, abdominal pain, nausea, vomiting, anorexia) in some.

- Cyclosporine A: Benefit in weeks to months. Nephrotoxicity and drug interactions. Contraindicated in pregnancy.
- Mycophenolate (CellCept): Unclear benefit in MG.
- Plasma exchange: Rapid benefits that last weeks. Risk of hypotension, bleeding, hypocalcemia, complications of IV access.
- IVIG: Improvement in days, benefit lasts weeks to months; 2 g/kg divided over 2–5 days for severe exacerbation. Expensive; headache and meningismus common. Can cause renal failure, rarely hyperviscosity (eg, stroke, myocardial infarction). Hypersensitivity/anaphylaxis risk is high in IgA deficiency.

- Thymectomy:
  - Clear indication in thymoma (all MG patients need CT).
  - Benefit of routine thymectomy less clear. Consider in young patients with moderate to severe seropositive generalized MG.
  - Avoid drugs known to exacerbate MG: Aminoglycoside antibiotics. Beta blockers. Calcium channel blockers. Antimalarials/antiarrhythmics (quinidine, procainamide). Thyroid replacement medications. Magnesium-containing preparations.
- Neonatal autoimmune MG:
  - Weakness (feeble cry, difficulty feeding) due to placental transfer of maternal IgG directed against the AChR.
  - Ten percent of babies born to mothers with MG; mother can be asymptomatic.
  - Typically resolves in weeks, responds to cholinesterase inhibitors.

Lambert-Eaton Myasthenic Syndrome (LEMS)

- **Epidemiology:**
  - Second most common NMJ disorder.
  - Most patients older than 40.
- **Symptoms and signs:**
  - Weakness and fatigability, usually proximal legs > arms > bulbar or ocular. Respiratory involvement rare.
  - Autonomic symptoms: Dry eyes, dry mouth, constipation, bladder/sexual dysfunction.
  - Weakness transiently improves after brief effort (facilitation): 10 seconds of exercise can cause a buildup of calcium in the motor nerve terminal, which briefly improves NMJ transmission.
- **Pathophysiology:**
  - Antibodies against P/Q type voltage-gated Ca^{2+} channels on motor axons interfere with binding and release of ACh-containing vesicles.
  - Paraneoplastic in about two-thirds; 90% of these related to small cell lung cancer (others include hematologic, ovarian, breast).

TOXIC/INFECTIOUS

Botulism

- **Symptoms/exam:**
  - Early nausea, vomiting. Initial diarrhea → constipation. Dry mouth, double vision, dysphagia and dysarthria, ptosis.
  - **Exam:** Generalized weakness, especially bulbar, hyporeflexia, and autonomic symptoms (eg, poorly responsive pupils).
  - **Foodborne botulism** develops over 12–36 hours.
  - **Wound botulism** develops over days to weeks; GI symptoms less common.

- **Infantile botulism** is on the differential for poor feeding and hypotonia.
- GI symptoms, autonomic symptoms, and pupillary abnormalities distinguish from myasthenia gravis.
- **Pathophysiology:** Caused by botulinum toxin produced by *Clostridium botulinum* in food, wounds, or intestinal flora (especially in neonates).
- **Treatment:**
  - Supportive, especially respiratory and management of ileus.
  - Antitoxin is helpful only within 24 hours after onset of symptoms.

Tick Paralysis

- Rapidly ascending weakness due to toxins produced by various ticks. In North America, common wood tick and dog tick.
- Some toxins block NMJ transmission, some block sodium channels at nodes of Ranvier.
- **Treatment:** Tick removal, supportive care.

Presynaptic Toxins

- Na^+ channels:
  - **Tetrodotoxin:** Na^+ channel blockade. Found in organs of Japanese pufferfish.
  - **Saxitoxin:** Na^+ channel blockade. Found in dinoflagellates (which cause red tide). Shellfish that feed on the dinoflagellates concentrate the toxin.
  - **Ciguatoxin:** Prolonged Na^+ channel opening. Found in dinoflagellates and accumulates in reef fish. Classic presentation is abdominal pain, oral and acral paresthesias, altered temperature sensation.
- K^+ channels:
  - **Aminopyridines:** Slow repolarization and promote ACh release (3,4 diaminopyridine used in LEMS).
  - **Dendrotoxin** (black mamba, green mamba).
  - **Notexin** (Australian tiger snake).
- Ca^{2+} channels:
  - **Ca^{2+}-channel blockers** (verapamil, diltiazem) can worsen myasthenia.
  - **Antibiotics,** especially aminoglycosides, can alter NMJ transmission presynaptically and postsynaptically.
  - Mg^{2+} inhibits calcium entry into nerve terminal.
  - **ω-conotoxin** (marine snail).

Synaptic Toxins (Anticholinesterases)

- Organophosphates:
  - Weaponized **nerve agents** (eg, tabun, sarin, soman, VX).
  - **Insecticides** (eg, parathion).
- **Symptoms related to cholinergic excess:**
  - Neurologic: Muscle twitching, flaccid paralysis, pinpoint pupils.
  - GI/autonomic: Salivation, sweating, nausea, vomiting, abdominal cramps, involuntary defecation/urination, bradycardia.
- **Treatment:**
  - Atropine (competes with ACh).
  - Pralidoxime (reactivates acetylcholinesterase).
  - Anticholinesterase medication overdose (pyridostigmine, neostigmine, edrophonium).

Postsynaptic Toxins

- NMJ-blocking toxins and medications:
  - **Curare:** Plant toxin that competitively blocks AChR.
  - Curare-related nondepolarizing NMJ-blocking medications (eg, pancuronium, vecuronium)—competitive blockade.
  - Depolarizing NMJ blockers (eg, succinlycholine): Bind and inactivate AChR.
  - Aminoglycosides.
  - Tetracyclines.
  - Procainamide.
  - Penicillamine.
- α-bungarotoxin/α-cobratoxin:
  - Bind to AChRs, used in research.
  - **α-bungarotoxin** produced by the banded krait.
  - **α-cobratoxin** produced by the Siamese cobra.

HEREDITARY NMJ DISORDERS

Symptoms

Congenital myasthenic syndromes present at birth or in infancy with hypotonia, weak cry, poor feeding.

Pathophysiology

Mutations affect various proteins important for NMJ transmission:

- **Presynaptic:**
  - Choline acetyltransferase deficiency.
  - Reduced synaptic vesicles and abnormal ACh release.
- **Synaptic:** End-plate acetylcholinesterase deficiency → increased ACh availability and end-plate desensitization (worsens with cholinesterase inhibitors).
- **Postsynaptic:**
  - Slow channel disorders: AD mutations of α-, β-, ε-subunits of AChR → prolonged opening of AChR channel.
  - Fast channel disorders: Either α-subunit mutation (AR inheritance), ε-subunit mutation (AD inheritance).
  - Primary AChR deficiency (AR mutation of ε-subunit → decreased number and abnormal density of AChRs).
  - Rapsyn deficiency.
  - Sodium channel myasthenia (mutation of Nav 1.4 Na^+ channel) interferes with action potential generation.
  - Plectin deficiency.
  - MuSK mutations.
  - Dok-7 mutation.

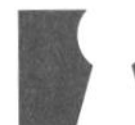

KEY FACT

Most congenital myasthenia syndromes can be improved by increasing availability of ACh in the neuromuscular junction. An important exception is acetylcholinesterase deficiency, in which the problem is the presence of too much acetylcholine in the NMJ.

Treatment

- No response to immunosuppression.
- Some respond to cholinesterase inhibitors or aminopyridines.
- End-plate AChE deficiency worsens with cholinesterase inhibitors.

Disorders of Muscle

Most myopathies present with painless proximal weakness. Muscle pain with normal strength, CK, and EMG is rarely due to muscle disease.

AUTOIMMUNE/INFLAMMATORY MYOPATHIES

Polymyositis/Dermatomyositis

Symptoms

- Subacute-chronic proximal > distal weakness (shoulder, hip girdle).
- Usually symmetric.
- Dysphagia common in both.
- DM: Childhood (juvenile DM) or adulthood (adult DM).
- PM: Rare before 18 years.
- Skin changes in dermatomyositis (DM):
  - Heliotrope rash (eyelid edema and purplish discoloration).
  - Erythematous photosensitive rash of upper trunk (shawl sign/V-neck rash).
  - Gottron papules (erythema, papular rash over knuckles).
  - Holster sign.
  - DM can manifest without rash (*sine dermatitis*).
- Associated with interstitial lung disease.

Laboratory

- CK moderately to severely elevated. Never normal in active PM, sometimes normal in DM.
- EMG myopathic.
- Ten percent have Jo-1 antibodies; 50% of Jo-1+ patients have interstitial lung disease (ILD).
- Pulmonary function tests:
  - In neuromuscular respiratory weakness, restrictive pattern, reduced MIP/MEP.
  - In ILD, reduced DL_{CO}.

Pathophysiology/Histopathology

- Associated with malignancy (6–45% in adult DM).
- Associated with other connective tissue disorders (SLE, Sjögrens, RA).
- Dermatomyositis:
  - Perifascicular atrophy: Fibers at outer edge of fascicles are atrophied/degenerating (specific).
  - Perivascular and perimysial inflammation (nonspecific).
  - Membrane attack complex (MAC) deposition on blood vessels.
  - Tubuloreticular inclusions in endothelial cells on EM.
- **Polymyositis:**
  - Endomysial inflammation invading non-necrotic muscle fibers (specific).
  - Endomysial $CD8^+$ T cells.

Treatment

Immunosuppression/immunomodulation: Corticosteroids, methotrexate, azathioprine, IVIG, plasma exchange, mycophenolate, rituximab.

Inclusion Body Myositis

- **Symptoms and signs:**
  - Onset usually > 30 (80% are older than 50).
  - Male predominance.
  - Subacute-chronic proximal > distal weakness and atrophy, usually asymmetric.
  - Predilection for finger flexors, wrist flexors, and quadriceps.
  - Dysphagia in one-third.
- **Laboratory:**
  - CK mildly to moderately elevated (< 10 times normal).
  - EMG myopathic/mixed neurogenic units; sensory nerve action potentials often reduced amplitude.
  - Can have antibodies against cytosolic 5′-nucleotidase.
- **Pathophysiology/histopathology:**
  - Some association with autoimmune diseases, but probably not a primary autoimmune disease.
  - Histopathology: Inclusion bodies (rimmed vacuoles), mononuclear invasion of non-necrotic fibers, intracellular amyloid deposits.
- **Treatment:** No effective treatment; does not respond to immune therapies.

OTHER ACQUIRED MYOPATHIES

A number of systemic conditions and toxicities can cause generalized, proximal > distal weakness.

- Associated with systemic disease:
  - Amyloidosis—usually light-chain amyloidosis, not familial. Accumulation of amyloid causes neuropathy (especially small-fiber/autonomic) and myopathy (symmetric proximal weakness).
  - Critical illness:
    - Risk factors: Prolonged severe illness, corticosteroids. Association with NMJ blocking agents is unclear. Common cause of failure to wean from ventilator.
    - Biopsy: Myofiber necrosis, absence of myosin thick filaments.
- Toxic/infectious myopathies:
  - Alcohol.
  - Medications: HMG-CoA reductase (statins), cyclosporine, amiodarone, antiretrovirals, corticosteroids, chloroquine/hydroxychloroquine, colchicine, vincristine.
  - Viral/bacterial/fungal/parasitic.
- Nutritional and endocrine myopathies:
  - Hyperthyroidism: Can be associated with hypokalemic periodic paralysis.
  - Hypothyroidism: Progressive proximal weakness and atrophy, myalgias, cramps, fatigue. Delayed relaxation of reflexes.
  - Diabetes can cause acute muscle infarction, usually in the thigh, presumably due to vasculopathy.
  - Hypercortisolism (Cushing syndrome) causes proximal weakness—CK and EMG usually normal.
  - Hyperparathyroidism.
  - Hypoparathyroidism.

KEY FACT

Absence of myosin thick filaments on EM is the board-exam clue to critical illness myopathy.

HEREDITARY MYOPATHIES

Classification confusing and semiarbitrary. Best classified by inheritance pattern and mutated gene/protein (see Table 11.12).

- **Muscular dystrophy:** Progressive hereditary myopathies with dystrophic histopathology (myofiber necrosis with fatty/connective tissue replacement).
- **Muscular dystrophy—congenital (MDC):** Muscular dystrophy clinically evident at birth or in infancy.
- **Congenital myopathies:** Hereditary myopathies lacking dystrophic histopathologic features. Most present at birth or infancy but can present in adulthood.

Muscular Dystrophies

X-Linked Dystrophies

- **Duchenne muscular dystrophy (DMD):**
  - X-linked recessive mutation → loss of dystrophin (sarcolemmal protein).
  - Frequently due to spontaneous mutation.
  - 1/3500 male births.
  - **Symptoms and signs:** Usually normal at birth, sit and stand at normal age. Age 2–6 develop waddling gait, slow running due to proximal weakness. Proximal weakness → **Gowers sign** (when getting up from the floor, patients "walk the hands up the thighs" to help raise the torso). Calf pseudohypertrophy due to fatty replacement. Frequent cardiomyopathy and conduction abnormalities. Scoliosis, joint contractures. Death commonly in second to third decade from respiratory or cardiac failure. Female carriers sometimes symptomatic.
  - **Laboratory:** CK usually 50–100 times normal. EMG is myopathic. DNA testing reveals deletions of dystrophin gene.
  - **Pathology:** Necrotic and regenerating muscle fibers, increased connective tissue, inflammation usually mild. Reduced or absent staining for dystrophin.
  - **Treatment:** Supportive—management of tendon contractures, scoliosis, cardiac disease, respiratory weakness. Corticosteroids temporarily increase strength and function, slow progression, but significant side effects.
- **Becker muscular dystrophy:**
  - X-linked recessive.
  - Truncation/partial loss of dystrophin.
  - Phenotype similar to Duchenne but less severe and more variable.
  - Walking until age 15 by definition; 40% cannot walk by age 30.
  - CK very elevated 20–200.
  - Histopathology similar to DMD but dystrophin staining can be relatively normal.
- **Emery-Dreifuss muscular dystrophy:**
  - X-linked recessive mutation affecting emerin, a nuclear membrane protein (see also the autosomal dominant forms, below).
  - Early tendon contractures—elbows, Achilles tendon, posterior cervical tendons.
  - Humeroperoneal weakness.
  - Cardiomyopathy and conduction abnormalities.
- **Limb girdle muscular dystrophies (LGMD):**
  - **Symptoms:** Variable age of onset, inheritance pattern, CK levels. Most have shoulder and hip girdle weakness and atrophy, with some excep-

TABLE 11.12. Genetic Classification of the Limb Girdle and Distal Muscular Dystrophies

Disease	Inheritance	Protein	Notes
X-linked dystrophies			
Duchenne	XR	Dystrophin	Onset 2–6 years, very high CK.
Becker	XR	Dystrophin	Similar to DMD but less severe.
Emery-Dreifuss	XR	Emerin	Joint contractures.
Limb girdle muscular dystrophies (LGMD)			
LGMD 1A	AD	Myotilin	Onset in adulthood, occasional distal predominance.
LGMD 1B	AD	Lamin A & C	Arryhythmias common.
LGMD 1C	AD	Caveolin-3	Some have "rippling muscle disease."
LGMD 1D	AD	DNAJB6	
LGMD 1E	AD	Desmin	
LGMD 1F	AD	TNPO3	
LGMD 2A	AR	Calpain-3	
LGMD 2B	AR	Dysferlin	Can have posterior calf atrophy (Miyoshi phenotype).
LGMD 2C	AR	γ-sarcoglycan	10% of LGMDs.
LGMD 2D	AR	α-sarcoglycan	
LGMD 2E	AR	β-sarcoglycan	
LGMD 2F	AR	δ-sarcoglycan	
LGMD 2G	AR	Telethonin	Quadriceps and anterior tibial atrophy/weakness.
LGMD 2H	AR	TRIM 32	
LGMD 2I	AR	FKRP	When severe = MDC 1C.
LGMD 2J	AR	Titin	Can be distal ("Udd distal myopathy").
LGMD 2K	AR	POMT1	When severe = Walker-Warburg MDC.
LGMD 2L	AR	ANO-5	
LGMD 2M	AR	Fukutin	
LGMD 2N	AR	POMT2	
LGMD 2O	AR	POMGnT1	
LGMD 2P	AR	α-dystroglycan	

TABLE 11.12. Genetic Classification of the Limb Girdle and Distal Muscular Dystrophies *(continued)*

Disease	Inheritance	Protein	Notes
LGMD 2Q	AR	Plectin	
LGMD 2R	AR	Desmin	
LGMD 2S	AR	TRAPC11	
Myofibrillar Myopathies			
	AD	Myotilin	Common feature: Disrupted Z-disk proteins → myofibrillar inclusions.
	AD	ZASP	
	AD	Filamin-c	
	AD	αB-crystallin	
	AD/AR	Desmin	
	AR	Titin	
	AD	DNAJB6	
	AD	TNPO3	
Hereditary IBM			
AR-Hereditary IBM	AR	GNE	
H-IBM with FTD and Paget disease	AD	VCP	
H-IBM 3	AD	MyHC IIa	
Distal dystrophies/myopathies			
Welander	AD	TIA	
Udd	AD	Titin	
Markesbery-Griggs	AD	ZASP	
Nonaka	AR	GNE	
Miyoshi	AR	Dysferlin	
Laing	AD	MyHC7	
Williams	AD	Filamin C	
Nebulin myopathy	AR	Nebulin	
Early-onset distal myopathy with Kelch-like 9 (*Drosophila*) mutation	AD	Kelch-like 9	

tions noted in Table 11.12. Historically categorized by inheritance type (AD for Type 1, or AR for Type 2).

- LGMDs of note:
  - **LGMD type 1** (autosomal dominant): LGMD1B (lamin A/C): cardiac conduction defects and contractures (also called autosomal dominant Emery-Dreifuss). LGMD1C (caveolin-3): Some patients have rippling muscle disease.
  - **LGMD type 2** (autosomal recessive): LGMD2A (calpain-3): Accounts for approximately one-fourth of dystrophies with normal dystrophin and sarcoglycans. LGMD2B (dysferlin): Atrophy and weakness of posterior calf is early and common (Miyoshi phenotype). LGMD2C, 2D, 2E, 2F (sarcoglycans γ, α, β, δ): About 10% of LGMDs. LGMD2J (titin): Usually causes distal (tibial) myopathy (Udd-type). Usually cause MDC but rarely cause milder LGMD phenotype: LGMD2K (POMT1) = Walker-Warburg. LGMD2L (fukutin) = Fukuyama. LGMD2M (POMGnT1) = muscle-eye-brain disease.

Other Dystrophies

- Most autosomal dominant with a few exceptions (see Table 11.13).
- **Facioscapulohumeral dystrophy (FSHD), types 1 and 2:**
  - **Symptoms and signs:** Facial weakness—transverse smile, incomplete eye closure. Scapular weakness and winging—often asymmetric. Pectoralis weakness—horizontal axillary crease. Biceps and triceps (humeral) weakness/atrophy ("Popeye arms"). Some lower-extremity weakness (distal or distal and proximal). Beevor sign (umbilicus moves up when contracting abdominal muscles, due to weaker lower abdominal muscles).
  - **Laboratory:** CK normal to moderately high. Histopathology is dystrophic (fiber size variability, large rounded myofibers, necrotic/regenerating fibers, increased connective tissue), and can include robust inflammation.

TABLE 11.13. Other Dystrophies

Myotonic dystrophy 1	AD	DMPK	Distal > proximal weakness, myotonia. Temporal wasting, frontal balding, diabetes, cataracts, cardiac abnormalities.
Myotonic dystrophy 2	AD	ZNF9	Proximal > distal weakness, atypical chest and muscle pains, diabetes, cataracts, cardiac abnormalities less common.
FSHD1	AD	DUX4	Facial, scapular, humeral weakness and atrophy. Peroneal weakness common. Often asymmetric.
FSHD2	AD	SMCHD1	
EDMD3	AD	Nesprin-1	
EDMD4	AD	Nesprin-2	
EDMD5	AD	LUMA	
OPMD	AD	PABP2	Onset ~30–60 years. Ptosis, 50% have EOM weakness but diplopia is uncommon. Dysphagia, dysarthria, dysphonia.
Scapuloperoneal dystrophy	AD	Desmin 2q35	Weakness/atrophy of proximal arms, distal legs.

    - **Pathophysiology:** Two mutations associated, defining type 1 and type 2: D4Z4 deletion affecting DUX4 on chromosome 4 and SMCHD1 on chromosome 18. Pathogenesis unclear.
- **Scapuloperoneal dystrophy:**
    - First 2 decades.
    - Foot drop, ankle contractures, scapular/shoulder girdle weakness similar to FSHD but humeral muscles spared.
- **Myotonic dystrophy type 1 (DM1):**
    - **Neuromuscular symptoms:** Presents at any age including congenital. Slowly progressive limb weakness: Distal → proximal. Temporal atrophy and jaw weakness → "hatchet face" appearance. Myotonia: Delayed muscular relaxation after forceful contraction (action myotonia). Often not bothersome. Myotonia improves with repetition (warm-up phenomenon).
    - **Non-neuromuscular symptoms:** Most adults with DM1 have mildly reduced intelligence, depression, or personality disorders. Congenital DM1 associated with severe mental retardation, cataracts, cardiac conduction abnormalities (90%) or cardiomyopathy, diabetes, male-pattern baldness, daytime fatigue, sleep apnea.
    - **Laboratory:** CK normal to mildly increased, EMG shows myotonic discharges.
    - **Pathophysiology:** AD trinucleotide (CTG) repeat expansion in DMPK gene on 19q13.2. Repeat is transcribed to mRNA, but mutant mRNA accumulates and interferes with transcription of many other genes. Expansion size proportional to severity. Expansion is unstable; increases over time and varies between tissues. Children born to mothers with DM1 often very severely affected.
    - **Treatment:** Prevention of arrhythmia, management of cardiomyopathy; prevention of cataracts, diabetes; when myotonia severe, mexiletine or phenytoin.
- **Myotonic dystrophy type 2 (DM2—aka proximal myotonic myopathy, PROMM):**
    - **Neuromuscular symptoms:** Presents at any age, including congenital. Proximal muscle stiffness and pain, especially thighs. Myotonia with warm-up phenomenon in some. Atypical stabbing pains in thighs, shoulders, chest, upper arms. Neck flexors, elbow extension, hip flexion/extension weakness most prominent.
    - **Non-neuromuscular symptoms:** Cataracts; cardiac conduction defects (20%) or cardiomyopathy (7%); fatigue, sleep apnea; hypogonadism in some.
    - **Laboratory:** CK normal to mildly increased. EMG shows myotonic discharges, less prominent than DM1.
    - **Pathophysiology:** AD tetranucleotide (CCTG) repeat expansion in ZNF9 gene on chromosome 3. Repeat is transcribed to mRNA, but mutant mRNA accumulates and interferes with transcription of many other genes. Expansion size proportional to severity. Expansion is unstable; increases over time and varies between tissues.
    - **Treatment:** As with DM1.
- **Oculopharyngeal muscular dystrophy (OPMD):**
    - Slowly progressive ptosis in 30s–50s—usually bilateral.
    - Approximately 50% have EOM weakness, rarely diplopia.
    - Approximately 25% pharyngeal weakness and dysphagia.
    - Neck weakness and proximal weakness can occur.
    - GCC repeat expansion PABN1 gene on 14q11.1.
- **Myofibrillar myopathy (MFM; despite name, best thought of as a dystrophy):**
    - Clinically heterogeneous group with common histopathology.

- Usually weakness begins 20s–40s, can be proximal/distal/generalized.
- Facial, pharyngeal muscles can be involved.
- Cardiac involvement can occur.
- Caused by mutations in various proteins; all AD inheritance except desmin mutations: Myotilin, ZASP, Filamin-c, B-crystallin, Desmin (AD/AR), Selenoprotein N1.
- Common characteristic: Myofibrillar disruption on EM and desmin protein accumulation (has been called desmin myopathy, spheroid body myopathy, cystoplasmic body myopathy, Mallory body myopathy, others).

Congenital Muscular Dystrophies (MDCs)

- Basal lamina/extracellular space:
  - MDC1A (Laminin α_2 [merosin] deficiency), also called classic merosin deficiency; generalized weakness/hypotonia at birth, especially neck, limb girdle; calf hypertrophy, cardiomyopathy; caused by mutations in α_2 subchain of laminin; reduced merosin on biopsy is also caused by other MDCs.
  - Ullrich/Bethlem myopathy: Weakness at birth or infancy; proximal joint contractures; hyperextensible fingers; high-arched palate; protuberant calcanei.
  - Transmembrane attached to laminin α_2:
  - α-dystroglycan/abnormal glycosylation of α-dystroglycan usually severe, cause fetal/neonatal weakness, malformations of brain and eyes, mental retardation.
    - **MDC1C:** Mutation in FKRP, allelic to LGMD 2I.
    - **Fukuyama MDC:** Mutation in Fukutin, allelic to LGMD 2L.
    - **Walker-Warburg syndrome:** Mutation in POMT1, allelic to LGMD 2K.
    - **Muscle-eye-brain (Santivouri) disease:** Mutation in POMGnT1, allelic to LGMD 2M.
  - Other transmembrane (integrin α7).
  - Thirty to 40% of MDCs are deficient in merosin (laminin α_2). Complete merosin deficiency is caused by mutations in merosin itself, partial often caused by glycosylation defects in α-dystroglycan. MDCs can be grouped by the disrupted cellular structure/function.

Congenital Nondystrophic Myopathies

Catch-all category of hereditary myopathies without dystrophic features, grouped by other histopathologic features (Table 11.14).

TABLE 11.14. Nondystrophic Congenital Myopathies

Central core	AD	RyR1	Central type I fiber cores (reduced NADH).
Multi/minicore	AD/AR	RyR1, selenoprotein N1, others	Multiple small type I fiber cores.
Nemaline	AD/AR	← tropomyosin, β-tropomyosin, nembulin, troponin T, ← actin	Disrupted Z-disc proteins → nemaline rods. Several protein mutations; variable age/severity.
Late-onset nemaline	?		> 40 years, neck and respiratory weakness. Sporadic, ?acquired.
Centronuclear	XR		
Others	—		

- **Central core myopathy:**
  - Onset: Infancy/early childhood.
  - Variable weakness and progression.
  - No ptosis or extraocular muscle (EOM) weakness (unlike myotubular and nemaline myopathies).
  - Type I fibers have central/eccentric "core" area of reduced NADH staining that runs the length of the myofiber.
  - AD mutation in ryanodine receptor (RYR1).
  - Risk of malignant hyperthermia.
- **Multicore/minicore myopathy:**
  - Onset: Infancy/childhood, occasionally adulthood.
  - Hypotonia, generalized weakness.
  - Skeletal abnormalities: Contractures, scoliosis, high palate, club feet.
  - Type I fibers have multiple small core areas of reduced NADH staining that don't run the length of the myofiber.
  - Polygenetic (RyR1, selenoprotein N1, others).
  - AD, AR inheritance.
  - Risk of malignant hyperthermia.
- **Nemaline myopathy:**
  - Onset: Infancy to childhood.
  - Generalized weakness and hypotonia.
  - Arthrogryposis and ventilatory failure in severe cases.
  - Heterogeneous group shares nemaline rods (subsarcolemmal inclusions that stain red on trichrome).
  - Disruption of Z-disk related proteins: α-tropomyosin, β-tropomyosin, nembulin, troponin T, α-actin.
  - AD or AR inheritance.
- **Centronuclear myopathy (formerly myotubular myopathy):**
  - Genetically and clinically heterogeneous disorders.
  - Infantile-early childhood onset of hypotonia, generalized weakness.
  - Narrow, elongated face, EOM weakness, ptosis common.
  - Common feature is central myonuclei. Type I fibers predominate but are hypotrophic.
  - Myotubularin (MTM1) → severe X-linked neonatal.
  - Dynamin-2 (DNM2) → some late onset.
- **Others:** Congenital fiber-type disproportion, reducing body myopathy, fingerprint body myopathy, sarcotubular myopathy, zebra body myopathy, more.

Channelopathies

Chloride Channelopathies

- **Myotonia congenita:**
  - Myotonia: Delayed muscle relaxation after forceful contraction, improves with repetition (warm-up).
  - Worsens with cold.
  - Can worsen with pregnancy.
  - Muscular hypertrophy → Herculean appearance.
  - **Pathogenesis:** Mutation in chloride channel gene CLCN1 on 7q35.
    - **Thomsen disease:** AD (onset first few years, little weakness).
    - **Becker disease:** AR (onset 4–12 years, weakness more severe). Myotonia improves with mexiletine, phenytoin, carbamazepine.

Sodium Channelopathies With Periodic Paralysis

- Also called hyperkalemic periodic paralysis (hyperKPP).
- **Symptoms:**
  - Typically presents in first decade.

    - Three forms, all with attacks of weakness and precipitating factors:
        - **HyperKPP with clinical/electrical myotonia:** Action and percussion myotonia that improves with repetition.
        - **HyperKPP without myotonia:** No myotonia.
        - **HyperKPP with paramyotonia congenita (PMC)** (Eulenberg disease): Paramyotonia—paradoxical mytonia that worsens with repetition.
    - Attacks of moderate generalized weakness, especially in AM—usually not severe as in hypoKPP.
    - Attacks last < 2 hours, sometimes followed by a few days of mild weakness.
    - Precipitated by rest following exercise, fasting, stress, and intake of K^+-rich foods.
- **Laboratory:**
    - CK normal to mildly elevated.
    - Serum K^+ levels often normal, can be high (5–6 mEq/L).
    - Genetic testing available—K^+ challenge usually unnecessary.
- **Pathogenesis:** AD mutations in Na^+ channel SCN4A (α-subunit).
- **Treatment:**
    - Low-K^+, high-carbohydrate diet.
    - Avoid fasting, strenuous activity, cold.
    - Mild exercise after strenuous activity helps prevent weakness.
    - Acetazolamide may reduce attack frequency.
    - Mexiletine for myotonia.
    - Severe attacks: Glucose, insulin (drives K^+ into cells), calcium gluconate.

Sodium Channelopathies Without Periodic Paralysis

- Acetazolamide-responsive myotonia congenita:
    - Painful muscle stiffness.
    - Begins in childhood, worsens with age.
    - Myotonia most severe in face and hands, aggravated by K^+, fasting, exercise.
    - Eyelid paramyotonia sometimes appreciated.
    - Mutations in SCN4A.
- Myotonia fluctuans:
    - Fluctuating myotonia.
    - Delayed onset myotonia after exercise.
    - Eyelid paramyotonia.
    - Warm-up phenomenon.
    - No weakness after K^+, exercise, cold.
    - Myotonia worsened by K^+, but not cold.
    - Mutations in SCN4A.
- Myotonia permanens:
    - Constant myotonia/stiffness.
    - Worsened by K^+, activity.
    - No episodic weakness.
    - Mutations in SCN4A.
- HypoKPP type 2:
    - No myotonia.
    - No fixed weakness over time (unlike hypoKPP 1).
    - Serum K^+ low during attacks.
    - SCN4A gene mutation—rare cause of hypoKPP.
    - Acetazolamide, K^+ used prophylactically.

Calcium Channelopathies

HypoKPP type 1 (primary hypoKPP):

- No myotonia.
- Seventy percent develop fixed proximal weakness over time.
- Mutation in calcium channel CACN1A3 most common cause of hypoKPP.
- AD but reduced penetrance in women.
- Attacks of generalized weakness, mostly in AM.
- Attacks of mild to severe flaccid paralysis, sparing face, respiratory, sphincter muscles.
- Precipitated by: Exercise followed by rest/sleep; high carbohydrate, high Na^+ meals; alcohol; stress, sleep deprivation; illness; beta agonists, corticosteroids, insulin (lower K^+).
- Serum K^+ usually < 3.0 during attacks, normal between.
- Avoid high-carbohydrate, high-Na^+ meals.
- Avoid strenuous exercise.
- Acetazolamide, K^+ used prophylactically.

Other Channelopathies

- Andersen-Tawil syndrome:
  - Triad: Periodic paralysis. Cardiac arrhythmias (ventricular tachycardia, torsades). Skeletal abnormalities (hypertelorism, syndactyly, scoliosis, low ears, mandibular hypoplasia).
  - Most due to mutations in KCNJ2 (inwardly rectifying K^+ channel, predominantly in heart, skeletal muscle, brain).
- Malignant hyperthermia:
  - Attacks provoked by depolarizing NMJ blockers and inhaled anesthetics; severe muscle rigidity; myoglobinuria; high fever, tachycardia, arrhythmias; can occur even when prior anesthesia successful.
  - Most common: Mutations in Ryanodine receptor RyR1 on 19q13.1.
  - **Treatment:** Dantrolene, aggressive cooling. Treat acidosis and maintain urine output.

Metabolic and Mitochondrial Myopathies

Inherited disorders of energy storage and processing that affect liver, muscle, and brain. Defects in: (1) carbohydrate (glycolytic/glycogenolytic) pathways, (2) lipid/fatty acid metabolism, (3) purine nucleotide metabolism, (4) mitochondrial metabolism. A schematic overview is seen in Figure 11.5.

Laboratory Testing for Suspected Metabolic/Mitochondrial Disorders

- Forearm exercise test:
  - Draw serum lactate and ammonia levels at baseline.
  - One-minute intense forearm exercise ("ischemia" with a tourniquet is unnecessary).
  - Draw NH3, lactate 1, 2, 5, and 10 minutes postexercise.
  - Normal: rise in NH3, lactate (3–4 times baseline).
  - Rise in NH3, no rise in lactate: McArdle, phosphofructokinase (PFK), phosphoglyceric acid mutase (PGAM), phosphoglycerine kinase (PGK), phosphorylase B kinase (PBK), debrancher, lactic dehydrogenase (LDH) deficiency.
  - Rise in lactate, no rise in NH3: Multiple acyl-CoA dehydrogenase (MAD) deficiency.
- Serum and urine tests:
  - CK, CBC.
  - Glucose.

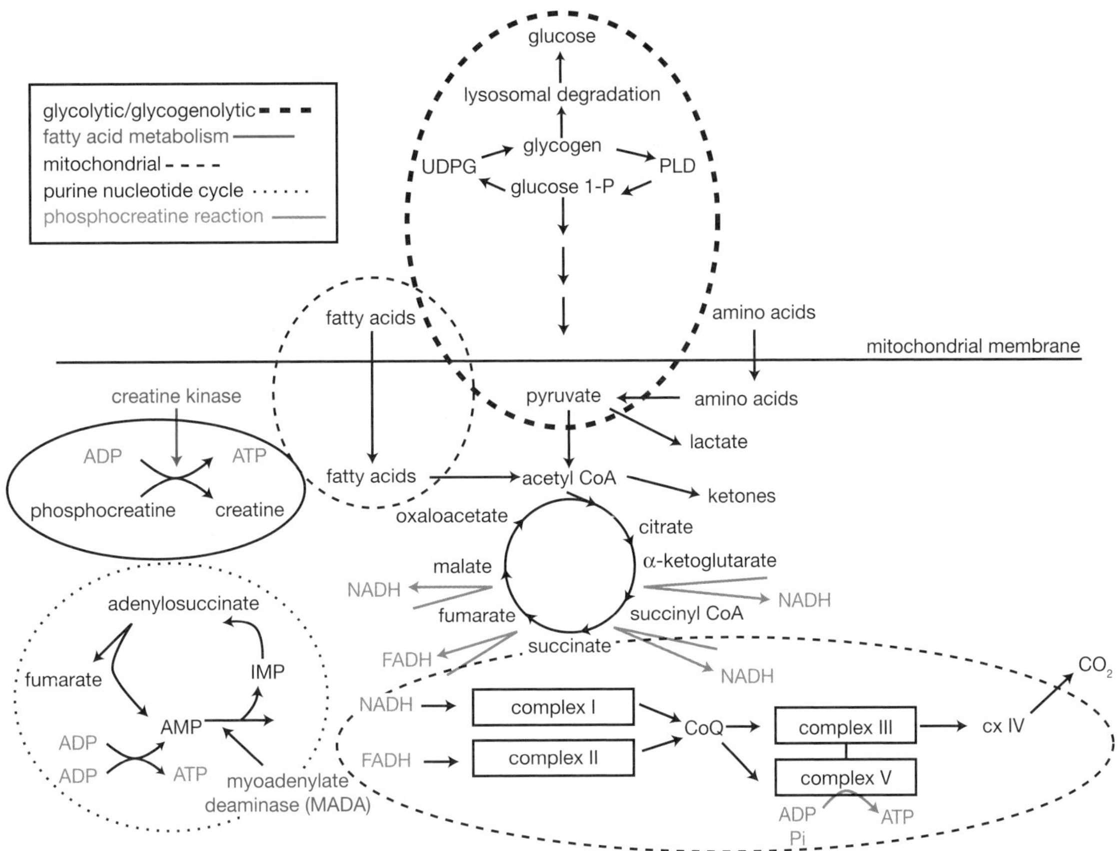

FIGURE 11.5. Metabolic and mitochondrial myopathies.

  - Ammonia.
  - Lactate, pyruvate, lactate/pyruvate (L/P) ratio.
  - LDH.
  - Transaminases.
  - Carnitine.
  - Ketones (serum and urine, especially during metabolic stress or hypoglycemia).
  - Myoglobin (serum and urine).
  - Acylcarnitines.
  - Free fatty acids.
  - Serum amino acids, organic acids.
  - Urine organic acids, acylglycines, dicarboxylic acids.
- Muscle biopsy:
  - Glycolytic/glycogenolytic disorders: Periodic acid-Schiff (PAS—stains glycogen, immunohistochemistry for PFK, PGAM, PGK, acid maltase, debrancher enzyme.
  - Lipid disorders: Oil red O stains accumulated lipid.
  - Mitochondrial defects: Succinate dehydrogenase (SDH), cytochrome oxidase (COX) stains, ragged red fibers on Gomori trichrome.

Glycolytic/Glycogenolytic

- Various defects in pathways converting glucose → glycogen → pyruvate → lactate (Figure 11.6).
- Liver and/or muscle affected; varying age and severity.
- Most cause exercise intolerance; only a few (II, III, IV) cause fixed weakness.

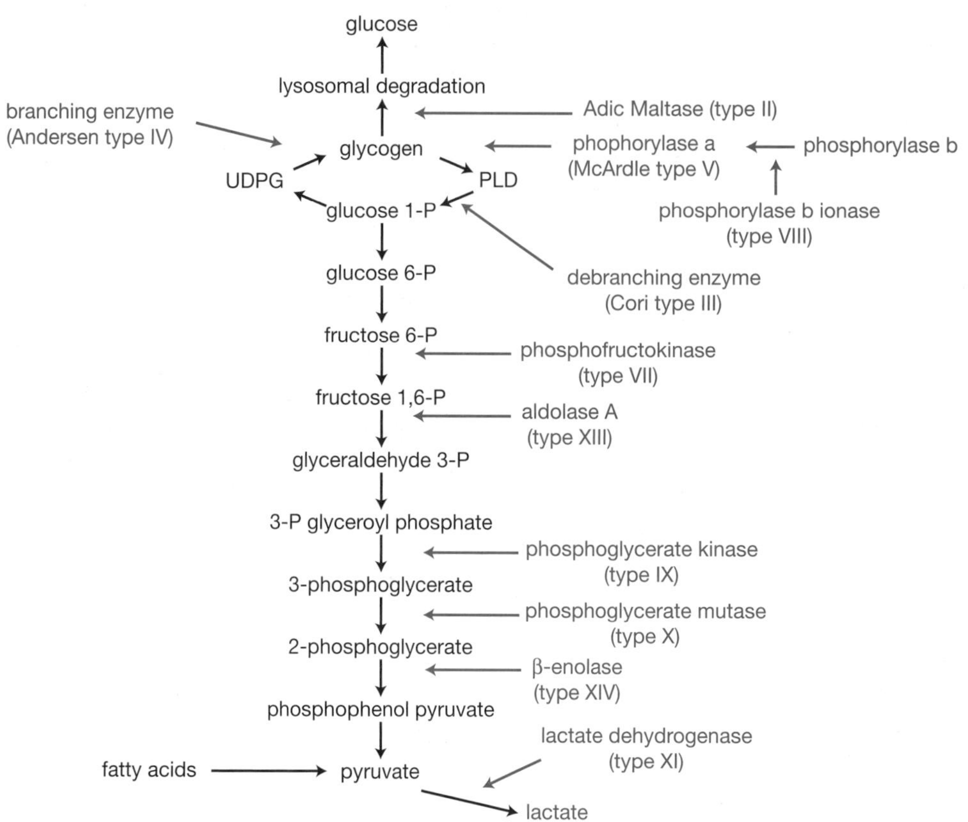

FIGURE 11.6. Glycolytic/glycogenolytic myopathies.

- **Laboratory diagnosis:**
  - Forearm exercise test: Lack normal increase in lactate.
  - Muscle biopsy: Subsarcolemmal/cytoplasmic glycogen accumulation.
- **Type II (Pompe disease):**
  - Severe infantile, juvenile, or adult onset.
  - Infants: Progressive generalized weakness/hypotonia, cardiomegaly, hepatomegaly, macroglossia, respiratory failure. Historically fatal within 2 years.
  - Juvenile (1–20 years): Delayed motor milestones, proximal weakness (Gower sign, waddling gait). Progressive weakness, hepatomegaly/cardiomegaly uncommon.
  - Adult (20s): Subacute/chronic proximal and axial weakness, respiratory failure. Hepatomegaly/cardiomegaly uncommon.
  - **Pathophysiology/Laboratory:**
    - AR defect in acid α-1,4-glucosidase → glycogen accumulation.
    - Muscle biopsy: Glycogen-filled (PAS+) subsarcolemmal vacuoles, cytoplasmic glycogen.
  - **Treatment:** IV recombinant α-glucosidase. Supportive care.
- **Type III (Cori-Forbes disease, debrancher deficiency):**
  - AR defect in a glycogen debranching enzyme → glycogen accumulation.
  - Type a: Liver and muscle → proximal weakness and atrophy, birth to 50 years.
  - Type b: Liver only.
- **Type IV (branching enzyme deficiency):**
  - Rare AR defect in glycogen branching enzyme → accumulation of polysaccharides (polyglucosan bodies) in muscle, nerve, brain, heart, liver, skin.
  - Liver transplant sometimes helpful.

- **Type V (McArdle disease, myophosphorylase deficiency):**
  - Most common glycolytic/glycogenolytic disorder.
  - AR deficiency of myophosphorylase (phosphorylase a kinase) → glycogen accumulation in muscle.
  - Exercise intolerance, muscle pain, cramps. Most noticeable with brief, intense exercise.
  - Second-wind phenomenon: Initial myalgias and cramping improve as blood glucose mobilized.
  - With heavy exertion, illness, can develop rhabdomyolysis → myoglobinuria.
  - Repeated rhabdo can cause fixed weakness.
  - Oral sucrose loading before exercise briefly improves tolerance.
  - Moderate intensity exercise is beneficial.
- **Type VII (Tarui disease, PFK deficiency):**
  - Rare AR defect in PFK → glycogen and polysaccharide accumulation in muscle and red blood cells.
  - Similar phenotype to McArdle but no second wind, and can have anemia.
- **Type VIII (PBK deficiency):**
  - AR defect in PBK → glycogen accumulation in muscles.
  - Exercise intolerance, cramps, myoglobinuria.
  - Sometimes childhood weakness, delayed early milestones, cardiomyopathy.
- **Type IX (PGK deficiency):**
  - X-linked defect in PGK → glycogen accumulation in muscles, RBCs, CNS.
  - Male children with hemolytic anemia, mental retardation, seizures, myopathy, exercise intolerance, myoglobinuria.
- **Type X (PGAM deficiency):**
  - AR defect in PGAM → glycogen accumulation in muscles.
  - Childhood to early adulthood.
  - Exercise intolerance, cramps, myoglobinuria.
- **Type XI (LDH deficiency):**
  - Rare AR defect in LDH → exercise intolerance, cramps, myoglobinuria, sometimes generalized rash.
  - Biopsy: Reduced LDH activity, but no glycogen accumulation.
- **Type XII (aldolase A deficiency):** Single case described → exercise intolerance, postexercise weakness, episodic hemolytic anemia.

Lipid/Free Fatty Acid (FFA) Metabolism

- FFAs → fatty acid oxidation (FAO) = primary source of muscle fuel after exercise > 1 hour.
- Long-chain FA (LCFAs) need enzymatic modification and transport into mitochondria.
- Short-chain (SCFAs) and medium-chain (MCFAs) diffuse freely into mitochondria.
- **CPT II deficiency:**
  - AR deficiency in CPT2 gene → impaired acylcarnitine transport and modification at inner mitochondrial membrane.
  - Second to third decade, myalgia and myoglobinuria provoked by prolonged/intense exercise, fasting, illness, cold.
  - EMG, CK, forearm exercise lactate tests usually normal.
  - High-protein, low-fat diet; avoid prolonged heavy exertion and fasting.
- **Carnitine transporter deficiency:**
  - Mutation in carnitine transporter protein OCTN2 → primary carnitine deficiency.

  - Most common disorder of lipid metabolism.
  - Recurrent attacks of vomiting, confusion, hypoglycemia, hepatic dysfunction resembling Reye syndrome. Myopathy relatively mild.
  - Secondary carnitine deficiency: Organ failure, malnutrition, medication, mitochondrial disorders.
- **Very long-chain (VLCAD), long-chain (LCAD), medium-chain (MCAD), short-chain (SCAD) acyl-CoA dehydrogenase deficiency:**
  - Mutations of acyl-CoA dehydrogenases → reduced fatty acid oxidation (Figure 11.7).
  - Variable phenotypes and ages of onset.
  - Cardiomyopathy, hepatomegaly, hypoketotic hypoglycemia, dicarboxylic aciduria, exercise-induced myoglobinuria.

Myoadenylate Deaminase Deficiency

- Exertional myalgias, fatigue.
- Common in patients with other neuromuscular disorders—may not be primary cause of disease.

Mitochondrial Myopathies

- Caused by defects in oxidative phosphorylation and adenosine triphosphate (ATP) production. Caused by mutations in nuclear or mitochondrial DNA (mtDNA)—can be AD, AR, X-linked, or maternal inheritance pattern. Onset usually childhood to early adulthood, but can present any time.

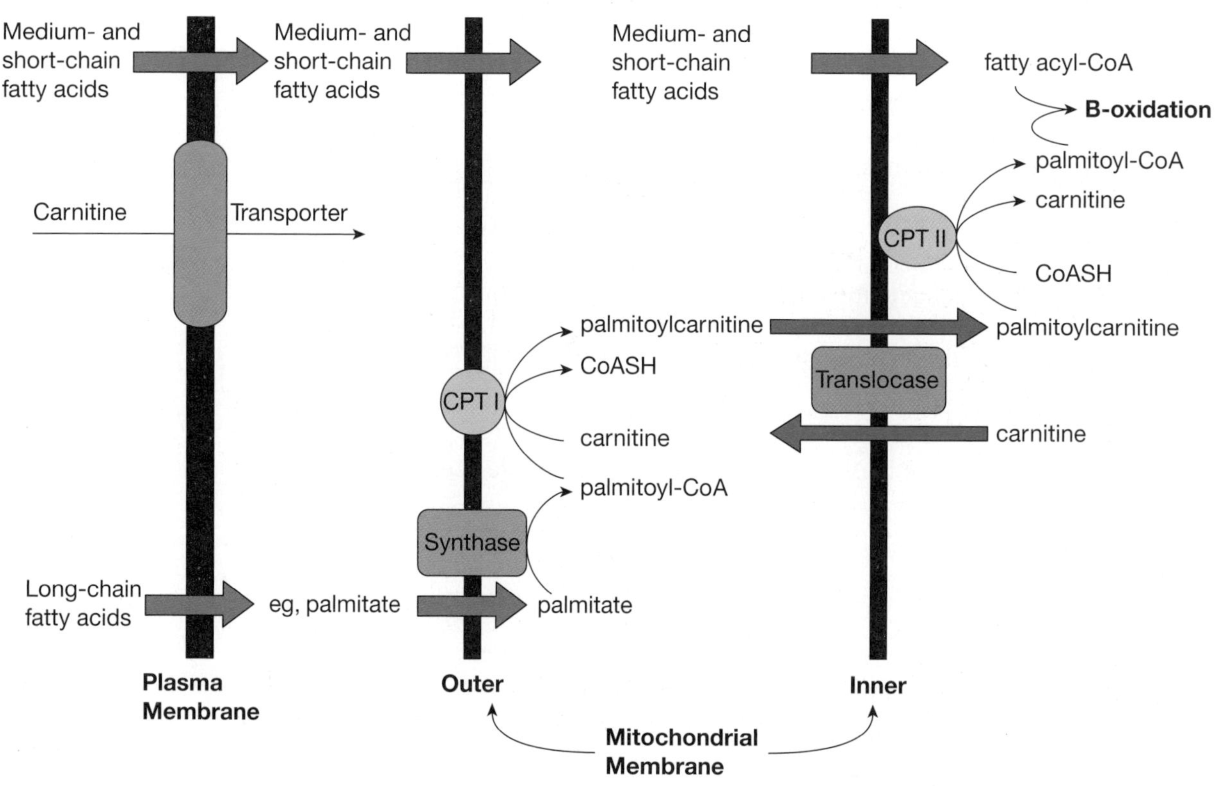

FIGURE 11.7. Free fatty acid metabolism. (Reproduced, with permission, from Walsh R. Metabolic myopathies. *Continuum.* 2006;12(3):76–120.)

- **Progressive external ophthalmoplegia (PEO):**
  - Ptosis and ophthalmoparesis.
  - mtDNA deletion or mutation, AD or maternal.
  - Muscle biopsy: Some ragged red fibers, COX fibers.
- **Kearns-Sayre syndrome (KSS):**
  - Triad: PEO, pigmentary retinopathy, cardiomyopathy.
  - Other features: Short stature, proximal weakness, hearing loss, dementia, ataxia, endocrine (DM, hypothyroid, hypogonadism).
  - Large mtDNA deletion, usually sporadic, AD.
  - Muscle biopsy: Some ragged red fibers, COX fibers.
- **Myoclonic epilepsy with ragged red fibers (MERRF):**
  - Myoclonus, generalized seizures, ataxia, dementia, hearing loss, optic atrophy, progressive weakness.
  - Multiple mtDNA mutations, AR or maternal inheritance.
- **Myo-neuro-gastrointestinal encephalopathy (MNGIE):**
  - POLIP syndrome: **P**olyneuropathy, **O**phthalmoplegia, **L**eukoencephalopathy, **I**ntestinal **P**seudoobstruction.
  - Nuclear mutations → mtDNA deletions.
  - AR or maternal inheritance.
- **Leigh syndrome:**
  - Usually presents in infancy to early childhood.
  - Subacute necrotizing encephalomyopathy.
  - Facial dysmorphism.
  - Recurrent vomiting, psychomotor retardation, hypotonia, generalized weakness/atrophy, ptosis/ophthalmoplegia, optic atrophy, ataxia, seizures, hearing loss.
  - Brain MRI: Thalamic, brain stem, cerebellum, spinal cord.
  - Nuclear or mtDNA mutations → mtDNA deletions.
  - AR, maternal, or X-linked inheritance.

Electromyography (EMG) and Nerve Conduction Studies (NCS)

- Extension of the neurological exam.
- Useful for localization (root, plexus, nerve, neuromuscular junction, muscle).
- Aids in localization of focal or multifocal neuropathies, and differentiates axonal and demyelinating nerve diseases.
- Can help quantify chronicity and severity of a nerve injury.

SENSORY NERVE ACTION POTENTIALS (SNAPs)

- Surface stimulator depolarizes a nerve, surface electrodes record SNAP.
- **Antidromic study:** Depolarizes sensory nerve proximally, records distally (stimulus travels opposite to the physiologic direction of depolarization).
- SNAPs preserved in lesions proximal to the DRG (cell body and distal axon are preserved). Most compressive radiculopathies have normal SNAPs.
- SNAP amplitudes nadir ~11 days after axonal injury distal to the DRG.

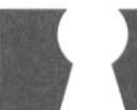

KEY FACT

SNAP amplitudes are typically preserved in radiculopathies, and abnormal in plexopathies or neuropathies.

COMPOUND MUSCLE ACTION POTENTIALS (CMAPs)

- Depolarization of motor axons → surface electrode over a muscle, recording CMAPs (a summation of the depolarization of individual muscle fibers).
- **Orthodromic study:** Proximal depolarization, distal recording.
- CMAP amplitudes nadir at approximately 7 days after an axonal injury.
- **F waves and H reflexes:**
  - **F waves:** Operator stimulates motor axon distally → antidromic depolarization → "backfiring" of some anterior horn cells → orthodromic depolarization and surface recording of late response. Motor fibers only, no synapses.
  - **H reflex:** Electrical correlate of tendon stretch reflexes. Activation of Ia afferent sensory fibers → oligosynaptic reflex arc in the spinal cord → surface recording of late motor response. Reflects sensory and motor limbs of the reflex.

NEEDLE EMG

Recording needle electrode is inserted into a muscle. Three types of information are obtained: spontaneous activity, motor unit morphology, and activation/recruitment pattern.

- **Spontaneous activity:** Electrical activity of a muscle at rest. Normally limited to brief activity after needle insertion. Decreased in chronic myopathies or neuropathies when muscle fibers are few and far between. Increased spontaneous activity in many disorders:
  - **Fibrillation potentials and positive sharp waves:** Spontaneous, usually rhythmic, membrane depolarizations of individual muscle fibers. Fibs/PSW represent "instability" of the muscle membrane and are seen in both myopathies and neuropathies.
  - **Fasciculation potentials:** Spontaneous depolarizations of a single motor unit and its muscle fibers—originates from a motor neuron; seen exclusively in neuropathic disorders.
  - **Complex repetitive discharge (CRD):** Caused by adjacent abnormal muscle fibers depolarizing each other in turn—most common in myopathies, but occasionally seen in acute/subacute neuropathies.
  - **Myotonia** is spontaneous rapid depolarization of an individual muscle fiber. Seen in myotonic disorders (eg, myotonic dystrophies, myotonia and paramyotonia congenita, some periodic paralyses).
  - **Myokymia:** Brief random bursts of electrical activity originating from the motor neuron. Seen in demyelinating neuropathies, radiation neuropathies.
- **Motor unit action potentials (MUAPs):** Summed potential of all the depolarizing muscle fibers in a single motor unit. Amplitude and duration decreased in myopathic disorders, increased in neuropathic disorders after reinnervation. Polyphasia typically occurs during reinnervation; sometimes seen in myopathic disorders.
- **Motor unit activation and recruitment:**
  - **Activation:** *Speed* at which motor units fire, determined by the upper motor neuron (UMN). Maximum volitional speed ~50 Hz. Decreased in disorders of UMN and when effort is poor.
  - **Recruitment:** *Number* of MUAPs firing at a given activation. Normal: 1 motor unit seen at ~5 Hz, 2 at 10 Hz, 3 units at 15 Hz, etc. **Reduced** in neuropathic disorders (eg, 1 unit seen at 30 Hz). **Early** in myopathic disorders (full recruitment pattern with reduced muscle force generated).

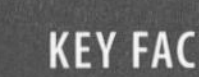

KEY FACT

Fibrillation potentials and positive sharp waves reflect muscle membrane instability, and are seen in both myopathic and neuropathic disorders. Do not reflexively think "neuropathy."

SINGLE-FIBER EMG (SFEMG)

- Measures synchrony of myofibers belonging to the same motor unit.
- Normally, fibers fire within a fixed time period (called the "jitter") of each other. Disorders of the NMJ (eg, myasthenia) cause the jitter to increase.
- Very sensitive for NMJ disorders, but jitter is frequently increased in nerve and muscle disorders—so nonspecific.

KEY FACT

Decrement of the CMAP with RNS is seen in both MG and LEMS at slow (2–3 Hz) rates of RNS. CMAP increment is seen in LEMS, but only with high (10–50 Hz) rates of RNS or for a short time after voluntary contraction.

REPETITIVE NERVE STIMULATION (RNS)

Repeated stimulation of a motor nerve at various rates, with recording of a CMAP. Measure of NMJ function. Approximately 75% sensitive in patients with generalized MG, ~50% in patients with ocular MG.

- **RNS at 2–3 Hz (slow):** In both *presynaptic and postsynaptic* disorders of NMJ, 2–3 Hz RNS results in decreasing CMAP amplitude ("decrement"). Decrement of more than 10% is considered abnormal.
- **RNS at 10–50 Hz (rapid):** In *presynaptic* NMJ disorders (eg, LEMS), CMAP amplitudes increase ("increment"). In LEMS, increment is large, usually > 100%.

Evoked Potentials

Electrophysiologic studies that evaluate central conduction pathways.

SOMATOSENSORY EVOKED POTENTIALS (SSEPs)

- Surface depolarization of a sensory nerve (typically median, tibial).
- Surface electrodes record from:
  - Erb point (median nerve EP), or popliteal fossa and lumbar spine (tibial nerve EP).
  - Cervical spine.
  - Scalp.
- Waveforms correspond to depolarization of groups of axons or neurons; labeled according to direction of deflection (N = negative, P = positive) and usual latency (in milliseconds) (Figure 11.8).

VISUAL EVOKED POTENTIALS (VEPs)

- Visual stimulus presented while recording from scalp in occipital region.
- Delay of the "P100" (positive deflection, ~100 milliseconds) signifies demyelination along visual pathways.

BRAIN STEM AUDITORY EVOKED POTENTIALS (BAERs)

- Auditory stimuli presented, recording cortical activity from the scalp.
- Five waves (I through V) reflects central conduction of auditory information:
  - CN VIII nerve and nucleus (waves I and II).
  - Pons → midbrain → cortex (waves III–V).

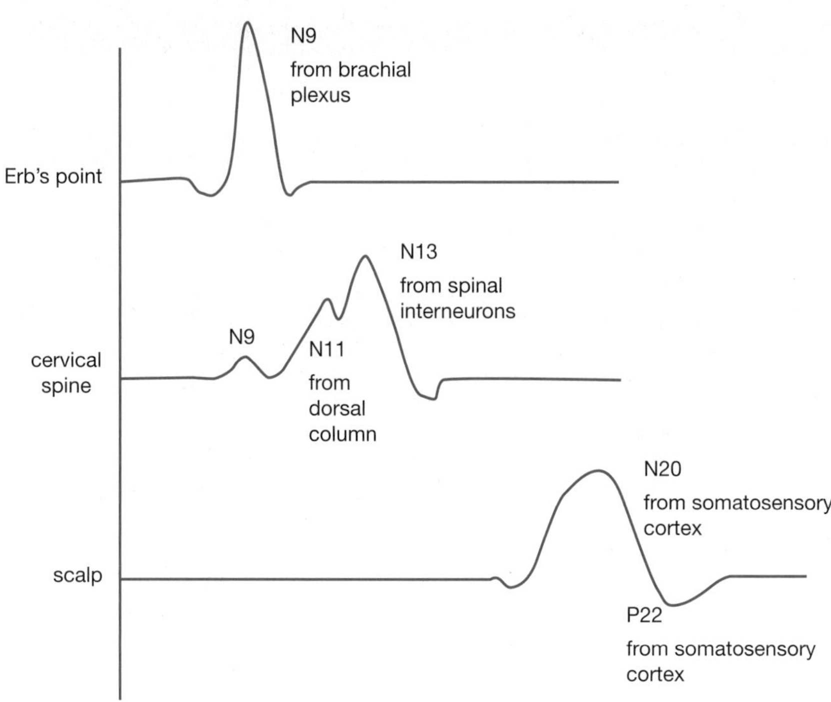

FIGURE 11.8. Median somatosensory evoked potentials. N, negative (upward) deflection. P, positive (downward) deflection.

MOTOR EVOKED POTENTIALS

- Motor cortex is stimulated electrically or magnetically, while recording at skin surface over muscles.
- Yields central and/or peripheral conduction times.
- Can be done transcranially or directly during surgery to monitor central motor pathways (eg, spine surgery).

CHAPTER 12

Pediatric Neurology and Neurogenetics

Lori C. Jordan, MD, PhD
W. Bryan Burnette, MD, MS
Ronald Cohn, MD, PhD

Childhood Epilepsies

FEBRILE SEIZURES (FS)

- Seizures occurring in a previously healthy child between the ages of 6 months and 5 years with no evidence of central nervous system (CNS) infection or other defined cause.
- Up to 5% of children will have febrile seizures.
- There is a family history of febrile seizures in approximately 10% of those affected.
- FSs are divided into 2 subtypes: simple and complex (Table 12.1).

Diagnosis

- In children with complex FSs, a prolonged postictal state, or abnormal neuro exam: Strongly consider lumbar puncture (LP) for cell counts, glucose, protein, and culture.
- In children with simple FS: No imaging or electroencephalogram (EEG) is recommended.

Treatment

- Anticonvulsants are rarely needed.
- The drugs with efficacy in FSs are phenobarbital and valproic acid.
- For children presenting with prolonged FSs or febrile status epilepticus, rectal valium may be prescribed for use on an as-needed basis.

Complications

- Recurrence risk after a single FS:
  - Children with a simple FS: 30%.
  - Children with a complex FS: 50%.
  - Antipyretics "around the clock" do *not* reduce the risk of recurrence.
  - Highest risk of recurrence is in children < 1 year of age and children with a family history of seizures.
- Risk of epilepsy in children with FSs:
  - With history of simple FSs: 2–4%.
  - With history of complex FSs: 6%.

TABLE 12.1. Febrile Seizure Subtypes

Simple Febrile Seizures[a]	Complex Febrile Seizures[b]
1 in 24 hours	More than 1 in 24 hours
Last < 15 minutes	Last > 15 minutes
Generalized seizure	Focal seizure
No residual neurologic deficits	Focal deficit (Todd paralysis) remains

[a] Must include all the variables in column 1.

[b] It includes any of the variables in column 2.

ABSENCE SEIZURES

Diagnosis

- EEG will show 3-Hz/sec spike-and-wave discharges.
- Hyperventilation may bring out seizures.

Treatment

- Ethosuximide (ETX).
- Valproic acid (VPA): Similar in efficacy to ETX but higher rate of attentional problems.
- Lamotrigine: Reduced efficacy compared to ETX and VPA.

Complications

Generalized tonic-clonic (GTC) seizures will occur in up to 40% but are usually infrequent and easily controlled.

Prognosis

Eighty to 95% remit by mid-adolescence.

NEONATAL SEIZURES—INFANTILE SPASMS (IS)

- Rapid tonic contractions of the trunk and limbs. Classically, these are flexor spasms, but can be flexor, extensor, and mixed.
- Usually occur in clusters upon awakening from sleep.
- Average age of onset is 5 months.

Diagnosis

- **West syndrome:** Triad of spasms, hypsarrhythmia on EEG, and developmental delay.
- Do skin exam with Woods (UV) lamp to assess for hypopigmented macules, as IS can be the presenting symptom of tuberous sclerosis.

Treatment

- Adrenocorticotropic hormone (ACTH) given as IM injections. Potential complication of ACTH is hypertrophic cardiomyopathy, which can be fatal. Should monitor blood pressure twice weekly for the duration of treatment.
- Other options that are considered second-line therapy: Topiramate, valproic acid, oral prednisolone, zonisamide, ketogenic diet.
- Vigabatrin: FDA approved in the United States for ISs related to tuberous sclerosis. Risk of retinal damage resulting in asymptomatic concentric visual field loss.

Complications

- Regression of skills.
- Complications of treatment with ACTH include hyperglycemia, hypertension, irritability, stomach ulcers from steroid use.

LENNOX-GASTAUT SYNDROME

Triad of (1) developmental delay/mental retardation, (2) multiple seizure types, and (3) characteristic EEG that shows generalized "slow spike-waves," typically at 1.5–2.5 Hz, superimposed on a slow and disorganized awake background.

Diagnosis

Seizures may be atonic, tonic, atypical absence, or GTC.

Treatment

- Multiple drugs may be effective for these children.
- One drug specifically studied in this group is felbamate. However, because of the risk of aplastic anemia, felbamate is not first-line therapy for difficult-to-control seizures.
- Recently approved AEDs that may be effective in LGS are rufinamide and clobazam. Clobazam seems particularly effective for atonic seizures.
- Other therapies: Ketogenic diet, vagus nerve stimulation, or corpus callosotomy.

Complications

Seizures are often difficult to control, continuing until adulthood.

JUVENILE MYOCLONIC EPILEPSY

- History often reveals myoclonic jerks in the mornings and GTC upon awakening.
- When inherited, this is an autosomal-dominant disorder.
- Life-long but very well controlled with AEDs.

Diagnosis

EEG shows characteristic 3- to 5-Hz spike-and-wave discharges.

Treatment

Valproic acid, lamotrigine, and levetiracetam are the most prescribed drugs.

Complications

Seizures may be lifelong.

EPILEPTIC APHASIA (LANDAU-KLEFFNER)

- Language disturbance in normally developing children between 3 and 8 years.
- Seizure semiology varies, and 20–30% of patients do not exhibit clinical seizure activity at all.
- Patients are much worse at producing language than with understanding it.

Diagnosis

History and EEG shows electrical status epilepticus of slow wave sleep (ESES).

Treatment

Several options: corticosteroids, levetiracetam, benzodiazepines, and valproic acid.

Complications

If the aphasia begins in early childhood and/or persists for more than 1–2 years, most will have long-term language deficits.

BENIGN OCCIPITAL EPILEPSY (PANAYIOTOPOULOS SYNDROME)

- Autonomic symptoms, including pallor, nausea, retching, and vomiting, sometimes associated with confusion and occasionally concluding in a focal clonic seizure event.
- Infrequent, often prolonged seizure events, usually nocturnal.
- Less than 10% have visual symptoms.

DIAGNOSIS

History; on EEG, interictal spikes are most likely to be located over the occipital regions.

TREATMENT

Valproic acid, carbamazepine and clobazam are first-line AED options.

COMPLICATIONS

Rare. Seizures are typically outgrown.

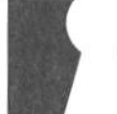

KEY FACT

Head circumference should **not** ↑ by more than 0.5 cm/week for the first 3 months of life.

Disorders of Head Growth

- Average head circumference—rule of 3s, 5s, and 9s.
- Head circumference ↑ by 5 cm at the following intervals from birth: 3 months, 9 months, 3 years, and 9 years (see Table 12.2).

MICROCEPHALY

An 8-month-old boy is evaluated for small head size, as small head circumference was noted at birth but was thought to be in proportion to his birth weight. Despite gaining weight postnatally, there was no concomitant head growth. In addition, the child is developmentally delayed. He has not begun rolling over and is unable to sit on his own. He has poor eye contact and he does not turn his head or his gaze toward any sounds. He does make gurgling noises but not necessarily in response to a voice that he should be familiar with, and he currently does not utter any words. His

TABLE 12.2. Head Circumference by Age

AGE	AVERAGE HEAD CIRCUMFERENCE[a]
Birth	35 cm
3 months	40 cm
9 months	45 cm
3 years	50 cm
9 years	55 cm

[a] Boys may have a head circumference 1 cm greater than these values; girls may be 1 cm less than these values.

past medical history is remarkable for a cardiac murmur at birth, which resolved on its own. He is taking no medications and has no known allergies. His mother was 19 years old when she gave birth.

The infant's examination is consistent with hyperreflexia and spasticity with poor visual tracking and poor acoustic blink reflex, which is suggestive of poor hearing. All of these findings in the context of microcephaly, which is defined as head circumference < 2 standard deviations from the mean, point to a disorder of cerebral origin. Microcephaly may in fact suggest intrauterine growth retardation when it is present at birth.

- Head circumference < 2 standard deviations the normal distribution for age and gender.
- A small head circumference indicates a small brain.
- Head circumference < 3 standard deviations below normal generally means the child will be mentally retarded.
- **Primary microcephaly** (typically genetic): Chromosomal abnormalities, genetic causes.
- **Secondary microcephaly** (typically nongenetic): Intrauterine infections (cytomegalovirus [CMV], toxoplasmosis, etc), toxins, perinatal brain injuries, hypoxic ischemic encephalopathy, postnatal systemic disease (ie, malnutrition, chronic cardiopulmonary, or renal disease).

Diagnosis

- Assess for positive family history.
- Consider karyotype.
- Obtain TORCH (toxoplasma, rubella, cytomegalovirus, herpes simplex) titers.
- Head CT/brain MRI.

Treatment

- Offer appropriate genetic counseling.
- Follow for possible mental retardation and connect family with appropriate services.

MACROCEPHALY

Head circumference > 2 standard deviations above the normal distribution for age and gender.

Differential Diagnosis

- Megalencephaly (abnormally large brain):
  - 1°: Sporadic or associated with neurofibromatosis, tuberous sclerosis, or achondroplasia.
  - 2°: Metabolic—classic examples include Alexander disease and Canavan disease.
- Thickening of skull.
- Hemorrhage into subdural or epidural space in a child with an open fontanelle.
- ↑ intracranial pressure (ICP) with hydrocephalus.

Diagnosis

- Assess of for positive family history, underlying disorder.
- Evaluate for ↑ ICP.

- If no ↑ ICP or neurologic abnormalities found, presumed diagnosis is benign familial macrocephaly.
- If any ↑ ICP or neurologic abnormalities found, consider head CT, brain MRI.

Treatment

- Treat underlying disorder.
- Connect family with appropriate services when indicated.

HYDROCEPHALUS

Abnormal accumulation of cerebrospinal fluid (CSF) within the ventricles.

- **Obstructive (noncommunicating) hydrocephalus:**
  - Obstruction of CSF flow the aqueduct of Sylvius or the fourth ventricle.
  - Occurs most commonly with congenital aqueductal stenosis, but also with posterior fossa tumor, Arnold-Chiari type II malformations, Dandy-Walker syndrome, and vein of Galen malformations.
- **Nonobstructive (communicating) hydrocephalus:**
  - Blood or infectious material obliterates the cisterns or archnoid villi and impedes CSF flow and reabsorption.
  - Typically occurs after subarachnoid hemorrhage (SAH), intraventricular hemorrhage in a preemie, meningitis, intrauterine infections, or leukemia.
- **Hydrocephalus ex vacuo:** Decreased brain parenchymal volume leads to ↑ CSF seen in ventricles, as well as increased prominence of sulci and gyri.

Symptoms/Exam

- Family history of aqueductal stenosis (may be X-linked recessive), signs of increased ICP: vomiting, altered mental status.
- Physical exam may show irritability, full fontanel, split sutures and rapid head growth in infants, eyes that deviate downward (sunset sign) or difficulty with upgaze, papilledema, and increased tone/reflexes.

Diagnosis

- Ultrasound may be helpful in infants.
- Head CT or MRI in infants, older children, and adults. MRI preferred.

Treatment

- Where possible, treat the underlying cause.
- Medical management with acetazolamide or furosemide may provide some relief.
- Definitive treatment is with a ventriculoperitoneal shunt; however, with meningitis or hemorrhage, this procedure often must be delayed until CSF viscosity is low enough that shunt tubing will not be obstructed.

CRANIOSYNOSTOSIS

- Craniosynostosis is the premature closure of one or more sutures.
- Incidence is approximately 1 in 2000 children.
- The majority of cases are idiopathic, but other etiologies include **genetic causes**—Crouzon, Apert, Carpenter, Chotzen, and Pfeiffer syndromes.

DIAGNOSIS

- Via inspection of the skull and palpation of the sutures.
- CT if surgery is contemplated.

TREATMENT

Surgery is used sparingly for cosmetic indications. For increased ICP, it is mandatory.

Malformations of the Brain

ARNOLD-CHIARI MALFORMATION

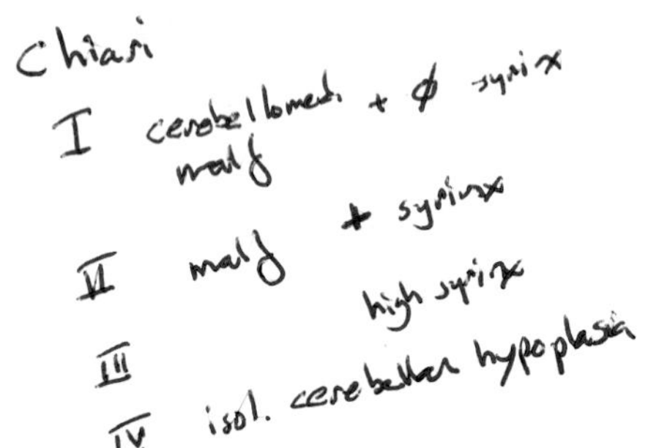

- Chiari recognized 4 types of abnormality. In recent years, the term has come to be restricted to Chiari types I and II—that is, to the cerebellomedullary malformation without and with a meningomyelocele, respectively.
- Type III Chiari malformation is simply a high cervical or occipitocervical meningomyelocele with cerebellar herniation.
- Type IV Chiari is isolated cerebellar hypoplasia.

Chiari I

SYMPTOMS/EXAM

- Headache, neck pain.
- If syrinx exists, numbness in a capelike distribution over the shoulders is typical.
- Urinary frequency.
- Progressive spasticity of the lower extremities.

DIAGNOSIS

- MRI sagittal views show tonsillar herniation through the foramen magnum into the cervical canal of typically > 5 mm.
- May have an associated spinal cord syrinx.

TREATMENT

Symptomatic patients may be treated with suboccipital craniectomy to remove the posterior arch of the foramen magnum, along with removal of the posterior ring of C1. Removal of these bony structures relieves the compression of the cerebellar tonsils and cervicomedullary junction, and may allow reestablishment of normal CSF flow patterns.

Chiari II

Cardinal features:

- Low cerebellar tonsils.
- Tectal "beaking."
- Kinking of the medulla.

SYMPTOMS/EXAM

- More than 95% will have associated myelomeningocele.
- Symptoms are typically those of progressive hydrocephalus.
- Approximately 10% of patients will present in infancy with apnea, stridor, and weak cry (symptoms of brain stem compression).

Diagnosis

Brain MRI shows protruding cerebellar tonsils and hindbrain abnormalities.

Treatment

- Ventricular shunting is often required to treat hydrocephalus.
- Surgical decompression may be required.

LISSENCEPHALY

"Smooth brain": Migrational disorder in which the cerebrum lacks sulci and gyri, though there is a spectrum of severity. Classic lissencephaly is associated with mutations in the *PAFAH1B1* gene (formerly *LIS1*) on chromosome 17p13.3.

Symptoms/Exam

- Severe neurologic impairment.
- Seizures, poor temperature regulation, failure to accept nourishment, and apneic attacks all combine to shorten life.
- Microcephaly, abnormal craniofacial features, and congenital heart disease may occur.
- Miller Dieker syndrome is classic lissencephaly with characteristic facial features that include a prominent forehead; midface hypoplasia, a small, upturned nose; low-set and abnormally shaped ears; a small jaw; and a thick upper lip.

Diagnosis

MRI.

Treatment

Supportive care.

SCHIZENCEPHALY

Congenital brain malformation characterized by a cleft extending from the pial surface of the cerebrum to the ventricle. The cleft is lined by polymicrogyric cortex (see p. 344). The most common location involves the insula and adjoining pre/post central gyri.

The etiology is heterogeneous and can be due to an early prenatal insult affecting the germinal zone prior to neuronal migration or can be genetic (mutation in the homeobox gene *Emx2* has been identified in some cases).

Symptoms/Exam

Seizures, hemiparesis, mental retardation if open lip.

Diagnosis

- MRI. The presence of gyri and sulci (gray matter) radiating into the cleft aids in differentiating this condition from a late intrauterine or early postnatal MCA infarction.
- The clefts can be unilateral or bilateral, "closed-lip" (small defect) or "open-lip" (large defect).

Treatment

Supportive care.

POLYMICROGYRIA

- Numerous small sulci on the surface of the brain, which is caused by abnormal migration of cortical neuroblasts.
- Gray matter heterotopias are often associated.
- **Symptoms/Exam:** Neurologic impairment. Seizures.
- **Diagnosis:** MRI.
- **Treatment:** Supportive care.

AGENESIS OF THE CORPUS CALLOSUM

- Agenesis or hypoplasia of the corpus callosum may occur if the crossing fibers fail to grow or are destroyed.
- Causes include chromosomal abnormalities, hereditary disorders (X-linked, autosomal dominant and recessive), inborn errors of metabolism, teratogens.

Symptoms/Exam

- If this is the only brain abnormality, development may be normal.
- Developmental delays, especially if other brain abnormalities are present.
- Retinal lacunes and vertebral abnormalities in girls (Aicardi syndrome).
- Hypo- or hypertelorism.
- Recurrent hypothermia (Shapiro syndrome).

Diagnosis

MRI. With complete agenesis, a "bat-wing" pattern of the ventricles is seen.

Treatment

Supportive care.

DANDY-WALKER MALFORMATION

- Cystic expansion of the fourth ventricle, with agenesis of the cerebellar vermis.
- Variants exist with hypoplasia of the cerebellar vermis that may have no clinical symptoms.

Symptoms/Exam

- Ninety percent of children with Dandy-Walker malformation have hydrocephalus.
- They may also have cerebellar ataxia and motor and cognitive delays.

Diagnosis

- Rapidly increasing head circumference, prominent occiput.
- MRI shows abnormalities described above.
- In babies, posterior skull may transilluminate.

Treatment

Shunt may be placed in the ventricles and/or the cystic cavity.

HYPOTONIA

- The spinal muscular atrophies (SMAs; Table 12.3) are disorders in which there is progressive loss of anterior horn cells in the spinal cord and motor nuclei in the brain stem.
- Autosomal recessive inheritance.
- Associated with deletion of exon 7 in the survival motor neuron (SMN) 1 gene on chromosome 5.
- Type of SMA depends on the number of copies of SMN 2 (ie, more SMN 2 allows less severe disease, copy number ranges from 0 to 5).

Symptoms/Exam

- Weakness of proximal > distal muscles.
- Hypotonia.
- Preserved extraocular and facial movement.
- Tongue fasiculations may be present.

Diagnosis

- DNA testing.
- Muscle biopsy is unnecessary, but has classic features—grouped atrophy of type I and II fibers.
- Electromyogram (EMG) will show abnormal spontaneous activity (fibrillations, positive sharp waves, fasciculations), reduced recruitment, and large-amplitude voluntary motor units.
- Creatine kinase (CK) is usually normal to mildly elevated.

Treatment

Supportive.

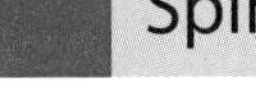

Spinal Cord Diseases of Childhood

TETHERED CORD

- Normally, during fetal life, the distal embryonic spinal cord regresses so that only a thin, threadlike filum terminale remains and stretches from the coccyx to the conus medullaris (located at L1).
- Tethered cord occurs when the filum terminale is thickened (> 2 mm) and anchors the conus medullaris at L2 or below.
- As the child grows, the spinal cord stretches and the lumbosacral segments become ischemic.

TABLE 12.3. Spinal Muscular Atrophies

SMA	Onset of Symptoms	Motor Function
I	0–6 months of age	Unable to sit
II	6–12 months of age	Sits but unable to walk
III	Childhood, after 12 months	Able to walk short distances
IV	Adult onset	Frequent falls

Symptoms/Exam

- Skin findings overlying the posterior spine are present in at least 70% of children (hair tuft, dermal pit, hyperpigmented patch, lipoma, or cutaneous hemangioma).
- Clinical presentation may occur anytime from infancy to adulthood.
- Constipation and urinary incontinence (detrusor hyperreflexia), progressive scoliosis, nonsegmental sensory loss, pain and/or spasticity in the lower extremities may be present.
- Young children may have asymmetric leg or foot growth. Pain in the lumbosacral region, perineum, and legs is the predominant symptom in older children.

Diagnosis

MRI of the lumbosacral spine shows the level of the conus medullaris (at or below L2) and filum terminale.

Treatment

Surgical—transect the filum terminale.

NEURAL TUBE DEFECTS (NTDs)

- Occur because the neural tube fails to close properly during weeks 3–4 of gestation.
- Severity ranges from very mild (ie, spina bifida occulta) to moderate (myelomeningocele) to severe (anencephaly).
- Causes include malnutrition (especially ↓ folate), radiation, drugs, chemical and genetic factors involving folate-dependent pathways.

Diagnosis

- Serum testing at 16–18 weeks shows a ↑ alpha-fetoprotein (AFP) level.
- Can often be confirmed via prenatal ultrasound.

Spina Bifida Occulta

Symptoms/Exam

- Midline sacral tuft of hair or dimple.
- No neurological symptoms.

Diagnosis

X-ray reveals nonfusion of the vertebral arches posteriorly.

Treatment

- Often none.
- Surgical if spine is unstable.

Meningocele

Symptoms/Exam

- Sac protruding from the back of an infant that does not contain neural elements, just meninges.
- Often pedunculated with a narrow base connecting the underlying spinal cord.

Diagnosis

- Exam and ultrasound.
- No neurologic symptoms.

Treatment

Surgical closure of the back.

Myelomeningocele

Symptoms/Exam

- Broad-based saclike defect in the back, typically oozing CSF and serum.
- Spinal cord is contained within the sac and remnants of the spinal cord are often fused to the dome of the sac.
- Exam depends on the spinal segments involved; should assess for sensory level, lower-extremity strength and reflexes, bladder distention, hip dislocation, head circumference, and level of alertness.

Diagnosis

- Clinical exam, though EMG may be helpful in precisely identifying segments involved.
- Head ultrasound should be done in all newborns with myelomeningocele.
- Only 15% have clinically evident hydrocephalus, but about 60% will have it via ultrasound and up to 80% develop hydrocephalus in time.

Treatment

Back closure and supportive care, including ventriculoperitoneal shunt if needed.

Prevention

- Folate supplementation (0.4 mg/day) is recommended for all women of childbearing age.
- For mothers who have had a child with an NTD, folate 4 mg/day is recommended, beginning at least 4 weeks prior to conception.

Neuromuscular Junction Diseases

BOTULISM

- *Clostridium botulinum* toxin prevents the release of acetylcholine, which causes cholinergic blockade of skeletal muscle and other cholinergic synapses.
- Disease is produced by ingesting *C botulinum* toxin from contaminated food in older children and adults.
- *C botulinum* spores may colonize the immature digestive tract in infants and produce toxin from this location.

Symptoms/Exam

- **Infantile:**
  - First symptom is usually constipation, followed by hypotonia in a previously healthy infant.
  - History may reveal exposure to honey, corn syrup, or soil that contains *C botulinum* spores. A clear exposure is found in approximately 20% of cases.

- **Older children and adults:** Bilateral cranial nerve palsies—swallowing difficulties and third nerve palsies with dilated, sluggishly reactive pupils are typical.

DIAGNOSIS

- EMG shows incremental response to high-rate (20–50 Hz) repetitive nerve stimulation.
- In infants, *C botulinum* toxin may be recovered from the stool.

TREATMENT

- Human botulinum immunoglobulin is available for use in the acute setting.
- Supportive care, particularly respiratory support, is often required.
- Antitoxin for older children and adults.

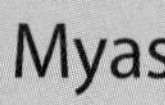

Myasthenic Syndromes in Childhood

NEONATAL MYASTHENIA

SYMPTOMS/EXAM

- Ptosis, difficulty feeding, fatigable weakness seen in a newborn infant of a myasthenic mother. Joint deformity (eg, club feet) occurs in severe cases.
- Due to passive, transplacental transfer of antibodies against nicotinic acetylcholine receptors (AChR), especially with high titers against *fetal* AChR.

DIAGNOSIS

History and exam are generally sufficient. AChR antibodies may be tested, though commercial assays do not detect antibodies against fetal AChR.

TREATMENT

Supportive care (more frequent, smaller oral feeds or nasogastric feeds, oral pyridostigmine or IM or SQ neostigmine prior to oral feeds) until antibodies disappear (may take days to weeks).

CONGENITAL MYASTHENIA

- Nonimmunologic, may be hereditary.
- Caused by defects in presynaptic, intrasynaptic, or postsynaptic NMJ. Examples: Endplate acetylcholinesterase deficiency, endplate ACh receptor defects, or defects in ACh synthesis or vesicle trafficking.
- Majority of forms are autosomal recessive with male predominance.

SYMPTOMS/EXAM

- Similar to neonatal myasthenia, though symptoms do not resolve.
- In addition to ptosis, babies have ophthalmoplegia.
- May develop generalized weakness.

DIAGNOSIS

Low-rate (2–3 Hz) repetitive stimulation on EMG produces a decremental response.

TREATMENT

Very difficult. Pyridostigmine (risk of worsening end plate acetylcholinesterase deficiency), 3,4-diaminopyridine (DAP), which increases release of ACh.

JUVENILE MYASTHENIA

- Post-synaptic ACh receptors are degraded, leading to muscle fatigue.
- Mechanism is autoimmune (immune-mediated neuromuscular blockade) and generally is not inherited.
- Onset is typically after age 10, females > males.
- Prepubertal children are rarely affected, but when myasthenia gravis occurs, males > females are affected.

SYMPTOMS/EXAM

- Ptosis and double vision a (weakness of extraocular muscles) are the earliest symptoms.
- Facial weakness and difficulty swallowing.
- Hallmark: Fatigable weakness.

DIAGNOSIS

- Based on 2 of 3 or more findings: EMG, improvement with edrophonium (Tensilon) test or response to pyridostigmine (Mestinon), and/or antibodies to ACh receptor.
- EMG shows decremental response with repetitive nerve stimulation (low-rate).
- ACh receptor–binding antibodies are detected in ~80% of cases.

TREATMENT

- Cholinesterase-inhibiting drugs are the mainstay of treatment.
- Oral steroids are often required for immunosuppression.
- Steroid sparing medications also may be used, though none have been proven effective (azathioprine).
- Thymectomy: No randomized trials prove effectiveness. Thought most effective in those with high titers of anti-ACh receptor antibodies.
- Test for and treat hypothyroidism if it exists.
- Myasthenic crisis is treated with intravenous immune globulin (IVIG) or plasma exchange.

COMPLICATIONS

Respiratory failure may occur during myasthenic crisis.

Myopathies

DUCHENNE MUSCULAR DYSTROPHY (DMD)

- The most common muscular dystrophy.
- X-linked with an incidence of 1 in 3500 live male births.
- Approximately 30% of cases are new mutations in the dystrophin gene.

SYMPTOMS/EXAM

- Gait disturbance before age 5.
- Pseudohypertrophy of the calves, toe walking, and frequent falls.

- Hip girdle weakness may be seen as early as 2 years of age.
- Affects proximal > distal strength.
- Gowers sign often seen by age 3 and always seen by age 5–6 years.
- Boys are usually unable to walk past 12 years of age.
- Other systemic involvement may include:
  - Cardiac: Cardiomyopathy.
  - Pulmonary: Decreased respiratory reserve, weak cough.
  - Genitourinary: Incontinence, if seen, is a late finding.
  - CNS: Mild intellectual impairment and learning disabilities.

DIAGNOSIS

- Genetic testing for mutation in the dystrophin gene on Xp21. Dystrophin content in muscle is < 3% of normal.
- Muscle biopsy will also be diagnostic with absent or reduced dystrophin immunostaining.
- ↑ CK.
- EMG will show myopathic features, but nerve conduction velocities are normal.
- At the time of diagnosis, electrocardiogram (ECG), echocardiogram, and chest x-ray should be done to evaluate cardiac function.

TREATMENT

- Steroids (prednisone in the United States and deflazacort in Europe) have been shown to prolong ambulation.
- Supportive care, including bracing and physical therapy.

COMPLICATIONS

Death usually occurs in the third decade.

BECKER MUSCULAR DYSTROPHY

- A genetic defect at the same locus as DMD, but patients have a milder course.
- Dystrophin content is 3–20% of normal.

SYMPTOMS/EXAM

- Onset of weakness is later than DMD.
- Boys ambulate until late adolescence/early adulthood.
- Same rate of cardiomyopathy as DMD.

DIAGNOSIS

- Genetic testing for mutation in the dystrophin gene.
- Muscle biopsy will also be diagnostic.
- ↑ creatine kinase.

TREATMENT

Supportive care. No evidence for benefit from steroid treatment.

COMPLICATIONS

Survival is to fourth decade or beyond.

MYOTONIC DYSTROPHY

A CTG trinucleotide repeat on chromosome 19 (type1) or CCTG tetranucleotide repeat on chromosome 3 (type 2); amplification increases with each generation, causing progressively more severe disease (anticipation). Patients may present either in the newborn period or in the first decade of life.

Symptoms/Exam

- **Neonatal/congenital myotonic dystrophy:** Hypotonia, facial diplegia, tenting of the upper lip, feeding problems, and respiratory distress due to weakness of intercostal and diaphragmatic muscles.
- **Juvenile myotonic dystrophy (childhood or adolescence):**
  - Myotonia (difficulty relaxing muscles after contraction).
  - Progressive weakness in the face, sternocleidomastoid muscles, shoulders, distal limbs.
  - Frontal baldness.
  - Facial muscle atrophy with bitemporal wasting.
  - Multiple endocrinopathies.
  - Impaired speech and hearing.
  - Cataracts.
  - Mental retardation may also be present.

Diagnosis

- Family history and exam (be sure to examine parents, as they may be undiagnosed).
- Genetic testing to assess the number of trinucleotide or tetranucleotide repeats is commercially available.

Treatment

- Supportive care such as leg braces for the progressive weakness.
- Myotonia may be treated by membrane-stabilizing drugs such as mexilitine, phenytoin, carbamazepine, etc.
- Cardiac evaluation for arrhythmia is recommended.

CENTRAL CORE DISEASE

Most common congenital myopathy. Defects in RYR1 gene, majority are autosomal dominant.

Symptoms/Exam

- Mild hyptonia in infancy, often congenital hip dislocation.
- Slowly progressive weakness after age 5 years, which doesn't affect extraocular or facial muscles.
- Affects proximal > distal muscles and arms > legs.
- Risk of malignant hyperthermia exists—avoid triggering anesthetic agents (succinylcholine, volatile anesthetics such as halothane, isoflurane, enflurane, etc).

Diagnosis

- Muscle biopsy.
- CK is normal, and EMG may be normal or myopathic.
- RYR1 sequencing identifies abnormalities in ~50–80%.

TREATMENT

Supportive.

NEMALINE MYOPATHY

There are 7 types of nemaline myopathy, neonatal to adult onset, with considerable overlap. The neonatal or congenital form may be severe, intermediate, or typical, with significant survival differences. Inheritance is complex and may be autosomal dominant or recessive.

SYMPTOMS/EXAM

- Weakness, hypotonia, and depressed or absent deep tendon reflexes.
- Muscle weakness is usually most severe in the face, the neck flexors, and the proximal limb muscles.

DIAGNOSIS

- Clinical findings and muscle biopsy: Characteristic rod-shaped structures (nemaline bodies) on muscle biopsy stained with Gomori trichrome.
- Disease-causing mutations have been identified in 7 different genes most encode proteins associated with the contractile elements (sarcomere).

TREATMENT

Supportive.

Developmental Disorders

PERVASIVE DEVELOPMENTAL DISORDERS

CDC is reporting autism occurs 1 in 68 (1 in 42 boys, 1 in 189 girls).

Asperger Disorder

Autism spectrum but:

- Individuals with Asperger disorder have better verbal expression, higher levels of cognitive function, and greater interest in interpersonal social activity.
- There is no clinically significant delay in cognitive development or in the development of age-appropriate self-help skills, adaptive behavior (other than social interaction), and curiosity about the environment in childhood.

Autism

Onset of symptoms is before age 3 years.

SYMPTOMS/EXAM

- Abnormal social interactions (impaired eye contact, other nonverbal behaviors).
- Language delays; stereotyped or repetitive use of language.

Diagnosis

Via *Diagnostic and Statistical Manual of Mental Disorders*, 4th edition (DSM-IV) diagnostic criteria.

Treatment

- No good treatment options.
- Behavioral therapy.

Rett Syndrome

- A neurodegenerative disorder that affects primarily girls.
- Triad: Microcephaly, hand wringing, and hyperventilation.

Symptoms/Exam

- Children initially develop normally until 12–18 months of age, then gradually lose speech and purposeful hand use.
- Deceleration of head growth, stereotypic hand movements, seizures, autistic features, ataxia, and breathing abnormalities (typically hyperventilation) subsequently develop.

Diagnosis

- Diagnosis is clinical.
- Many but not all children will have mutations in the *MECP2* gene, which maps to Xq28.
- Almost all cases are sporadic.
- If no *MECP2* mutation is found, additional workup for other neurodegenerative disorders should be undertaken before the child is called *MECP2*-negative Rett.
- Brain MRI, serum amino acids, urine organic acids, chromosome analysis, with specific attention to chromosome 15, and fluorescence in situ hybridization (FISH) for Angelman syndrome, hearing test, ophthalmologic evaluation.

Treatment

Anticonvulsants for seizures.

Cerebral Palsy (CP) (Table 12.4)

- Incidence is 2–3 in 1000 children.
- Nonprogressive disorder of the motor system due to brain injury.
- Causes include prematurity; prenatal, peripartum, or other asphyxia; early infection and kernictus.
- In many cases of CP, the cause of the brain injury is unknown. History should explore the pregnancy, delivery, and postpartum periods.

Symptoms/Exam

- CP is purely a motor disorder and does not imply lack of intellectual ability.
- No loss of skills.
- Exam shows hypertonia, hyperreflexia, and possibly choreoathetosis or dystonia.

Diagnosis

MRI may show periventricular leukomalacia, cystic encephalomalacia, stroke (particularly with hemiplegic CP), and pathology of the basal ganglia. MRI is abnormal in 80–90% with CP.

TABLE 12.4. Types of Cerebral Palsy

Motor Syndrome	Clinical Findings	Neuropathology
Spastic diplegia	Bilateral spasticity of the legs more than the arms. Often first noticed when the infant is learning to crawl. If severe, spasticity may make it difficult to put on diapers. Scissoring of the legs. Usually associated with normal intellectual development and a low risk of seizures.	Periventricular leukomalacia (PVL).
Spastic quadriplegia	The most severe form, affecting all extremities. Has a strong association with mental retardation and seizures. Evidence of athetosis is often seen; may be diagnosed with mixed CP.	PVL, multicystic encephalomalacia.
Spastic hemiplegia	One-sided CP; the arms are more frequently affected than the legs. Hand preference is seen at an early age. Delayed walking. Patients often walk on tiptoes owing to ↑ tone. Associated with a positive family history of thrombophilic states or strokes.	Stroke.
Dyskinesia/ataxia	Less common than spastic CP. Infants are hypotonic with poor head control; feeding and speech are affected. Intellectual problems and seizures are uncommon.	Basal ganglia pathology involving the putamen, globus pallidus, and thalamus.

Reproduced, with permission, from Le T, Lam W, Rabizadeh S, Schroeder A, Vera K. *First Aid for the Pediatric Boards,* 1st ed. New York: McGraw-Hill, 2006: 465.

Treatment

- A multidisciplinary team will maximize function. Team should include physicians, physical and occupational therapists, speech and language pathologists, and educational specialists.
- Treat spasticity with medication (baclofen, trihexyphenidyl, benzodiazepines, tizanidine), physical therapy, botulinum toxin, and surgery in some cases.

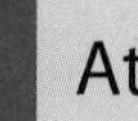

Ataxia

ACUTE CEREBELLAR ATAXIA

Thought to be an immune response against a virus, which then recognizes a "self" epitope in the cerebellum. Age at onset: typically 1–3 years. Often follows a viral infection by 2–3 weeks.

Symptoms/Exam

- Acute onset of ataxia, often upon awakening.
- Ataxia often is truncal.
- Horizontal nystagmus is present in 50% of cases.

Diagnosis

- A diagnosis of exclusion.
- LP should be done to exclude encephalitis.

Treatment

Supportive. Typically children recover within 2 months.

FRIEDREICH ATAXIA

Symptoms/Exam

- Slowly progressive ataxia with mean age of onset between age 10 and 15 years.
- Typically associated with depressed tendon reflexes.
- Other symptoms include: dysarthria, muscle weakness, spasticity in the lower limbs, optic nerve atrophy, scoliosis, bladder dysfunction, and loss of position and vibration sense in the lower > upper extremites.
- Two-thirds of individuals will have cardiomyopathy.
- Thirty percent have diabetes mellitus.
- About 25% have an "atypical" presentation with later onset, retained tendon reflexes, or unusually slow progression of disease.
- Autosomal recessive.

Diagnosis

The most common mutation, seen in more than 96% of individuals with Friedreich ataxia, is homozygous GAA triplet-repeat expansion located on chromosome 9. Testing is commercially available.

Treatment

Supportive.

ATAXIA-TELANGECTASIA

- An autosomal recessive disorder characterized by progressive cerebellar ataxia beginning between 1 and 4 years of age, oculomotor apraxia, frequent infections, choreoathetosis, telangiectasias of the conjunctivae, immunodeficiency, and an increased risk for malignancy, particularly leukemia and lymphoma.
- Individuals with ataxia-telangectasia are unusually sensitive to ionizing radiation.

Symptoms/Exam

Slurred speech, truncal ataxia, oculomotor apraxia, telangiectasias of the conjunctivae, premature aging.

Diagnosis

- ↑ AFP.
- Identification of a 7;14 chromosomal translocation on routine karyotype of peripheral blood is found in 5–15%.
- Testing for the *ATM* gene.
- A small cerebellum is often seen on MRI, but may not be apparent in young children.

Treatment

- Supportive.
- IVIG replacement therapy appears to reduce the number of infections and should be considered for individuals with frequent and severe infections.
- Surveillance for malignancy with regular medical visits.

Movement Disorders

TICS

- Involuntary, brief, stereotyped movements that typically involve the face, eyes, mouth, head, and neck.
- Tics may be motor or vocal, and simple or complex.
- May be transient (symptoms for < 1 year) or chronic (symptoms persist for ≥ 1 year).

Symptoms/Exam

- **Motor:**
  - **Simple tics:** Involve 1 muscle group.
  - **Complex:** A combination of simple tics or involving multiple muscle groups.
- **Vocal:**
  - **Simple tics:** Produced by moving air through the nose and mouth: grunting, barking, throat clearing.
  - **Complex tics:** May involve words, phrases, or sentences.

Diagnosis

- Observation.
- Tics are associated with a number of disorders: mental retardation, autism, CNS infections (encephalitis), and medications (stimulants and anticonvulsants).

Treatment

- Medication is usually unnecessary in transient tic disorder. See Treatment section of "Tourette Syndrome" below for pharmacotherapy.
- Relaxation techniques may help.

TOURETTE SYNDROME

Affects boys > girls and children > adults. Onset of symptoms must be before 18 years of age.

Diagnosis

- Multiple motor and vocal tics occurring for > 1 year.
- No tic-free period for > 4 months.
- Attention-deficit hyperactivity disorder (ADHD), obsessive-compulsive disorder (OCD), mood disorders, and learning disabilities may all be associated with Tourette syndrome.

Treatment

- Treatment is recommended when there is impairment in social functioning.
- Treatment is not curative and does not alter the course of the disease.
- Medications include: clonidine, risperidone, haloperidol, and pimozide.

SYDENHAM CHOREA

- Movement disorder that appears weeks to months after group A strep infection.
- Girls > boys.
- Average age at onset 8–12 years.

Symptoms/Exam

- Choreiform movements, "St. Vitus dance" hypotonia, emotional lability, dysarthria.
- Emotional and behavioral disturbance may be more troublesome than chorea.
- Difficulty with writing is common.

Diagnosis

- Recent positive strep culture, ASO titer, or anti-DNase B.
- History and physical exam looking for other major manifestation of rheumatic fever, including echocardiogram to evaluate for carditis.
- Check serum electrolytes, including calcium, erythrocyte sedimentation rate (ESR), thyroid-stimulating hormone (TSH), antinuclear antibodies (ANA), anticardiolipin antibodies, ceruloplasmin, and urine copper.
- MRI of the brain is normal.

Treatment

- Penicillin should be given for prophylaxis against recurrence of rheumatic fever.
- Additional treatment is symptomatic not curative and options include:
  - Anticonvulsant: Both valproic acid and carbamazepine have been shown to be beneficial in small studies.
  - Benzodiazepines: Clonazepam.
  - Dopamine agonists such as haloperidol and pimozide.
  - Immunomodulatory therapies: Steroids, IVIG, and plasmapheresis, though none have been well studied. In particular, coritcosteroids may shorten the time to recovery.

Complications

Recurrence rate may be as high as 20%.

Neurocutaneous Disorders

NEUROFIBROMATOSIS (NF)

NF1

- Autosomal dominant, chromosome 17q11.2.
- Approximately 50% of cases are new mutations.
- Incidence: 1 in 3000.
- Onset is in childhood.
- NF1 is approximately 10 times more common than NF2.

Symptoms/Exam

Symptoms may be limited to skin or eye markings or may include more serious complications. Which symptoms people with NF1 develop varies widely—even within families—but at least some symptoms are usually present by age 10 and may include:

- Café au lait ("coffee with milk") spots on the skin usually appear in the first few years of a person's life and increase in number and size over time. They can occur on most parts of the body other than the scalp, palms of the hands, and soles of the feet. They often increase in number during puberty and may darken with exposure to sunlight. While helpful in diagnosing NF1, these spots don't cause health problems.
- Freckles may appear in places not typically exposed to the sun, such as the underarm (axillary freckling) or groin (inguinal freckling). Freckles may not develop until puberty. They are not a health problem, though they may sometimes itch.
- Lisch nodules—pigmented bumps on the eye's iris (also called iris hamartomas)—can help diagnose NF1 but don't affect vision. They often don't appear until later in childhood.
- Neurofibromas (sometimes called fibroneuromas) are slow-growing benign tumors that can develop along nerves almost anywhere in the body. They often appear as small, fleshy, pea-sized nodules within the skin, called dermal or cutaneous neurofibromas. People with NF1 may develop a few or many. People who do not have NF1 sometimes have neurofibromas, though usually no more than several.
- Plexiform neurofibromas are larger, more ropelike tumors that can wrap in and around nerves, blood vessels, and other structures almost anywhere in the body.
- Neurofibromas can affect appearance, cause pain or affect function, depending on their location and size. Neurofibromas that affect large nerves or the spinal cord are the most likely to cause serious problems.
- Pheochromocytomas (tumors of the adrenal gland) also sometimes occur in people with NF1 and can cause high blood pressure (as can a neurofibroma that presses on the kidneys or renal artery).
- In rare instances, a neurofibroma (usually a plexiform neurofibroma) mutates into a malignant tumor (called a neurofibrosarcoma, malignant schwannoma, neurogenic sarcoma, or malignant peripheral nerve sheath tumor).
- Optic pathway gliomas (also called optic nerve gliomas or juvenile pilocytic astrocytomas) occur in about 20% of people with NF1. The optic pathway includes the optic nerve, which sends messages from the eye to the brain, and the optic chiasm, where the optic nerves from each eye cross before entering the 2 hemispheres of the brain. A glioma is a tumor that arises from glial cells (supporting cells of the nervous system).
- Optic pathway gliomas usually develop by age 10, but sometimes may not be detected until later. While many people with optic gliomas have no symptoms, signs might include:
  - Impaired vision (which can lead to eventual blindness without treatment).
  - Protrusion of the eyeball.
  - Early puberty (rare and due to the tumor pressing on the hypothalamus, the hormone center of the brain).
- Weakness of the dura (covering of the brain and spinal cord) is associated with NF1 and can sometimes cause problems such as a meningocele (herniation of the spinal cord through the vertebrae) or hydrocephalus (excess fluid accumulation in the brain).
- Skeletal abnormalities:
  - Abnormal development of the temple bone (sphenoid dyplasia) occurs in about 1% of people with NF1 and can lead to eye displacement or herniation of part of the brain.

- Thinning of the tibia in the shin or the radius in the arm is found at birth in about 1% of people with NF1. It can result in pseudarthrosis, meaning "false joint," because unhealed fractures resulting from bone loss can cause the bone to bow, bend, and eventually break. It usually only occurs on 1 side of the body, and males are more likely than females to have the problem.

DIAGNOSIS

Two or more of the following:

- Six or more café-au-lait macules > 5 mm in diameter (prepubertal) and > 15 mm in diameter after puberty.
- Two or more neurofibromas of any type or 1 plexiform neurofibroma.
- Axillary or inguinal freckling.
- Optic pathway glioma.
- Two or more Lisch nodules.
- An osseous lesion: Sphenoid wing dysplasia or thinning of the cortex of the long bones (with or without a pseudoarthrosis "false joint").
- A first-degree relative who meets criteria for NF1.

MANAGEMENT

- Biannual physicals in childhood and annually in adulthood.
- Blood pressure should be checked twice a year due to risk of renal artery stenosis and pheochromocytoma.
- Spine should be checked for the early detection of scoliosis.
- Limbs should be examined for bowing and pseudoarthosis.
- Yearly ophthalmologic exams (risk of an optic pathway glioma is highest in the first decade).
- Screening exams such as MRI, EEG, and x-rays are no longer routinely recommended. Instead, there should be careful attention for symptoms and signs with appropriate testing ordered.
- Genetic counseling and consideration of screening for first-degree relatives.

COMPLICATIONS

- Attentional problems and learning disabilities are more common in individuals with NF1.
- Plexiform neurofibromas have the potential to become malignant peripheral nerve sheath tumors.
- Macrocephaly is generally due to increased brain size, but can be due to hydrocephalus related to aqueductal stenosis.
- Patients are at ↑ risk for other CNS tumors (astrocytomas and meningiomas).

NF2

- Autosomal-dominant, chromosome 22q12.2.
- Approximately 50% of cases are new mutations.
- Incidence: 1 in 40,000.
- Onset is in adolescence.

SYMPTOMS/EXAM

The most common symptoms of NF2 are tinnitus (ringing in the ears), hearing loss and loss of balance. Other symptoms include:

- Headaches.
- Nausea or vomiting.

- Facial or muscle weakness.
- Pain in the face or ear.
- Problems with vision.
- A lump or swelling under the skin caused by the development of a neurofibroma or schwannoma (tumor on a nerve).

Patients with neurofibromatosis type 2 may develop multiple tumors on nerves associated with swallowing, speech, eye movements, and facial sensation and on the spinal nerves going to the arms and legs. A type of cataract (juvenile posterior subcapsular cataract) may also be present in children.

Diagnosis

Either of the following:

- Bilateral eighth nerve masses (vestibular schwanommas).
- A first-degree relative with NF2 and either a unilateral eighth nerve mass or 2 of the following: glioma, meningioma, schwannoma, neurofibroma, juvenile posterior subcapsular lenticular opacities.

Management

- **Initial evaluation:**
  - Careful neurologic and ophthalmologic exams.
  - Auditory testing.
  - MRI of the brain with gadolinium, with thin cuts through the internal auditory canals.
  - MRI of the spine if there are signs or symptoms of myelopathy.
  - Genetic counseling and consideration of screening for first-degree relatives.
- **Annual evaluations:**
  - Thorough neurological exam.
  - Auditory testing.
  - Brain MRI.
- Vestibular schwanommas may be treated surgically, but there is significant risk of deafness. They are generally followed until they cause significant symptoms.

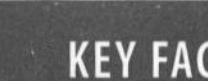

KEY FACT

The classic triad of seizures, mental retardation, and facial angiofibromas is present in < 50% of patients with TS.

TUBEROUS SCLEROSIS (TS)

- Autosomal dominant and associated with chromosome 9 or 16.
- More than half of all cases are new mutations.
- Incidence: 1 in 6000.

Symptoms/Exam

- Severity varies widely and ranges from normal intelligence with no seizures to severe mental retardation and intractable epilepsy.
- Generally, earlier presentation signals more severe disease, for example, infantile spasms in infancy.
- Up to 70% of children with TS get infantile spasms.

Diagnosis

- A definite diagnosis of TS requires 2 major features or 1 major and 2 minor features (see Table 12.5).
- Careful skin exam (see Table 12.6).
- Head CT or MRI shows calcified tubers in the periventricular area (may not be seen until mid-childhood).
- Baseline studies include echocardiogram, chest x-ray, and renal ultrasound.

TABLE 12.5. Diagnostic Criteria for TS

Major features:

- Facial angiofibromas or forehead plaques
- Shagreen patch (connective tissue nevus)
- Three or more hypomelanotic macules
- Nontraumatic ungula or periungual fibromas
- Lymphangioleiomyomatosis (also known as lymphangiomyomatosis)
- Renal angiomyolipoma
- Cardiac rhabdomyoma
- Multiple retinal nodular hamartomas
- Cortical tuber
- Subependymal nodules
- Subependymal giant cell astrocytoma

Minor features:

- Confetti skin lesions (multiple 1- to 2-mm hypomelanotic macules)
- Gingival fibromas
- Multiple randomly distributed pits in dental enamel
- Hamartomatous rectal polyps
- Multiple renal cysts
- Nonrenal hamartomas
- Bone cysts
- Retinal achromic patch
- Cerebral white matter radial migration lines

TREATMENT

Seizure control. Rapamycin therapy may induce partial regression of SEGAs.

COMPLICATIONS

Subependymal giant cell astrocytomas may obstruct the foramen of Monro causing hydrocephalus.

TABLE 12.6. Dermatologic Manifestations of TS

LESION	DESCRIPTION	PERCENTAGE
Ash leaf spot	Hypopigmented macules seen best with Wood's lamp. May be seen in infancy.	90%
Sebaceous adenoma	Begin as tiny red nodule over the nose and cheeks usually in late childhood. They grow, coalesce, and become flesh colored.	75%
Shagreen patch	Roughened patch of skin often located in the lumbosacral region.	25% (< 5 years) 50% (> 5 years)
Ungual fibromas	Red to flesh colored benign tumors located underneath or adjacent to the nails. More frequent around toes than fingers.	

STURGE-WEBER SYNDROME

Incidence is 1 in 50,000 and is not familial.

SYMPTOMS/EXAM

Triad: Facial port-wine stain, leptomeningeal venous angioma, glaucoma.

DIAGNOSIS

- Eye exam.
- Skull x-ray/head CT will show calcification of the cortex underlying the angioma, called "tram-track" calcifications.
- MRI with contrast will show angioma and underlying atrophy of affected hemisphere.
- Imaging may be negative in young children. Consider repeating MRI after age 2 in children with facial port-wine stain.
- Angioma typically affects the occipital > parietal > frontotemporal lobes.

TREATMENT

- Anticonvulsants.
- Aspirin is controversial.
- Surgical treatment of epilepsy may be necessary.

COMPLICATIONS

Often have progressive hemiparesis and visual field cut.

INCONTINENTIA PIGMENTI

X-linked dominant disorder that typically is lethal in males prenatally.

SYMPTOMS/EXAM

The skin lesions develop in 4 stages:

- Affected newborns have linear papules and vesicles.
- These lesions progress within weeks or months to verrucous streaks, which typically resolve.
- At 3–6 months of age, hyperpigmented whorls and swirls appear along Blaschko lines.
- By the second or third decade of life or sooner, the hyperpigmented whorls may gradually become hypopigmented and may atrophy.

DIAGNOSIS

- Characteristic skin lesions.
- Skin biopsy shows abundant eosinophils.
- Peripheral eosinophilia is typically present in early infancy.
- Molecular-based diagnosis is available by demonstrating mutations in NEMO (NF-κB essential modulator) in ~85% of affected patients.

MANAGEMENT

CNS manifestations that occur in approximately one-third of affected patients include seizures; mental retardation; spastic paralysis; and ophthalmologic problems, such as strabismus, cataracts, and retinal vascular changes leading to blindness.

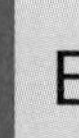

Eye Movement Abnormalities

SPASMUS NUTANS

Symptoms/Exam

- Triad of acquired nystagmus, head nodding, and torticollis.
- All 3 features are not necessary for diagnosis; head nodding and nystagmus are most common, with torticollis in only 30%.
- Age at onset is usually 6–12 months.

Diagnosis

- Brain MRI should be done to rule out an underlying tumor.
- Tumor is present in about 1% of cases (usually gliomas of the intracranial visual system or ependymomas of the fourth ventricle).
- Ophthalmologic exam for retinal problems that may be associated.

Treatment

None. Symptoms are generally outgrown.

OPSOCLONUS MYOCLONUS SYNDROME (OMS)

Symptoms/Exam

- Rapid, dancing, erratic eye movements along with and rhythmic, lightning-like jerks.
- Typically with associated ataxia.

Diagnosis

- May be the presenting manifestation of an occult neuroblastoma (OMS is then a paraneoplastic syndrome). As many as half of children with opsoclonus-myoclonus have a neuroblastoma.
- Brain MRI to look for structural lesions.
- Chest and abdominal imaging with CT or MRI.
- Measurement of urinary vanillylmandelic acid (VMA) and homovanillic acid (HVA).
- ^{131}I-metaiodobenzylguanidine (MIBG) scan also for neuroblastoma.
- Elevated concentrations of urinary VMA and HVA are diagnostic, but low levels do not exclude neuroblastoma. In several series, urinary VMA and HVA were normal in up to one-third of children with neuroblastoma in association with paraneoplastic opsoclonus.
- Neuroblastomas that are associated with OMA are usually of lower stage and have a more favorable prognosis for survival.

Treatment

Immunomodulatory therapies such as IVIG, steroids, and immunosuppression have been reported.

Strokes in Children

- Incidence is 2–3 in 100,000 children with a prevalence of 1 in 4000 neonates. In contrast to adults, childhood stroke is 50% ischemic and 50% hemorrhagic.

- Despite a thorough evaluation, the cause of stroke remains idiopathic in approximately 25% of children.
- Ischemic stroke may be caused by congenital heart disease, sickle cell disease, arterial dissection, coagulation disorders, infections such as meningitis and varicella zoster, as well as intracranial vasculopathy, including moyamoya.
- Hemorrhagic stroke may be caused by arteriovenous malformation (AVM), cerebral cavernous malformation, aneurysm, tumor, bleeding disorder, etc.
- Cerebral sinovenous thrombosis may also lead to ischemic or hemorrhagic complications.

SYMPTOMS/EXAM

Sudden onset of hemiparesis, focal seizure with "Todd paralysis," altered mental status.

DIAGNOSIS

- Head CT, brain MRI/MRA (magnetic resonance angiography), imaging of the neck vessels via MRA or computed tomography angiography (CTA).
- Cerebral angiogram if etiology is unclear and noninvasive studies are unrevealing.
- Echocardiogram with saline contrast injection to look for intracardiac shunting.
- Hypercoaguable evaluation.

TREATMENT

- Depends on underlying cause of stroke.
- Chronic transfusion therapy in sickle cell disease is the only evidence-based therapy in childhood stroke. Goal is to reduce the %HgbS to under 30%.
- Aspirin appears to be modestly protective.
- Anticoagulants are controversial, except in arterial dissection and cardioembolic stroke.
- Surgical treatment may be indicated for moyamoya, AVM, and aneurysm.

COMPLICATIONS

- Recurrence after neonatal stroke is very rare (< 5%).
- Recurrence after childhood stroke is on the order of 25% (higher in HgbSS) unless underlying cause is identified and treated.

Vein of Galen Malformation (VGAM)

Arteriovenous shunt between cerebral arteries and the vein of Galen, which occurs because there is failure to regress of a fetal midline venous structure, at about 11–14 weeks' gestation.

SYMPTOMS/EXAM

There are 2 presentations:

- **Neonatal/prenatal:** High-output congestive heart failure (CHF) and failure to thrive.
- **Later in infancy:** Often presents with rapidly ↑ head circumference, hydrocephalus, and cerebral ischemia.

- In both presentations, a loud cranial bruit is present. Facial and scalp veins are often prominent.

Diagnosis

CT and MRI show the abnormal venous structures.

Treatment

Embolization or rarely surgical treatment of the VGAM. Mortality is up to 50%.

Neurogenetics

A full-term infant is delivered with significant hypotonia, weakness, respiratory insufficiency, and feeding issues. The mother is noted to have mild mental retardation but no significant weakness. The clinical suspicion was myotonic dystrophy. What is the inheritance pattern? Myotonic dystrophy is an autosomal-dominant disorder with evidence of genetic anticipation.

INHERITANCE PATTERNS

Autosomal-Dominant Inheritance

- If 1 parent displays a dominant condition and is heterozygous for the gene, then each child has a **50% chance** of receiving the gene's single allele and of manifesting the condition. **Not all patients** with the affected gene may be symptomatic (see Figure 12.1 and Table 12.7).
- **Penetrance:** Reflects the percentage of patients with the gene who manifest symptoms or signs.
- **Expressivity:** The spectrum of severity among patients having clinical manifestations.
- **Anticipation:** Evident if the severity of the disease ↑ with each subsequent generation. An example of anticipation is **myotonic dystrophy,** an autosomal-dominant disorder that is unusual in that a severe congenital form occurs by transmission from the **mother only** and not from the father. The

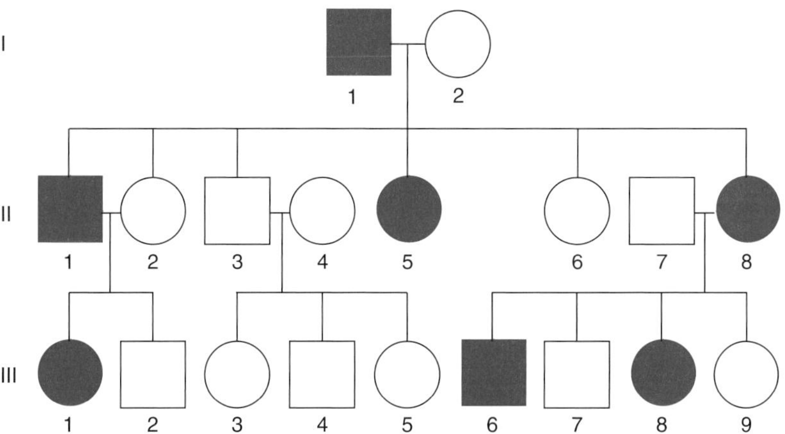

FIGURE 12.1. Example of an autosomal-dominant pedigree.

TABLE 12.7. Common Autosomal-Dominant Diseases

Disorder	Characteristics
Huntington disease	Chromosome 4p, 1 in 2500.
Neurofibromatosis Type 1 (NF1)	Chromosome 17, 50% new mutations.
Neurofibromatosis Type 2 (NF2)	Chromosome 22q, 1 in 1×10^6.
Myotonic dystrophy	Chromosome 19q, 1 in 25,000.
Tuberous sclerosis	Chromosome 9 and 16, tuberin and hamartin genes.
Hereditary hemorrhagic telangiectasia (Osler-Weber-Rendu disease)	1–2 in 100,000; angiodysplasia.

expansion of the mutational **CTG trinucleotide repeat** in a 3′ untranslated region of the myotonic protein kinase gene develops with each meiosis (mainly maternal), thereby explaining the genetic anticipation and ↑ severity in the next generation.

Autosomal-Recessive Inheritance

- The phenotype is expressed when **identical alleles** are present. Consanguinity ↑ the risk of expressing an autosomal-recessive disorder (see Figure 12.2 and Table 12.8).
- The risk of 2 carriers having a child with an autosomal-recessive disorder is 1 in 4 (25%).

X-Linked Recessive Inheritance

- The incidence of the trait is much **higher in males** than in females.
- Heterozygous females are usually unaffected, but some may express the condition with variable severity, as determined by the pattern of X-inactivation **(Lyon hypothesis or Lyonization).**
- The gene responsible for the condition is transmitted from an affected male to **all** his daughters. Any of the daughters will then have a **50% chance** of transmitting it further.
- Ordinarily the gene is **never** transmitted directly from father to son.
- The gene may be transmitted through a series of carrier females; if so, the affected males in a kindred are related through females.
- A significant proportion of isolated cases (about 90%) are due to new mutations.

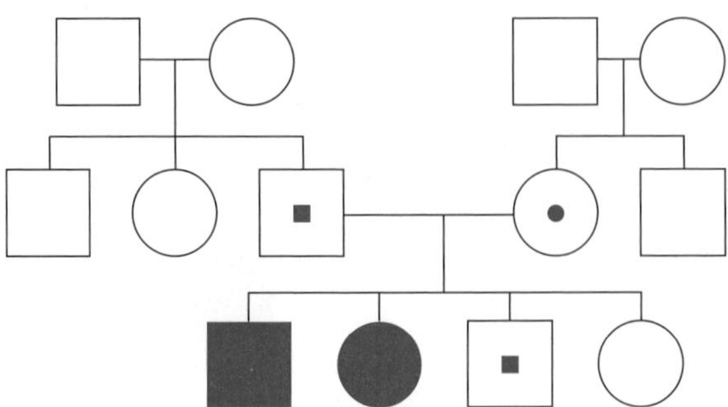

FIGURE 12.2. Example of an autosomal-recessive pedigree.

TABLE 12.8. Autosomal-Recessive Diseases

DISORDER	CHARACTERISTICS
Phenylketonuria (PKU)	Chromosome 12q, 1 in 14,000.
Sickle cell disease	Chromosome 11, 1 in 625 African-Americans.
Gaucher disease	Chromosome 1q, 1 in 2500 Ashkenazi Jews.
Tay-Sachs disease	Chromosome 15q, 1 in 3000 Ashkenazi Jews.
Galactosemia	Chromosome 9p, 1 in 60,000.
Wilson disease	Chromosome 1q, 1 in 200,000.

- Figure 12.3 gives an example of an X-linked recessive pedigree; Table 12.9 outlines common disorders associated with this mode of inheritance.

X-Linked Dominant Inheritance

- Daughters of affected males with normal mates are **all affected** but **sons are not.**
- **Both male and female** offspring of female carriers have a 50% chance of inheriting the phenotype. The pedigree pattern is the same as that seen with autosomal-dominant inheritance (see Figure 12.4).
- For rare phenotypes, affected females are about twice as common as affected males, but affected females typically have milder (though variable) expression of the phenotype.
- Example: **Hypophosphatemic** (vitamin D–resistant) rickets.

Mitochondrial Inheritance

- Mitochondrial proteins and enzymes are encoded by nuclear genes, and 37 are encoded by **mitochondrial (mt) circular DNA.**
- Mitochondria are derived **exclusively from the mother;** defects in mtDNA therefore demonstrate **maternal inheritance** (see Figure 12.5).
- All children of a **female** with a mutation in mtDNA will inherit the mutation, whereas none of the offspring of a **male** carrying the same mutation will inherit defective DNA.
- **Mitochondrial syndromes** include the following:
  - **Leber hereditary optic neuropathy:** Characterized by rapid optic nerve death and blindness; usually **homoplasmic** (cells contain mostly abnormal mtDNA).

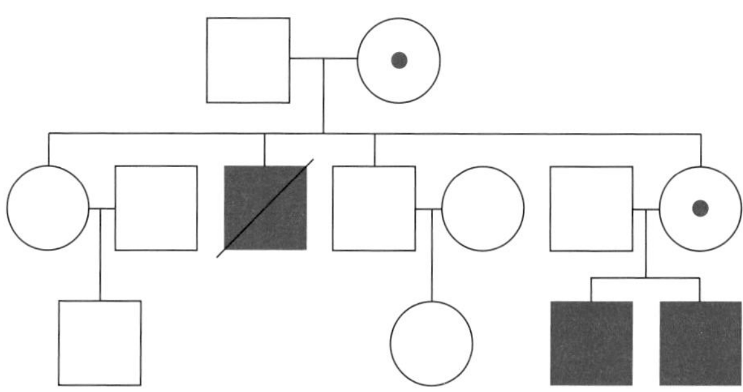

FIGURE 12.3. Example of an X-linked recessive pedigree.

TABLE 12.9. X-Linked Recessive Diseases

Disorder	Characteristics
Duchenne muscular dystrophy	Dystrophin gene, 1 in 3500–5000.
Lesch-Nyhan syndrome	Hypoxanthine-phosphoribosyl transferase, 1 in 100,000.
Ornithine transcarbamoylase (OTC) deficiency	Hyperammonemia, urea cycle defect, females often affected.
Adrenoleukodystrophy	1:17,000.
Fragile X syndrome	Affects 25% of mentally retarded males with macrocephaly and macro-orchidism; demonstrates anticipation.

KEY FACT

Heteroplasmy is defined as the presence of > 1 type of mitochondrial DNA in the mitochondria of a single individual. Heteroplasmy is responsible for significant variation of the phenotype.

- **NARP (Leigh disease):** **N**europathy, **A**taxia, **R**etinitis **P**igmentosa, developmental delay, mental retardation, lactic acidosis; heteroplasmic.
- **MELAS:** **M**itochondrial **E**ncephalomyopathy, **L**actic **A**cidosis, and **S**trokelike episodes; may manifest only as DM; heteroplasmic.
- **MERRF:** **M**yoclonic **E**pilepsy, **R**agged **R**ed **F**ibers in skeletal muscle, ataxia, sensorineural deafness; heteroplasmic.
- **Kearns-Sayre syndrome:** Progressive external ophthalmoplegia, heart block, retinal pigmentation; heteroplasmic with sporadic mutations.
- Of note, mitochondrial diseases in children are more frequently caused by mutations in nuclear DNA then in mtDNA.

Inheritance of Complex Multifactorial Diseases

- **Not single-gene** disorders; recurrence risk is not based on mendelian genetic laws.
- Demonstrate **familial aggregation** because relatives of an affected individual are more likely than are unrelated individuals to have disease-predisposing alleles in common with the affected person.
- Pairs of relatives who share disease-predisposing genotypes at relevant loci

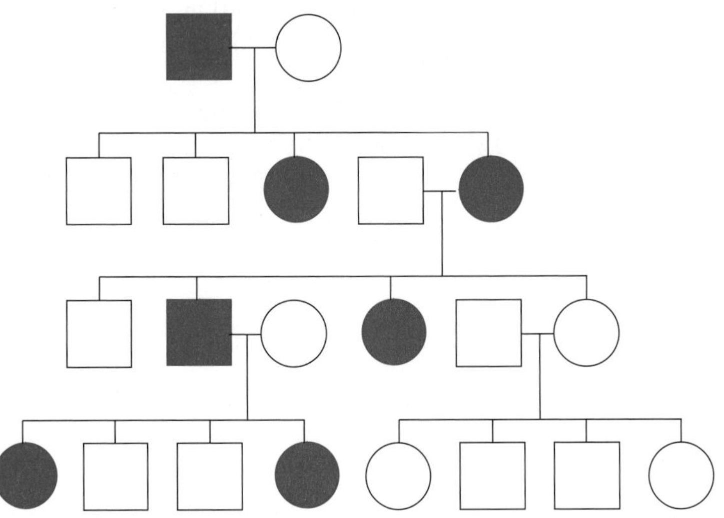

FIGURE 12.4. Example of an X-linked dominant pedigree.

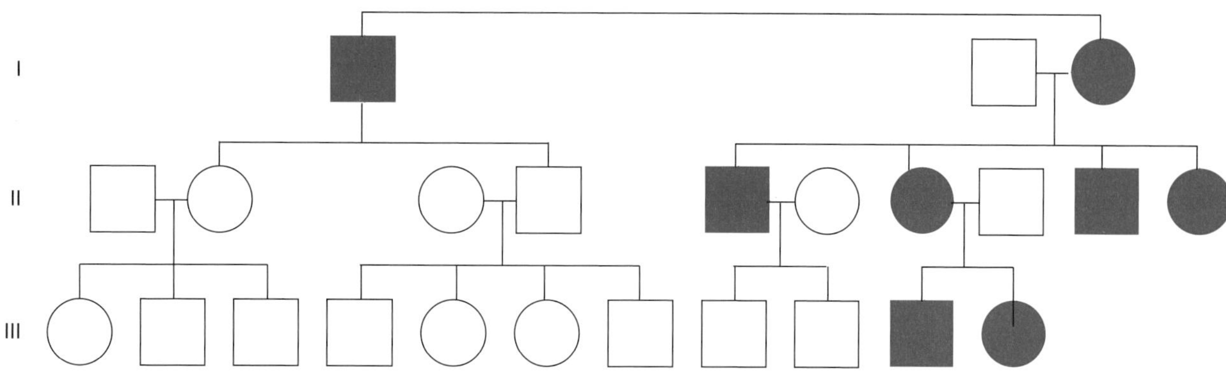

FIGURE 12.5. Example of a maternal inheritance pedigree.

may still show lack of penetrance because of the crucial role of **nongenetic factors** in disease causation.

- **Example: Coronary artery disease.**
  - **Environmental factors:** Smoking, lack of exercise, obesity.
  - **Genetic factors:** LDL receptor mutations in familial hypercholesterolemia.

Genetic Imprinting

- **Different expression of alleles can cause different diseases depending on the parent of origin. Examples:** Prader-Willi syndrome and Angelman syndrome on chromosome 15q11-q13.
- **Prader-Willi syndrome:**
  - Some 70% of cases are caused by a deletion of chromosome 15q11-q13 that is inherited by the patient's **father (missing paternal part).**
  - Can also be caused by **uniparental disomy** (no deletion, but **2 inherited copies of chromosome 15 from the mother**).
  - **Symptoms/Exam:** Hypotonia and failure to thrive during infancy, and subsequent hyperphagia; small hands and feet; mental retardation; hypogonadism.
- **Angelman syndrome:**
  - Some 70% of cases are caused by a deletion of chromosome 15q11-q13 that is inherited by the patient's **mother (missing maternal part).**
  - Can also be caused by **uniparental disomy** (no deletion, but **2 inherited copies of chromosome 15 from the father**).
  - Single-gene mutations have also been described.
  - **Symptoms/Exam:** Early speech delay, distinctive facial appearance, seizures, mental retardation, laughter outbursts.

Common Neurogenetic Syndromes

TRINUCLEOTIDE REPEAT DISORDERS

Fragile X

- The most common form of familial mental retardation. Both males and females can be affected.
- There is an increased number of CGG trinucleotide repeats (typically > 200) in the *FMR1* gene accompanied by aberrant methylation of the *FMR1* gene.
- **Symptoms/Exam:** Moderate mental retardation in affected males and

mild mental retardation in affected females. Characteristic appearance in males: large head, long face, prominent forehead and chin, protuding ears, joint laxity, and large testes (postpubertally). Behavioral abnormalities include autism spectrum disorders.

- **Diagnosis:** DNA analysis.
- **Treatment:** Supportive.

Fragile X–Associated Tremor/Ataxia Syndrome

- Occurs in males who have an *FMR1* premutation (61–200 CGG repeats).
- Characterized by late-onset (typically > 50 years of age), progressive cerebellar ataxia and intention tremor.
- *FMR1*-related premature ovarian failure occurs in approximately 20% of females who have an *FMR1* premutation.

Myotonic Dystrophy

See Myopathies section.

Friedreich Ataxia

See Ataxia section.

CHANNELOPATHIES

Periodic Paralysis

- **Hypokalemic periodic paralysis:** Defect in a sodium or a calcium channel.
  - **Symptoms/Exam:** Attacks of reversible flaccid paralysis with concomitant hypokalemia, usually leading to paraparesis or tetraparesis but sparing the respiratory muscles and heart. Triggering factors are carbohydrate-rich meals and rest after exercise; rarely, cold temperature. Frequency of attacks is highest between ages 15 and 35 and then decreases with age.
  - **Treatment:** Acetazolamide and potassium supplements.
- **Hyperkalemic periodic paralysis:** Point mutation in gene encoding the voltage-gated skeletal muscle sodium channel.
  - **Symptoms/Exam:** Attacks of reversible flaccid paralysis with concomitant hyperkalemia, usually leading to paraparesis or tetraparesis but sparing the respiratory muscles and heart. Potassium-rich food or rest after exercise may precipitate an attack. A cold environment, emotional stress, glucocorticoids, and pregnancy provoke or worsen the attacks. Between attacks, hyperkalemic periodic paralysis is usually associated with mild myotonia (muscle stiffness) that does not impede voluntary movements.
  - **Treatment:** High-carbohydrate meal may abort an attack. Other treatments include inhaled salbutamol and IV calcium gluconate.

Episodic Ataxia

- Type I (EA1) and type II (EA2) are autosomal-dominant diseases associated with abnormalities of voltage-gated ion channels (Table 12.10).
- **Symptoms/Exam:** Paroxysmal attacks of ataxia, vertigo, and nausea. Attacks can be associated with dysarthria, diplopia, tinnitus, dystonia, hemiplegia, and headache. Triggered by stress, exertion, caffeine, alcohol, and phenytoin.
- **Treatment:** Acetazolamide.

TABLE 12.10. Comparison of Episodic Ataxia Types 1 and 2

	EA1	EA2
Ion channel	Potassium	Calcium
Duration of attack	Minutes to hours	Hours to days
EMG	Myokymia	None
MRI	Normal	Cerebellar atrophy
Associated conditions	Epilepsy	Migraine
Course of disease	Attacks lessen with age	Progressive

INBORN ERRORS OF METABOLISM

Newborn Metabolic Screening

- All states screen for phenylketonuria (PKU) and hypothyroidism; tandem mass spectrometry is currently available that ↑ the number of diseases detected (eg, fatty acid oxidation disorders, organic acidurias, urea cycle defects).
- Additional conditions for which screening can be conducted include the following:
  - Galactosemia
  - Hemoglobinopathy
  - Tyrosinemia
  - Biotinidase deficiency
  - Congenital adrenal hyperplasia
  - Maple syrup urine disease
  - Homocystinuria
  - Cystic fibrosis

Laboratory Tests

- **Initial testing:**
  - CBC with differential.
  - Serum electrolytes **(calculate anion gap).**
  - Blood glucose.
  - Liver enzymes, ALT, AST.
  - Total and direct bilirubin.
  - Blood gas.
  - Plasma ammonium.
  - Plasma lactate.
  - Acylcarnitine profile.
  - Urine dipstick: pH, ketones, glucose.
  - Urine odor: **Acute disease—maple syrup urine disease:** maple syrup, burned sugar; **isovaleric acidemia:** cheesy; sweaty feet; **multiple carboxylase deficiency:** cat urine. **Nonacute disease—PKU:** musty; **hypermethioninemia:** rancid butter, rotten cabbage; **trimethylaminuria:** fishy.
  - Urine-reducing substances (positive in galactosemia, hereditary fructose intolerance, DM, tyrosinemia).

- **Further testing:** Plasma amino acids, urine organic acids. If lactate is ↑, pyruvate levels should be obtained.
- Additional tools for the differential diagnosis of metabolic disease are listed in Table 12.11 and Figure 12.6.

OVERVIEW OF METABOLIC DISEASES

Phenylketonuria (PKU)

KEY FACT

Pregnant women with PKU require rigorous management prior to conception and throughout pregnancy to prevent fetal brain damage and microcephaly.

- An autosomal-recessive disorder caused by a defect in the hydroxylation of phenylalanine to tyrosine in the liver. Incidence is 1 in 10,000–15,000.
- **Symptoms/Exam:**
  - Affected infants are normal at birth but develop severe mental retardation if not treated.
  - Children may have blond hair, blue eyes, eczema, and a mousy urine odor.
- **Treatment:** A phenylalanine-restricted diet can prevent mental retardation.

Homocystinuria

- An autosomal-recessive disease caused by a deficiency of the enzyme cystathionine β-synthase → accumulation of homocysteine in the serum and urine → enhanced reconversion to **methionine** (newborn screening).
- Incidence is 1 in 200,000 live births.
- **Symptoms/Exam:**
  - **Marfanoid habitus:** Dislocated lenses, arachnodactyly, scoliosis, pectus deformities.
  - **Mental retardation.**
  - **Arterial and venous thrombosis.**
- **Treatment:** Special diet and folate/pyridoxine supplementation.

TABLE 12.11. Differential Diagnosis of Suspected Metabolic Disease

	Maple Syrup Urine Disease	Type 1 Glycogen Storage Disease	Medium-Chain Acyl-CoA Dehydrogenase Deficiency	Propionic Acidemia	OTC Deficiency
Mechanism	Amino acid metabolism	Carbohydrate metabolism	Fatty acid oxidation	Organic acid metabolism	Urea cycle defect
Test					
Blood pH	Acidosis	Acidosis	Variable	Acidosis	Alkalosis
Anion gap	↑	↑	↑/Normal	↑	Normal
Ketones	↑	↑	Low	↑↑	Negative
Lactate	Normal	↑	Slightly ↑	Normal or ↑	Normal
Glucose	Variable	↓	↓	Normal, ↑, or ↓	Normal
NH_4^+	Slightly ↑	Normal	Moderately ↑	Normal or ↑	↑↑↑
Neurologic findings	Lethargy, coma, developmental delay	Hypoglycemic seizures, normal development	Lethargy, coma, normal development	Lethargy, coma, developmental delay	Irritability, combative, coma, developmental delay

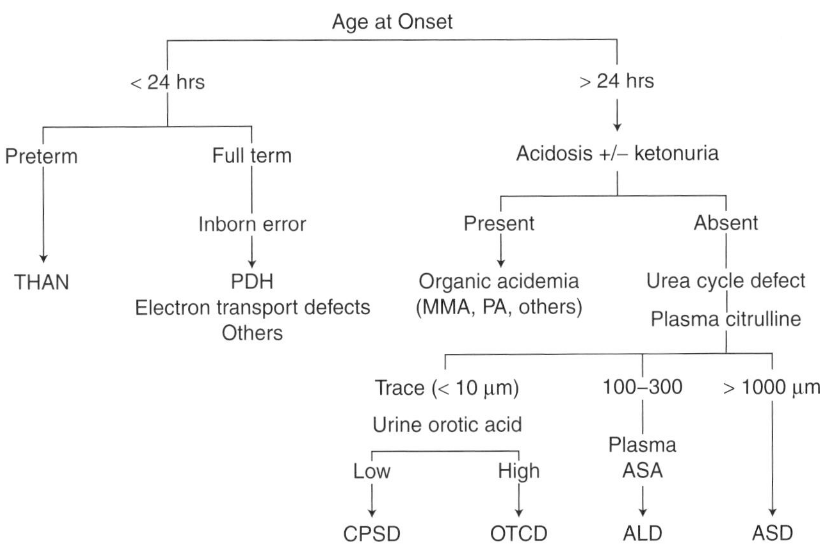

FIGURE 12.6. Differential diagnosis of a hyperammonemic newborn (NH4 > 50 μm). THAN, transitory hyperammonemia of the newborn; PDH, pyruvate dehydrogenase deficiency; MMA, methylmalonic acidemia; PA, propionic acidemia; CPSD, carbamyl phosphate synthetase deficiency; OTCD, ornithine transcarbamoylase deficiency; ALD, argininosuccinic acid lyase deficiency; ASD, argininosuccinic acid synthetase.

Galactosemia

- An autosomal-recessive disorder caused by a deficiency of galactose-1-phosphate uridyltransferase.
- Incidence is 1 in 60,000 live births.

KEY FACT

Galactosemia is associated with an ↑ risk of *E coli* sepsis and positive urine-reducing substances.

Maple Syrup Urine Disease

- An autosomal-recessive, branched-chain ketoaciduria caused by a deficiency of decarboxylase that initiates the degradation of leucine, isoleucine, and valine.
- Incidence is 1 in 250,000.
- **Symptoms/Exam:** Clinical manifestations usually occur within the first 10–14 days of life and include lethargy, irritability, seizures, opisthotonus, and coma.
- **Diagnosis:** Definitive diagnosis is made through the measurement of plasma leucine concentration.
- **Treatment:** Dietary restriction of leucine, isoleucine, and valine.

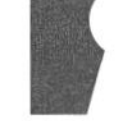

KEY FACT

During acute episodes of decompensation, patients with an organic aciduria can present with pancytopenia and hypocalcemia.

Organic Acidurias

- Include methylmalonic acidemia (MMA), propionic acidemia (PPA), and isovaleric acidemia (IVA).
- **Symptoms/Exam:**
  - May have early or late onset.
  - Presentation usually involves anion-gap metabolic acidosis, hypo- or hyperglycemia, large ketones in urine, and mild hyperammonemia.
- **Diagnosis:** Suspected diagnosis should be confirmed through analysis of plasma amino acids *and* urine organic acids (plus an acylcarnitine profile).
- **Treatment:**
  - Amino acids must be restricted in MMA and PPA.
  - Treatment during acute decompensation is intended to **stop catabolism.** Give high caloric glucose by day 10 at 1.5 or 2 times maintenance plus Na/K as needed. Do not give any protein. Provide IV car-

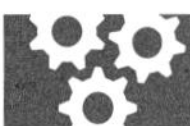

MNEMONIC

Dietary restrictions in MMA and PPA—

VOMIT

Valine
Odd-chain fatty acids
Methionine
Isoleucine
Threonine

nitine (a detoxifying agent). Replace HCO_3^- if necessary (pH < 7.1). Long-term treatment consists of dietary restriction of relevant amino acids and carnitine supplementation.
- **Complications:** Patients are at risk of basal ganglia infarction during acute metabolic decompensation.

Urea Cycle Defects

- An **X-linked recessive** disorder with many clinically affected females.
- The most common form is OTC deficiency.
- The liver is a mosaic of affected versus unaffected cells → variable severity of the phenotype.
- **Symptoms/Exam:**
  - Clinical manifestations range from neonatal onset (some lethal) to late onset in adulthood.
  - Features encompass emesis, irritability, lethargy, and psychiatric problems.
- **Diagnosis:** Made by hyperammonemia and excretion of **orotic acid in urine** detected by urine organic acid chromatography.
- **Treatment:** Generalized protein restriction during acute episodes to halt catabolism.

Nonketotic Hyperglycinemia

- An autosomal-recessive disorder caused by a defect in glycine cleavage.
- **Symptoms/Exam:** Characterized by clinically profound deterioration of the CNS in the neonatal period, as evidenced by seizures → respiratory depression, lethargy, and coma within the first few weeks of life.
- **Diagnosis:** Made by **simultaneous** determination of glycine in both plasma amino acids and CSF.
- **Treatment:**
  - No effective treatment is currently available.
  - Symptomatic treatment consists of administration of agents that ↓ glycine concentration (eg, sodium benzoate) and dextromethorphan as an anticonvulsant.

Biotinidase Deficiency

- An autosomal-recessive disorder.
- **Symptoms/Exam:** Clinical presentation may include intractable seizures, hypotonia, alopecia, skin rashes, metabolic acidosis, and immunodeficiency.
- **Treatment:** If provided early, oral supplementation of biotin ensures completely normal development and life.

Glutaric Aciduria

- **Type I:**
  - **Symptoms/Exam:** Macrocephaly (at birth), dystonia, recurrent episodes of liver dysfunction with metabolic acidosis, hypoglycemia, and hyperammonemia. Idiopathic subdural hematomas may occur.
  - **Diagnosis:** Requires plasma amino acids and urine organic acids. MRI shows very wide CSF spaces and open Sylvian fissures and this gives the characteristic "bat-wings" appearance.
  - **Treatment:** Consists of a low-protein diet, riboflavin, and agents that ↑ gamma-aminobutyric acid in the brain, such as valproic acid and baclofen.

- **Type II:**
  - A defect in the transfer of electrons from flavine-adenine nucleotides to the electron transport chain.
  - Associated with an ↑ risk of cardiomyopathy.
  - **Symptoms/Exam:** Congenital anomalies include renal cysts, facial dysmorphism, rocker-bottom feet, and hypospadias. Infants may show **hypoglycemia without ketosis,** an odor of sweaty feet, and metabolic acidosis.
  - **Treatment:** Riboflavin has not been effective.

Peroxisomal Diseases

- **Zellweger syndrome:**
  - An autosomal-recessive disorder with an incidence of 1 in 100,000.
  - Also known as cerebrohepatorenal syndrome.
  - **Symptoms/Exam:** Dysmorphic features include high forehead, flat orbital ridges, and widely open fontanelles. Also associated with hepatomegaly, hypotonia and seizures, and migration disorders of the brain.
  - **Diagnosis:** ↑ **very long chain fatty acids** in plasma. Lack of peroxisomal function.
  - **Treatment:** No treatment is available. Death usually occurs at 6–12 months of age.
- **Adrenoleukodystrophy:**
  - An X-linked peroxisomal disorder of beta-oxidation that results in accumulation of very long chain fatty acids (VLCFA) in all tissues. ALD consists of a spectrum of phenotypes (including adrenomyeloneuropathy, AMN) that vary in the age and severity of clinical presentation.
  - Childhood ALD is most common and typically presents between ages 4 and 8 years.
  - **Symptoms/Exam:** Boys typically present with learning disabilities and behavior problems, followed by neurologic deterioration, increasing cognitive and behavioral abnormalities, blindness, and quadriparesis. Approximately 20 percent of affected boys have seizures.
  - Most boys have adrenal insufficiency and some may have hyperpigmented skin.
  - **Diagnosis:** ↑ VLCFA. MRI typically shows demyelination, primarily of the posterior white matter, with enhancement along the peripheral edge of these demyelinating lesions.
  - **Treatment:** Treat adrenal insufficiency if present. Dietary therapy, "Lorenzo's oil" has been tried but results are conflicting. Bone marrow transplantation may be effective for those with mild neurologic manifestations. Mortality has been approximately 20%.
- **Adrenomyeloneuropathy (AMN):**
  - Typically presents in adult males between 20 and 40 years of age.
  - The primary manifestation is spinal cord dysfunction with progressive stiffness and weakness of the legs (spastic paraparesis), abnormal sphincter control, and sexual dysfunction. AMN may also present as a progressive cerebellar disorder.

Glycogen Storage Diseases

Table 12.12 outlines the presentation of common glycogen storage diseases.

Lysosomal Storage Diseases—Mucopolysaccharidoses (MPS)

The mucopolysaccharidoses are a heterogeneous group of lysosomal storage disorders, each caused by deficiency of an enzyme involved in the degradation of glycosaminoglycans (previously called mucopolysaccharides). The MPS disorders are inherited in an autosomal recessive manner, with the exception of MPS II (Hunter syndrome), which is X-linked recessive.

TABLE 12.12. Overview of Glycogen Storage Disease

Disease	Enzyme Defect	Organs Involved	Phenotype	Management
Type I—von Gierke disease	Glucose-6-phosphatase	Liver, kidney, platelets, bones.	Hypoglycemia, lactic acidosis, doll-like face, hepatomegaly with risk of hepatic adenomas, hypotonia, ↑ uric acid, ↑ triglycerides, xanthomas.	Prevention of hypoglycemia with cornstarch and frequent meals.
Type II—Pompe disease	α-glucosidase **(lysosomal)**	Liver, skeletal muscle, cardiac muscle, peripheral nerves.	Profound hypotonia, enlarged tongue, cardiomegaly with short PR interval. The late-onset form is rare.	Enzyme replacement therapy is available; if no therapy is given, death occurs within the first year of life.
Type III—Forbes disease, Cori disease	Debranching enzyme	**IIIa:** Liver, skeletal muscle. **IIIb:** Only liver.	Hypoglycemia, ketosis, **no lactic acidosis, normal uric acid,** muscle weakness, risk of hepatic fibrosis and cardiomyopathy.	Liver symptoms improve with age; muscle weakness may persist.
Type IV—Andersen disease	Branching enzyme	Liver, skeletal and cardiac muscle, CNS.	Failure to thrive, liver cirrhosis, cardiomyopathy, muscle weakness, hypotonia, absent DTRs.	Symptomatic management of liver failure and cardiomyopathy.
Type V—McArdle disease	Muscle phosphorylase	Skeletal muscle.	Exercise-induced rhabdomyolysis; muscle weakness beginning in adolescence.	Sucrose supplementation may be beneficial.
Type VI—Hers disease	Liver phosphorylase	Liver.	Mild hypoglycemia and ketosis; hepatomegaly.	Good prognosis.
Type VII—Tarui disease	Muscle phosphofructokinase	Skeletal muscle.	Exercise-induced rhabdomyolysis; muscle weakness beginning in adolescence.	Avoid strenuous exercise.
Type VIII	Phosphorylase kinase	Liver.	Hypoglycemia, ketosis, **no lactic acidosis, normal uric acid.**	Good prognosis.

- **MPS I (Hurler disease):**
  - A deficiency of α-L-iduronidase.
  - A mild form is called Scheie syndrome.
  - **Symptoms/Exam:** Patients are normal at birth but subsequently present with **coarse facies, corneal clouding,** mental retardation, hernias, **dysostosis multiplex,** and hepatosplenomegaly.
  - **Diagnosis:** Made by the detection of abnormal glycosaminoglycans in urine and confirmation of enzyme defect.
  - **Treatment:** Bone marrow transplantation and enzyme replacement provide therapeutic benefit. Enzyme replacement has been shown to improve pulmonary function and walking ability.
- **MPS II (Hunter disease):**
  - An **X-linked recessive** iduronate-2-sulfatase deficiency.
  - **Symptoms/Exam:** Mild dwarfism, coarse facial features, macroceph-

KEY FACT

MPS I is associated with an ↑ risk of upper airway obstruction.

aly, **no corneal opacities,** hepatosplenomegaly, dysostosis multiplex, neurodegeneration → profound mental retardation.
- **Diagnosis:** Diagnosed by dermatan and heparan sulfate excretion in urine.

- **MPS III (Sanfilippo disease):**
  - A heparan N-sulfatase deficiency; various types exist.
  - **Symptoms/Exam:** The presenting symptoms may include marked overactivity, destructive tendencies, and other behavioral aberrations in a child 4–6 years of age. Also presents with visceromegaly, mild corneal clouding, and claw hands.
  - **Diagnosis:** Heparan sulfate excretion in urine.
- **MPS IV (Morquio disease):**
  - An N-acetylgalactosamine-6-sulfatase deficiency.
  - **Symptoms/Exam:** Short-trunked dwarfism characterized by mild coarse features, corneal clouding, restrictive lung disease, **no dysostosis multiplex,** and **normal intelligence.**
  - **Diagnosis:** Chondroitin 6-sulfate excretion in urine.
- **MPS VI (Maroteaux-Lamy disease):**
  - An arylsulfatase B deficiency.
  - **Symptoms/Exam:** A short-trunked dwarfism that presents with corneal clouding, infantile cardiomyopathy, hepatosplenomegaly, dysostosis multiplex, and claw-hand deformities.
  - **Diagnosis:** Dermatan sulfate excretion in urine.
  - **Treatment:** Bone marrow transplantation.
- **MPS VII (Sly disease):**
  - A beta-glucuronidase enzyme deficiency.
  - **Symptoms/Exam:** Short stature, mental retardation, coarse facial features, variable degree of corneal clouding, visceromegaly, anterior beaking of vertebrae. Sometimes presents as hydrops fetalis.
  - **Diagnosis:** Dermatan and heparan sulfate, chondroitin 4-,6-sulfate excretion in urine. Coarse metachromatic granules in WBCs.

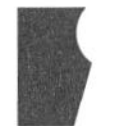

KEY FACT

Patients with MPS IV have normal intelligence.

Lysosomal Storage Diseases—Lipidoses

A 7-month-old boy has been healthy and developing normally since birth. His mother now reports that he has ↓ eye contact and startles very easily. Which diagnostic test is most likely to reveal a diagnosis in this case? This case describes a child with Tay-Sachs disease. The diagnosis is confirmed by enzyme activity measurement in leukocytes.

- **Type I Gaucher disease:**
  - A glucocerebrosidase enzyme deficiency.
  - **Symptoms/Exam:** Accumulation of Gaucher cells at the corneoscleral limbus; **hepatosplenomegaly, osteolytic lesions, anemia and thrombocytopenia,** ↑ risk of pathologic fractures.
  - **Diagnosis:** Gaucher cells in the bone marrow.
  - **Treatment:** Enzyme replacement therapy is available.
- **Type A Niemann-Pick disease:**
  - A sphingomyelinase deficiency that is more common among Ashkenazi Jews.
  - **Symptoms/Exam: Hypotonia, hyperreflexia, cherry-red spots,** hepatosplenomegaly, failure to thrive, profound loss of CNS function over time.
  - **Diagnosis:** Multiple organs show foam cells, including the brain, lung, and bone marrow.

- **Type B Niemann-Pick disease:**
  - A sphingomyelinase deficiency that is also most commonly found among Ashkenazi Jews.
  - **Symptoms/Exam: Visceral form** has **no neurologic manifestations.** Hepatosplenomegaly and cherry-red spot are less common; frequent respiratory infections.
  - **Diagnosis:** Large vacuolated foam cells ("NP cells") on bone marrow biopsy. Laboratory findings include ↑ LDL, ↑ triglycerides, and ↓ HDL.

KEY FACT

Limited upgaze is found often in Niemann-Pick, type C.

- **Type C Niemann-Pick disease:**
  - Intracellular accumulation of cholesterol.
  - Highly variable phenotype with NPC-1 mutations.
  - **Symptoms/Exam:** Vertical supranuclear gaze palsy, hepatosplenomegaly, hypotonia, developmental delay, cerebellar ataxia, mental retardation, poor school performance and behavioral abnormalities.
  - **Diagnosis:** Foam cells on bone marrow biopsy.
- **Tay-Sachs disease (GM2 gangliosidosis):**
  - A hexosaminidase A deficiency that is more common among Ashkenazi Jews and French Canadians.
  - The infantile form is fatal by age 5.
  - **Symptoms/Exam: Cherry-red spot and blindness,** ↑ startle response, hypotonia and poor head control, later spasticity.
  - **Diagnosis:** GM2-ganglioside accumulation.
- **Metachromatic leukodystrophy:**
  - An arylsulfatase A deficiency.
  - Age of onset may vary; adult onset may present as psychiatric illness.
  - **Symptoms/Exam: Optic atrophy, biliary tract abnormalities,** severe CNS disease including hypotonia progressing to spasticity, seizures, loss of mental function, progressive polyneuropathy. Loss or depression of deep tendon reflexes.
  - **Diagnosis:** ↑ protein in CSF; ↓ arylsulfatase A activity in urine, leukocytes, and fibroblasts; ↑ urinary sulfatide excretion. MRI brain with evidence of leukodystrophy.
- **Fabry disease:**
  - An X-linked recessive α-galactosidase deficiency.
  - **Symptoms/Exam:** Delayed puberty; whorl-like corneal dystrophy in heterozygous females and hemizygous males; heart abnormalities, including coronary artery disease (CAD) and cardiomyopathy; renal failure; Autonomic dysfunction, **acroparesthesia,** ↑ risk for strokes.
  - **Diagnosis:** Lipid-laden macrophages in bone marrow; glycosphingolipid deposition in all areas of the body.
  - **Treatment:** Enzyme replacement therapy is available.

KEY FACT

Loss of deep tendon reflexes and involvement of the peripheral as well as the CNS is a distinguishing feature of Krabbe disease and metachromatic leukodystrophy.

- **Krabbe disease:**
  - A beta-galactosidase deficiency that takes 4 clinical forms: infantile, late infantile, juvenile, and adult.
  - **Symptoms/Exam:** Failure to thrive; **optic atrophy, blindness; hyperirritability,** hypersensitivity to stimuli, mental deterioration, neurodegeneration, loss of deep tendon reflexes, hypertonicity in early stage, seizures, decerebrate posturing in late stages.
  - **Diagnosis:** Diffuse cerebral atrophy on CT and MRI, ↓ nerve conduction velocity, ↑ **protein in CSF;** galactocerebroside beta-galactosidase deficiency in serum, leukocytes, and fibroblasts.

Disorders of Copper Metabolism

- **Wilson disease:**
  - Classic triad: liver disease, movement disorder, and Kayser-Fleischer rings on the cornea.

- May present with neurologic disease, psychiatric disease, or liver disease.
- Neurologic symptoms may include: tremors, poor coordination, loss of fine-motor control, chorea, choreoathetosis, and rigid dystonia including masklike facies.
- **Diagnosis:** Made by ↓ serum ceruloplasmin and ↑ urinary copper (age-appropriate norms). Also, a high hepatic copper concentration will be seen if liver biopsy is performed.
- **Treatment:** Penicillamine for copper chelation.

- **Menkes disease:**
  - An X-linked disorder of copper transport caused by mutations in the copper-transporting ATPase gene (*ATP7A*). The result is copper deficiency.
  - Infants appear healthy until age 2 to 3 months, when loss of developmental milestones, hypotonia, seizures, and failure to thrive occur.
  - Changes of the hair (short, sparse, coarse, twisted, often lightly pigmented). Temperature instability and hypoglycemia may be present in the neonatal period. Death usually occurs by 3 years of age.
  - **Diagnosis:** Serum copper concentration and serum ceruloplasmin concentration are ↓.
  - **Treatment:** Subcutaneous injections of copper histidine or copper chloride before 10 days of age may improve neurologic outcome. Supportive care including gastrostomy tube placement may be helpful.

Genetic Disorders with Macrocephaly

- **Alexander disease:**
  - Autosomal dominant inheritance, most are de novo mutations. There are infantile, juvenile, and adult forms. Infantile is the most common and is described below.
  - **Symptoms/Exam:** Onset is anytime from birth to early childhood. Neurologic regression is seen. Macrocephaly, spasticity and seizure develop. Typically death occurs by 2 years of age.
  - MRI shows progressive leukodystrophy affecting the deep white matter, sparing the perventricular region with a frontal predominance.
  - **Diagnosis:** Made by the detection of a mutation in the glial fibrillary acidic protein gene (*GFAP*). Brain biopsy demonstrating Rosenthal fibers is practically never needed.
  - **Treatment:** Supportive therapy, particularly anticonvulsants for seizures.
- **Canavan disease:**
  - Autosomal recessive neurodegenerative disorder. More common in those of Jewish descent.
  - **Symptoms/Exam:** Macrocephaly, lack of head control, and developmental delays by the age of 3–5 months.
  - Severe hypotonia, and failure to achieve independent sitting, ambulation, or speech.
  - Hypotonia eventually changes to spasticity. Assistance with feeding becomes necessary. Life expectancy is usually into the teens.
  - **Diagnosis:** Demonstration of very high concentration of *N*-acetyl aspartic acid (NAA) in the urine.
  - MRI shows diffuse, symmetrical white matter changes are observed in the subcortical areas and in the cerebral cortex. MR spectroscopy shows NAA peak.
  - **Treatment:** Supportive care.
- **Neurofibromatosis Type 1:** See Neurocutaneous Disorders section.

Leukodystrophies

- **Krabbe disease:** See above.
- **Metachromatic leukodystrophy:** See above.
- **Pelizaeus-Merzbacher disease:**
  - X-linked dysmyelinating disorder (normal myelination never occurs). If unfavorable X chromosome inactivation occurs, females carriers may be symptomatic.
  - **Symptoms/Exam:** Present in early childhood with roving nystagmus, hypotonia, and cognitive impairment; and progress to severe spasticity and ataxia.
  - **MRI:** Increased signal intensity in the cerebral hemispheres, cerebellum, and brain stem on T2-weighted or fluid-attenuated inversion recovery (FLAIR) sequences.
  - **Diagnosis:** Molecular testing for mutations in the proteolipid protein (PLP) gene, Xq22.
  - **Treatment:** Supportive.
  - **Other:** The same gene also causes X-linked spastic paraplegia.
- **Vanishing white matter disease:**
  - Autosomal recessive inheritance, age of onset is variable.
  - **Symptoms/Exam:** Episodes of rapid deterioration that follow an infection or head trauma. The patient may have a partial recovery following these episodes, or the episode may lead to coma and death.
  - Neurologic signs are primarily cerebellar ataxia and spasticity.
  - Seizures may develop.
  - MRI shows extensive white matter disease and cystic degenerative changes. Spares the temporal lobes.
  - Life expectancy is reduced.
  - **Diagnosis:** Based on clinical criteria. Testing for mutations in 1 of the 5 genes that are collectively called eIF2B, or eukaryotic initiation factor is not commercially available.
  - **Treatment:** Supportive.

CHAPTER 13

Seizures, Epilepsy, and Sleep Disorders

Tracey A. Milligan, MD, MS

Seizures and Epilepsy

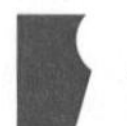

KEY FACT

Epilepsy should usually be diagnosed only after 2 or more unprovoked seizures separated by at least 24 hours.

- A **seizure** is a temporary alteration in brain function due to excessive or synchronized neuronal activity.
- **Epilepsy** is a group of disorders characterized by a tendency toward recurrent unprovoked seizures, typically diagnosed after 2 or more unprovoked seizures. Epilepsy is occasionally diagnosed after 1 unprovoked seizure and a high probability (> 60%) of seizure recurrence.

EPIDEMIOLOGY

- Ten percent of individuals will have 1 seizure in their lifetime.
- Sixty-five million people in the world, including 2.2 million people in the United States, have epilepsy.
- There is a 0.4–1% point prevalence of epilepsy (higher in developing countries).
- Incidence varies with age, with high rates in early childhood and a second peak in people over 65. Incidence of epilepsy is highest in the elderly.
- Thirty to 40% of patients with epilepsy continue to experience occasional seizures despite treatment.
- Recurrence rate after a single generalized tonic-clonic (GTC) seizure is 30–70% within 3–4 years in untreated patients.
- Fourth most common neurological disorder in the United States after migraine, stroke, and Alzheimer disease.

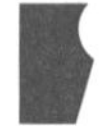

KEY FACT

The incidence of epilepsy is highest in the elderly.

DESCRIPTION OF SEIZURES

- Epilepsy is not a single condition but a symptom of various disorders that cause brain dysfunction.
- Description of a seizure helps classify the seizure, determine diagnostic evaluation, choice of medication, prognosis, and possible genetic transmission.
- **Focal:** Focal seizures involving networks limited to 1 hemisphere of the brain. They may be discretely localized or more widely distributed.
- **Focal with no impairment in consciousness or awareness (simple partial seizures).** Usually associated with "positive" symptoms (eg, tingling rather than numbness). Manifestation depends on localization: can include motor and subjective sensory (visual, gustatory, olfactory, auditory, somatosensory) or psychic phenomena (déjà vu, jamais vu, fear, panic, euphoria), These subjective sensory and psychic seizures are also referred to as auras.
- **Focal with alteration in consciousness (complex partial seizures):** Alteration in consciousness (dyscognitive), and may include automatisms (lip smacking, chewing, picking at clothing).
- Evolving to bilateral, convulsive seizure **(secondarily generalized):** A convulsion preceded by focal onset (the focal onset is sometimes not apparent clinically).
- **Generalized:** Seizures originating at some point within, and rapidly engaging, bilaterally distributed networks.
- **Myoclonic:** Shortest generalized seizure; may consist of a single jerk, and shows generalized spike or polyspike wave discharge on electroencephalogram (EEG).
- **Clonic:** Rhythmic jerking.

- **Tonic:** Sustained muscle contraction; may → "drop seizures."
- **Tonic-clonic:** Tonic period, followed by clonic jerking. Commonly referred to as "convulsion" or "grand mal."
- **Absence, typical:** 3-Hz spike-and-wave discharges on EEG associated with brief (usually < 30 seconds) episode of unresponsiveness, may be accompanied by eyelid fluttering, ↓ tone, ↑ tone, or automatisms (petit mal).
- **Absence, atypical:** 1.5- to 2.5-Hz spike wave discharges on EEG; longer in duration and associated with more automatisms and motor signs than typical absence.
- **Atonic (astatic):** Loss of muscle tone; may → "drop seizures."

KEY FACT

Seizures are classified as focal or generalized. **Generalized** seizures begin in networks involving both hemispheres at the same time. **Focal** seizures begin in networks limited to 1 hemisphere, but can spread so rapidly that clinically they resemble primary generalized seizures. Focal seizures can spread to become generalized seizures.

CLASSIFICATION OF EPILEPSIES

Subdivisions of focal and generalized epilepsy (previously used terms were *idiopathic, cryptogenic, symptomatic*).

- **Genetic:** The epilepsy is, as best understood, the direct result of a known or presumed genetic defect(s). Seizures are the core symptoms of the disorder. Does not exclude possibility of environmental factors contributing.
- **Structural-metabolic:** A distinct other structural or metabolic condition or disease is present and associated with a substantially increased risk of epilepsy. May be acquired or genetic in origin.
- **Unknown:** The nature of the underlying cause is as yet unknown. Idiopathic is not used because in the prior classification system, it was sometimes used for presumed genetic causes.

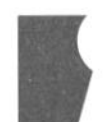

KEY FACT

Focal seizures with alteration of cognition (complex partial) often can be distinguished from absence seizures by presence of an aura, longer duration (90 seconds vs 15 seconds), and postictal confusion.

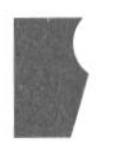

KEY FACT

Generalized epilepsy often has a genetic predisposition and begins in childhood or young adulthood. There is not a well-defined aura.

ELECTROCLINICAL SYNDROMES

Neonatal

- **Benign neonatal seizures ("fifth day fits")** (not traditionally diagnosed as epilepsy):
  - Healthy infant, typically occur on day 5 of life.
  - Focal tonic or focal clonic.
  - Can be treated with phenobarbital, but remit spontaneously after 1–2 days.
- **Benign familial neonatal epilepsy (BFNE):**
  - Rare; seizures begin on days 2–7 of life, with spontaneous remission.
  - Focal tonic or clonic.
  - AD, incomplete penetrance.
  - Defect in voltage-dependent potassium channel.
  - Treat with phenobarbital.
- **Ohtahara syndrome:**
  - Also known as early infantile epileptic encephalopathy with burst-suppression (EIEE).
  - Seizures begin within the first 3 months of life (most often within the first 10 days).
  - Primarily **tonic** seizures (can also include fragmentary myoclonic jerks and focal seizures).
  - Etiologies include brain malformations and metabolic syndromes (eg, glycine encephalopathy, mitochondrial disorders).
  - EEG shows **burst suppression.**
  - Severely progressive, with mental retardation and may evolve into West syndrome and Lennox-Gastaut syndrome.

Infancy

- **Infantile spasms:**
  - "Jack-knifing" with sudden flexion, extension, or mixed flexion-extension movements of the trunk and proximal muscles; often occur in clusters.
  - Often have mental retardation (West syndrome).
  - EEG is diffusely abnormal with high-amplitude sharp and slow waves (hypsarrhythmia).
  - Causes include inborn errors of metabolism, structural brain abnormalities, tuberous sclerosis (TS).
  - Treatment with adrenocortropic hormone (ACTH; vigabatrin is often used with TS but can cause of visual loss); resection can be considered if there is a focal lesion.
- **Generalized epilepsy with febrile seizures plus (GEFS+):**
  - Autosomal dominant epilepsy syndrome, with variable penetrance.
  - Encompasses severe myoclonic epilepsy of infancy (Dravet syndrome).
  - Febrile seizures in infancy and other seizures usually start in the first decade of life.
  - Several different seizure types may be found within the same family.
  - Genetically heterogeneous (including sodium channel and GABAa receptor mutations).
  - **Benign myoclonic epilepsy of infancy:**
  - First or second year of life.
  - Males > females 2:1.
  - Thirty percent have family history of epilepsy.
  - Brief generalized myoclonic seizures.
  - Treated with valproate.

Childhood

> The teacher of a 5-year-old girl refers her for evaluation of "spacing out." She is not paying attention and seems to be daydreaming during class. Her neurological exam is normal. During hyperventilation, she stares and becomes unresponsive for 10 seconds. She then is completely back to her baseline. What is her diagnosis? Childhood absence epilepsy.

- **Childhood epilepsy with occipital paroxysms (Panayiotopoulos syndrome):**
  - Onset at age 1–14; peak at age 5; girls and boys equally affected.
  - Principal seizure type is autonomic and autonomic status epilepticus.
  - Clinically, child is conscious but complains about feeling sick, turns pale, and vomits (headaches may occur at onset).
  - Twenty percent progress into loss of consciousness (LOC), ictal syncope.
  - Neurological exam and imaging normal, multifocal spike and slow waves; misdiagnosis is common; overall prognosis is benign.
- **Childhood absence epilepsy (CAE):**
  - Ten to 15% of childhood epilepsy cases.
  - Age range 2–13; typical age 7.
  - Girls > boys 3:2.
  - Family history of epilepsy in 15–45% of cases (complex inheritance pattern).
  - Only seizure type in 90% (10% develop GTC seizures).
  - Frequent seizures (often > 100 a day) consisting of staring, arrest of activity, eye fluttering; may also have automatisms, change in tone, clonic component.

  - EEG shows 3-Hz frontally predominant generalized spike-and-wave discharges.
  - Provoked by hyperventilation.
  - Spontaneous remission in 70% during adolescence.
  - Treated with ethosuximide (absences only); valproic acid or lamotrigine could also be used.
- **Benign epilepsy with centrotemporal spikes (BECTS) (Rolandic epilepsy):**
  - Found in school-age, otherwise healthy children and usually resolves by puberty.
  - Most common focal epilepsy of childhood (two-thirds of all idiopathic focal epilepsy).
  - Onset at age 3–16 (peak at 5–8).
  - Complex genetic inheritance.
  - **Symptoms/Exam:** Nocturnal seizures with excessive salivation, gurgling or choking sounds, and clonic contractions of upper face and upper extremity.
  - Twenty percent of patients will have only 1 seizure; two-thirds have infrequent seizures; can be treated with antiepileptic drugs (AEDs) used for focal seizures (eg, carbamazepine).
  - Patients are neurologically normal and outgrow the disorder.
- **Idiopathic childhood occipital epilepsy (Gastaut type):**
  - Range age 3–16; average age 8 years.
  - Equal gender.
  - Fifty percent have family history of epilepsy.
  - Symptoms of episodic blindness or colored luminous discs, visual hallucinations lasting seconds or minutes; postictal migraine in one-third.
  - Interictal EEG shows high-amplitude spike-and-wave complexes occurring with the eyes closed.
  - Treated with medications used for focal seizures, such as carbamazepine.
  - Good prognosis.
- **Lennox-Gastaut syndrome:**
  - Appears between the ages of 1 and 10 years, sometimes de novo and sometimes following infantile spasms.
  - Most are mentally retarded; approximately 70% have an identifiable cause for the retardation and epilepsy.
  - Multiple seizure types (tonic, atypical absence, atonic).
  - No single etiology.
  - Diffusely abnormal EEG, becomes more abnormal in sleep; slow spike-and-wave discharges of 1.5–2 Hz.
  - Difficult to control. Treated with broad-spectrum agent; felbamate may be used and runinamide is a recently FDA approved medication for this syndrome. VNS can also be helpful.
- **Epileptic encephalopathy with continuous spike-and-wave during sleep (CSWS) or status epilepticus in slow-wave sleep (ESES):**
  - Begins during early childhood, peaking between 4 and 5 years of age.
  - Associated with cognitive impairment, particularly language, and behavioral disturbances.
  - An EEG diagnosis with generalized spike-and-wave activity as the dominant pattern during sleep (> 85% of slow-wave sleep time).
- **Acquired epileptic aphasia (Landau-Kleffner syndrome):**
  - Rare childhood disorder.
  - Acquired aphasia and epileptiform discharges.
  - Typically develops in healthy children who acutely or progressively lose receptive and expressive language ability coincident with the appearance of paroxysmal EEG changes usually in sleep.

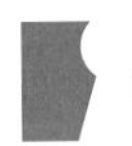

KEY FACT

Lennox-Gastaut syndrome is a triad of (1) multiple seizure types refractory to AEDs, (2) mental retardation, and (3) slow spike-and-wave activity on EEG.

Adolescence-Adult

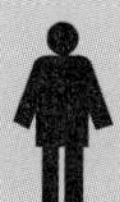

An 18-year-old boy presents with early morning myoclonic seizures. EEG shows fast (4- to 6-Hz) spike-and-wave complexes. How is he treated, and what is his prognosis? Juvenile myoclonic epilepsy. Valproic acid is the treatment of choice and seizures will recur if treatment is stopped.

- **Juvenile absence epilepsy:**
  - Onset later than CAE—on average 10–17 years; peak 10–12 years.
  - Occur equally in boys and girls.
  - Often have occasional GTC seizures.
  - Tend to cluster in the morning.
  - May be mild and unnoticed.
  - EEG shows 4- to 5-Hz generalized spike-and-wave discharges.
  - Treated with broad-spectrum AEDs.
- **Juvenile myoclonic epilepsy (JME):**
  - Most common form of idiopathic epilepsy; 18% of all IGEs.
  - Onset at age 12–18; peak at 15 years; gender distribution is equal.
  - Usually developmentally and neurologically normal.
  - Positive family history in one-third; complex inheritance.
  - Myoclonus is required for diagnosis; typically occurs in the morning.
  - GTC +/– absence.
  - Seizures may be precipitated by alcohol or sleep deprivation.
  - EEG shows bursts of 4 Hz to 6 Hz spike-and-wave discharges.
  - Broad spectrum agents used to treat (eg, valproic acid, lamotrigine, levetiracetam).
- **Epilepsy with grand mal seizures on awakening:**
  - Usually begin in childhood, peak onset at 15 years.
  - Slightly higher incidence in girls; family history in 12%; complex inheritance.
  - GTC seizures almost exclusively within 30 minutes of awakening, regardless of the time of day.

Variable Age at Onset

- **Frontal lobe epilepsies:**
  - Frequent seizures, often in stage 2 sleep.
  - Short seizure duration.
  - Minimal or no postictal confusion.
  - Rapid secondary generalization.
  - Prominent motor manifestations.
  - Complex gestural automatisms.
  - Supplementary motor seizures: Brief, lasting 10–40 seconds, bilateral tonic or clonic movements in association with preserved consciousness.
  - Bicycling movements and other asynchronous bilateral movements may occur (pelvic thrusting and side-to-side head movements are suggestive of psychogenic nonepileptic seizure [PNES]).
  - Autosomal-dominant (AD) frontal lobe nocturnal epilepsy: Onset in first 2 decades of life; usually occur during sleep. Clinically similar to other types of frontal lobe seizures. Mutations in gene coding for neuronal nicotinic acetylcholine receptors.
- **Temporal lobe epilepsies (TLEs):**
  - Mesial temporal seizures are the most common form of TLE.
  - Seizures may consist of rising epigastric discomfort, nausea, autonomic signs, fear, and olfactory hallucinations, followed by loss of awareness,

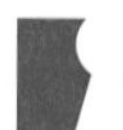

KEY FACT

Frontal lobe seizures are clinically variable, little or no impairment of consciousness, hyperkinetic automatisms, rapid secondary generalization, little postictal period.

oral or manual automatisms (ipsilateral to ictal focus), dystonic postures (contralateral to ictal focus).
- Patients often have a history of prolonged, severe, febrile seizures.
- **Autosomal-dominant focal epilepsy with auditory features (ADPEAF):** Onset in second decade of life. Auditory hallucinations of monotonous buzzing, voices from the past, specific singers, or distortions of sounds in the environment. May have other focal seizure types. Mutations in the LGI1 gene (leucine-rich gene, glioma inactivated).

KEY FACT

Mesial temporal lobe epilepsy with hippocampal sclerosis shows MRI-apparent hippocampal atrophy and ↑ T2-weighted signal changes.

- **Progressive myoclonic epilepsies:**
  - Rare group of disorders characterized by severe myoclonus and other generalized seizure types, progressive dementia, ataxia.
  - **Unverricht-Lundborg disease (Baltic myoclonus):** Autosomal recessive (AR); mutation cystatin B on chromosome 21. Onset between ages 8 and 13; at onset may be indistinguishable from JME. Ataxia and dementia occur late and are usually mild. Markedly photosensitive; may have giant somatosensory evoked potentials.
  - **Lafora disease:** AR; 80% of cases due to mutations in the laforin gene on chromosome 6. Seizures begin between 10 and 18 years of age. Rapid progression resulting in quadriparesis, dementia, and death in 2–20 years. Marked photosensitivity.
  - **Myoclonic epilepsy with ragged red fibers (MERRF):** Mitochondrial inheritance, wide phenotypic variability. Symptoms may begin in childhood or adulthood. Seizures, dementia, ataxia, and may have myopathy, neuropathy, deafness, optic atrophy, exercise intolerance, short stature, lactic acidosis.

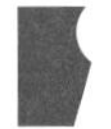

KEY FACT

Progressive myoclonic epilepsies are characterized by severe myoclonus, other generalized seizures, ataxia, and progressive dementia.

- **Reflex epilepsy:**
  - Seizures are regularly elicited by some specific stimulus or event (visual, thinking, music, eating, reading, exercise, praxis, somatosensory).
  - Flickering light, patterns.
  - Treat with trigger avoidance, desensitization therapy, AEDs.

Surgical Syndromes

- **Mesial temporal lobe epilepsy with hippocampal sclerosis (MTLE with HS):** Hippocampal (Ammon horn) sclerosis is the most common pathology seen with gliosis and neuronal loss in the CA1 pyramidal cell layer (CA3, CA4 less involved, CA2 is relatively spared, and subiculum typically uninvolved).
- **Rasmussen encephalitis:**
  - Usually presents in childhood.
  - Typically 6–10 years of age with uncontrollable focal seizures.
  - May present with epilepsia focalis continua (EPC)—focal motor status epilepticus.
  - Progressive; usually involves only 1 hemisphere.
  - Antiglutamate receptor antibodies are seen in some cases.
  - **Neuropathology:** Perivascular lymphocystic infiltrates with vascular injury, astrogliosis, neuronal loss, and cortical atrophy.
  - Hemispherectomy is the best established treatment (see Table 13.1); high-dose intravenous human immunoglobulin (IVIG) may be helpful.
- **Gelastic seizures with hypothalamic hamartoma:**
  - Seizures involve sudden bursts of sardonic laughing or crying.
  - Hamartoma is a benign mass of glial tissue on or near the hypothalamus; endocrine effects are uncommon, but precocious puberty may occur.

TABLE 13.1. Surgical Epilepsy Treatments and Indications

Treatment	Indication
Vagus nerve stimulator	Medically intractable epilepsy
Focal resection	Partial-onset seizures arising from resectable cortex (good for mesial temporal sclerosis)
Corpus callosotomy	Drop attacks
Hemispherectomy	Rasmussen syndrome
Subpial transactions	Partial-onset seizures arising from unresectable cortex
Neuropace RNS	Medically intractable focal epilepsy
Deep brain stimulation	Experimental anterior thalamic stimulation

SPECIAL SYNDROMES/SITUATION-RELATED SEIZURES

A 55-year-old university professor presents with a GTC seizure. He has a normal examination. He drinks 4 glasses of scotch every night, but did not drink last night because he was babysitting his grandson. What is the likely etiology, and how should he be treated? Alcohol withdrawal seizure treated with benzodiazepines.

Not necessarily associated with a diagnosis of epilepsy (see Tables 13.2 and 13.3).

- **Febrile seizures:**
  - Seizures associated with fever in children 6 months to 5 years of age without intracranial infection; average age 18–22 months; boys > girls.
  - Approximately 1 in 25 children have febrile seizure and one-third will have a recurrence.
  - Usually occurs the first day of a fever, sometimes before a fever is recognized.
  - Seizures of any type—usually tonic-clonic or tonic.
  - Complex if seizure lasts > 15 minutes, more than 1 seizure in 24 hours, or focal features.
  - EEG is generally not useful; epileptiform activity is not predictive of eventual development of epilepsy.
  - ↑ risk of developing epilepsy (3% by age 7 vs 0.5% in the general population).

TABLE 13.2. Nonepileptic Disorders That Mimic Epilepsy

Syncope: Vasovagal/neurocardiogenic, ↓ cardiac output, volume depletion, arrhythmia
Migraine: Classic, basilar, confusional, acephalgic
Cerebrovascular: Transient ischemic attack, amyloid angiopathy
Sleep disorders: REM behavior disorder, narcolepsy, cataplexy, parasomnias
Movement disorders: Tics, nonepileptic myoclonus, tremor
Transient global amnesia
Psychiatric: Panic, dissociation, conversion, malingering

TABLE 13.3. Common Causes of Provoked Seizures

Metabolic ■ Hyponatremia ■ Hypoglycemia ■ Hyperthyroidism ■ Nonketotic hyperglycemia ■ Hypocalcemia ■ Hypomagnesemia ■ Renal failure
Porphyria
Hypoxia
Medications ■ Benzodiazepine withdrawal ■ Barbiturate withdrawal ■ Phenothiazines ■ Buproprion ■ Tramadol
Substance abuse ■ Alcohol withdrawal ■ Cocaine ■ Amphetamine ■ Phencyclidine ■ Methylenedioxymethamphetatime (MDMA, "ecstasy")

- **Management:**
  - Identify underlying illness and do lumbar puncture if there is clinical concern about meningitis.
  - No neuroimaging is necessary unless the physical exam points to possible structural lesion.
  - No treatment is necessary; for children who have frequent or prolonged febrile seizures, oral or rectal diazepam during fevers can be used.
- **Alcohol withdrawal:**
  - Ninety percent occur 7–48 hours after cessation of drinking; 50% 13–24 hours after drinking has ceased; can occur up to 7 days after stopping drinking. Tremulousness and some myoclonic jerks of extremities.
  - Risk of delirium tremens (DTs) and status epilepticus.
  - EEG may show heightened excitability to photic stimulation that resolves with benzodiazepines.
  - **Nonketotic hyperglycemia.**
  - **Focal motor seizures, epilepsia partialis continua, and occipital seizures with visual hallucinations are the most frequent seizure types.**
  - **Management:**
    - Administer thiamine before glucose, correct fluid and electrolyte abnormalities; administer magnesium. Lorazepam and additional doses every 4 hours as needed. Phenytoin has no value for alcohol withdrawal seizures.
    - **Treated by rehydration and normalization of glucose.**

- **Eclampsia:**
  - Occurrence of focal or secondarily generalized seizures, not caused by another neurological disease, in a woman who meets the criteria for preeclampsia (pregnancy-induced proteinuria and edema after the 20th week of gestation).
  - Headache, confusion, hyperreflexia, visual hallucinations, or blindness may occur.
  - Seizures may occur even when few signs of preeclampsia are present.
  - Occur before, during, or after childbirth.
  - EEG with focal or diffuse slowing and epileptiform activity.
  - Treat with magnesium sulfate.

Investigations

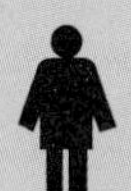

An 18-year-old woman presents to the emergency room after her boyfriend witnessed a convulsion (her first), from which she has recovered fully. What investigations should she have in the emergency room?

An eyewitness account of the event, physical and neurologic examination, screening for drugs and alcohol use or withdrawal, electrolytes, blood urea nitrogen (BUN), creatinine, glucose, complete blood count, pregnancy test, electrocardiogram (ECG), head computed tomography (CT).

KEY FACT

The most valuable tool in evaluating a history of possible seizure is a good eyewitness account.

- History, including:
  - Medication and drug exposure.
  - Previous seizures: Screen for myoclonus, odd behaviors, loss of time, staring spells.
  - Risk factors: History of febrile seizures, developmental delay, head injury resulting in loss of consciousness, brain infection, brain lesions, family history of seizures.
- General physical exam:
  - Assess for signs of other systemic disease.
  - Skin findings suggestive of tuberous sclerosis, neurofibromatosis, or Sturge-Weber syndrome.
  - Complete neurologic exam.
  - Blood tests to check for metabolic and toxic disorders (see Table 13.3).
- EEG:
  - Positive in 20–59% of people with epilepsy—a normal EEG never excludes the diagnosis of seizure.
  - Ninety-five percent abnormal in absence epilepsy.
  - Repeated EEGs are positive in 59–92% of people with epilepsy; three 30-minute EEGs should diagnose 90% of cases with epilepsy.
  - Photic stimulation, hyperventilation, and sleep are all activating procedures used to ↑ the yield of EEG in finding abnormalities.
  - Sleep-deprived EEG is a more sensitive measurement.
  - Epilepsy is suggested by abnormal spikes, polyspike discharges, spike-and-wave complexes.
  - EEG may distinguish between focal and generalized epilepsies. The interictal EEG of generalized seizures is frontally predominant, generalized spike, or polyspike wave discharges.
  - Ambulatory EEG can be helpful to obtain a longer sample, monitor frequency of seizures, or diagnosis events of unclear etiology.

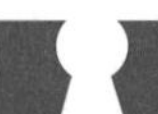

KEY FACT

A normal or nonspecifically abnormal EEG never excludes the diagnosis of seizures.

KEY FACT

Between 60% and 75% of children with epilepsy who have been seizure free for > 2 years on medications will remain seizure free for 2 years when AEDs are withdrawn.

- Video-EEG monitoring in an epilepsy monitoring unit may be necessary to diagnose events of unclear etiology or obtain information for surgical planning.
- **Neuroimaging:** MRI with thin (0.5-mm) cuts through the temporal lobes is the preferred neuroimaging technique in epilepsy.

Treatment

Selection of AEDs depends on seizure type, medical comorbidities, and in women with contraceptive and pregnancy issues (see Tables 13.4 and 13.5).

SUDDEN UNEXPLAINED DEATH IN EPILEPSY (SUDEP)

- Sudden, unexpected, witnessed or unwitnessed, nontraumatic and non-drowning death in patients with epilepsy, with or without evidence for a seizure and excluding documented status epilepticus.
- Cause is unknown; many cases occur after a seizure. May be cardiac and/or pulmonary.
- Higher risk in candidates for epilepsy surgery (more severe epilepsy).
- Other risk factors are early age of onset, long duration of epilepsy, higher number of AEDs, frequent GTCs, poor adherence with AED regimen, frequent medication changes.

TABLE 13.4. Epilepsy Management in Pregnancy

Preconception
■ Evaluate need for continued AED therapy.
■ Attempt to ↓ pharmacotherapy to monotherapy.
■ Taper AEDs to the lowest possible dose(s).
■ Establish the level of total and free AEDs necessary for achieving good clinical control.
■ Review family history for birth defects and consider genetic counseling.
■ Begin folate supplementation (4 mg/day).
During pregnancy
■ Do not switch to an alternate AED solely to reduce teratogenic risk.
■ Check total and free levels of AEDs monthly (many AEDs will require significant ↑ during pregnancy).
■ Consider early genetic counseling.
■ Check maternal serum AFP levels at 16 weeks' gestation.
■ Perform a level II fetal survey and ultrasonography at 18–20 weeks' gestation.
■ Consider amniocentesis for AFP and acetylcholinesterase.
Postpartum
■ Encourage breast-feeding, but counsel about avoiding sleep deprivation.
■ Continue to monitor AED blood concentrations closely; anticipate adjustments over the next several months.
■ Counsel about extra safety tips for infant care as appropriate (eg, changing clothing and diapers on the floor).
■ Monitor for development of postpartum depression.

AED, antiepileptic drug; AFP, alpha-fetoprotein.

TABLE 13.5. High-Yield Facts About Antiepileptic Drugs

All AEDs have potential for increased risk of depression and suicidality.

Carbamazepine

- May exacerbate seizures in generalized epilepsies.
- Many drug-drug interactions; eg, increasing levels caused by isoniazid, erythromycin, clarithromycin, fluoxetine, simvastatin, cimetidine, calcium channel blockers, grapefruit juice.
- Serious and sometimes fatal dematologic reactions, especially in patients with HLA-B*1502 (patients of Asian descent); screen genetically at-risk patients prior to prescribing and do not prescribe if positive for this allele. Carbamazepine directly binds to HLA-B molecules on antigen presenting T cells and contributes to cell death mediated by cytotoxic T cells in persons with Stevens-Johnson syndrome.
- Aplastic anemia and agranulocytosis have been reported; obtain pretreatment CBC and periodically monitor.
- Hyponatremia due to syndrome of inappropriate antidiuretic hormone secreation (SIADH).
- Decreases efficacy of hormonal contraceptives.
- Osteopenia.
- Also treats pain; mood stabilizer.

Clobazam

- Has a 1,5 substitution instead of the usual 1,4-diazepine.
- Decreased anxiolytic and sedative properties compared to other benzodiazepines.
- Decreases efficacy of hormonal contraceptives.
- FDA approved for treatment of Lennox-Gastaut syndrome.
- Eslicarbazepine acetate.
- Prodrug that is activated to S-licarbazepine the major active metabolite of oxcarbazepine.
- FDA approved in 2013 for adjunctive therapy in partial seizures in adults.

Ethosuximide

- T-type calcium channel blocker.
- Treats absence seizures only.

Ezogabine

- Potassium channel opener.
- Black box warning: retinal abnormalities that can progress to vision loss in about one-third of patients.
- Can also cause bladder dysfunction and blue nails and lips.

Felbamate

- Risk of aplastic anemia and hepatic failure.

Fosphenytoin

- Prodrug intended for parenteral administration.
- Active metabolite is phenytoin.
- Can be administered intramuscularly as well.

Gabapentin

- No drug-drug interactions.
- May be used in patients with HIV and porphyria.
- Safe in the setting of liver disease.
- Also treats neuropathic pain.
- May cause weight gain, pedal edema.

TABLE 13.5. High-Yield Facts About Antiepileptic Drugs *(continued)*

Lacosamide

- Associated with risk of A-V block and syncope.
- No drug-drug interactions.
- IV formulation.

Lamotrigine

- Primarily metabolized by hepatic glucuronidation. This system is induced by oral hormone contraception (OHC).
- Level decreased by OHC and pregnancy.
- Associated with the lowest risk of major congenital malformations during exposure in the first trimester compared to other AEDs.
- No increased risk of OHC failure.
- Also treats mood stabilizer and mild antidepressant.
- Slow titration due to risk of rash.
- Drug interactions with valproate (decreases metabolism)and enzyme inducers (increases metabolism).
- If rash develops, must stop.

Levetiracetam

- No drug-drug interactions.
- May cause depression and hostile behavior.
- IV formulation available.

Oxcarbazepine

- Hyponatremia more common than with carbamazepine.
- Decreases efficacy of hormonal contraception.
- Also used as mood stabilizer.
- Does not metabolize to the epoxide metabolite (less side effects).

Perampanel

- AMPA antagonist.
- Can have serious or life-threatening psychiatric and behavioral adverse reactions including homicidal ideation.

Phenytoin

- Zero order kinetics.
- Many drug-drug interactions.
- Osteopenia, cerebellar dysfunction, neuropathy, gingival hyperplasia, hirsutism.

Phenobarbital/primidone

- Osteopenia, connective tissue dysfunction.
- Decreases efficacy of hormonal contraception.
- Teratogenicity.
- Primidone is also used to treat essential tremor.
- Acute treatment of neonatal seizures.

Pregabalin

- Safe in setting of liver disease.
- Also used to treat neuropathic pain.

Rufinimide

- Treats seizures in Lennox-Gastaut syndrome.
- Avoid in familial H9 short Q-T syndrome.

TABLE 13.5. High-Yield Facts About Antiepileptic Drugs *(continued)*

Tiagabine
■ Can cause new onset seizures and status epilepticus in patients without epilepsy.
Topiramate
■ Weight loss, renal stones (calcium phosphate), oligohydrosis, confusion, and disorders of language, open-angle glaucoma, metabolic acidosis. ■ May decrease efficacy of hormonal contraception. ■ Also treats migraines.
Valproate
■ Highest teratogenicity. ■ Also treats migraines and mood stabilizer. ■ Cause weight gain, hair loss, tremor, platelet dysfunction, drug-drug interactions. ■ Low risk of skin hypersensitivity. ■ Good for JME, absence seizures. ■ VPA may also cause impairments in fatty-acid metabolism and disrupt the urea cycle, leading to hyperammonemia. VPA also alters fatty acid. ■ Risk of hepatotoxicity, pancreatitis.
Zonisamide
■ Weight loss, renal stones, oligohydrosis (increased risk of heat stroke, particularly in children).

PSYCHIATRIC COMORBIDITIES

Treatment of the patient with epilepsy also requires attention to the psychological and social consequences of epilepsy:

- Twenty to 30% of patients with epilepsy have a psychiatric comorbidity.
- Depression is the most common psychiatric diagnosis and occurs in 30–40% of patients with epilepsy.
- There is an approximately 5- to 10-fold ↑ risk of suicide.
- Anxiety and psychosis are also more common than in the general population.
- Neuropsychiatric symptoms reported with temporal lobe epilepsy include psychosis, fear, anxiety, hypergraphia, hypermorality, and altered sexual function.

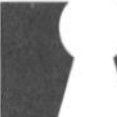

PSYCHOGENIC NONEPILEPTIC SEIZURES (PNES; "PSEUDOSEIZURES")

- Paroxysmal changes in behavior that resemble epileptic seizures but are without organic cause and EEG changes, usually due to a conversion disorder.
- Many have comorbid psychiatric illness or a history of abuse.
- Ten to 30% of patients evaluated at tertiary referral centers for medically refractory epilepsy actually have PNES.
- Differential diagnosis includes frontal lobe seizures that may have unusual movements and very brief postictal state.
- Video-EEG monitoring is generally necessary for diagnosis.

KEY FACT

Elevated serum prolactin, when measured at 10–20 minutes after an event, is a useful adjunct for the differentiation of GTC or complex focal seizures from PNES.

WOMEN'S ISSUES

- **Conception:**
  - Up to 20% of women with epilepsy have abnormal ovarian function, including anovulatory menstrual cycles, polycystic ovaries.
  - More common in women taking valproic acid.
  - Several AEDs induce metabolism of female sex hormones, ↓ efficacy of hormonal contraception (see Table 13.4).
- **Pregnancy:**
  - Most pregnant women with treated epilepsy have uneventful pregnancies and deliver healthy babies.
  - There is an ↑ incidence of minor and major fetal malformations, even if untreated. The risk is 2–3% in the general population and 4–6% in women with epilepsy.
  - The risk of birth defects ↑ with the use of more AEDs (see Table 13.4).
  - Lamotrigine has lowest reported incidence of major congenital malformations.
- **Bone health:**
  - Osteopenia and osteoporosis occur at a higher frequency in both men and women after long-term exposure to certain AEDs.
  - Induced vitamin D metabolism may play a role.
  - Vitamin D supplementation and dual-energy x-ray absorptiometry (DEXA) screening.

EPILEPSY IN THE ELDERLY

A 75-year-old man is brought to the emergency department having a GTC seizure. He has been having seizures for over 30 minutes without interval recovery. How should he be treated? Circulation, airway, and breathing; drugs (lorazepam and intravenous fosphenytoin).

- Most common time to develop epilepsy.
- Seizures may be difficult to recognize, and postictal confusion can be prolonged.
- May be secondary to vascular events, neurodegenerative condition, or other structural etiology, but often are idiopathic.

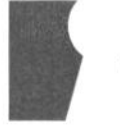

KEY FACT

Status epilepticus is 30 minutes of either continuous seizure activity or repetitive seizures without recovery in between.

MANAGEMENT OF STATUS EPILEPTICUS

A life-threatening condition in which the brain is in a state of persistent seizure. Definitions vary, but traditionally it is defined as 1 continuous unremitting seizure lasting longer than 30 minutes, or recurrent seizures without regaining consciousness between seizures for > 30 minutes. See Figure 13.1.

- Most seizures last less than 2–3 minutes. If a seizure lasts > 5 minutes, begin treatment for status epilepticus.
- Approximately 10% of people with epilepsy will go into status epilepticus at some point in their life.
- Most common in young children and the elderly.
- Approximately 80% of prolonged seizures are stopped with combination of a benzodiazepine and phenytoin.
- AEDs with IV formulation are phenytoin, valproate, phenobarbital, levetiracetam, lacosamide.

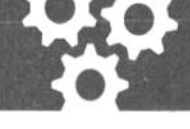

MNEMONIC

***Management of status epilepticus*—**

ABCD DEFG:

Airway
Breathing (administer oxygen)
Circulation
Drugs (lorazepam and intravenous fosphenytoin)
DEFG: "**D**on't **E**ver **F**orget **G**lucose—and thiamine"

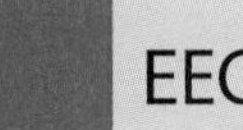

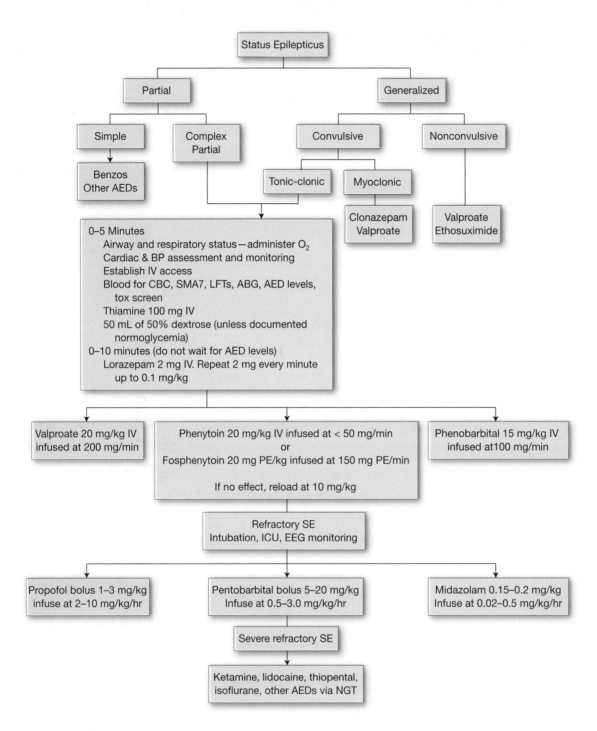

FIGURE 13.1. Management of status epilepticus.

EEG

- Electrical fields that generate EEG signals are the result of inhibitory and excitatory postsynaptic potentials (IPSPSs and EPSPs) on the apical dendrites of cortical neurons.
- The EEG record is generated by recording electrical potential differences between pairs of electrodes. Negative potential differences = deflection above the baseline (up).

- Bipolar montages compare an electrode to an adjacent electrode in a specified pattern. Signals are localized by phase reversal.
- Referential montages compare all electrodes to a specified reference electrode. Signals are localized by amplitude.

NORMAL EEG PATTERNS

- **Alpha:** 8–13 Hz; attenuates with eye opening and concentration; maximal occipitally.
- **Beta:** > 13 Hz; frontocentral maximum; ↑ with benzodiazepines, barbiturates, anxiety, hyperthyroidism; ↑ over skull defect (part of breach rhythm).
- **Theta:** 4–7 Hz; normal during drowsiness and sleep.
- **Delta:** < 4 Hz; normal during sleep, ↑ with slow-wave sleep.
- **Normal variants:**
    - **Mu:** 7–11 Hz, archiform centroparietal rhythm that attenuates with contralateral hand movement.
    - **Lambda:** Occipital positive sharp transients that occur with visual scanning.
    - **Small sharp spikes or benign epileptiform transients of sleep (BETS):** Benign EEG pattern in adults, usually occurs during drowsiness and light sleep.
    - **"14 and 6" positive spikes:** Sharply contoured discharges at 14 Hz and 6 Hz. Occur in the posterior head regions during light sleep; best demonstrated on referential EEG montages; most common in adolescent patients.
    - **Wicket waves** (Figure 13.2): Benign pattern of uncertain clinical significance, occurring predominantly in the temporal region in the EEG of older adults during light sleep. Can be mistaken for epileptiform discharges.

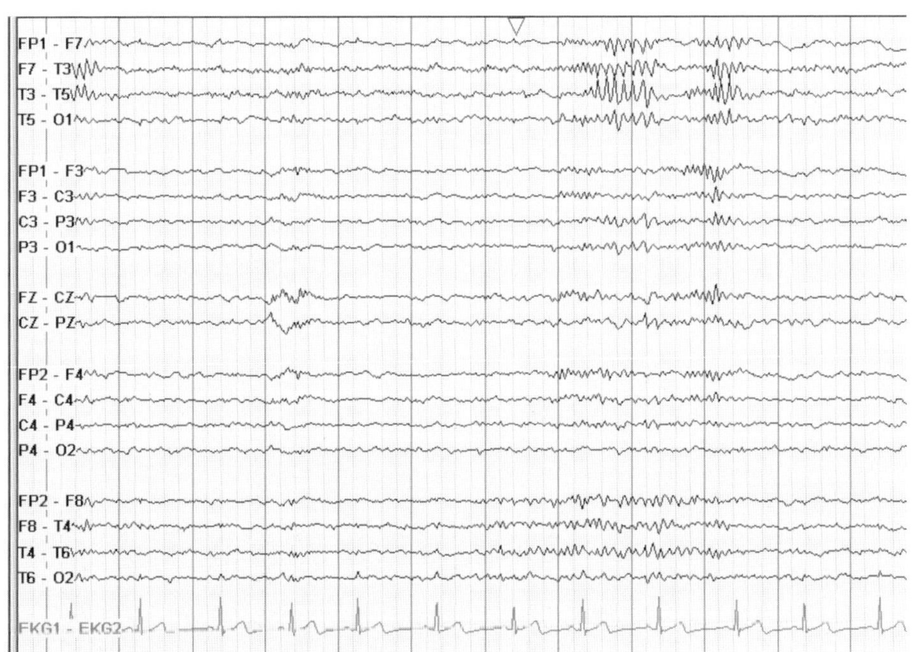

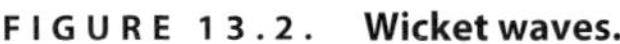
FIGURE 13.2. Wicket waves.

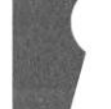
KEY FACT

Normal EEG variants during drowsiness and sleep include 14- and 6-Hz positive waves, small sharp spikes, wickets, 6-Hz spike and wave, and rhythmic temporal theta.

MNEMONIC

Sleep stages:

Features **DE**lta waves during **DE**epest sleep (stage 3 slow-wave).
d**REaM** during **REM** sleep.

REM:

Rapid pulse/**R**espiratory rate
Erection
Mental activity ↑/**M**uscle paralysis

EEG PATTERNS OF SLEEP

- **Stage N1:** Roving eye movements, waxing and waning of the posterior alpha rhythm; may see vertex waves. Positive occipital sharp transients of sleep (POSTS) are a normal phenomenon in drowsiness and sleep.
- **Stage N2:** Sleep spindles, 11–15 Hz, < 0.5-second bursts, maximal centrally.
  - Vertex waves, POSTS, and K complexes also occur.
  - K complexes: Negative sharp wave followed immediately by a slower positive component, maximal at vertex.
- **Stage N3 (slow-wave sleep):**
  - Slow waves (0.5–2 Hz) in greater than 20% of the epoch.
  - Delta spindles, K complexes, POSTS.
- **Stage R REM:** Rapid eye movement.
  - May see sawtooth waves, mixed-frequency EEG; electromyogram (EMG) drops to the lowest level of recording; ↑ heart rate.
  - Low-voltage desynchronized EEG.

KEY FACT

Breach rhythm consists of EEG activity that is ↑ in amplitude and prominence recorded over the area of a skull defect. It is most prominent when seen over the central and temporal regions.

ABNORMAL ADULT EEG (TABLE 13.6)

- **Triphasic waves** (Figure 13.3):
  - Rhythmic and bilaterally synchronous/symmetrical with a fronto-occipital or occipitofrontal time lag; usually have a frontal predominance.
  - Consistent with a metabolic encephalopathy, most commonly hepatic encephalopathy.

TABLE 13.6. Disease-EEG Associations

Disorder	EEG Finding
Hepatic encephalopathy	Triphasic waves.
Focal epilepsy	Focal spikes, sharp waves, slowing.
Generalized epilepsy	Bilateral spike-and-wave discharges.
Brain lesion	Focal slowing.
Alzheimer disease	Normal or background slowing.
Prion disease	Periodic, short-interval (0.5–1 sec) generalized, bisynchronous discharges on EEG.
Subacute sclerosing panencephalitis	Periodic slow-wave complexes in the EEG that recur every 4–15 seconds.
Anoxia	Burst suppression; intermittent sharp complexes interrupted by delta or no activity for 2 seconds to many minutes.
Brain death	Electrocerebral inactivity.
History of brain surgery	Breach rhythm.
Drug overdose	Delta and beta activity.
Herpes simplex encephalitis	Lateralized periodic discharges (LPDs) (aka periodic lateralized epileptiform discharges [PLEDs]).
Huntington disease	Low-amplitude EEG.

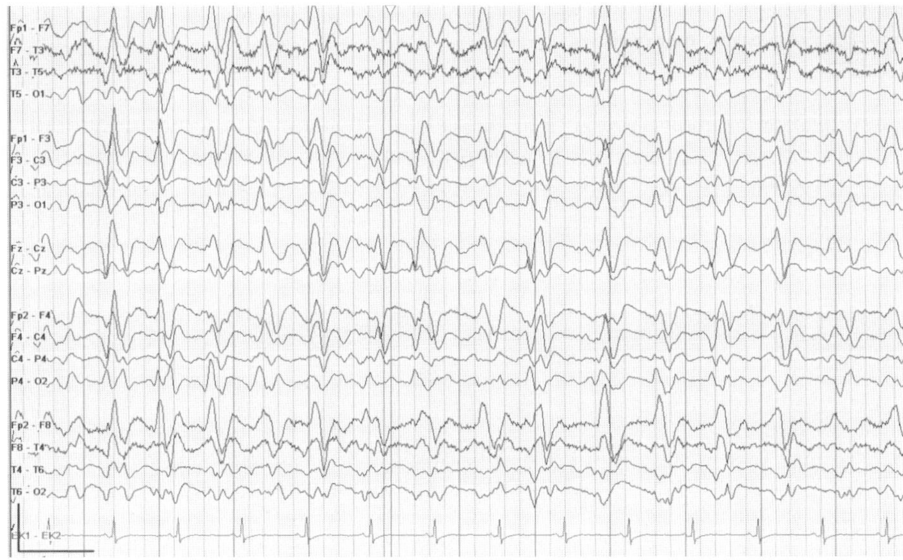

FIGURE 13.3. Triphasic waves.

- **Epileptiform discharge:**
  - Spike < 70 msec.
  - Sharp wave 70–200 msec.
- **Electrocerebral inactivity (ECI):**
  - No brain electric activity or reactivity seen on EEG with sensitivity 2 uV; interelectrode distance 10 cm; impedance 100–10,000 ohms; minimum of 8 scalp electrodes; low-frequency filter < 1 Hz; high-frequency filter > 30 Hz, at least 30 minutes long.
  - Does not exclude potential for recovery; can be seen after drug overdoses.
- **Frontal intermittent rhythmic delta activity (FIRDA)** (Figure 13.4): Seen with a variety of lesions, including posterior fossa lesions, encephalopathy, intracranial lesions, and ↑ intraventricular pressure.

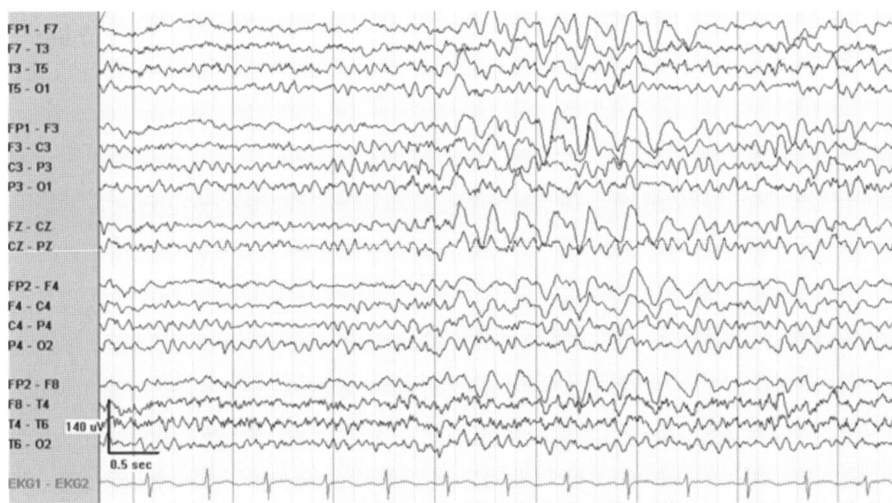

FIGURE 13.4. Frontal intermittent rhythmic delta activity (FIRDA).

Sleep Disorders

Sleep disorders involve any difficulties related to sleeping, including difficulty falling or staying asleep, falling asleep at inappropriate times, excessive total sleep time, or abnormal behaviors associated with sleep. Some sleep disorders are serious enough to interfere with normal physical, cognitive, and emotional functioning.

INSOMNIA

- Difficulty with sleep initiation, maintenance, duration, or subjective quality of sleep.
- Primary insomnias include psychophsyiologic insomnia, paradoxical insomnia (sleep state misperception), idiopathic insomnia, behavioral insomnia of childhood.
- Secondary insomnia results from a medical condition, drug, or psychiatric disorder.

SLEEP-RELATED BREATHING DISORDERS

- **Central sleep apnea:** Respiratory effort is intermittently diminished or absent.
- **Cheyne-Stokes breathing pattern:** Recurrent central apnea alternating with prolonged hyperpnea; usually seen in non-REM (NREM) sleep; seen in medical disorders (congestive heart failure), cerebrovascular disorders, renal failure.
- **Primary central sleep apnea:** Idiopathic recurrent episodes of cessation of breathing without associated ventilatory effort.
- **Secondary** due to drugs such as opioids.
- **Primary sleep apnea of infancy:** Most often seen in preterm infants.
- **Obstructive sleep apnea (OSA):** Airway obstruction resulting in ↑ breathing effort and inadequate ventilation.
  - At least 5 apneas and/or hypopneas per hour as identified by polysomnography, in addition to symptoms.
  - Continuous positive airway pressure (CPAP), if used appropriately, is 100% effective. Surgery has success rate of 50% with a high relapse rate. A dental appliance is good for only mild OSA. Weight loss for all with body mass index > 25; hypnotic use may worsen OSA.

> **KEY FACT**
>
> The minimum duration required for a respiratory event to be called obstructive apnea or hypopnea is 10 seconds in an adult.

HYPERSOMNIAS

- Daytime sleepiness not due to disturbed nocturnal sleep.
- Narcolepsy with or without cataplexy:
- Males = females, prevalence ~1 in 2000.
- **Symptoms:** Excessive daytime somnolence ≥ 3 months, sleep attacks, cataplexy (pathognomonic, abrupt onset of REM atonia triggered by strong emotional stimuli or physical exercise, occurs in 67–80% of narcoleptics)—varying severity, weakness most frequent at the knee, sleep paralysis (64% of narcoleptics), hypnogogic hallucinations.
- Onset at any age—usually second decade of life.
- **Diagnosis:** Overnight polysomnogram and multiple sleep latency test showing mean sleep latency of < 8 minutes and 2 or more sleep-onset REM periods.

- Narcolepsy with cataplexy: Loss of hypocretin-containing neurons in the hypothalamus, cerebrospinal fluid hypocretin level of < 110 pg/mL. Over 90% of patients with narcolepsy-cataplexy carry HLA-DQB1*0602. Treat cataplexy with SSRI or sodium oxybate (can lead to dramatic slow wave sleep).

CIRCADIAN RHYTHM DISORDERS

Patient unable to sleep when sleep is desired or expected. Examples: delayed or advanced sleep-phase type, shift work, jet lag.

PARASOMNIAS

Undesirable phenomena that occur during sleep (Table 13.7):

- Non-REM sleep: Confusional arousals, sleepwalking, sleep terrors.
- REM sleep: REM sleep behavioral disorder, recurrent isolated sleep paralysis, nightmares.

SLEEP-RELATED MOVEMENT DISORDERS

- Sleep-related leg cramps, bruxism, rhythmic movement disorder; restless leg syndrome (RLS).
- **RLS:** Urge to move the legs, often associated with sensory discomfort, worsening at rest with relief by activity, worsening at night.
  - Often inherited in AD fashion.
  - Periodic limb movements in sleep occur frequently with RLS but are not specific or sensitive for RLS.

TABLE 13.7. Parasomnias and Other Nocturnal Events

	Sleep Terror	Nightmare	Confusional Arousal	Sleepwalking/ Somnambulism	REM Sleep Behavior Disorder	Nocturnal Seizure	Rhythmic Movement Disorder	Hypnic Jerks
Behavior	Autonomic arousal, screaming, motor activity	Less intense vocalization, fear, motor activity	Confused; semipurposeful, complex behavior with eyes open	Complex behaviors not limited to walking	Acting out dreams, sometimes combative, may be violent	Variable, but stereotyped	Head banging or body rocking that occurs prior to or in light sleep	Brief movement, sound, or sensation at sleep onset
Age of onset	Childhood	Any age	Childhood/adolescence	Any age; peak incidence in early adolescence	Older adult (may herald a neurodegenerative disorder such as Parkinson disease or Lewy body dementia)	Anytime	Early childhood	Any age
Time of occurrence	First 90 min of sleep	Second half of night	First third of night	First third of night	Last third of night	Anytime	Prior to sleep onset	Sleep onset
Duration	Usually < 3 min	< 30 min	Minutes	Variable; can be long	Seconds to minutes	< 3 min	Minutes to hours	< 1 sec
Memory of event	No	Yes	No	No	Dream recall	No	Yes	Yes
Polysomnogram findings	Slow-wave sleep	REM	Slow-wave sleep	Slow-wave sleep	REM sleep but with ↑ EMG tone	Potentially epileptiform activity	Light sleep	Brief ↓ in EMG prior to myoclonus
Treatment	Behavioral	Behavioral	Benzodiazepines	Benzodiazepines; tricyclics	Clonazepam, carbamazepine	Antiepileptic drug	Behavioral	Behavioral

- Exacerbated by pregnancy, iron deficiency, renal failure, rheumatoid arthritis, and fibromyalgia; associated with attention deficit disorder, depression, and anxiety.
- Treated with dopamine agonists, levadopa (tolerance develops), opioids, gabapentin, benzodiazepines.

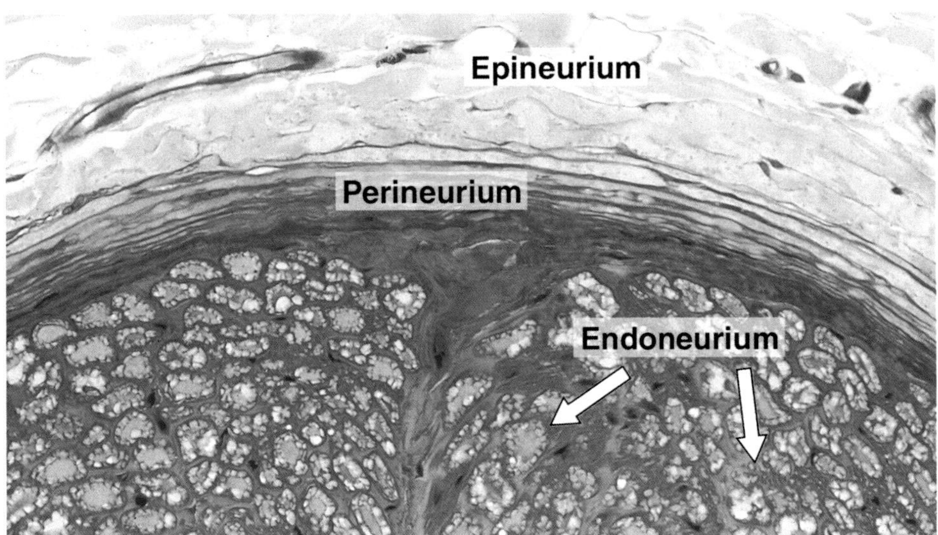

COLOR PLATE 1. Peripheral nerve anatomy.

Cross-section of a thick nerve showing the epineurium, perineurium, and endoneurium. The myelin sheath that envelops each axon was partially removed by the histological technique. PT stain. Medium magnification. (Reproduced, with permission, from Junqueria LC. *Basic Histology Text & Atlas*, 11th ed. New York: McGraw-Hill, 2005: Figure 9-34.)

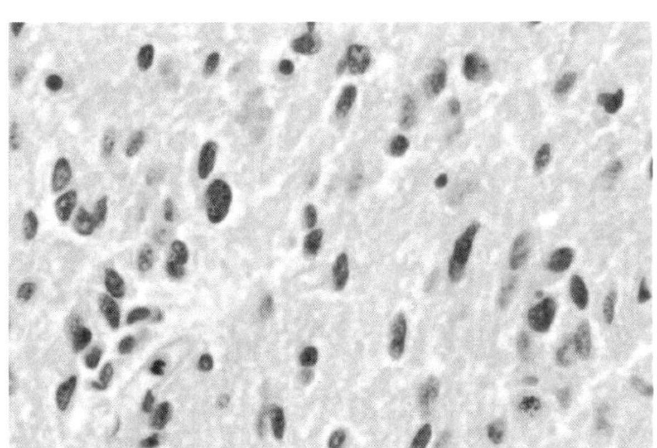

COLOR PLATE 2. Low-grade glioma, WHO-grade II (x 400).

Diffuse infiltration of the brain parenchyma by neoplastic glial cells. (Reproduced, with permission, from Kantarjian HM, Wolff RA, Koller CA. *MD Anderson Manual of Medical Oncology*. New York: McGraw-Hill, 2006: Fig. 30-12.)

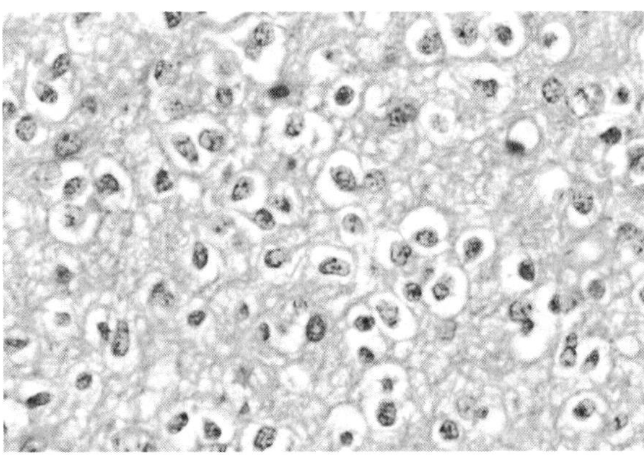

COLOR PLATE 3. Oligodendroglioma (x 400).

Characteristic "fried-egg" appearance due to clearing of the cytoplasm around the nuclei. (Reproduced, with permission, from Kantarjian HM, Wolff RA, Koller CA. *MD Anderson Manual of Medical Oncology*. New York: McGraw-Hill, 2006: Fig. 30-14.)

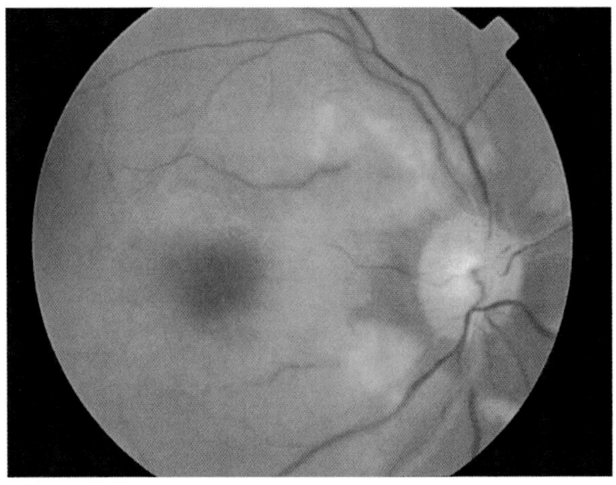

COLOR PLATE 4. Central retinal artery occlusion.

Note the lack of blood column in retinal arteries (veins still have blood inside), cherry red spot, and retinal whitening. (Reproduced, with permission, from Tintinalli JE, Kelen GD, Stapczynski JS. *Tintinalli's Emergency Medicine: A Comprehensive Study Guide*, 6th ed. New York: McGraw-Hill, 2004: Figure 238-17.)

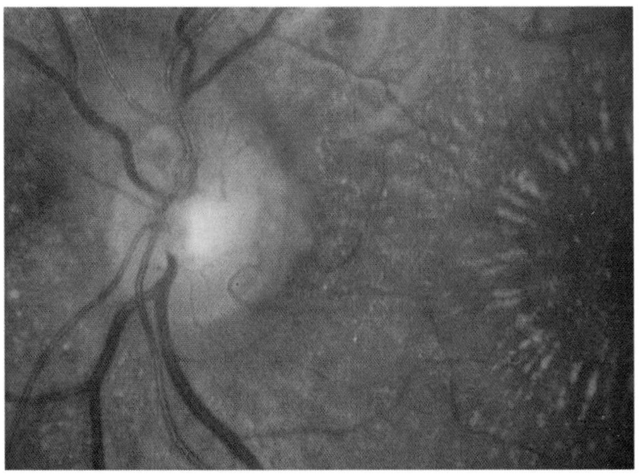

COLOR PLATE 5. Neuroretinitis.

Note the mild optic nerve head edema and the exudates in a starlike pattern in the macula.

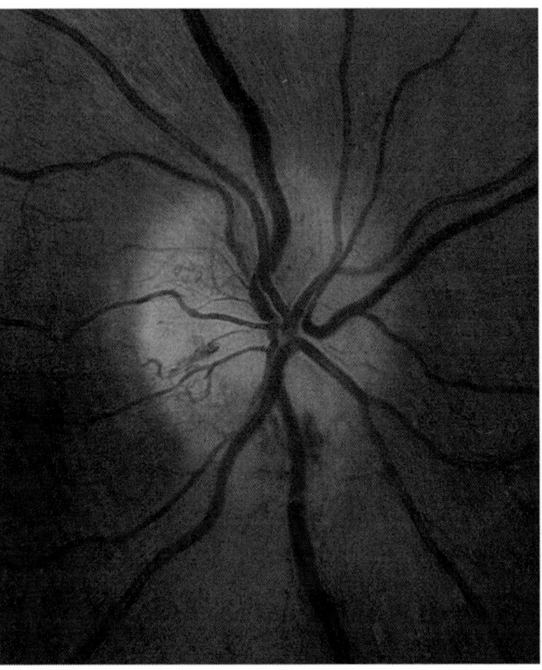

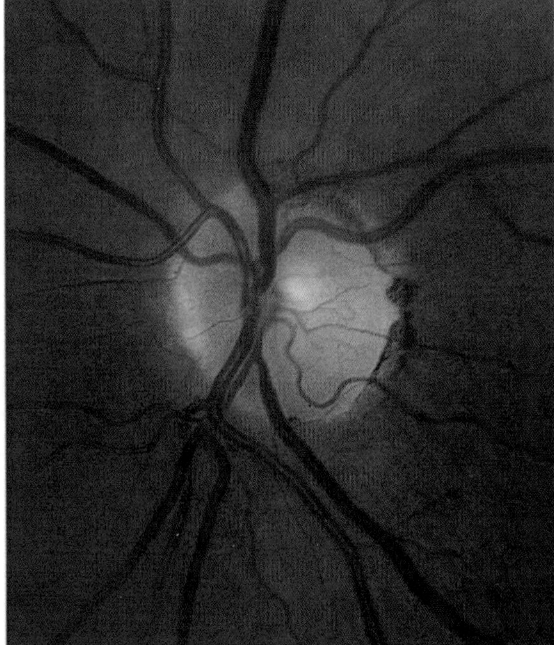

COLOR PLATE 6. Optic neuropathy and altitudinal defect.

Right anterior ischemic optic neuropathy: The right eye (photo on the left above) shows optic disc edema with disc hemorrhages. The left optic nerve has a small cup-to-disc ratio (0.1) seen in most cases of nonartertic AION. (Reproduced, with permission, from Biousse V, Newman NJ. *Neuro-ophthalmology Illustrated.* New York: Thieme, 2009: 197.)

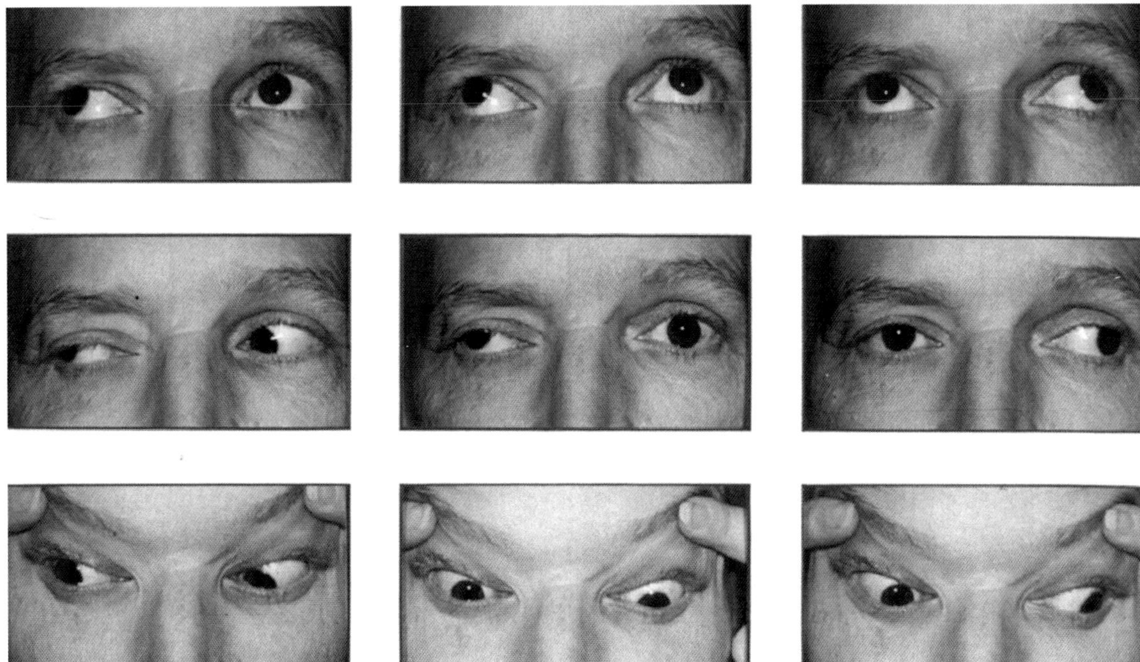

COLOR PLATE 7. Right third nerve palsy.

Note the ptosis and limitation in the movement of the right eye upward, downward, and inward. (Reproduced, with permission, from Biousse V, Newman NJ. *Neuro-ophthalmology Illustrated.* New York: Thieme Medical Publishers, 2009: 392.)

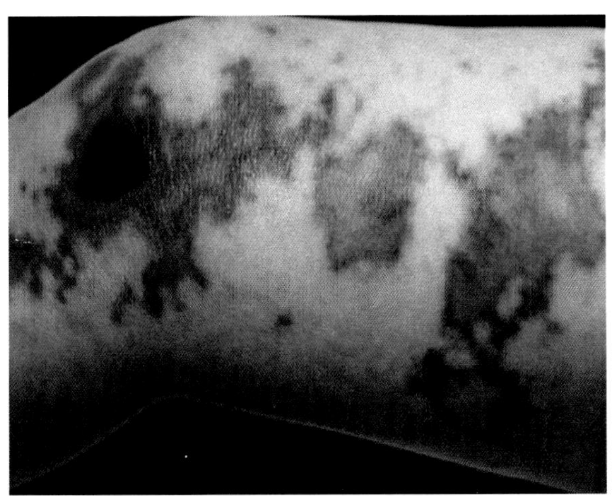

COLOR PLATE 8. Acute meningococcal rash.

(Reproduced, with permission, from Wolff K, Johnson RA, Saavedra AP. *Fitzpatrick's Color Atlas & Synopsis of Clinical Dermatology*, 7th ed. New York: McGraw-Hill Education, 2013. Figure 25-57.)

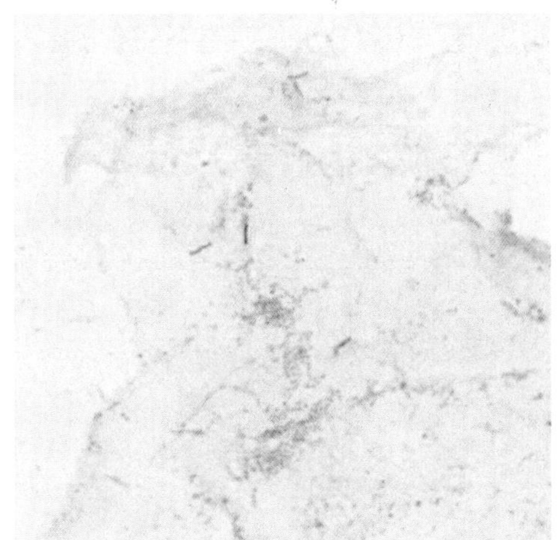

COLOR PLATE 9. Acid-fast bacillus smear showing *M tuberculosis.*

(Courtesy of the CDC, Atlanta. Reproduced, with permission, from Kasper DL, Braunwald E, Fauci AS, et al. *Harrison's Principles of Internal Medicine*, 16th ed. New York: McGraw-Hill, 2005: 954.)

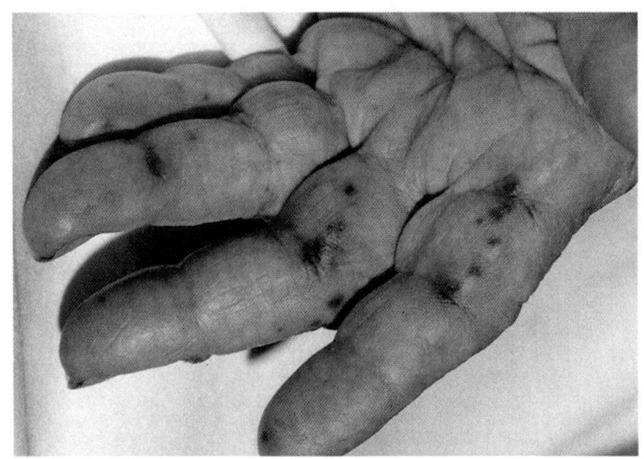

COLOR PLATE 10. Janeway lesions.

(Reproduced, with permission, from Wolff K, Johnson RA. *Fitzpatrick's Color Atlas and Synopsis of Clinical Dermatology*, 5th ed. New York: McGraw-Hill, 2005: 636.)

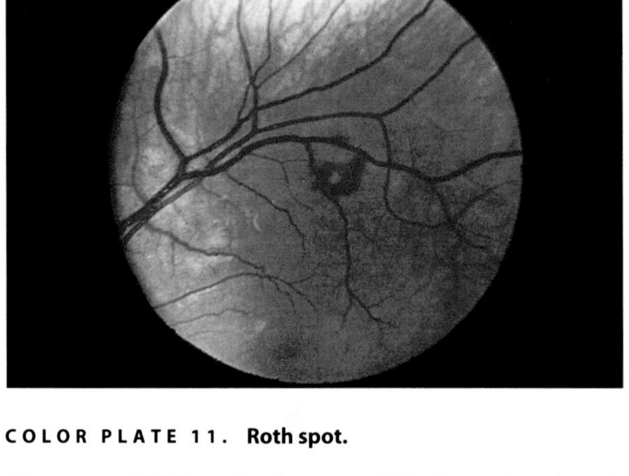

COLOR PLATE 11. Roth spot.

(Courtesy of William E. Cappaert, MD. Reproduced, with permission, from Knoop KJ, Stack LB, Storrow AB. *Atlas of Emergency Medicine*, 2nd ed. New York: McGraw-Hill, 2002: 80.)

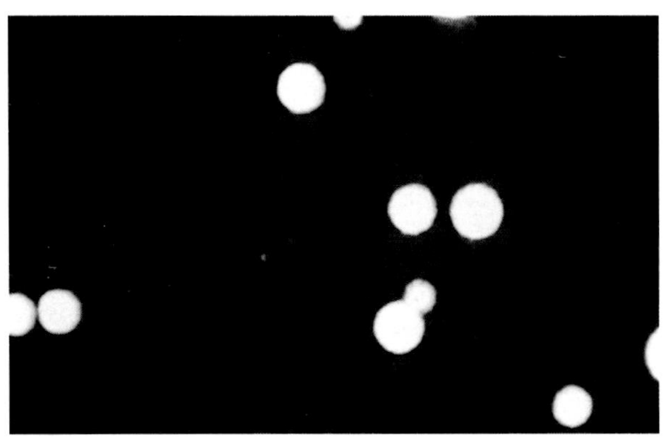

COLOR PLATE 12. India ink preparation from a patient with cryptococcal meningitis demonstrating the budding yeast form with prominent capsule.

(Courtesy of Morse et al. *Atlas of Sexually Transmitted Diseases*. London: Mosby-Wolfe; 1990. Reproduced, with permission, from Knoop KJ, Stack LB, Storrow AB. *Atlas of Emergency Medicine*, 2nd ed. New York: McGraw-Hill, 2002: 688.)

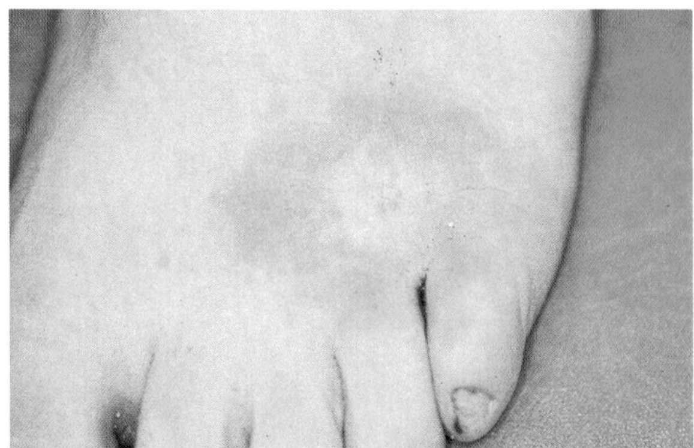

COLOR PLATE 13. Erythema migrans.

This pathognomonic enlarging rash of Lyme disease forms at the site of the tick bite and consists of an outer ring where spirochetes can be found, an inner ring of clearing, and sometimes an area of central erythema as well. (Courtesy of Timothy Hinman, MD. Reproduced, with permission, from Knoop KJ, Stack LB, Storrow AB. *Atlas of Emergency Medicine*, 2nd ed. New York: McGraw-Hill, 2002: 399.)

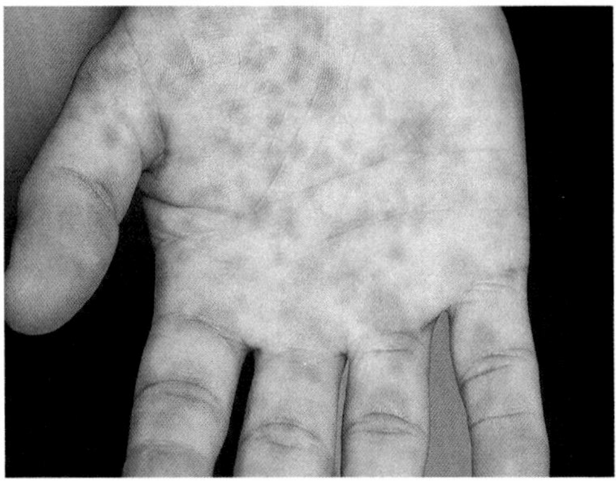

COLOR PLATE 14. The rash of Rocky Mountain spotted fever starts in the distal extremities and spread centripetally.

(Reproduced, with permission, from Knoop KJ, Stack LB, Storrow AB, Thurman RJ. *The Atlas of Emergency Medicine*, 3rd ed. New York, McGraw-Hill Education, 2010. Photographer: Daniel Noltkamper, MD.)

SECTION II

Psychiatry Topics

CHAPTER 14

Substance Abuse and Dependence

Timothy Scarella, MD

Substance-Related Disorders

Substance use disorders (SUDs) relate to the use and abuse of substances (ie, alcohol, cocaine, opiates, etc) that result in psychological distress, social dysfunction, and medical consequences. The *Diagnostic and Statistical Manual of Mental Disorders*, 5th edition (DSM-5) divides this category into disorders of the pattern of use of substances (substance use disorder) and conditions directly attributable to the ingestion of or withdrawal from a substance.

SUBSTANCE USE DISORDER

- Describes the set of physiological, cognitive, and behavioral symptoms that occur as a result of the continued use of any substance, despite a pattern of negative consequences.
- In DSM-IV, there was a distinction made between substance abuse and substance dependence. However, based on data that this distinction is problematic in terms of ability, prognostic implications, and treatment planning significance, these 2 diagnoses have been combined into the DSM-5 diagnosis of substance use disorder.
- To meet DSM-5 criteria for diagnosis of substance use disorder, one must have a **problematic pattern** of use that causes **clinically significant impairment or distress.** The patient must also meet 2 of the following symptoms at some point within a 12-month period:
  - Tolerance (needing greater amounts of the substance to achieve the same effect or markedly reduced effect with a previously effective drug dose).
  - Withdrawal (either a characteristic withdrawal syndrome *or* a pattern of using the substance to avoid a withdrawal).
  - Pattern of using more of a substance *or* using it over a longer period than intended.
  - Persistent desire *or* a history of unsuccessful attempts to ↓ use of the substance.
  - Large amount of time spent acquiring, using, *or* recovering from the effects of the substance.
  - Cravings to use the substance.
  - Use of substance causes failure to fill necessary obligations (work, school, home).
  - Continued use despite recurrent problems caused by the substance use.
  - Important activities are given up in order to use.
  - Recurrent use at times when it is physically hazardous to do so.
  - Continued use despite knowledge of a physical or psychological problem caused or made worse by use.

INTOXICATION

- Intoxication is a reversible, substance-specific syndrome that occurs due to the recent ingestion of a substance, directly attributable to the physiologic effects of the substance.
- Repeated intoxication is present in substance use disorders. However, the presence of repeated intoxication does not necessarily represent a diagnosis of substance use disorder.

- Intoxication syndromes vary, depending on the particular substance, and the effects are generally reversible with time. They rarely require medical intervention except for certain acute situations that involve severe dangerousness.

WITHDRAWAL

- Withdrawal is a substance-specific syndrome with both physiologic and cognitive components that is directly due to cessation or reduction of substance use.
- Withdrawal symptoms are typically characterized by the *opposite* effects of the substance one is withdrawing from.

SUBSTANCE-INDUCED MENTAL DISORDERS

There are certain individuals who present with depression, anxiety, mania, or psychosis, where a last psychiatric syndrome is thought to be the effect of the acute or chronic use of a substance. The category of substance-induced mental disorder is then made rather than of the corresponding primary psychiatric problem (ie, major depressive disorder).

Case Example 1: A 32-year-old man relapses on alcohol after 5 years of sobriety. He reports that, after 3 days of heavy drinking, he had depressed mood, low energy, poor sleep, severe guilt about his drinking relapse, and was having thoughts of killing himself by alcohol poisoning. These persisted for 4 weeks while he continued to drink heavily on a daily basis. After checking into a detoxification center, he reported improvement in his mood within 1 week. He was followed for over 20 years after this, during which he remained sober and never had a recurrence of depression.

In this case, a diagnosis of alcohol-induced depressive disorder is more appropriate than major depressive disorder.

Case Example 2: A 19-year-old college student presents with anxiety. He reports that he spends all day feeling anxious and nervous about various things, including whether or not his grades will be good enough to get into medical school, whether people in his classes like him, and whether he will have enough time to study. He has trouble sleeping at night and lies awake ruminating. He has noticed that he is so anxious that he trembles at times. This has been going on since the semester started. On further questioning, you learn he has been buying stimulants from his roommate and using up to 100 mg of methylphenidate daily. Once confronted, he stops using the drug and symptoms resolve.

In this case, a diagnosis of stimulant-induced anxiety disorder is more appropriate than generalized anxiety disorder.

ASSESSMENT OF SUBSTANCE DISORDERS

- Take a detailed history: What do they use? When was the last time they used? How much do they use? How much money do they spend? How often do they use? What is the route of administration?
- Ask about every drug, and don't forget about tobacco.
- Collect collateral information (eg, family, friends, workplace, if available).
- Screen for mood, anxiety, psychotic, and personality disorder, with which substance use disorders are highly comorbid.
- Perform appropriate laboratory tests (see Table 14.1).

TABLE 14.1. Substance Abuse Laboratory Tests and Detection Periods

Substance	Urine	Hair	Blood	Potential False Positives
Alcohol	3–5 days via ethyl gluconoride (EtG) metabolite or 10–12 hours via traditional method	Can detect use over long period of time	Up to 12 hours	Mouthwash, some sugarless candies
Amphetamines, MDMA (except methamphetamine)	1–2 days	Up to 90 days	12 hours	Pseudoephedrine, bupropion, amantadine, chloroquine, chlorpromazine, desipramine, ephedrine, labetalol, phenylephrine, ranitidine, selegiline, trazodone, tyramine
Methamphetamine	2–4 days	Up to 90 days	24 hours	Pseudoephedrine
Barbiturates (except phenobarbital)	2–3 days	Up to 90 days	1–2 days	Phenytoin, primidone
Phenobarbital	7–14 days	Up to 90 days	4–7 days	None
Benzodiazepines	Short-term use use: 3 days Chronic use (over 1 year): 4–6 weeks	Up to 90 days	6–48 hours	Sertraline, oxaprozin
Cocaine	2–4 days	Up to 90 days	24 hours	Topical anesthetics containing cocaine (TAC)
Heroin	2–5 days	Up to 90 days	6 hours	Poppy seeds (depending on assay sensitivity), rifampin, floroquinolones

Note: Drug testing itself is not treatment. It is part of monitoring to assess treatment efficacy. Reinforcement with drug testing is best used when patients have negative urine drug screens versus punishing patients with positive toxicology tests.

TREATMENT OF SUBSTANCE USE DISORDERS

General principles:

- Substance use disorders are chronic relapsing disorders like hypertension, diabetes, and asthma. They should be managed as such (eg, do not discharge patients for relapse). Relapses are symptoms of the disorder.
- Detoxification is only a preparatory step for further treatment; it treats withdrawal and established abstinence but does not treat the underlying substance use disorder.
- Relapse prevention interventions tend to have small effect sizes individually, but when combined can help a patient maintain abstinence.

Caffeine

Caffeine is the most commonly used substance worldwide. It is found in coffee, caffeinated sodas, tea, and a number of medications (Fioricet, Excedrin).

Pharmacology and Mechanism

- Half-life 3–7 hours.
- Competitive antagonist at adenosine binding sites.

Effects/Intoxication

- Psychological: Enhanced concentration, alertness, insomnia, feeling of well-being, anxiety, irritability.
- Physical: ↑ cardiac contractility, ↓ vascular resistance (at low doses), ↑ vascular resistance (at higher doses).
- Overdose is rare; symptoms of intoxication include restlessness, nervousness, insomnia, flushing, diuresis, gastrointestinal (GI) disturbance, muscle twitches, racing thoughts, rapid speech, arrhythmia or tachycardia, psychomotor agitation.

Withdrawal

- Symptoms: Headaches, lethargy, irritability, fatigue, muscle tension.
- Peaks at 48–96 hours and resolves within a week.

Tobacco

Tobacco use is the number-one preventable cause of morbidity and mortality worldwide. The principal psychoactive ingredient in tobacco is nicotine. Tobacco is most commonly smoked in the form of cigarettes or chewed. Tobacco smoke contains nearly 4000 different substances, including tar, ammonia, benzene, carbon monoxide, and polyaromatic hydrocarbons.

Pharmacology and Mechanism

- Binds primarily at the $\alpha4\beta2$ nicotinic receptor, which is distributed heavily throughout the central nervous system (CNS).
- Effects on dopamine, norepinephrine, acetylcholine, glutamate, vasopressin, serotonin, gamma-aminobutyric acid (GABA), and beta-endorphin systems are all seen with tobacco use.

Epidemiology

- Prevalence of about 20% in the United States with significant regional variation.
- Not all smokers, even if heavy smokers, meet DSM-5 criteria for tobacco use disorder; nevertheless, all smokers should be counselled to quit and treated appropriately.
- Historically, there have been more male than female smokers. However they are now almost equal.
- More than 80% of smokers are daily smokers.
- Most smokers begin prior to age 18.
- More than one-third of smokers will die prematurely from smoking-related illness.

Nicotine Effects

- Nicotine improves memory and cognition, reduces appetite, modulates mood, and reduces anxiety.
- Adverse physical effects of tobacco smoke (not nicotine, per se): ↑ risk of cancer, cardiovascular disease, respiratory disease, impotence, cataracts.
- Nicotine tolerance develops rapidly and reliably.

Nicotine Withdrawal

- Nicotine-dependent individuals experience nicotine withdrawal within hours of last use.
- Common withdrawal symptoms include anxiety, irritability, anger, difficulty concentrating, appetite ↑, depression, and poor sleep.
- Withdrawal symptoms from attempts to quit "cold turkey" peak at 12–24 hours and typically resolve within 72 hours.

Pharmacologic Treatment

- **Nicotine replacement:**
  - Goal is to replace "dirty" nicotine with "clean" nicotine.
  - Nicotine preparations: Patches, gum, lozenges, nasal spray, inhaler.
  - Patients may use multiple preparations at the same time; for example, wearing a patch for baseline cravings and using gum or lozenge as needed for more intense cravings.
- **Bupropion:**
  - A norepinephrine/dopamine reuptake inhibiting antidepressant. Its mechanism of efficacy in smoking cessation is unclear.
  - Side effects: Anxiety, insomnia.
  - Most head-to-head trials suggest varenicline may be more effective, though magnitude of difference varies.
- **Varenicline:**
  - Mechanism: $\alpha 4\beta 2$—nicotine receptor partial agonist.
  - Side effects: Nausea, abnormal sleep/dreams, dizziness, fatigue.
  - Advantage is that patient may continue smoking after they take it; typically, a quit date is set for about a week after the medication is started.

Alcohol

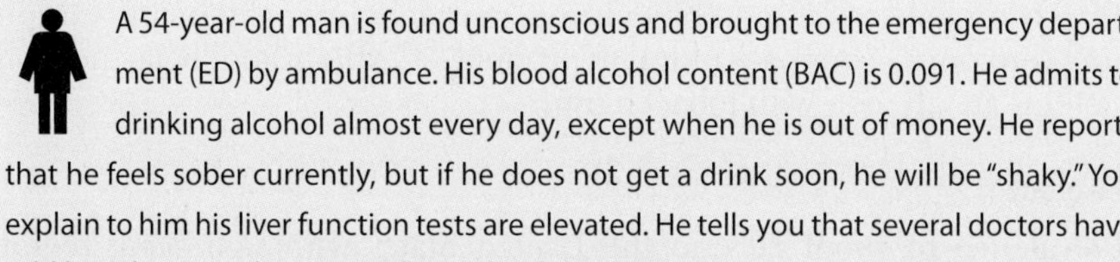

A 54-year-old man is found unconscious and brought to the emergency department (ED) by ambulance. His blood alcohol content (BAC) is 0.091. He admits to drinking alcohol almost every day, except when he is out of money. He reports that he feels sober currently, but if he does not get a drink soon, he will be "shaky." You explain to him his liver function tests are elevated. He tells you that several doctors have told him that over the years. What is the diagnosis?

Alcohol use disorder. He has symptoms of alcohol use for most of the time, tolerance (feeling sober at 0.091% BAC). He also reports a withdrawal history if he does not drink. He has continued use despite medical consequences of elevated liver enzymes.

- Alcohol has CNS effects at almost every neurotransmitter system. Alcohol, acutely administered, ↑ serotonin, dopamine, and GABA transmission and inhibits N-methyl-D-aspartate (NMDA) system activity.
- Alcohol causes behavioral changes that are influenced by age, weight, gender, food consumption, and prior experience with alcohol.

Epidemiology

- Alcohol use disorders have 12-month prevalence of about 12% in adult men and 5% in adult women. Rates are highest for Native Americans, and higher in whites and Hispanics than African Americans.
- Early development of high tolerance is predictive of alcohol dependence.

Medical Consequences

- Medical side effects: Liver damage (including alcoholic hepatitis [reversible if drinking stops], fatty liver [usually reversible], and cirrhosis [not reversible]), pancreatitis, refractory hypertension, hypertriglyceridemia, and alcoholic gastritis/ulcers.
- Alcohol affects the production of all types of blood cells; early signs of bone marrow effects include thrombocytopenia and macrocytosis.
- Alcohol's effects on the CNS typically occur in the setting of mental clouding during intoxication.
- Alcoholic dementia is an area of controversy. It is unclear whether the direct effects of alcohol or, rather, related nutritional deficiencies or neglect of chronic medical conditions cause the most damage.

Wernicke-Korsakoff Syndrome

A 43-year-old man presents to the ED complaining of "the shakes." He drinks 1 liter of vodka per day and has minimal additional PO consumption. His last drink was 5 hours earlier. He was started on 5% dextrose in normal saline solution (D_5NS). He rapidly developed ophthalmoplegia, amnesia, and confusion. What happened? What is the next step in management?

Wernicke-Korsakoff sydrome was probably precipitated in this patient due to receiving dextrose in the setting of thiamine deficiency. The patient should receive thiamine immediately, although this condition may not be reversible.

- Wernicke-Korsakoff syndrome is a consequence of thiamine deficiency in susceptible individuals (especially those with transketolase deficiency).
- Wernicke encephalopathy results from acute administration of glucose in a thiamine deficient individual; if caught early, there is possibility of reversal. Korsakoff syndrome consists of chronic, usually irreversible changes:
  - Wernicke encephalopathy: Typically diagnosed by the clinical triad of delirium, occulomotor abnormalities (opthalmoplegia or nystagmus), and ataxia, though full triad is present in a minority of cases. May progress to coma and death.
  - Korsakoff psychosis: Anterograde and retrograde amnesia, confabulation.
- Treatment consists of giving supplemental thiamine; if Wernicke is suspected, high-dose parenteral thiamine repletion is indicated. This must be started prior to administration of glucose, or the condition can be worsened.

Alcohol Withdrawal

- Mild to moderate symptoms: Anxiety, shakiness, emotional volatility, irritability, depression, fatigue, confusion, headache, nausea, vomiting, loss of appetite, insomnia, palpitations, hand tremor.
- Severe symptoms: Delirium, vital sign instability, seizures.
- **Alcoholic hallucinosis:** Rare, develops 12–24 hours after drinking, usually involves auditory hallucinations, no physical symptoms, resolves on its own. May persist for weeks after cessation; reliably goes away if drinking is reinitiated. The presence of a normal sensorium distinguishes alcoholic hallucinosis from delirium tremens.
- **Withdrawal seizures:** Generalized tonic clonic seizures that usually occur 12–48 hours after the last drink. Treat with benzodiazepenes or phenobarbital; there is some evidence that phenytoin is less effective for withdrawal seizures than idiopathic epileptic seizures.

- **Delirium tremens (DTs):** Severe form of alcohol withdrawal. The hallmark of DTs is the presence of delirium, regardless of other signs/symptoms of withdrawal.
  - Besides past history of DT, the best predictor of impending DT is presence of withdrawal seizures; one-third of patients who have a withdrawal seizure will progress to DTs.
  - DTs can show up 72–96 hours after last drink.
  - Even when treated, DTs carry 10–15% mortality, usually secondary to wild swings in blood pressure, heart rate, and associated arrhythmia due to sympathetic hyperactivity.
  - Prevent DTs with the use of benzodiazepines (eg, diazepam, chlordiazepoxide, lorazepam). May choose either fixed-dose regimen and taper (using conversion between reported amount of alcohol use daily and benzodiazepenes) or symptom-based treatment using monitoring scales. Studies have not found consistent advantage to either method other than reduced total dose of benzodiazepenes in patients with symptom-triggered treatment.

Treatment for Dependence

- Assess for chronic use primarily by taking a history and obtaining collateral information if possible. May also test for these findings:
  - Elevated liver functions which indicate alcoholic hepatitis: Aspartate transaminase (AST) at twice the level of alanine transaminase (ALT) is a classic ratio but has poor specificity.
  - Elevated gamma-glutamyl (GGT): 70–80% sensitive and specific.
  - Elevated % CDT (carbohydrate deficient transferring): 70–80% specific.
  - Macrocytic anemia or thrombocytopenia.
- Most do not seek treatment until into their late 40s or 50s.
- Alcoholism requires chronic management. Detoxification is not a cure.
- Psychosocial treatment:
  - Brief intervention: Counseling and education about medical consequences of drinking.
  - Cognitive-behavioral therapy: Founded on learning theory, focuses on situations and triggers for use.
  - Alcoholics Anonymous: 12-step model with a dose-response curve (eg, more meetings predicts greater sobriety).
  - Relapse prevention therapy: Helps patients identify and cope effectively with high-risk situations, manage urges and craving, and implement damage control procedures during relapses.
- Medication treatment: See Table 14.2.

Cocaine

Cocaine is a central nervous system stimulant. Because of its direct effect on the mesolimbic reward pathway, it is highly addictive.

Mechanism and Metabolism

- Rapid dopamine and norepinephrine reuptake inhibition.
- Increases dopaminergic activity in the mesolimbic and mesocortical areas of the brain.
- Given norepinephrine reuptake inhibition, concomitant use of beta blockers can cause a dangerous unopposed alpha-adrenergic stimulation and hypertensive crisis.

TABLE 14.2. Medications for the Treatment of Alcohol Abuse

MEDICATION	CONTRAINDICATIONS	SIDE EFFECTS	COMMENTS
Disulfiram	Continuing alcohol use, metronidazole	Disulfiram-alcohol reaction, heptatitis, peripheral neuropathy, psychosis, metallic aftertaste, drowsiness	Contraindicated with warfarin; isoniazid; metronidazole; any nonprescription drug containing alcohol; phenytoin. Requires motivated patient; if they want to drink, they can just skip pill.
Naltrexone	Opioid use, acute hepatitis or liver failure	Hepatotoxicity, nausea, anxiety, fatigue	Data suggests increased efficacy if initiated after at least 4 days abstinence.
Acamprosate	Severe renal failure	Diarrhea, drowsiness, rare suicidal ideation	No clinically relevant interactions known.
Topiramite	No absolute contraindications	Cognitive dulling, kidney stones	No FDA indication for this but increasingly used. May be more effective in Caucasian due to prevalence of certain genetic polymorphisms.

- Half-life: 2 hours although duration of intoxication is very brief: intranasal 15–30 minutes, smoked/injected 5–10 minutes.
- Primarily processed by the liver and excreted in urine and feces.
- Can be detected in urine typically up to 3–4 days (but as high as 10 days in heavy users).

Intoxication and Long-Term Use

- Psychological: Euphoria, ↑ energy, hypersexuality, improved concentration and ↓ need for sleep, anxiety, irritability, impaired judgment.
- Physiological: Tachycardia, blood vessel constriction, hypertension, hyperthermia, diaphoresis, tremor, pupillary dilation.
- Seizures are possible with heavy doses of cocaine use.
- Psychosis, characterized by the rapid onset of hallucinations (both visual and auditory), paranoia, and delusions. Psychosis may persist for days to weeks beyond period of initial intoxication especially with chronic users.
- Snorting cocaine causes blood vessel constriction in nasal passages over time, preventing further drug absorption.

Tolerance and Withdrawal

- Tolerance to the effects of cocaine develop rapidly, and users will self-administer cocaine repeatedly to avoid withdrawal.
- Withdrawal begins shortly after the cessation of use.
- Withdrawal is characterized by fatigue, depressed mood, hunger, irritability, uncontrollable sleepiness, and waves of cocaine craving.
- Duration of withdrawal is greater with longer duration of use.

Treatment for Overdose

- Treat hyperthermia with cold water, ice packs, hypothermic blanket.
- Treat seizures with IV diazepam.

- Treat malignant hypertension with IV phentolamine (remember: administering beta blockers can cause unopposed alpha-adrenergic agonism and worsen hypertension.
- Treat agitation with haloperidol or lorazepam.

Treatment for Dependence

Disulfiram, modafinil, topiramate, tiagabine have shown some limited efficacy for cocaine abstinence. However, no medications have shown consistent evidence of effectiveness in treating cocaine dependence.

Amphetamines

This category includes amphetamines and amphetamine-like substances (dextroamphetamine, methamphetamine). Amphetamine compounds are produced both pharmaceutically and illicitly.

Pharmacology

- Chemically similar to dopamine.
- Promotes rapid release and reuptake inhibition of biogenic amines (dopamine and norepinephrine) from vesicular and cystosolic stores.
- Promotes release of serotonin at higher doses.

Effects

- Euphoria, elevated mood, alertness, ↑ energy, "crystal clear thinking."
- Adverse effects: Anxiety, paranoia, insomnia, anorexia, diaphoresis, hypersexuality, elevated blood pressure and heart rate, dilated pupils, tremor.
- Mood disturbances can occur with chronic use.
- Psychosis may occur, with delusions of persecution, ideas of reference, visual and auditory hallucinations.

Treatment

- **Psychosocial:** Similar psychotherapies and psychosocial interventions to other substance use disorders.
- **Medications:** Small literature for use of topiramte or modafinil but off label. Use antipsychotics for hallucinations and severe agitation in acute intoxication.

Opiates

This class includes natural opioids (morphine), semisynthetics (heroin, hydrocodone), and synthetics that behave like natural opioids (methadone, propoxyphene, fentanyl).

- Naturally occurring opioids are derived from the opium poppy plant.
- Opioids are indicated in the treatment of pain, cough, diarrhea, and anesthesia.
- Opioids can be administered in by oral ingestion, snorting, smoking, and injecting.

Pharmacology

- Categorized into agonists (morphine, heroin, codeine, methadone) and partial agonists (buprenorphine, pentazocine).
- There are three major subtypes of opioid receptors: delta, kappa, mu (see Table 14.3).
- Full agonists exert their effects at all receptor sites.
- Partial agonists, such as buprenorphine, bind tightly to the mu opiate receptors but activate them less than full agonists.
- Buprenorphine is an antagonist at the kappa receptor site.
- Opioid antagonists (naloxone, naltrexone) block the effects of opiates at all three types of receptor sites.

Facts About Specific Opioids

- **Heroin:** A semisynthetic opiate that rapidly crosses the blood-brain barrier when administered, where it is cleaved into morphine. Rapid rise in blood and CNS levels after administration lead to high addictive potential.
- **Oxycodone:** Synthetic opioid prescribed as lone agent or in pharmaceutical preparation with acetaminophen. Poor cross-reactivity with urine opiate assays and is generally tested for separately.
- **Meperidine:** Used medically in GI procedures, especially endoscopy, due to its specific activity in dilating the sphincter of Oddi, making it favorable for endoscopic retrograde cholangiopancreatography (ERCP). Has risks of seizure at higher doses and serotonin syndrome when combined with other serotenergic agents.

TABLE 14.3. Opioid Receptors

Receptor	Subtypes	Location	Function
Delta	Delta 1,2		
		Pontine nuclei	Antidepressant effects
		Amygdala	Analgesia
		Olfactory bulbs	
		Deep cortex	
Kappa	Kappa 1,2,3		
		Hypothalamus	Analgesia
		Periaqueductal gray	Sedation
		Claustrum	Pupillary miosis
		Substantia gelatinosa of spinal cord	Inhibition of ADH release
Mu	Mu 1,2		*Mu 1*
		Cortex	Analgesia
		Thalamus	
		Periaqueductal gray	
			Mu 2
		Substantia gelatinosa of spinal cord	Respiratory depression
			Pupillary miosis
			Euphoria
			Reduced gastrointestinal motility

- **Fentanyl:** Synthetic opioid, 80–100 times as potent as morphine. Available IV or in transdermal patch. Poor cross reactivity with general urine opioid assays.
- **Methadone:** Used in pain management, as well as treatment of opioid dependence. Has extremely long half-life (18–36 hours) and is extensively plasma bound and liver stored. Given slow time to peak blood level and long half-life has lower propensity to cause psychologic "high" but still can be abused. Methadone overdoses occur more in pain treatment settings where patients have lower tolerances.
- **Morphine:** Metabolized by liver to morphine-3-glucuronide (inactive) and morphine-6-glucuronide (active at mu receptor with about 50% the potency of morphine). This is important because those with cirrhosis will metabolize morphine very slowly and are at risk for overdose. Those with renal failure will clear morphine-6-glucoronide slowly and are at risk of opiate overdose effects due to build-up of the metabolite.

Intoxication and Overdose

- Intoxication symptoms include euphoria, sedation, cognitive slowing, slurred speech, pupillary miosis, itching, nausea, respiratory depression, constipation.
- Overdose results in respiratory suppression, coma, and death.
- Treat with intravenous administration of naloxone (opiate antagonist). Nalxone has a very short half-life, where many opiates (eg, methadone, sustained-release morphine preparations) have very long half-lives. Be cautious not to discharge a patient too early.

Withdrawal

- Highly uncomfortable, rarely lethal without co-occurring medical conditions or concomitant substance use.
- Symptoms: Dilated pupils, goosebumps, rhinorrhea, subjective anxiety and discomfort, diarrhea and GI distress, bony pain, fatigue (which is usually last symptom to resolve).
- Higher-potency/shorter-acting opioids have greater withdrawal symptoms over a shorter duration.
- Withdrawal management: Treat the symptoms.
  - Clonidine addresses most withdrawal symptoms.
  - Antihistamines such as diphenhydramine or trazodone helpful for sleep.
  - Nonsteroidal anti-inflammatory drugs (NSAIDs) for bone pain.
  - Loperamide for diarrhea.

Treatment for Abuse and Dependence

- **Methadone maintenance:**
  - Highly effective in short-term and long-term outcome data. It is the single most empirically validated treatment in all of addiction treatment.
  - Works by competitive blockade of the opioid receptor.
  - Usually administered on a once-a-day basis.
  - Can be legally prescribed for opioid dependence only in specially certified narcotic treatment programs.
  - Methadone doses for opiate dependence tend to be higher than methadone for pain. Patient taking at least 60 mg/day are more successful in maintaining abstinence.
  - When patients are at stable doses, methadone produces no euphoria and no analgesia.
  - Methadone maintenance causes 10× reduction in death rates, criminal behavior, infectious disease transmission.

    - Recommended for use in pregnant opioid addicts by American College of Obstetrics and Gynecology.
- **Buprenorphine maintenance:**
    - Highly effective in short-term and long-term efficacy data.
    - Also works by competitive blockade of the opioid receptor while partially activating the receptor.
    - Outcome data for buprenorphine shows that it is as efficacious as high-dose methadone for treating opiate dependence.
    - Buprenorphine can be prescribed only by physicians with Drug Addiction Treatment Act of 2000 (DATA) waivers.
    - Prior to starting buprenorphine, it is important to ensure that a patient evidences some withdrawal symptoms or else withdrawal can be precipitated by buprenorphine administration; be sure to ask if patient has used any long-acting opiates (methadone or extended-release morphine/oxycodone preparations).
    - Buprenorphine has a far greater safety profile than methadone in that its partial agonist effects provide a ceiling against overdose, even in naïve users.
- **Naltrexone maintenance:**
    - Long-acting opioid antagonist.
    - Numerous studies show poor results in opioid dependence in patient retention and overall efficacy.
    - It is theorized that naltrexone can cause dysphoria in opioid-dependent individuals.

NOTES

CHAPTER 15

Delirium

William Z. Barnard, MD

Delirium is a common syndrome found across many medical specialties and has many other names (ie, encephalopathy, acute brain syndrome, acute brain failure, toxic psychosis, etc).

Symptoms

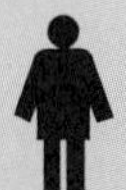

A 75-year-old man presents with a change in mental status over the course of a week. He recently underwent a hip replacement and has since been having visual hallucinations. What is the most likely clinical diagnosis for this patient?

The diagnosis is delirium because of the acute onset and predisposing factor of undergoing a hip replacement. Visual hallucinations are also more common in delirium than in other acute psychiatric diagnoses.

Clinical symptoms include:

- **Disruption of consciousness,** resulting in impaired focus and attention.
- Global **cognitive impairment,** → poor memory and language, disorientation, and disorganized thinking.
- **Perceptual abnormalities** (ie, illusions, hallucinations, and delusions).
- **Emotional changes** (ie, fear, changes in mood, affective instability, and anxiety, irritability, anger, euphoria, apathy).
- **Sleep disturbance,** often causing disruption of diurnal rhythms.
- Changes happen **acutely** (hours to days), and symptoms are generally worse at night (ie, **sundowning**).
- The clinical course often **fluctuates** between lucidity and disorientation, making the diagnosis difficult.
- There are several subtypes of delirium:
  - Hypoactive/hypoalert: Psychomotor retardation, lethargy, ↓ arousal.
  - Hyperactive/hyperalert: Hyperactivity, agitation.
  - Mixed: Both hyperactive and hypoactive activity.
  - Normal: No psychomotor retardation or agitation present.

KEY FACT

Key hallmarks of delirium are inattention and disorientation.

Exam

The physical exam is aimed at discovering the underlying cause of delirium:

- Vital signs: blood pressure, heart rate, temperature, respiratory rate.
- Neuro: Mental status exam, mini-mental state exam (MMSE), cranial nerves II–XII, upper and lower motor abnormalities, sensory deficits, primitive reflexes, gait, cerebellar dysfunction.
- Head and neck: Look for evidence of trauma, impairments in hearing or seeing, papilledema, inspection of tongue for lacerations (from seizure), carotid bruits, thyromegaly, nuchal rigidity.
- Lungs: Crackles, wheezing, rales, areas dull to percussion.
- Cardio: Rhythm, rate, evidence of murmurs.
- Abdomen: Hepatomegaly, splenomegaly, masses, bowel sounds, rebound tenderness.
- Back: Costovertebral angle tenderness.
- Musculoskeletal: Evidence of fractures/trauma.

Predisposing Factors

- Age > 65.
- Dementia.
- Depression.
- Brain injury.
- History of neurologic disease.

- History of cardiac disease.
- History of alcohol abuse.
- Previous episodes of delirium.
- Sensory impairment (visual or auditory).
- Malnutrition or dehydration.
- Postoperative stated or intensive care unit (ICU) stay.
- Prolonged sleep deprivation.
- Polypharmacy.
- Chronic renal or hepatic disease.

DIFFERENTIAL DIAGNOSIS

- The differential diagnosis of delirium includes dementia, depression, and psychotic disorders. Table 15.1 compares and contrasts these diagnoses.
- Delirium always has an **underlying cause(s)** (medical condition, drugs, or procedure). Table 15.2 lists the differential diagnoses of the causes of delirium.

DIAGNOSIS

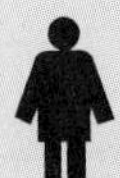

A 36-year-old man seen in the emergency department (ED) is disoriented. He has tachycardia, hypertension, a fever, and is very tremulous. You smell alcohol on his breath. How should this patient be managed?

The patient should be given benzodiazepines as he is in delirium tremens from alcohol withdrawal. He should also be given thiamine to prevent Wernicke-Korsakoff syndrome.

- Delirium is a clinical diagnosis. The **MMSE** can aid in discovering cognitive dysfunction and is useful for following the fluctuating course of delirium.
- An electroencephalogram (EEG) can be helpful to rule out seizure activity as contributing to altered mental status and will usually show diffuse slow background activity.

TABLE 15.1. Differential Diagnosis of Delirium

DISORDER	PRIMARY FEATURE	LEVEL OF CONSCIOUSNESS	HALLUCINATIONS	ASSOCIATED SYMPTOMS	CLINICAL COURSE
Delirium	Fluctuation in consciousness, impaired attention, disorientation.	Impaired.	Usually visual.	Cognitive impairment, emotional disturbances.	Acute onset, fluctuates, improvement with resolution of underlying cause.
Dementia	Persistent impairment.	Normal until late stages.	Often absent with some exceptions.	Disorientation, agitation.	Insidious onset, progressive.
Depression	Low mood, anhedonia.	Normal.	Often absent.	Sleep disturbance, hopelessness, ↓ concentration and appetite.	May have multiple episodes or be chronic.
Psychotic disorders	Impairment in reality testing.	Normal.	Usually auditory.	Negative symptoms.	Prodromal with chronic course.

TABLE 15.2. Causes of Delirium

CATEGORY	EXAMPLES
CNS processes	Traumatic brain injury, intracranial neoplasm, seizure (ictal, peri-ictal, postictal), stroke, meningitis, encephalitis, brain abscess, hypertensive encephalopathy.
Organ failure	Cardiac failure (myocardial infarction), respiratory failure (hypoxia, hypercarbia), hepatic encephalopathy, uremic encephalopathy.
Drugs and toxins	Anticholinergic drugs, benzodiazepines, narcotics, antihistamines, anticonvulsants, antihypertensives, antiparkinsonian drugs, cardiac glycosides, cimetidine and ranitidine, disulfuram, insulin, salicylates, sedatives (hypnotics), antipsychotics. Heavy metals, carbon monoxide, organophosphates. Alcohol, cocaine, heroin.
Endocrinology disorders	Hypopituitarism, hypothyroidism, hyperthyroidism, hypoparathyroidism, hyperparathyroidism, Addison disease, pancreatic insufficiency.
Miscellaneous	Sepsis, electrolyte imbalances, hypoglycemia, hypotension, acid-base disturbances, postoperative states, urinary catheters, nutritional deficiencies (thiamine, nicotinic acid, folate, vitamin B_{12}), anemia.

- Once delirium has been identified, its underlying cause must be determined.
- Useful tests for detecting conditions that can cause delirium are listed in Table 15.3.
- Alcohol withdrawal can result in **delirium tremens** (DTs), which can be fatal if not diagnosed and treated. See the substance use chapter for

TABLE 15.3. Diagnostic Workup of the Delirious Patient

STANDARD WORKUP	ADDITIONAL TESTS
Complete metabolic panel	Ammonia level
CBC	Arterial blood gas
Urine and blood tox screen	HIV test Blood cultures Erythrocyte sedimentation rate Cardiac enzymes Lumbar puncture Urine culture
Chest x-ray	Thyroid function tests RPR or VDRL Vitamin B_{12} and folate
Electrocardiogram	Head CT/MRI ANA/ESR Electroencephalogram

ANA, antinuclear antibody; CBC, complete blood count; CT, computed tomography; ESR, erythrocyte sedimentation rate; MRI, magnetic resonance imaging; RPR, rapid plasma reagin; VDRL, Venereal Disease Research Laboratory.

TABLE 15.4. Management Strategies for Delirium

INTERVENTION	EXAMPLES
Prevention	Identify those at risk: Elderly, dementia, preexisting medical illness, history of alcohol abuse, sensory impairment, males, sleep deprived, immobile, dehydration.
Pharmacologic: Antipsychotics	*Haloperidol:* Initial dose of 0.5–10 mg IV/IM repeated every hour as needed. When giving PO, give 1.5× parenteral dose BID with two-thirds of dose in PM. *Droperidol:* Initial dose of 2.5 mg IV/IM. Monitor ECG. *Quetiapine:* Initial dose of 25–50 mg daily. *Risperidone:* Initial dose of 0.25–0.5 mg bid. *Olanzapine:* Initial dose of 2.5–5 mg at bedtime.
Benzodiazepines	*Lorazepam:* Used very judiciously for insomnia 1–2 mg at bedtime. Preferred drug for those with hepatic insufficiency. Use higher doses for alcohol withdrawal. *Chlordiazepoxide:* Initial dose of 50–100 mg IM/IV q2–4 hours. *Diazepam:* Initial dose 5–10 mg q4 hours. Use for alcohol withdrawal.
Electroconvulsive therapy (ECT)	Helpful in medically refractory cases.

more details. Symptoms include ↑ **temperature, heart rate, and blood pressure;** change in level of consciousness; hallucinations; agitation; and **tremors.** Although DTs are the result of alcohol withdrawal, patients with chronic alcoholism can have DTs even with a positive blood alcohol level.

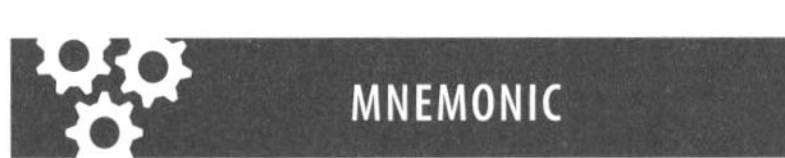

Symptoms of alcohol withdrawal/delirium tremens—

HITS

Hallucinosis
Increased vitals (temp, BP, HR)/**I**nsomnia
Tremors
Shakes/**S**eizures/**S**weats/**S**tomach (nausea/vomiting)

TREATMENT

Treatment should first be directed at the underlying cause of delirium. In the interim, there are other ways to manage delirium prior to its resolution (see Table 15.4):

- **Environmental support:** Provide the patient with frequent reorientation (clocks, calendars, pictures), turn the lights on during the day and off at nighttime, use sitters, remedy any sensory impairment (glasses for poor eyesight, hearing aids), avoid over- or understimulation.
- **Pharmacotherapy** includes the use of antipsychotics in certain circumstances. Haloperidol is the treatment of choice for behavioral agitation and psychiatric symptoms (ie, hallucinations) in delirium because of its low rate of anticholinergic side effects. Atypical antipsychotics and rarely benzodiazepines are also used. Benzodiazepines are the treatment of choice for alcohol withdrawal (DTs). Sample doses of several pharmacological agents are in Table 15.4.

COMPLICATIONS

There are numerous complications of delirium, including:

- **↑ in morbidity and mortality** (it is estimated that the 1-year mortality rate for delirious patients is as high as 50%).
- **Institutionalization** is three times more likely in delirious patients who are 65 years of age or older compared to nondelirious patients in this age group.
- **↑ length of stay** in the hospital.
- Frequent falls, pressure ulcers, pneumonia, malnutrition, and ↓ functioning.

NOTES

CHAPTER 16

Anxiety and Related Disorders

Timothy Scarella, MD

Generalized Anxiety Disorder (GAD)

A 45-year-old man is referred to your practice "because of my nerves." He feels anxious about his career and his relationship, and finds himself worrying that he will die prematurely, leaving his wife and children uncared for. He notes that when he can step back and look at the state of his life, there isn't serious cause for concern, but he can't help worrying. For several months he has been having difficulties concentrating at work and has not slept well. Further questioning reveals that the symptoms have been going on for 9 months, and that during that time he has been trying acupuncture to relieve shoulder tension and headaches. He doesn't describe himself as depressed, nor has he experienced a loss of interest in things he usually enjoys. What is the most likely diagnosis?

A diagnosis of generalized anxiety disorder should be entertained.

Symptoms

- A sense of constant worry over a wide range of events or activities.
- There is considerable comorbidity and symptom overlap with major depression, dysthymic disorder, other anxiety disorders, and personality disorders.

Diagnosis

First, establish the presence of excessive anxiety or worry (eg, over a number of activities, for more days than not, and at least 6 months' duration). Then check that the worry is difficult to control, and confirm the accompanying presence of at least 3 of the following 6 symptoms:

- Restlessness/feeling keyed up.
- Difficulty concentrating/mind going blank.
- Irritability.
- Easily fatigued.
- Muscle tension.
- Sleep disturbance.

As with all other disorders, be sure that another Axis I disorder is not better suited, that substances and/or medical problems are not primary, and that there is actual impairment in important areas of function.

Differential Diagnosis

- The main task is to distinguish from (or diagnose alongside) depressive disorders and other anxiety disorders. Tips for differentiating GAD from other psychiatric disorders are provided in Table 16.1.
- Like other Axis I diagnoses, it is important to consider the role of substances. Consider anxiety secondary to substance use (amphetamines, caffeine) or withdrawal (alcohol, opiates, sedatives, nicotine).
- Substance use may be a form of self-medicating anxiety, but this is difficult to establish without a good history.

Treatment

Therapy, medications, or both may be used. GAD is often chronic and people often have chronic nervousness/anxiety even if medication treatment brings their symptoms below threshold for diagnosis.

Cognitive-behavioral therapy is often used, as the cognitive component

TABLE 16.1. Differentiating GAD from Other Primary Psychiatric Conditions

Other Illness	Common Symptoms with GAD	Tips to Differentiate
Mania	Racing thoughts Irritability Trouble sleeping	Presence of grandiosity, increased goal directed behavior, or psychotic features suggests bipolar disorder.
Adjustment disorder with anxious mood	Anxiety	Limited in scope and symptoms, occurs in the presence of a stressor, and resolves relatively quickly after stressor resolves.
Depressive disorders	Anxiety Fatigue Sleep difficulty Concentration Irritability	Focus on the hallmark symptom: worry (constant mind spinning, often involving future events) versus sadness (a more withdrawn negative mood state). Individuals with major depression tend to be self critical and focus on the past. Individuals with GAD tend to worry about possible future events. Early morning awakening, diurnal mood variation, and suicidal thoughts are uncommon in GAD.
Social anxiety disorder	Anxiety	Anxiety is linked solely to social/interpersonal settings.
PTSD	Chronic anxiety Sleep difficulty Concentration Irritability	History of trauma and presence of intrusive and avoidant symptoms.
Psychotic disorders	Anxiety	Is the content focus of the worry delusional or bizarre in nature?[a]
Somatoform disorders	Anxiety	Is the focus of worry based on physical symptoms or body imagery? Individuals with GAD tend to worry about multiple and various things. Individuals with hypochondriasis for example worry principally about illness.

[a] Constant worry about symptoms of a diagnosed Axis I disorder do not count toward the diagnosis of GAD (eg, a paranoid schizophrenic with delusions of being chased by the CIA may be very anxious, but this is not GAD).

involves correcting cognitive distortions (eg, catastrophizing), while the behavioral component includes progressive deep muscle relaxation and desensitization. Psychodynamic therapy is also often used both for people fully meeting GAD criteria and those complaining of generalized anxiety who may not meet GAD criteria.

Medications used in treatment are provided in Table 16.2. If medications are discontinued, patients are at high risk for relapse if some form of therapy has not addressed core cognitive distortions and beliefs that lead to anxiety.

Specific Phobias

A young man in his 30s is referred to you for "panic attacks." His firm has recently changed office locations, and now instead of the ground floor, he is situated on the 10th floor. He relates that he has always been afraid of heights, and as a result he never drives across bridges or flies in airplanes. Since his office has several windows, he has been avoiding going to work because he is afraid of the view; the couple of times he has been in his office, he has had such intense anxiety that he had to

TABLE 16.2. Medications for the Treatment of GAD

Type	Description	Comments
SSRIs and SNRIs (most frequently used)	FDA-approved SSRIs for GAD (in practice, any SSRI/SNRI may be used): Lexapro (escitalopram): 10–20 mg daily Paxil (paroxetine): 20–50 mg daily FDA-approved SNRIs: Cymbalta (duloxetine): 60–120 mg daily Effexor XR (venlafaxine): 75–225 mg daily	Warning to patient: Initial ↑ in anxiety may result! (Consider initial short-term use of benzodiazepine.) Will also help if you suspect a concurrent depressive disorder.
Buspirone	FDA approved Starting dose 5 mg tid, max 60 mg total/day	Non-benzodiazepine anxiolytic. Slow onset moderate efficacy. Common side effects: Initial anxiety/nervousness, headache, nausea. Will *not* help a concurrent depressive disorder. Advantage over SSRIs: No sexual side effects, few drug-drug interactions (useful in elderly or medically complicated).
Benzodiazepines	Clonazepam (1–6 mg total daily) Lorazepam (1–10 mg total daily)	Useful for rapid symptom reduction. Note that tolerance should not develop to anxiolytic effect, so if patient requesting dose increase after long time on stable dose, investigate what is going on (change in life circumstance, onset of depression, substance abuse). Long acting (eg, clonazepam) is preferable, as short acting (eg, alprazolam) has a higher probability of causing withdrawal-induced anxiety. As always, abuse potential; not first choice for those with history of substance use.
Atypical antipsychotics	None are FDA approved.	Some evidence for quetiapine (a second-generation antipsychotic), in doses ranging from 50 to 300 mg daily. Potential augmentation choice for partial response to antidepressant or alternate as monotherapy.
Anticonvulstants	Valproic acid, gabapentin, pregabalin may be used but no antiepileptic is FDA approved for this purpose.	Some evidence for efficacy of pregabalin (a GABA analog calcium channel modulator anticonvulsant) in GAD in randomized trials, dose range 50–300 mg in divided daily doses.

GABA, gamma-aminobutyric acid; SNRI, serotonin-norepinephrine reuptake inhibitor; SSRI, selective serotonin reuptake inhibitor.

leave. He is does not report excess anxiety in any other situation and does not have panic attacks. What is the most likely diagnosis?

This patient has a fear of heights that causes him to have immediate fear on exposure and leads to avoidance of heights; a diagnosis of specific phobia is warranted.

Symptoms

- The hallmark is fear of something very specific, to the point of either avoiding the exposure or enduring it with great distress.
- These are among the most common of all psychiatric disorders, affecting 7–9% of the general population. It is common for individuals with a specific phobia to have more than one.
- Onset is usually during childhood, with persistence across the life span.

Diagnosis

- There must be a marked and persistent fear that is excessive and unreasonable cued by a specific object or situation.
- Exposure always leads to anxiety. (*Note:* This may be in the form of a panic attack)
- The anxiety-provoking stimulus is avoided or endured with great duress, and the resultant avoidance, endurance, or anxious anticipation interferes significantly with functioning.
- Subtypes in the *Diagnostic and Statistical Manual of Mental Disorders*, 5th edition (DSM-5) include animal, natural environment, blood/injection/injury, situational, or other.

Differential Diagnosis

Tips for differentiating specific phobias from other primary psychiatric conditions are provided in Table 16.3.

Treatment

- The mainstay of treatment is psychotherapy, though medications may be used if individual must endure a situation prior to their ability to complete needed therapy.
- The psychotherapy of choice is cognitive-behavioral therapy, particularly exposure therapy, and it is extremely effective.
- Medications used in the treatment include benzodiazepines for times when exposure to stimulus is necessary (such as prior to MRIs for claustrophobic people) and propranolol (for performance situations).

Social Anxiety Disorder

A 17-year-old boy is referred for help with "shyness." His parents are concerned because he has stopped participating in after school activities and never seems to go out with his friends. He reports that he previously enjoyed these activities but for the past year or so has felt that whenever he is around people he is being scrutinized and judged by his peers. Therefore, he avoids peer interactions so that others don't make fun of him. He notes, "I've never heard anyone actually say anything mean to me; I just can't shake the feeling that everyone is talking behind my back." He recognizes that his worries are unfounded but cannot shake the anxiety. What is the diagnosis?

TABLE 16.3. Differentiating Specific Phobias from Other Primary Psychiatric Conditions

Other Illness	Common Symptoms with Phobias	Tips to Differentiate
OCD	Intrusive thought that is repetitive.	In OCD it is the *thought* of something that causes anxiety; compulsive behaviors are a mechanism to stop the thought.
PTSD	Avoidance of places/activities that remind the person of a trauma and severe distress with triggers.	Look for the presence (PTSD) of a Criterion A traumatic event.
Panic disorder	Panic attacks.	*Context driven* for phobia; *recurrent and unexpected* for panic disorder.

Though further questions may elicit other anxious symptoms, a diagnosis of social anxiety disorder is possible.

Symptoms

The hallmark of social anxiety disorder is fear and anxiety in social situations. This was previously a subtype of specific phobia in DSM-IV but is considered a separate disorder in DSM-5.

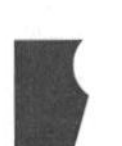

KEY FACT

Social anxiety disorder is highly comorbid with other anxiety disorders, so be sure to screen for them!

Diagnosis

To make the diagnosis, an individual most reports intense anxiety or fear in social situations where they may be judged by others, such as social outings, occasions where they are being directly observed (being out in public places), or performing. The person feels as if his anxiety will be noticed by others and judged negatively, and he either avoids the situation or endures it with distress.

Differential Diagnosis

- If social situations are avoided due to the fear of having panic attacks or the fear of being unable to escape or get help in the event of a panic attack, consider panic disorder or agoraphobia.
- Feelings that others are watching, judging, and in general behaving in a negative way toward the patient that are not based in reality may also be part of a psychotic disorder; in general, those with social anxiety disorder have insight that their fears are excessive or unwarranted but they have no control over them.
- If objective reports are found to say the patient does in fact behave awkwardly in social interactions and has trouble reading other people socially, consider diagnosis of an autism spectrum disorder.

Treatment

- Both medication and therapy are used to treat social anxiety disorder. Selective serotonin reuptake inhibitors (SSRIs) are the most commonly used medication, and while paroxetine and sertraline have received an FDA indication, any SSRI may be used. Venlafaxine, a serotonin-norepinephrine reuptake inhibitor (SNRI), has also been approved for social anxiety disorder treatment.
- Psychotherapy commonly involves a cognitive-behavioral therapy (CBT) approach. Group CBT psychotherapy can be effective, as the group setting provides an environment to explore and expose a person to anxiety in social situations.

Panic Disorder

A 28-year-old student presents at the drop-in clinic complaining of "stress." It turns out next month she has her oral thesis presentation, for which she has been preparing over the past several months. She reports feeling more anxious in general during this time, with occasional bouts of insomnia. Your questions reveal that at least 3 times weekly over the past 2 months she has suffered from 15-minute bouts of intense anxiety, with shortness of breath, sweating, dizziness, palpitations, and a sense that she is "separate from my body." These come out of nowhere and have happened in many public situations. She has found herself avoiding going to class and sending her boyfriend to do the grocery shopping out of fear of having an attack in public. What is the most likely diagnosis?

This patient has recurrent and unexpected panic attacks that have led to avoidance behaviors and trouble with daily functioning. A diagnosis of panic disorder should be considered.

Symptoms

The hallmark of panic disorder is recurrent, unexpected panic attacks. In interview, one must be careful to ask what patients mean if they volunteer that they have panic attacks, as this has become a common colloquial expression with wide variation in meaning. A **panic attack** is defined as a *discrete* period of intense fear or discomfort, reaching a peak within 10 minutes, with at least 4 of the following (broken down into 4 main categories):

- Subjective psychologic experience (3): Fear of losing control or going crazy; fear of dying; derealization or depersonalization.
- Chest (4): Palpitations (pounding heart, accelerated heart rate); chest pain/discomfort; shortness of breath/smothering; feeling of choking.
- Gastrointestinal (1): Nausea/abdominal distress.
- Autonomic (5): Sweating; chills/hot flashes; trembling/shaking; dizzy/lightheaded; paresthesias.

Diagnosis

- It is important to note that the mere presence of panic attacks does not automatically mean panic disorder is the diagnosis. Panic attacks may also be present in other anxiety disorders, post-traumatic stress disorder (PTSD), or mood disorders; a person with panic attacks may not even meet criteria for a DSM defined mental illness.
- In panic disorder, panic attacks are recurrent and unexpected, and there must be persistent concern about having additional attacks or the consequences of the attacks or a maladaptive change in behavior due to the attacks.
- As with all disorders, rule out substances/medical disorder, as well as other Axis I disorders that better fit the symptom pattern.

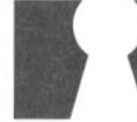

KEY FACT

Remember, panic attacks may be a symptom of many psychiatric disorders, not just panic disorder.

Differential Diagnosis

- If attacks are predictable and in relation to a specific trigger, consider specific phobia or PTSD.
- Tips for differentiating panic disorder from other primary psychiatric conditions are provided in Table 16.4.

Treatment

- Treatment includes both pharmacotherapy and/or psychotherapy. Treatment of panic disorder can result in dramatic improvement, and goal should be remission.
- Common medications used in treatment are provided in Table 16.5.
- Cognitive-behavioral therapy is extremely effective. The cognitive component addresses automatic thoughts that cause the person to fear the bodily sensations associated with panic, while behavioral therapy usually involves exposure to situation that lead to panic and interoceptive exposure (forced hyperventilation, spinning in a chair to induce dizziness) to decrease reactivity to bodily sensations.

TABLE 16.4. Differentiating Panic Disorder from Other Primary Psychiatric Conditions

Other Illness	Tips to Differentiate
Specific phobia	May involve a panic attack but has a specific trigger. Key feature of panic disorder is its unexpectedness.
Generalized anxiety disorder	More persistent, less discrete time boundaries. Has exacerbations that patient might describe (mistakenly or not) as a panic attack.
PTSD	Reexperiencing symptoms may have similar suddenness, but they should reference a specific past event.
Substance related	Intoxication or withdrawal.
Medical disorders	Cardiac, pulmonary, endocrine (hyperthyroid, hypoglycemia, Cushing, etc). Let history and presentation guide the appropriate medical workup.

Complications

In general, there is a good long-term prognosis if treatment is initiated. However, there is a significant comorbidity with depression and substance abuse (particularly alcohol).

Agoraphobia

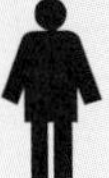

The student from the vignette on panic disorder decides not to initiate therapy because her school and work schedule are too busy. She is brought to clinic 6 months later by her boyfriend, who explains that the patient now will only

TABLE 16.5. Medications Most Commonly Used in the Treatment of Panic Disorder

Type	Description	Comments
SSRIs	Fluoxetine: Start at 10 mg daily, target 20–40 mg. Citalopram: Start at 10 mg, target 20–40 mg. Sertraline: Start at 25 mg daily, target 50–150 mg.	Considered to be first-line agents. SSRIs commonly cause an increase in anxiety in the first week or two, so initiate at lower dosage, warn your patient, and consider adding a benzodiazepine short term.
Other antidepressants	SNRIs, tricyclics, and MAOIs have all been shown to be effective.	Use SSRI or SNRI first due to better safety profile.
Benzodiazepines	Alprazolam 1–4 mg total daily, may require higher doses.	Short-acting agents like alprazolam are effective at reducing anxiety, but there is a risk of dependence/rebound anxiety. Benzodiazepines may interfere with safety learning and decrease efficacy of therapy.
	Clonazepam 1–4 mg total daily. Lorazepam 1–10 mg total daily.	Consider if panic attacks are relatively infrequent.

MAOI, monoamine oxidase inhibitor; SNRI, serotonin-norepinephrine reuptake inhibitor; SSRI, selective serotonin reuptake inhibitor.

leave the house once or twice per week, and even then she frequently has to return home. On the rare occasions she goes to class, she demands to sit at the end of the row. She explains to you that she refuses to go to supermarkets, sit on trains, or sit in class because if she had a panic attack there would be no way to escape. She is okay with the coffee shop down the street because she knows where the bathroom is and knows where all the doors are located. What additional diagnosis is now warranted?

The patient has developed a fear of putting herself in any situation where escape would be difficult in the event of a panic attack. A diagnosis of agoraphobia is warranted.

Symptoms

Agoraphobia is anxiety about being in places or situations from which escape is difficult or embarrassing. These situations are avoided altogether or endured with great distress, and they may trigger panic attacks.

In DSM-IV, the presence or absence of agoraphobia was used as a modifier for the diagnosis of panic disorder; however, the finding that many patients have agoraphobia without meeting criteria for panic disorder has led to it being a separate diagnostic entity in DSM-5.

Diagnosis

To make the diagnosis, a person has anxiety about specific situations and avoids those situations *due to the idea that escape or obtaining help would be difficult in the event of panic-like symptoms.* Being in these situations must reliable provoke the fear, which is out of proportion to any actual danger or cultural context.

DSM-5 defines 5 different agoraphobic situations, of which an individual must have anxiety about 2 in order to make the diagnosis:

- Public transportation
- Open spaces
- Enclosed spaces (including types of buildings)
- Waiting in lines or being in crowds
- Being outside of one's home while alone

Differential Diagnosis

Depending on what is being avoided, consider PTSD (person avoids situations that trigger memories/flashbacks of trauma), specific phobia (avoidance is not generalized), and panic disorder (fear of the panic attack itself as opposed to worry about being able to escape the situation).

Untreated, agoraphobia has a poor prognosis and may result in serious functional impairment. When agoraphobia develops during the course of panic disorder, the prognosis is significantly worse than for panic disorder alone.

Treatment

Few studies have addressed treatment for agoraphobia outside of the context of panic disorder. In general, treatment mirrors that of panic disorder with both pharmacotherapy and psychotherapy.

Complications

Untreated, agoraphobia has a poor prognosis and may result in serious functional impairment. When agoraphobia develops during the course of panic disorder, the prognosis is significantly worse than for panic disorder alone.

Obsessive-Compulsive Disorder (OCD)

A 28-year-old woman is referred to the clinic by her work supervisor for "odd behavior." Her supervisor had noticed she was frequently over an hour late to work, then noticed one day that she saw the patient repeatedly driving around the block without pulling into the parking lot. The patient tells you that when driving she is overcome with the fear that she has run over and killed a pedestrian; therefore, she finds herself driving back around streets to check to see if she hurt anyone. She is unable to stop herself from repeatedly checking because she becomes too afraid that she has hit someone. When she finally stops driving, she spends most of the day worrying about whether or not she hit someone. She estimates she spends 2–3 hours every day driving in circles. What is the diagnosis?

Obsessive-compulsive disorder should be considered.

Obsessive-compulsive disorder was previously listed with anxiety disorders in DSM-IV but has been given its own chapter, "Obsessive-Compulsive and Related Disorders," in DSM-5. It is presented here with anxiety disorders for convenience.

Symptoms

OCD is defined by the presence of obsessions and/or compulsions.

- **Obsessions** are recurrent thoughts, mental images, or urges that are experienced as intrusive and unwanted and cause subjective distress. An individual will frequently attempt to suppress these with a mental or physical action.
- **Compulsions** are repetitive acts that may be physical (hand washing) or mental (counting) that a person feels must be performed in response either to an obsession or to some rigid rule system. The purpose of the acts is alleviation of anxiety, and they are clearly excessive and out of proportion to the anxiety.

Diagnosis

- To make the diagnosis of OCD, a person must have either obsessions or compulsions, and they must occupy at least 1 hour per day and cause impairment in functioning.
- OCD is highly comorbid with tic disorders; if a patient has tic disorder, consider asking questions to rule out OCD.

Differential Diagnosis

- The sometimes bizarre and idiosyncratic nature of both obsessions and compulsions can sometimes sounds like part of a psychotic disorder. Importantly, patient with OCD often retain insight into the unreasonable nature of their symptoms, yet are powerless to stop them.
- Patients with schizoid, schizotypal, and obsessive-compulsive personality disorders may also apply rigid rule systems to their lives that can sometimes look like OCD.
- If food or feeding patterns are the topic of either obsessions or compulsions, primary eating disorder should be ruled out.

Treatment

Both medications and therapy are used to treat OCD. Medications are listed in Table 16.6. The mainstay of therapy is CBT, specifically behavioral interventions where the person is exposed to the anxiety-provoking stimulus and prevented from performing the compulsion (exposure-response prevention therapy).

Post-Traumatic Stress Disorder (PTSD)

A 26-year-old woman presents for evaluation of anxiety. She reports constant anxiety during the day that is worse when she is walking around in public. When in public, she feels that she has to constantly scan her environment and experiences racing heart, flushing, and sweating. She describes feeling "constantly on guard" and has trouble leaving her house at night. She goes on to describe that she was raped in college, but says "it was pretty much my fault"; since then, she avoids sexual encounters, as they cause flashbacks where she feels like she is experiencing the attacks again. She has nightmares about the attack most nights of the week, significantly interfering with sleep. She describes herself as feeling "emotionally numb" and unable to enjoy the company of others. She frequently has episodes where she explodes in anger at friends.

The patient's stated complaint is anxiety; however, when trauma is part of the history, one can elicit other symptoms of PTSD, including intrusive symptoms, avoidance, negative cognitions, and hyperarousal, which show that her anxiety is part of a cluster of post-traumatic symptoms.

Symptoms

The years following the Vietnam War witnessed official DSM recognition of the diagnosis of PTSD, but the syndrome had been recognized well before this. Though originally formulated in terms of combat veterans, civilian traumas are frequently the culprit. Patients' chief complaints may be primar-

TABLE 16.6. Medications Used in Treatment of Obsessive-Compulsive Disorder

Type	Description	Comments
SSRIs	Fluoxetine, fluvoxamine, sertraline, and paroxetine have FDA indications. In practice, any SSRI may be used.	Considered to be first-line agents.
Serotonergic Tricylclic Antidepressants	Clomipramine 25–100 mg daily.	Clomipramine is the gold standard in OCD treatment; however, not first line due to less favorable side effect profile.
SNRI	Venlafaxine, 225–300 mg daily.	Less evidence for efficacy than SSRIs.
Antipsychotics	Risperidone and haloperidol most studied.	Used to augment 1 of the above agents if incomplete symptom remission; generally not useful as monotherapy.

SNRI, serotonin-norepinephrine reuptake inhibitor; SSRI, selective serotonin reuptake inhibitor.

ily mood disturbance, anxiety, or sleep disturbance, but careful history taking will reveal not only the history of a traumatic event but the instrusive symptoms, avoidance, negative cognitions, and hyperarousal that distinguish PTSD from primary disorders of mood and anxiety.

In DSM-IV, PTSD was grouped with anxiety disorders; however, in DSM-5 trauma-related disorders have been given their own chapter. PTSD is presented with anxiety disorders here for convenience.

DIAGNOSIS

It is important to note that the presence of trauma and the presence of psychiatric symptoms do not automatically warrant a diagnosis of PTSD.

First, a trauma must be identified that fulfills Criterion A of the DSM-5 definition of PTSD, which requires exposure to actual or threatened death, injury, or sexual violence. This may be experienced directly, witnessed by the person, learning of a traumatic event occurring to a close family member or friend, or repeated and extreme exposure to aversive details of the event (ie, medical examiner seeing several murdered bodies).

If criterion A is present, then patient must have the symptoms in Table 16.7 to qualify for diagnosis. Symptoms must occur for at least 1 month, and they must include all 4 categories. The qualifying symptoms *must* have had onset after the trauma.

TABLE 16.7. Symptoms of PTSD

SYMPTOM CATEGORY	SYMPTOMS
Intrusion (diagnosis requires at least 1 symptom from this category)	Recurrent, involuntary distressing memories. Recurrent and distressing dreams related to the event (ie, may not be of the actual event but may have related content or affect). Feeling as if the event were recurring (eg, flashbacks). Intense *psychological* distress at cues that recall or symbolize the event. Intense *physiological* distress at cues that recall or symbolize the event.
Avoidance (diagnosis requires at least one symptom from this category)	Avoiding thoughts, memories, or associated with the trauma. Avoiding activities, places, people, or other things associated with the trauma.
Negative alternations in cognition (diagnosis requires at least 2 symptoms from this category)	Inability to remember important aspects of the event. Exaggerated negative beliefs about oneself or the world ("I am evil"; "People cannot be trusted"; "I am damaged forever"). Distorted thoughts about the cause event or its consequences leading to self-blame or inappropriate blaming of others. Persistent negative emotional state (including persistent sadness, anger, guilt). Persistent decreased interest in significant activities. Feelings of being unattached and unrelated to others. Inability to have positive emotions (love, satisfaction, enjoyment).
Increased arousal (diagnosis requires at least 2 symptoms from this category)	Sleep disturbance. Irritability or outbursts of anger and aggressiveness. Difficulty with concentration. Hypervigilance. Exaggerated startle response. Reckless or self-destructive behavior.

TABLE 16.8. Differential Diagnosis of PTSD Symptoms

PTSD Symptom Cluster	Diagnostic Considerations
Intrusion	Differentiate flashbacks from hallucinations (as in psychotic disorders, organic brain injury, delirium, intoxication). Differentiate psychologic/physiologic distress from panic disorder, agoraphobia, specific phobia.
Avoidance	Differentiate from stimulus avoidance as in panic disorder, specific phobia, social anxiety disorder. Differentiate from low motivation for activities as in depressive disorders.
Negative alterations in cognition	Differentiate negative beliefs about self and others from depressive disorders and personality disorders. Differentiate persistent negative emotional state, decreased interest in activities, lack of positive emotions from depressive disorders.
Hypervigilance	Differentiate irritability, aggressive outbursts, reckless and self-destructive behavior from (hypo)mania, personality disorder. Differentiate concentration problems from depressive disorders, attention-deficit hyperactivity disorder. Consider wide range of etiologies for sleep disturbance.

Differential Diagnosis

The differential is extensive due to the particularly broad nature of the symptoms. Table 16.8 lists other psychiatric illnesses with similar symptoms to PTSD. Keep in mind that there is a high comorbidity of mood, anxiety, and substance abuse disorders with PTSD.

TABLE 16.9. Medications Used in the Treatment of PTSD

Type	Description	Comments
Selective serotonin reuptake inhibitors (SSRIs)	Paxil (paroxetine; 20–50 mg daily) and Zoloft (sertraline; 50–200 mg daily) are FDA approved for this indication but any SSRI may be used.	Studies suggest overall positive effect on illness with lower effect sizes than seen in depression or other anxiety disorders.
Prazosin	Alpha-1-adrenergic antagonist. Specifically targets nightmares. Start at 1 mg at night and titrate to effective dose. May use morning doses as well to target daytime hyperarousal.	Quickly becoming a widely prescribed and effective drug for nightmares. Higher doses (up to 16 mg nightly) used in studies with military populations.
Clonidine	Alpha-2-adrenergic agonist. Start at 0.1 mg at bedtime or bid, titrate as needed; average effective dose up to 0.6 mg total daily.	Used to treat hyperarousal symptoms. Check blood pressure (hypotension, orthostasis).
Beta blockers	Possibly blocks the hyperarousal reaction and prevents the later development of PTSD if utilized in the immediate hours of the trauma.	Emerging evidence, but not yet widespread community use for this purpose.
Antipsychotics	Hyperarousal and reexperiencing symptoms.	Off-label use, only small studies into effectiveness.
Benzodiazepines	Commonly prescribed, most often alprazolam, lorazepam, clonazepam.	Some evidence that benzodiazepines are harmful in PTSD due to inhibition of safety learning, though this is controversial. If used, time-limited course is best. Abuse potential, especially for short-acting (alprazolam).

TABLE 16.10. Psychotherapies Used in the Treatment of PTSD

TYPE	DESCRIPTION	COMMENTS
Cognitive-behavioral therapy	Can take the form of cognitive restructuring or exposure therapy via revisiting the experience in a safe setting.	Most validated among various therapies.
Eye movement desensitization and reprocessing	Clients focus on traumatic memory while their eyes track side-to-side movements of another object. The therapist supplies positive associations in an effort to replace the negative ones.	Evidence of effectiveness.
Debriefing prophylaxis	Provides support and therapy immediately after the traumatic event.	Available evidence suggests debriefing does not significantly lower rate of PTSD development after trauma.

If a person has exposure to a Criterion A event and has onset of symptoms after the event lasting at least 3 days but with complete resolution within 1 month, a diagnosis of acute stress disorder is warranted. For this diagnosis, patient must have at least 9 of 14 symptoms that are nearly identical to the symptoms in Table 16.7.

TREATMENT

- Most patients with PTSD will end up receiving a combination of medications and psychotherapy.
- Treatment guidelines tend to recommend psychotherapy as first-line therapy over medications; however, if a comorbid disorder such as major depression or bipolar disorder is present, that should be treated with medications as per guidelines for that disorder.
- Common medications used in treatment are provided in Table 16.9, and common psychotherapies used are provided in Table 16.10.

CHAPTER 17

Somatic Symptom and Related Disorders (formerly Somatoform Disorders)

Ryan C. W. Hall, MD

Historically somatoform disorders involve complaints of physical symptoms suggestive of a general medical condition that were **not** explained by an identifiable cause. The categorical name for these conditions has changed to Somatic Symptom and Related Disorders in DSM-5. The diagnostic criteria and names of some of the disorders were reformulated in an attempt to reduce stigma, improve diagnostic accuracy, and to reduce the frequency of not otherwise specified (NOS) diagnosis. DSM-5 criteria emphasize the degree to which a patient's thoughts, feelings, and behaviors about their somatic symptoms are disproportionate or excessive rather than the unexplained nature of the symptoms.

There are 7 conditions that make up this diagnostic grouping:

1. Somatic symptom disorder
2. Illness anxiety disorder
3. Conversion disorder (aka functional neurological symptom disorder)
4. Psychological factors affecting other medical conditions
5. Factitious disorder
6. Other specified somatic symptom and related disorder
7. Unspecified somatic symptom disorder

Features

- Prominence of somatic symptoms, abnormal thoughts, feelings, behaviors.
- Can occur with real comorbid physical illness.
- **No** longer biased on unexplained nature of symptoms.
- Marked distress and/or impairment in social, occupational, or other areas of function usually lasting for months.
- Often results in excessive or unnecessary diagnostic testing and medical treatments.
- Generally **not** delusional beliefs (rare case may approach that).
- Somatization ≠ malingering (see Table 17.1).

Treatment

Keys to successful treatment:

- Strong doctor-patient relationship.
- Patient believes his concerns are taken seriously.
- Teamwork between the neurologist, primary medical doctor, and psychiatrist.
- Treatment of comorbid psychiatric conditions (eg, depression/anxiety).
- Insight-oriented psychotherapy, supportive psychotherapy, and cognitive-behavioral therapy (CBT).
- **Never** tell patients that their symptoms are "all in their head."

TABLE 17.1. When to Suspect Malingering

■ Patient presents for treatment shortly before or during a legal issue.
■ Clear secondary gains from having the illness.
■ Marked discrepancy between symptoms complained of and objective findings.
■ Lack of cooperation with diagnostic examinations.
■ Presence of personality disorder, particularly antisocial personality disorder.
■ No improvement occurs from any type of intervention or with the passage of time.
■ History of previous lawsuits and/or poor work record.

Somatic Symptom Disorder (SSD)

A 31-year-old woman is referred to a neurologist by her primary care doctor due to concerns of an unknown neurologic condition after having multiple exploratory surgeries for abdominal pain and gynecologic concerns. Her primary care doctor is concerned about the patient's anxious mental state regarding her pain and gastric symptoms thought to possibly be due to delayed gastric emptying. However no major problems were found following an extensive GI workup. The patient has also been referred to a psychiatrist but refuses to go since her problem is physical not mental. The patient reports that she has always had medical issues dating back to adolescence. She reports periods of extreme abdominal pain, vomiting, diarrhea, and possible food intolerances. The primary care doctor is her fourth care provider because "my other doctors were not able to help me."

The patient states her problems got worse in college, which was the first time she was operated on. She reports that due to her health problems and severe lack of energy, it took her 5½ years to graduate from college. She did better for a year or two after college but then had a return of symptoms. She reports recently feeling very lonely and isolated because she has not been able to find a boyfriend who can tolerate her frequent illnesses. Additionally, she is concerned that she might lose her job due to the number of days she has missed from work because of her abdominal pain, fatigue, and weakness. Review of symptom also noted other complaints such as headaches and shakes. What is the likely diagnosis?

Somatic symptom disorder. The patient has a history of one or more somatic symptoms that are distressing beyond what would be expected and result in significant disruption of her daily life. She demonstrates persistent anxiety. She devotes excessive time and energy to her health concerns potentially interfering with relationships and employment. Her concerns have been ongoing for longer than 6 months.

SSD often presents with multiple current somatic symptoms that are distressing. Symptoms may be either specific—like regional pain—or general such as fatigue. It is the level of concern expressed (eg, consistent overwhelming fear of developing or having a disease) which is diagnostically important, not whether a cause can be found. Individuals with this disorder view body symptoms, sometimes even normal sensations, as unduly threating or problematic. The level of distress can reach a point where a person may view themselves as an invalid, be unwilling to engage in normal activities such as exercises, or disregard evidence of no significant medical problem. Often these patients have a high level of medical utilization and tend to be "very sensitive to medication side effects."

Features

- Patients report one or more exaggerated, vague, and inconsistent symptoms for 6 months.
- Have excessive thoughts, feelings, or behaviors related to the somatic symptoms or health concerns.
- Often referred to psychiatrist after seeing multiple physicians without improvement.
- Often have high levels of neuroticism and comorbid anxiety/depressed mood.

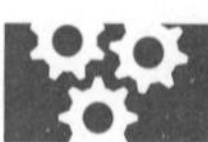

MNEMONIC

Seven-Symptom Screening Test for SSD—

***Somatic Symptom Disorder* Besets *Ladies And Vexes* Physicians**

SOB
Dysmenorrhea
Burning in sexual organs
Lump in throat
Amnesia
Vomiting
Painful extremities

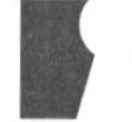

KEY FACT

SSD can have a fluctuating pattern of symptom severity.

- Often have chaotic lives marked by marital discord, employment problems, suicidal ideation, and other impairments of social function.
- SSD is often a chronic condition which can have a fluctuating pattern of exacerbation often during times of stress.

Epidemiology

- Prevalence estimated at 5–7% of general population.
- Prevalence thought to be greater in women.
- Historically having either biological or adoptive parent with a similar concern over somatic symptoms ↑ the risk of developing SSD like conditions.

Diagnosis

- Can be diagnosed when no condition to describe symptoms is evident (but not required).
- Can be diagnosed in presence of a somatic illness if physical complaints or impairments are grossly in excess of what would be expected by history, physical examination, and laboratory findings.
- Excessive concern or behavior over somatic symptoms (potential multiple fluctuating symptoms) persist for 6 months or longer.
- There are no laboratory findings that are associated with this disorder.
- A diagnosis of SSD should **not** be made if symptoms are clearly intentionally produced (ie, malingering or fractious disorder).
- Patients with SSD tend to "doctor shop" to find an answer to their symptoms. They are often given unnecessary and often harmful treatments. Some SSD patients have "checkerboard abdomens" due to exploratory surgeries undergone in an attempt to find a cause for vague abdominal or gynecologic symptoms.
- A checklist approach or detailed review of symptoms often results in multiple complaints and can → create additional diagnostic confusion.
- Care must be taken when making this diagnosis because historically 5–33% of individuals diagnosed with SSD like conditions will eventually be diagnosed with a specific medical condition that appropriately explains their symptoms.
- Common medical conditions, with vague presentation, such as thyroid disease, lupus, Lyme disease, and multiple sclerosis should be ruled out in many individuals with SSD.
- At times may be difficult to different from fibromyalgia, RSD, and irritable bowel.

Treatment

Psychiatric consultation reduces medical costs/frequency of hospitalization (see Table 17.2).

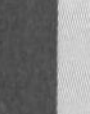

Illness Anxiety Disorder

- Preoccupation (eg, excessive or disproportion anxiety) with having or acquiring an illness for at least 6 months or longer.
- Somatic symptoms only mild if present at all.
- Excessive behavior such a frequent body/ health checks or excessive avoidance such as never seeing a doctor although is extremely worried is sick.

TABLE 17.2. **Psychiatric Approach for Treating Patients with Somatic Symptom Disorder**

Therapeutic Relationship	Education	Consistent Reassurance/Treatment
■ Acknowledge patient concerns about symptoms and illness. ■ Conduct a thorough review of previous medical record. ■ Perform careful physical and psychiatric examination.	■ Educate the patient and his family about the nature of the disorder. ■ Frame symptoms in a positive light. (eg, can have improvement). ■ Define realistic treatment expectations (eg, reduction in hospitalizations, testing, and anxiety).	■ Discourage doctor shopping. ■ Encourage the notion that the patient is being "continuously evaluated." ■ Change in care will result in a delay in treatment, not an improvement in treatment. ■ Highlight relationship between stress and physical symptom presentation. ■ Treat comorbid psychiatric disorders. ■ Involve family members in the treatment process.

Conversion Disorder (Functional Neurological Symptom Disorder)

A neurology consult team is asked to see a 34-year-old man by an emergency department physician to see if it is appropriate to admit the patient to a monitored electroencephalogram (EEG) unit. The patient has a documented history of seizures, which until recently had been well controlled. His lab work is normal, and his epileptic medications are in the therapeutic range. Over the past 10 days, the patient has been experiencing several seizures a day. His internist ordered an EEG since his regular neurologist was out of town and the patient did not want to see the covering neurologist who he did not like. In the process of obtaining an outpatient EEG he had an episode with no corresponding EEG findings. His wife was able to diminish the seizure activity by talking to him during the "fit." The patient reports that he and his wife have recently been having marital difficulties and he was worried that she would divorce him. In a strange way, he is grateful for the return of the seizures because it has helped to repair the relationship with his wife. He knows she will not leave him if he is sick. What is the diagnosis?

Either malingering, factitious disorder, or conversion disorder. Not enough information is given to make a clear diagnosis. The patient could be diagnosed as a conversion disorder based on his recent psychological distress, which seems to correlate with symptoms incompatible with seizures (no activity on EEG, responsive to wife during seizure). Although the patient has secondary gain from having the seizures (wife not leaving), he also potentially has primary gain of reduced anxiety (eg, less fighting, improved relationship). If **definite evidence** of intentional production may consider factitious disorder if wanting to be in the sick role or malingering if done just so wife did not leave. Individuals with seizure disorders can also experience "pseudo seizures" (aka nonelectrical seizure or psychogenic seizure). This episode does not negate the original diagnosis of epilepsy if appropriately diagnosed.

Conversion disorder (aka functional neurological symptom disorder) is a condition in which patients usually present with neurological complains such as perceived paralysis or seizures incompatible with recognized neurological or medical condition. This disorder was formerly known as *acute hysteria*.

The term *conversion disorder* is derived from a hypothesis that a patient's somatic symptoms are due to unconscious psychological conflict. Since the stress of the conflict is too great for the patient, they "convert" the psychological stress to physical manifestations thus reducing their anxiety.

Conversion symptoms function as a form of primary gain (positive internal motivations) usually resulting in reduction or avoidance of anxiety. The individual may also derive secondary gain (external benefits) from their condition, which reinforces their symptoms and supports the continuation of their condition but is not the primary motivator.

The diagnosis of conversion disorder no longer requires the determination that the symptoms are unconsciously produced since judgment on conscious intention is at times subjective.

KEY FACT

"Pseudoneurological symptoms" are symptoms that appear to affect voluntary motor or sensory function but are not caused by a neurological condition.

Features

- Patients often come to medical attention when they present with "pseudoneurological" symptoms.
- Often confused with SSD, factitious disorder, or malingering.
- Individuals with greater medical sophistication (eg, health care providers) tend to present with more subtle symptoms and deficits that more closely mimic actual neurological or medical conditions.
- Many suffers of conversion disorder will also present with symptoms similar to past or current illness (eg, seizures) or symptoms witnessed in a family member or friend who has a "real illness."
- Onset is usually acute (eg, acute blindness, acute paralysis).
- Most conversion symptoms are of short duration with the majority resolving within 2 weeks of their appearance.
- Individual episodes usually only involve 1 symptom but over the course of the disorder multiple deficits may present.
- High rate of recurrence.

Epidemiology

KEY FACT

Women are 2–3 times more likely to suffer from conversion disorder than are men.

- Five percent of referrals to neurology clinics have conversion symptoms.
- Can appear in any age group (individuals younger than 10 usually present with gait disturbances or pseudoseizures).
- No significant gender preference in children.
- In adolescents and adults, occurrence is 2–3 times more likely in females than males.
- Common comorbid disorder with somatic symptom disorder, anxiety disorders, depressive disorders, and personality disorders.

KEY FACT

Roughly 25% of individuals who have had an episode of conversion disorder will have a second episode with new symptoms or a relapse of previous symptoms within 1 year.

Diagnosis

- Presence of symptoms or deficits that affect voluntary motor or sensory function, which appear to be related to a neurological or general medical condition (Table 17.3).
- Clinical findings and symptoms are incompatible with recognized neurological or medical conditions (more than lack of a cause being found).
- Frequently psychologic factors appear to coincide with initiation or exacerbation of symptoms.
- Symptoms must be clinically significant and cause marked social or occupational impairment.
- Diagnosis cannot be made if the symptoms are sanctioned by an individual's cultural or spiritual beliefs (eg, "speaking in tongues," and having "spells" during religious ceremonies).
- Symptoms are usually based on what the patient believes a neurological condition would look like. This may explain why naïve patients have more fantastic presentations.

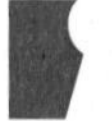

KEY FACT

If the disturbance involves a sensory symptom without other organ involvement, conversion disorder is more likely than SSD.

TABLE 17.3. Common Categories of Conversion Disorder and Corresponding Symptoms

Conversion Disorder with Motor Symptoms	Conversion Disorder with Sensory Symptoms	Conversion Disorder with Convulsions	Conversion Disorder with Mixed Presentations
Aphonia	Blindness	Pseudoseizures	Presents with combination from previous rows
Difficulty swallowing	Deafness	Tremor	
Gait disturbance	Double vision		
Localized weakness	Globus hystericus (lump in throat)		
Paralysis (partial or full)	Hallucinations		
Unstable balance	Loss of pain sensation		
Impaired coordination	Loss of proprioception		
Urinary retention	Loss of tactile sensation		
	Hyperesthesia (hypersensitivity to touch)		
	Tunnel vision		

- There are various methods to determine whether deficits are true neurological disorders vs. a conversion disorder or malingering (Table 17.4). For example, a classic diagnostic technique for a paralyzed upper limb is to try and drop the limb onto the patient's face. With conversion disorder there is a momentary hesitation before the limb falls to the side of the patient's face, not striking the individual as would a truly paralyzed flaccid limb. Another classic sign found with both conversion disorder and malingering is the lack of antagonistic muscle activity in cases of paralysis of the lower limbs.
- The **Hoover sign** for non-neurological lower-extremity paralysis is based on "complementary oppositional muscle activity." It is positive when there is less pressure felt under the good leg/heel than the paralyzed leg when the patient attempts to raise each limb separately.
- Individuals with conversion disorder may show a relative lack of concern about significant deficits. This phenomenon is called *la belle indifference.*
- *La belle indifference* is a French term that translates to "the beautiful/good indifference." It defines the patient's relative lack of concern and bland emotional reaction to alarming or extreme symptoms such as paralysis or blindness.
- La belle indifference is **not** pathognomonic for the condition. Some patients with conversion disorder will seem overly concerned, just as some patients with a physical illness may be stoic in presentation.

TABLE 17.4. Common Tests or Observations that May Suggest Conversion Disorder

- Arm drop (avoids hitting face).
- Testing for missing antagonistic muscle activity (Hoover sign).
- Normal muscle tone.
- Intact reflexes.
- Weakness on ankle planter flexion in individual able to walk on tiptoes.
- Positive findings on the tremor entrainment test.
- In cases of swallowing difficulties, no difference between liquids or solids.
- Stocking glove sensory loss, which affects all sensory modalities (touch and temperature) with no gradient of loss.
- Sensory landmarks at anatomical markers, not dermatologic markers (loss of facial sensation at midline of forehead).
- Seizures that don't follow a consistent pattern.
- Seizures whose course is influenced by observer suggestions.
- Seizures with no abnormal EEG activity.
- Tunnel vision with lack of radiologic support for symptom.

TABLE 17.5. Conversion Disorder: Prognostic Indicators for Recovery

Positive Indicators	Negative Indicators
Above average intelligence	Maladaptive personality traits
Acute onset	Low or low-normal intelligences
Good premorbid functioning	Symptoms of pseudoseizures
Presence of a clearly identifiably stressor	Symptoms of tremor
Short interval between onset and treatment	Lack of acceptance of the diagnosis
Symptoms of aphonia	Comorbid physical disease
Symptoms of blindness	Receipt of disability benefits
Symptoms of paralysis	

KEY FACT

Roughly 10–25% of patients with proven epileptic seizures will also experience pseudoseizures, a form of conversion disorder.

- It is common for conversion disorder patients to present with other comorbid psychiatric disorders such as dissociative disorder; major depressive disorder; histrionic, antisocial social, or dependent personality disorders.

Treatment

- Focuses on regaining function.
- Direct confrontation is **not** recommended (eg, "you are not sick" frequently results in the symptoms worsening).
- Reassure patients that they will have improvement if not fully recover. (See Table 17.5 for prognostic indicators for recovery.)
- Educate patient about illness—suggest that course of the impairment is brief.
- Face-saving interventions such as physical therapy.
- Behavioral interventions focus on ↑ self-esteem, ability to express emotion, assertiveness training, and enhancing communication and coping skills.
- Behavioral interventions focus on ↑ self-esteem, ability to express emotion, treatment of conversion disorder focuses on addressing the 3 P's:
  - **Predisposing factors** (eg, limited education or understanding).
  - **Precipitating stressors** (eg, marital stress).
  - **Perpetuating factors** (eg, conflict management, dependency issues, secondary gain).

Psychological Factors Affecting Other Medical Conditions

- Diagnosed medical condition clearly exists.
- Psychological factors or behavior adversely impacts the condition by affecting treatment (eg, compliance), worsening underling condition (eg, anxiety worsening asthma) or continuation of behavior which exacerbates condition (eg, denial resulting in continued smoking, poor diet) to the point of suffering, disability, or death (Table 17.6).
- **Not** just anxiety over having the disease.

TABLE 17.6. Examples of Psychological Factors Affecting Other Medical Conditions

Anxiety worsening asthma
Misusing insulin for weight control
Denial of treatment for symptoms of acute chest pain
Stress worsening Irritable bowel syndrome
Depression worsening chronic pain or fibromyalgia

TABLE 17.7. Classic Presentations of Factious Disorder

Fake seizure and bite tongue or blood capsule in front of others.
Inject unclean substances sub-q like feces or contaminated water.
Inject exogenous insulin to cause hypoglycemia.
Prick finger to add blood to urine sample.
Take medications like warfin to cause symptoms such as bleeding and create abnormal labs.
Use of ipecac to induces emesis.
Excess use of over the counter medications to cause diarrhea.

Factitious Disorder

- Intentionally causing an illness or falsification of physical or psychological symptoms to assume the patient role not directly for secondary gain (Table 17.7).
- Factitious disorder ≠ malingering.
- Often willing to undergo diagnostic testing because is part of being in the patient role.
- Behavior is not do to other psychiatric condition such as delusional disorder or body dysmorphic disorder.
- Can also present as producing a false illness in another (aka by proxy) where goal is usually to be perceived as a concerned caretaker or parent.

Other Specified Somatic Symptom and Related Disorders

Includes disorders which are similar to existing conditions but may not meet certain limiting criteria such as length of time (Table 17.8).

UNSPECIFIED SOMATIC SYMPTOM AND RELATED DISORDER

- Symptoms suggestive of a somatic symptom disorder which does not meet criteria for existing diagnosis.
- Historically known as "not otherwise specified."

TABLE 17.8. Examples of Other Specified Somatic Symptom and Related Disorder

Brief somatic symptom disorder (less than six months).
Brief illness anxiety disorder (less than six months).
Illness anxiety disorder without excessive health behaviors.
Pseudocyesis (false belief is pregnant with presenting "signs" and symptoms).

NOTES

CHAPTER 18

Bipolar Disorder

Priti Ojha, MD

Bipolar Affective Disorder (BPAD)

A 22-year-old white man presents to the emergency department complaining of feeling depressed for the past week. He reports that he also has experienced difficulty sleeping, lack of appetite, ↓ energy, ↓ concentration, a loss of interest in socializing, and suicidal thoughts.

When probed further, the patient reports similar episodes of depression "on and off" for the past few years. He says that his depressive episodes usually last for approximately 1 month.

The patient also reported that on 2–3 occasions in the past few years, he has also experienced episodes marked by an elevated mood and ↑ energy lasting 4–5 days. During these episodes, the patient felt great despite sleeping 2–3 hours per night. He was able to complete his schoolwork and even wrote a novel in 2 nights. The patient recalled that during these episodes, he had "nonstop ideas circling through my head." He said that he drank heavily, engaged in sexual intercourse indiscriminately, and gambled excessively. Although he recognized that these behaviors were odd for him, he insisted that he was able to function well during these episodes.

When asked about substance use, the patient acknowledged heavy drinking twice a month. He also reported occasional marijuana and cocaine use. He clarified that his marijuana and cocaine use was an attempt to "self-medicate" during periods of depression and anxiety. What is this patient's diagnosis?

Bipolar disorder type II, currently depressed. The differential diagnosis is bipolar type I, substance-induced mood disorder, and cyclothymia. A history of depressive episodes in addition to hypomanic episodes warrant a diagnosis of bipolar disorder type II. Indications of hypomania include inflated self-esteem, ↓ need for sleep, ↑ goal-directed activity, excessive involvement in goal-directed activities, racing thoughts, and pressured speech. The patient's substance use does not seem to be temporally related to his onset of hypomania. He does not meet criteria for cyclothymia because he has been free of depression and hypomania for more than 2 months at a time.

- BPAD, also referred to as **manic-depression,** is a psychiatric diagnosis in the category of mood disorders. It is defined by extreme mood swings that can range from the high pole of mania to the low pole of depression. There are 2 main variants of BPAD, bipolar I and bipolar II, which have different diagnostic criteria as outlined below.
- Symptoms of mania or hypomania may alternate with depressive episodes.
- Some patients may experience **mixed episodes** during which symptoms of mania/hypomania and symptoms of depression occur at the same time. In most individuals, bipolar mood episodes are separated by periods of normal or euthymic mood. However, in some patients with particularly severe illness, this time between episodes can be relatively short, with patients experiencing 4 or more mood episodes in a year. These patients are referred to as rapid cyclers, and can often be more difficult to treat.
- In both mania and depression, severe episodes may be complicated by psychosis.

Epidemiology

- Bipolar I and II: 3.5–4% of population. (per DSM-5, prevalence is 1.8%.
- Male-to-female ratio is 1:1.

- Mean age of onset: 21.
- Peak age at onset of first symptoms: 15–24, with males typically presenting at a younger age than females.
- Onset after age 60 is more likely secondary to general medical condition.
- Highly heritable:
  - Up to 80% concordance in monozygotic twins.
  - Up to 25% concordance in dizygotic twins.
- Environment/stress impact severity and course.
- Suicide rates: 10–15%.

Etiology and Biological Findings

- Psychosocial stressors may precede mania.
- "Kindling" is when repeated episodes cause ↑ disease severity and poorer outcome. Better outcome with early/aggressive treatment.
- Biologic: Metabolites/hormones/neurotransmitters theorized to be involved include 5-hydroxyindoleacetic acid (5-HIAA), homovanillic acid (HVA), 3-methoxy-4-hydroxyphenylglycol (MHPG), norepinephrine, serotonin, gamma-aminobutyric acid (GABA), vasopressin, endogenous opiates, N-methyl-D-aspartate (NMDA).
- ↑ plasma cortisol levels (abnormal dexamethasone suppression test).
- Attenuated nocturnal thyroid-stimulating hormone (TSH) peak and blunted TSH response to administration of thyrotropin-releasing hormone (TRH).
- Associated hypothyroidism in many patients.
- Frontotemporal/left parieto-occipital lesions associated with mania.

Diagnosis/Criteria

BPAD is broken down into:

- Bipolar I:
  - ≥ 1 mixed or manic episode.
  - Depressive episode **not** required.
- Bipolar II:
  - ≥ 1 major depressive episode.
  - ≥ 1 hypomanic episode.

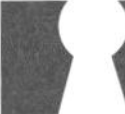

KEY FACT

At least 1 episode of mania is necessary for a diagnosis of bipolar disorder type I.

MANIC EPISODE

Diagnosis

- A distinct period of persistently elevated, expansive, or irritable mood for at least 1 week (or any duration if hospitalization is necessary), during which 3 or more of the following symptoms have persisted to a significant degree (4 if the mood is only irritable):
  - Inflated self-esteem or grandiosity.
  - ↓ need for sleep (eg, feels rested after only 3 hours of sleep).
  - More talkative than usual or pressure to keep talking.
  - Flight of ideas or subjective experience that thoughts are racing.
  - Distractibility (ie, attention too easily drawn to unimportant or irrelevant external stimuli).
  - ↑ in goal-directed activity (either socially, at work or school, or sexually) or psychomotor agitation.
  - Excessive involvement in pleasurable activities that have a high potential for painful consequences (eg, engaging in unrestrained buying sprees, sexual indiscretions, or foolish business investments). See Table 18.1 for clinical features of mania vs. depression.

MNEMONIC

Symptoms of mania:

DIGFAST

Distractibility, **I**nsomnia, **G**randiosity, **F**light of ideas, **A**ctivity increase goal-directed activity, **S**peech- pressured, **T**houghtlessness

TABLE 18.1. Clinical Features of Mania versus Depression

	MANIA	DEPRESSION
Mood/Affect/Feelings	Classically euphoric, also irritable, low frustration tolerance, easily angered and hostile, emotionally labile.	Depression, social withdrawal, dysphoria, crying spells, blunted affect, anhedonic.
Speech	Verbose, fast, pressured at times. As mania worsens, speech can become incomprehensible, with loosening of associations, word salad, flight of ideas, and neologisms.	↓ rate/volume, one-word responses, delayed response to questions, ↓ elaboration.
Perceptual disturbances	Delusions present in up to 75% of patients. Mood-congruent manic delusions often of grandiose nature concerning great wealth, extraordinary abilities, super powers, sense of entitlement, but delusions can also be bizarre and incongruent.	In psychotic depression, grossly regressed and depressed patients with mood-congruent/incongruent delusions/hallucinations.
Thought	Themes of grandiosity and inflated self-esteem, distractible, racing thoughts.	Negative views of world/self, pessimistic, ruminate over loss/guilt/suicide/death, ~10% with evidence of thought disorder/thought blocking/poverty of content.
Sensorium/Cognition	May have some minor cognitive deficits in severe depression/mania but grossly intact in orientation/memory.	Usually fully oriented, impaired concentration/forgetfulness.
Impulse control	About 75% are threatening, sometimes → assaultiveness. Completed suicide rate up to 10–15%.	~10–15% attempt suicide and two-thirds have suicidal ideations. ↑ risk of suicide as energy improves.
Insight/Judgment	Impaired judgment is hallmark; little insight into disorder, especially when off medication.	In midst of depressive episode, patient often forgets the importance of treatment and past success.

KEY FACT

Manic-like episodes that are clearly caused by somatic antidepressant treatment (eg, medication, electroconvulsive therapy, light therapy) do not count as a diagnosis of BPAD unless they persist at a fully syndromal level beyond the physiological effect of the treatment.

- Must be severe enough to cause marked impairment in occupational or social functioning, require hospitalization, or be accompanied by psychotic features.
- Must not be due to the direct physiological effects of a substance (eg, a drug of abuse, a medication, or other treatment) or a general medical condition (eg, hyperthyroidism).

HYPOMANIC EPISODE

DIAGNOSIS

- A distinct period of persistently elevated, expansive, or irritable mood, lasting throughout **at least 4 days,** that is clearly different from the usual nondepressed mood and causes a change in functioning. This change must be observable by other people.
- Must be 3 or more of the same symptoms listed for manic episodes.
- Main difference between mania is that hypomanic episodes are not severe enough to cause *marked* impairment in social or occupational functioning, or to necessitate hospitalization, and there are no psychotic features.
- Symptoms not due to medical conditions or substances.

DIFFERENTIAL DIAGNOSIS

- Cyclothymia.
- Mood disorder due to a general medical condition.

- Substance-induced mood disorder.
- Other psychiatric diagnoses with mood components (ie, schizophrenia and schizoaffective disorder).
- Personality disorders (particularly Cluster B). Impulsivity is a common feature of BPII.

Treatment

- For acute symptoms *and* maintenance treatment:
  - Mood stabilizers.
  - Antipsychotics.
  - Antidepressants (with caution).
- Factors guiding selection of medications:
  - Severity of symptoms.
  - Presence of psychotic features.
  - Presence of rapid cycling.
  - Associated medical conditions (ie, pregnancy).
  - Side effects of medication.
- See Table 18.2 for bipolar disorder pharmacotherapy.
- See Table 18.3 for bipolar medication side effects and usage.
- ECT has shown improvement in severe mania with psychosis and in pregnant patients who cannot take medications.
- Psychosocial/other:
  - Maintain therapeutic alliance.
  - Educate patient and family.
  - Provide psychotherapy.

KEY FACT

Difference between mania and hypomania depends on duration (1 week vs 4 days), severity (requiring hospitalization), and functional impairment.

- There are manic, hypomanic, or depressed episodes, and any of them can be further specified as having "mixed features."
- Symptoms of mania/hypomania and symptoms of depression occur at the same time.

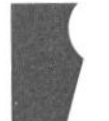

KEY FACT

Antidepressant therapy without mood stabilization may ↑ the risk of hypomania/mania.

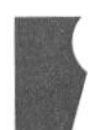

KEY FACT

When treating bipolar disorder pharmacologically, don't forget to monitor for metabolic syndrome and counsel females of reproductive age.

COMORBID DISORDERS

- Bipolar patients are at greater risk than the general population for comorbid anxiety disorders, especially panic disorder and obsessive-compulsive disorder (OCD).

TABLE 18.2. Bipolar Pharmacotherapy

Episode	Preferred Treatment According to APA Guidelines
Manic	Lithium + atypical antipsychotic. Valproate + atypical antipsychotic (good for mixed state). Alternatives: Carbamazepine, oxcarbazepine, but optimize original med dose first before switching or adding. Other: Electroconvulsive therapy (ECT) is a potential treatment for those with severe symptoms and pregnant women. Clozapine may be useful in refractory illness. For hypomania, monotherapy with lithium, valproate, or olanzapine is usually sufficient.
Depressive	Lithium or lamotrigine second line, antidepressant monotherapy not recommended. Olanzapine + fluoxetine received FDA approval for combination treatment of acute bipolar depression. Quetiapine monotherapy has evidence behind it for treatment of bipolar I/II depression. If no response to optimal doses, can add lamotrigine or second-line bupropion or paroxetine. Alternatively, newer agents such as venlafaxine, citalopram, or a monoamine oxidase inhibitor (MAOI) may be added. Other: ECT is a potential treatment for those with severe symptoms and pregnant women. May need atypical if psychosis involved.
Rapid cycling	Identify and correct any medical condition, medication, or substance use that may be contributing to rapid cycling (ie, hypothyroidism, alcohol/illicit substance use, antidepressants). Initial treatment is lithium or valproate, alternatively lamotrigine. Combination is sometimes needed.

TABLE 18.3. Bipolar Medication Side Effects and Usage

Medication	Common Side Effects	Dosing, Monitoring, and Toxicity
Lithium	Thirst Polyuria Fine tremor Weight gain Diarrhea Nausea Acne Hypothyroidism Benign leukocytosis Edema Cognitive slowing Diabetes insipidus **Teratogenic effects:** Ebstein anomaly	Baseline renal/cardiac/thyroid function and pregnancy test should be obtained. Start at 300 mg bid-tid and titrate upward to therapeutic level. First level after 5 days and levels every 3 months thereafter along with renal/TSH. Therapeutic index: 0.5–1.2 mEq/mL. Toxicity is usually experienced above 1.5 mEq and includes coarse tremor, ataxia, vomiting, confusion, seizures, arrhythmias. Hemodialysis is usually needed for levels > 4 mEq in chronic treatment and > 6–8 mEq in acute overdose (OD). Watch for renal failure with concurrent use of diuretics and ibuprofen.
Valproate	Sedation Weight gain Hair loss Tremor Ataxia Gastrointestinal distress Pancreatitis Associated with polycystic ovarian syndrome in adolescent females **Teratogenic effects:** Neural tube defects Fatal clotting defects and hepatic failure in infants Associated with acute hepatic failure in children under 2 years old	Get baseline liver function tests (LFTs), complete blood count (CBC), and pregnancy test. Start inpatients at 20–30 mg/kg and outpatients at 250 mg tid. Titrate up to maximum of 60 mg/kg. Wide therapeutic window: 50–125 µg/mL. Monitor LFTs every 6 months and valproate levels every 3 months. May raise lamictal blood level if given concurrently. May displace protein-bound drugs. Unintentional OD is rare. Signs include heart block, coma, somnolence. Treat OD with hemodialysis.
Carbamazepine	Nausea Diplopia Ataxia Fatigue Weight gain Sedation Rash Rare hepatic toxicity Bone marrow suppression Hyponatremia Pancreatitis Stevens-Johnson syndrome **Teratogenic effects:** Associated with congential malformations (fingertip hypoplasia, low-set ears)	Get baseline CBC/LFTs and pregnancy test. Begin at total daily dose of 200–600 mg divided tid-qid. CBC/LFT every 2 weeks for first 2 month then every 3 months thereafter. Be aware of autoinduction of its own metabolism (↓ levels of other drugs). Carbamazepine may ↑ when coadministered with 3A3/4 P450 inhibitors. Narrow therapeutic index of 4–12 µg/mL. May be fatal in OD. Symptoms include dizziness, ataxia, sedation, diplopia, nystagmus, convulsions, respiratory difficulty, stupor, coma.

TABLE 18.3. Bipolar Medication Side Effects and Usage *(continued)*

Medication	Common Side Effects	Dosing, Monitoring, and Toxicity
Other anticonvulsants (lamotrigine, gabapentin, topiramate, and oxcarbazepine)	Lamotrigine: Stevens-Johnson syndrome (0.1%), nausea, sedation, ataxia, insomnia Gabapentin: Sedation, dizziness, fatigue Topiramate: Fatigue, cognitive dulling, kidney stones, weight loss Oxcarbazepine: Somnolence, dizziness, diplopia, nausea, vomiting, rash, hyponatremia **Teratogenic effects:** Unknown	No lab tests needed with any. Lamotrigine: Slow weekly titration initiated at 25–50 mg qd ↑ by 50 mg/week to 15–200 mg qd. Gabapentin: Can start at 300 mg tid and titrate aggressively up to 3600 mg/day. May need dose ↓ in renal impairment. Topiramate: Starting dose 25–50 mg qd up to maximum of 400 mg/day. Oxcarbazepine: Start 300 mg bid ↑ by 600 mg/week up to 1200–2400 mg/day.
Olanzapine and risperidone	Olanzapine: Drowsiness, dry mouth, akathisia, insomnia, weight gain, constipation Risperidone: Somnolence, hyperkinesias, nausea **Teratogenic effects:** Unknown	Check baseline total cholesterol, HbA1c. No levels needed, but monitor sugars and lipids. Associated with metabolic syndrome. Monitor for extrapyramidal symptoms. Olanzapine: Initial dose 5–10 mg/day up to 40 mg/day. Risperidone: Initial 3 mg/day titrated up to 6 mg/day.
Other antipsychotics (quetiapine, aripiprazole, ziprasidone)	Quetiapine: Dry mouth, somnolence, weight gain, dizziness Aripiprazole: Nausea, dyspepsia, somnolence, vomiting, insomnia, akathisia Ziprasidone: Somnolence, dizziness, extrapyramidal symptoms, nausea, akathisia, tremor **Teratogenic effects:** Unknown	Baseline total cholesterol, HbA1c. Quetiapine: Start at 100 mg qd and titrate up to 800 mg/day. Aripiprazole: 15–30 mg/day. Ziprasidone: Starting dose 40 mg bid. No levels needed, but monitor sugars and lipids. Monitor QTc with ziprasidone. Associated with metabolic syndrome. Monitor for extrapyramidal symptoms.

- Patients with comorbid personality disorders generally have lower functioning and recovery.

Prognosis

- Chronic and disabling illness.
- Earlier onset, more frequent episodes, and presence of psychosis suggest poorer prognosis.
- Elevated risk of completed suicide of 10–15%.
- Comorbidity with substance use disorders, antisocial behavior, and other personality disorders has been associated with poorer outcome.
- Substantial psychosocial stressors impact outcome.

Cyclothymia

Epidemiology/Statistics

- Lifetime prevalence is 0.4–1% but can be as high as 3–5% in clinics.
- Approximately 10% of outpatients and ~20% of inpatients with borderline personality disorder may also have cyclothymia.

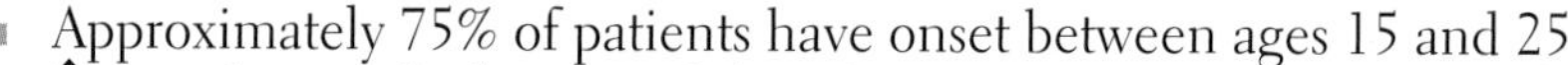

- Approximately 75% of patients have onset between ages 15 and 25.
- ↑ prevalence of other mood disorders (~30%) in family members of those diagnosed with cyclothymia.

Diagnosis/Criteria

For at least 2 years, the presence of numerous periods with hypomanic symptoms and numerous periods with depressive symptoms cause significant distress and impairment.

KEY FACT

Cyclothymia symptoms are not as severe as those in bipolar disorder and do not meet criteria for a major depressive disorder or manic episode.

- Must not meet criteria for a major depressive, manic, or mixed episode.
- The symptoms must not remit for > 2 months at a time.
- Must not be caused by schizophrenia or schizoaffective disorder.
- Must not be due to medical condition or substance.
- In children and adolescents, the duration must be at least 1 year.

Clinical Features

- Alternating periods of depression and hypomania.
- More rapid shifts in mood than BPAD (less time between depressive episode switching to hypomanic episode).
- More than 50% of episodes are depressive episodes.
- Many patients experience periods of mixed symptoms of both hypomania and depressive symptoms concurrently.
- Patients often have a history of impulsive actions (changes in career, etc).
- Episodes often related/coincide with psychosocial stressors.
- Moods often unpredictable in nature.
- Approximately 5–10% have substance dependence disorder.

KEY FACT

Symptoms of cyclothymia may look like borderline personality disorder.

Differential Diagnosis

- General medical condition.
- Bipolar I/II.
- Personality disorder (especially borderline personality disorder).
- Attention-deficit hyperactivity disorder (ADHD).

Treatment

See Table 18.4.

TABLE 18.4. Treatment of Cyclothymia

Pharmacologic	Psychosocial
■ Lithium has been used to treat labile and irritable moods.	■ Psychoeducation.
■ Buproprion, MAOIs, low-dose SSRIs used in conjunction with lithium or other mood stabilizer.	■ Psychotherapy focusing on interpersonal issues has been beneficial.
■ Thyroid augmentation has been found to be helpful in females.	
■ Note not to treat with solely SSRIs/TCAs as this can flip patient into a hypomanic state.	
■ Dosages/blood levels should be the same as those used for bipolar disorder.	

Complications

- Patients may go on to meet criteria for bipolar disorder I/II.
- Personality disorders worsen prognosis.
- Substance abuse confounds diagnosis and worsens prognosis.

Prognosis

- Fair prognosis.
- Chronic course, usually insidious in onset.
- There is a 15–50% chance of cyclothymia developing/progressing into bipolar I/II.

NOTES

CHAPTER 19

Major Depressive Disorder

William Z. Barnard, MD

Major Depressive Disorder (MDD)

A 33-year-old woman is brought to the emergency department (ED) by her spouse, who reports that the patient previously has always been healthy, but for the past several weeks her mood has been deteriorating. She has not been eating regularly and seems to have trouble getting out of bed in the morning and engaging in activities. Her energy is poor, and she has had difficulty concentrating lately. She also has symptoms of severe anxiety. She has been worried that she is a bad mother and is not deserving of her children. Her spouse brought her to the ED when he began to notice her increasingly paranoid behavior. Her spouse reports that she tried calling the police to turn herself in for bad parenting and causing psychological damage to her 4-month-old daughter. She describes having thoughts that her family would be better off without her, but denies having suicidal ideation, intent, or plan. What is this patient's diagnosis?

Major depressive disorder, recurrent, with psychotic features. This patient's symptoms have lasted more than 2 weeks and include depressed mood, anhedonia, decreased appetite, poor concentration, and low energy.

Often, depression decreases a patient's self-attitude in such a way that they lose confidence in aspects of themselves that they value the most. In this case, the patient valued being a mother. When her depression set in, she became preoccupied with thoughts that she was a bad parent. These thoughts escalated until they rose to a delusional level.

As part of the differential diagnosis, one may consider other mental disorders such as postpartum depression. However, most cases of postpartum depression show signs within the first 2 months after childbirth. This patient's daughter was born 4 months ago, but her symptoms did not begin until a few weeks ago. Also important to rule out is postpartum psychosis, however, the onset of this is usually within the first couple of days after delivery with a much more acute onset, typically associated with a history of bipolar disorder.

It is also important to consider other disorders such as schizophrenia or schizoaffective disorder. However, these are less likely in this case because the patient's symptoms began with a depressive episode that escalated until she had a **mood-congruent delusion.** Although the patient had a clear delusion that she was a criminal due to her poor parenting, this delusion appears to have been a product of her depressed mood.

KEY FACT

Diagnosis requires > **5 symptoms** for **2 weeks** (and 1 must be anhedonia or low mood).

Major depressive disorder, the clinical version of depression as defined by the *Diagnostic and Statistical Manual of Mental Disorders* (DSM) is one of the most common mental conditions that you will see both in practice and on exams. More than half of all people who commit suicide suffered from clinical depression or another mood disorder.

Diagnosis

In order to meet criteria for MDD, a patient must meet criteria for at least 1 major depressive episode (MDE):

- Must cause impairment in social, occupational, or other important areas of functioning.
- Must include either **depressed mood** or **anhedonia.**
- Sxs must not be explained by a medical condition or substance use.

- Sxs must not meet criteria for schizophrenia, schizoaffective disorder, schizophreniform disorder, delusional disorder.
- Must never have had a manic or hypomanic episode.
- Must have 5 or more of the following 9 symptoms most of the day for at least **2 weeks:**
  - Depressed mood.
  - Anhedonia (↓ interest or pleasure in activities).
  - Weight loss/gain (change of > 5% body weight in a month) **or** loss of appetite (when not dieting).
  - Insomnia **or** hypersomnia.
  - Psychomotor agitation **or** retardation.
  - Fatigue **or** ↓ energy.
  - Feelings of worthlessness **or** inappropriate guilt.
  - ↓ concentration **or** indecisiveness.
  - Suicidal thoughts.

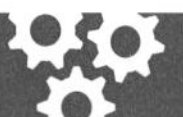

MNEMONIC

Symptoms of Major Depression Episode—

SIG EM CAPS

Sleep increase
Interest or pleasure loss (anhedonia)
Guilt or worthlessness
Energy loss (fatigue)
Mood low
Concentration problems
Appetite increased or decreased
Psychomotor retardation or agitation
Suicidal ideation (thoughts of death)

Differential Diagnosis of MDD

- Medical disorders (that may precipitate or perpetuate symptoms).
- Thyroid disorders.
- Diabetes mellitus.
- Adrenal disorders.
- Metabolic disturbances (↑Ca, ↓Na).
- Nutritional deficiencies (vitamin B_{12}, folate).
- Medication-induced (beta-blockers, CCB, barbiturates, cholinergic medications, corticosteroids, estrogens).
- HIV/AIDS.
- Neurological conditions (CVA, subdural hematoma, MS, tumor).

Other psychiatric disorders:

- Bipolar disorder (Patient with bipolar disorder can also have major depressive episodes, distinguishing between unipolar and bipolar depression can guide treatment. Bipolar I: history of at least 1 episode of mania, patients may have major depressive episodes. Bipolar II: history of hypomania/depressive episodes, no episodes of mania).
- Dysthymic disorder (chronic depression > 2 years).
- Schizophrenia/Schizoaffective disorder. (Psychotic symptoms can and do occur in the absence of major depressive symptoms, in unipolar major depression with psychotic symptoms, delusions, and hallucinations only occur during episode of major depression.)
- Premenstrual dysphoric disorder (temporally related to menstrual cycle, dysphoric mood in final week before onset of menses, improves in few days after onset of menses, minimal/absent postmenses).
- Adjustment disorder with depressed mood (depressive symptoms that occur in response to stressor and do not meet all criteria for MDD).
- Mood disorder due to general medical condition (requires presence of an etiological medical condition, eg, hypothyroidism).
- Substance-induced mood disorder (due to direct physiological effects of substance including medication).
- Bereavement (response to loss of loved one, generally less severe than MDE, characterized by persistent depressed mood and diminished ability to experience pleasure).

Epidemiology

- Incidence:
  - Primary care patients: 5–10%.
  - Medical inpatients: 15%.

KEY FACT

The prevalence of depression is about twice as high in women than in men.

- Prevalence (in adults):
  - Lifetime prevalence: 10–25% for women and 5–12% for men.
  - The point prevalence: 5–9% for women and 2–5% for men.
- Sex differences:
  - In prepubertal children, rate of depression is equal for boys and girls.
  - Between puberty and age 50 years, rate in women approximately 2 times rate in men.
  - After age of 50 years, the rates in women are equal to rates in men.
- Socioeconomic and cultural factors:
  - No correlation has been found between socioeconomic status and MDD.
  - MDD is more common in rural areas than in urban areas.

Prognosis and Course

- Onset:
  - Mean age at onset of MDD: 26.
  - Onset of 50% of all cases is between ages 20 and 50.
- Duration:
  - Most episodes last ~3 months.
  - Untreated episode can last 4–13 months.
- Recurrence:
  - MDD is a chronic illness.
  - Patients tend to relapse.
  - ↑ number of previous episodes = ↑ probability of relapse.
  - Mean number of depressive episodes: 5–6 in 20 years (5–9 lifetime).
  - After 1 MDE, relapse rate = 50%.
  - After 3 episodes, relapse rate ≥ 80%.
  - After hospitalization, relapse risk: 25% in 6 months, 30–50% in 2 years, 50–75% in 5 years. Risk of relapse ↓ if patient given continuous psychopharmacologic therapy.
  - Recovery after 1 year: 40% meet diagnostic criteria for MDD; 20% in partial remission; 40% in complete remission.

Treatment

Major depressive disorder is best treated with a combination of medications and psychotherapy. In severe or treatment-refractory cases, electroconvulsive therapy (ECT) may be indicated. Medication categories (see Table 19.1) include:

TABLE 19.1. Antidepressants by Category

Tricyclic Antidepressants (TCAs)	Monoamine Oxidase Inhibitors (MAOIs)	Selective Serotonin Reuptake Inhibitors (SSRIs)	Atypical/Mixed Receptor Antidepressants
Tertiary amines:	Isocarboxazid	Fluoxetine	Venlafaxine
Amitriptyline	Moclobemide	Citalopram	Nefazodone
Clomipramine	Phenelzine	Escitalopram	Trazadone
Doxepin	Tranylcypromine	Fluvoxamine	Desipramine
Imipramine	Iproniazid	Paroxetine	Duloxetine
Trimipramine	Selegiline	Sertaline	Mirtazapine
Secondary amines:			Buproprion
Nortriptyline			
Desipramine			
Protriptyline			
Amoxapine			

- Selective serotonin reuptake inhibitors (SSRIs). Atypical/mixed receptor antidepressants (including serotonin-norepinephrine reuptake inhibitors [SNRIs]).
- Tricyclic antidepressants (TCAs).
- Monoamine oxidase inhibitors (MAOIs).
- Psychotherapy (best evidence for cognitive behavioral therapy, CBT, and interpersonal therapy, IPT).
- Electroconvulsive therapy (ECT), for severe or treatment-refractory cases.

NOTES

CHAPTER 20

Primary Psychotic Disorders

Priti Ojha, MD

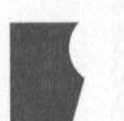

KEY FACT

In primary psychosis, auditory and visual hallucinations are more common than other sensory modalities (exception: delusional disorder, where olfactory and tactile hallucinations are often present).

Psychosis is defined as *a significant break with normal reality or functioning*. Primary psychoses are those not associated with mood episodes or the effects of a substance or discrete physiological condition. Regardless of etiology, all of the psychotic disorders are defined by abnormalities in 1 or more of the following domains: hallucinations, delusions, disorganized thinking or speech, grossly disorganized or abnormal motor behavior, and negative symptoms.

1. *Hallucinations* are sensory perceptions that occur in the absence of any stimuli. They can be of any sensory modality—sight, sound, touch, taste, smell—although auditory and visual are more common in primary psychosis. Tactile, gustatory, or olfactory hallucinations are more common in psychosis secondary to a neurological condition. Hallucinations that occur at the time of sleep onset (hypnogogic) or awakening (hypnopompic) are common and are generally not considered to be clinically significant psychotic symptoms, unless they are frequent and negatively impact functioning. considered within the normal spectrum of experience. *Illusions* (ie, sensory misperceptions of actual stimuli) are similarly not generally considered to be psychotic symptoms, unless they are frequent and negatively impact functioning. Neurologic causes of hallucinations include seizures, migraines, narcolepsy, visual pathology.
2. *Delusions* are fixed beliefs that are not amenable to change despite conflicting evidence. Themes include persecutory (one is going to be harmed by an individual/organization), most common; referential (certain gestures or environmental cues are directed at oneself); grandiose (exceptional abilities); erotomanic (another person is in love with him or her); somatic (preoccupied with health); and nihilistic (major catastrophe is coming). Delusions are further differentiated between bizarre and non-bizarre. Bizarre delusions are clearly implausible and not understandable by peers of the same culture (thought withdrawal, thought insertion, delusions of control are secondary to an outside force). Nonbizarre delusions are conceivable but there is a lack of convincing evidence (ie, one is under surveillance by the police).
3. *Disorganized thinking or speech*, often referred to as *formal thought disorder*, represents a collection of deficits in the ability to produce logical and linear communication. It often manifests as a tangential thought process or the inability to stay focused on pertinent topics (loose associations), as measured by speech or writing. In extreme cases, people with disorganization lose all connection between language and meaning, inventing new words ("neologisms") or violating basic rules of grammar ("word salad").
4. *Disorganized behavior* represents an inability to complete basic physical tasks that require coordination and/or manipulation. It often manifests in bizarre postures or movements and can lead to difficulty performing activities of daily living (as evidenced by extremely cluttered clothing or living environment). *Catatonia* is the absence of frequent movement coupled with rigidity of posture. In extreme cases, this is described as *waxy flexibility*, referring to the ability of others to "move" the sufferer's limbs into any position, which will then be "held" in that position. Presentation of catatonia varies from resistance to instructions to complete lack of verbal and motor response. Catatonic excitement can include stereotyped movements and echolalia.
5. *Negative symptoms* are a reduction in the level of one's activity, including speech output, experience of pleasure, and social interactions. In schizophrenia, the 2 most prominent manifestations are reductions in the emotional emphasis to speech and in motivated, self-initiated purposeful activities.

DIFFERENTIAL DIAGNOSIS

The differential diagnosis for isolated psychotic symptoms is large (Table 20.1), and any new onset of psychotic symptoms demands a careful and thorough medical workup. Magnetic resonance imaging (MRI) is recommended in cases of first psychotic presentation, especially when motor signs, impaired level of consciousness, or personality change is seen.

Schizophrenia

Schizophrenia is the prototypical disease of *chronic primary psychosis.*

- Estimates of the lifetime prevalence of schizophrenia vary from approximately 0.3% to 0.7%.
- According to the World Health Organization, schizophrenia is one of the leading causes of functional impairment worldwide.
- Risk for schizophrenia is highly genetic, with first-degree relatives having a prevalence of approximately 10% and monozygotic twins having a 50% concordance rate.
- There is growing evidence that certain drugs of abuse ↑ the risk for developing schizophrenia, especially when used heavily during adolescence. The current evidence is strongest for marijuana—some studies suggest with heavy use before the age of 16, the relative risk of schizophrenia is up to 6 times that of the general population.
- Onset of schizophrenia typically occurs in late adolescence or early adulthood, with women having a slightly later age of onset than men. The male-to-female prevalence ratio is slightly higher than 1:1.

TABLE 20.1. Differential Diagnosis for Nonprimary Psychotic Symptoms

AIDS
Autoimmune disease—especially systemic lupus erythematosus
B_{12} deficiency
Carbon monoxide poisoning
Delirium
Dementia
Epilepsy—especially temporal lobe epilepsy
Factitious disorder
Heavy metal poisoning
Herpes encephalitis
Huntington disease
Malingering
Mood disorders
Neurosyphilis
Obsessive-compulsive disorder
Pellagra
Personality disorders—especially schizotypal, schizoid, borderline, paranoid
Pervasive developmental delay—especially autism
Substance intoxication—especially alcohol, psychostimulants, and hallucinogens
Substance withdrawal—especially alcohol, barbiturates, and benzodiazepines
Tumor, stroke, or trauma—especially with damage to frontal or limbic areas
Wilson disease

- Families of people with schizophrenia tend to have higher rates of schizotypal and schizoid personality traits.

Diagnosis

- Schizophrenia requires that at least 1 primary psychotic symptom (hallucinations, delusions, disorganized speech) coupled with a second symptom (disorganized/catatonic behavior, negative symptoms, or a second primary symptom) have been present most of the time for at least 1 month.
- Level of functioning is markedly affected (ie, in work, interpersonal relations, self-care).
- Continuous signs of some level of disturbance for at least 6 months.

Differential Diagnosis

- Always remember: for new-onset psychosis, it is important to rule out psychosis secondary to substances or a general medical condition. One month of psychosis and 6 months of dysfunction are required to meet criteria for schizophrenia. If criteria is met, but dysfunction has been present for < 6 months, the correct diagnosis is *schizophreniform disorder.*

  In schizoaffective disorder, patients meet criteria for schizophrenia, have at least 2 weeks of psychosis without mood symptoms, and the mood symptoms have to be present for the majority of the duration of the psychotic symptoms. For example, if the psychotic episode is 1 year long, the patient has to have mood symptoms for at least 6 of those months to have schizoaffective disorder.
- Psychosis that persists for > 1 month but does not meet criteria for schizophrenia may be *delusional disorder, other specified psychotic disorder, or other unspecified psychotic disorder.*
  - For delusional disorder, the delusion should be fixed, and no hallucinations should be present, with the exception of tactile and olfactory hallucinations associated with themes of infestation or a lack of cleanliness.
  - For *other (specified vs unspecified) psychotic disorders,* the psychotic symptom(s) can be any combination that does not meet criteria for delusional disorder or criteria for schizophrenia (eg, persistent visual hallucinations without other symptoms or dysfunction).
- Psychosis that lasts 1 day to 1 month is either *brief psychotic disorder* or *other (specified vs unspecified) psychotic disorder.*
- Psychosis that lasts < 1 day is by definition other unspecified psychotic disorder.
- Many of the criteria for diagnosing *schizotypal personality disorder* can be thought of as attenuated psychotic symptoms. A good history may therefore be necessary to differentiate schizophrenia, residual type, from schizotypal personality disorder.

Treatment

Antipsychotic medications remain the mainstay for both acute and maintenance treatment of schizophrenia. All antipsychotics act as dopamine receptor antagonists, in particular binding strongly to D2 and D4 receptors. This has led to the *dopamine theory of psychosis,* which is also supported by the fact that many psychosis-inducing agents (eg, amphetamines, cocaine, carbidopa) act to ↑ dopamine release. The newer atypical antipsychotics also act as antagonists at the 5-HT2 postsynaptic serotonin receptor. The one exception to this is aripiprazole (Abilify), which is a partial agonist at the D2 receptor. (But like other atypicals, it is a 5HT2 receptor antagonist.) See Table 20.2 for commonly prescribed antipsychotics and their rough dose equivalents.

TABLE 20.2. Common Medications Used in Schizophrenia

Antipsychotic	Therapeutic Dose	Common Side Effects
Haloperidol (Haldol)	5–15 mg/day	EPS, TD, blunting
Risperidone (Risperdal)	2–6 mg	EPS, TD, blunting
Olanzapine (Zyprexa)	5–20 mg	Sedation, weight gain
Quetiapine (Seroquel)	200–600 mg	Sedation, weight gain
Ziprasidone (Geodon)	80–200 mg	Sedation, cardiac effects
Aripiprazole (Abilify)	10–30 mg	Restlessness, headache

EPS, extrapyramidal side effects; TD, tardive dyskinesia (with chronic use).

Data from Woods SW. Chlorpromazine equivalent doses for the newer atypical antipsychotics. *J Clin Psychiatry* 2003;64(6):663–667.

Complications

- Schizophrenia is associated with a 5% suicide rate, most of which occurs within the first few years after diagnosis.
- Many common chronic medical illnesses, such as diabetes, hypertension, and heart disease, exist at higher rates in people with schizophrenia than in the general population. These conditions are often exacerbated by heavy tobacco, alcohol, and/or drug use, as well as the side effects of antipsychotic medications. In particular, several of the atypical antipsychotics are associated with significant weight gain and the risk of developing *metabolic syndrome* followed eventually by *type 2 diabetes (all of them carry a warning for these side effects, but the risk varies depending on the drug).*

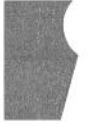

KEY FACT

The definition of a "nonbizarre" delusion includes situations or perceptions that could conceivably occur in real life, though by definition they will have no evidence to support them.

Delusional Disorder

Delusional disorder represents the chronic (> 1 month) presence of 1 or more delusions in a person who has never met criteria for *schizophrenia*. Psychosocial functioning is not significantly impaired outside of the direct impact of the delusion itself.

Diagnosis

- The diagnosis of *delusional disorder* requires that the delusion(s) in question have been persistent for at least 1 month in a person who has never met *Criterion* A for *schizophrenia.*
- Tactile, gustatory, or olfactory hallucinations may be present if they relate directly to the delusional theme, but auditory or visual hallucinations should not be prominent.
- Any mood symptoms associated with the delusion must have been brief relative to the duration of the delusion itself.

Differential Diagnosis

- Delusions often occur in people with *dementia*, especially that of Alzheimer's type, so be sure to assess for memory impairment.

- Delusions are common during depression and mania, but the diagnosis if *delusional disorder* requires the persistence of the delusion in the absence of a major mood episode.
- If a person has had a persistent delusion *and* another psychotic symptom or 1 or more negative symptoms, then the correct diagnosis is either *schizophreniform disorder* or *schizophrenia*, depending on the length of time the symptoms have been present.

TREATMENT

- Antipsychotic medications are generally less effective in *delusional disorder* than in other types of chronic psychosis, though they may be helpful in some cases.
- Psychotherapeutic approaches recommend avoiding directly confrontation of the delusion and instead focusing on its negative behavioral consequences.

Brief Psychotic Disorder

Brief psychotic disorder is defined by the sudden onset of at least 1 primary psychotic symptom (delusions, hallucinations, disorganized speech) for at least 1 day but less than 1 month. There is full return to premorbid function.

DIAGNOSIS

Brief psychotic disorder often occurs in the context of an obvious stressor, or soon after birth (postpartum onset), but it need not have an obvious trigger.

DIFFERENTIAL DIAGNOSIS

- Depending on the type of psychotic symptom, the level of functional impairment and the speed at which symptoms remit, it may be difficult to distinguish onset of a *brief psychotic disorder* from an eventual course of *schizophrenia, schizoaffective disorder,* or *delusional disorder.*

TREATMENT

- Antipsychotic medications are indicated for the acute reduction of the psychotic symptoms themselves. In general, doses listed in Table 20.2 are indicated, with medication use expected to continue only until the symptoms have fully remitted.
- Special attention should be paid toward working to resolve any stressors that seem associated with the onset of psychotic symptoms.

COMPLICATIONS

By definition, there are no long-term psychiatric sequelae to *brief psychotic disorder.*

Index

D

I

J

K

L

M

O

P

R

S

T

U

V

W

X

Z

NOTES

NOTES

NOTES

NOTES

NOTES

NOTES

NOTES

NOTES

NOTES

NOTES

NOTES

NOTES

NOTES

NOTES